Autotransplantation of Teeth

Mitsuhiro Tsukiboshi, DDS, PhD
Amagun, Aichi, Japan

Nozomu Yamauchi, DDS, MS
Oahu, Hawaii, USA

Yosuke Tsukiboshi, DDS, PhD
Amagun, Aichi, Japan

Taisuke Tsukiboshi, DDS, PhD
Amagun, Aichi, Japan

with contributions from

Jens Ove Andreasen, DDS, Odont Dr
Copenhagen, Denmark

Yasuhiro Asai, DDS
Tokyo, Japan

Takeyasu Maeda, DDS
Niigata, Japan

Leif K. Bakland, DDS
Loma Linda, California

クインテッセンス出版株式会社　2024

QUINTESSENCE PUBLISHING

Berlin | Chicago | Tokyo
Barcelona | London | Milan | Mexico City | Paris | Prague | Seoul | Warsaw
Beijing | Istanbul | Sao Paulo | Zagreb

Foreword

The second edition of *Autotransplantation of Teeth* adds to the many contributions Dr. Mitsuhiro Tsukiboshi has made to this surgical field of dentistry. Beginning with the first edition in 2001 and his numerous clinical articles, he has shown that when performed and based on the proper indications and improved surgical techniques, autotransplantation of teeth is a predictable procedure that usually results in a good prognosis.

Surgical transplantation of teeth has a long history. Ambroise Paré (1519-1590), a French Army surgeon described a technique that was used from the 1500s to the early 1800s to transplant teeth between individuals. Intentional replantation began to be used by dentists in the late 1800s. Of more recent origin is autotransplantation, but this procedure did not initially become commonly used because of its unpredictable outcome.

In recent decades, however, autotransplantation has gained increasing interest because of the development of precise clinical techniques by the late Dr. Jens Ove Andreasen and his colleagues in Copenhagen, Denmark and Dr. Mitsuhiro Tsukiboshi in Japan. They developed procedures that have improved the outcomes of autotransplantation based on advances in recognition of suitable clinical indications, understanding wound healing, and application of improved surgical techniques.

One of the valuable components of this textbook are the many clinical cases followed over time. They illustrate the clinical techniques and show the long-term results of these surgical procedures. In addition to autotransplantation, surgical extrusion and intentional replantation are also included. The second edition of *Autotransplantation of Teeth* can be expected to contribute to what one can now consider a valuable and predictable dental treatment procedure.

Leif K. Bakland, DDS
Distinguished Emeritus Professor of Endodontics
Loma Linda University School of Dentistry
Loma Linda, California

Preface

More than 70 years have passed since the introduction of autotransplantation of teeth (transplantation) in mainstream dentistry. Even in the 21st century, some dentists may associate the term transplantation with a heroic and unpredictable treatment modality. The reason for this is probably due to higher failure rates seen early on at a time when there was limited knowledge, research, and evidence available, which results often in pessimism that can be long lasting and difficult to change. Another reason is that transplantation is not something that is done with high frequency in most dental practices because the patient must have the right criteria and conditions available (i.e. there must be an available donor tooth). Also, before implant supported treatment was available, transplantation was attempted in cases that it was not indicated for (poor selection criteria). It is unfortunate that many dentists are not exposed and properly educated about transplantation, or if so, are not willing to be open-minded about understanding more about it because it can be a treatment of great benefit for the patient,

In June of 1992 Dr. Mitsuhiro Tsukiboshi, who was interested in dental traumatology and tooth transplantation, visited Dr. Jens Ove Andreasen in Copenhagen, Denmark. Dr. Andreasen is considered by many to be the most influential figure when it comes to these two fields of dentistry. By some luck and synchronicity, he saw Dr. Andreasen was working on the original (draft) of "Atlas of replantation and transplantation of teeth" (published by Saunders). Dr. M. Tsukiboshi was inspired and was given permission to translate the work into Japanese and publish it. With the help of colleagues, Dr. M. Tsukiboshi was able to publish the Japanese edition (Quintessence Publishing, 1993), which brought transplantation to the forefront in Japan.

Dr. M. Tsukiboshi published his own transplantation book six years later (1999) which was published in several languages, including English, and has served as a reference book for many dentists interested in transplantation around the world for nearly 15 years. The second edition was published in 2014, but only in Japanese. However, in response to the growing interest and enthusiasm for transplantation in recent years, it was decided to publish a revised second edition in English.

The purpose of this book is to provide an easy-to-understand summary of wound healing, indications, surgical procedures, and prognosis (follow-up results) of transplantation, that will help dentist develop further knowledge and understanding about the topic. In the chapter on wound healing, we have attempted to explain the basic healing mechanisms necessary to understand transplantation, using diagrams that are easy to understand. For indications and surgical procedures (treatment flow), we have designed atlas formats so that the indications and detailed surgical procedures can be more easily viewed and understood. We have tried to present many different case types and clinical situations with long-term follow-up results so that the reader can appreciate the great patient benefit and favorable prognosis of transplantation.

We hope that this book will contribute to the growth and further use of autotransplantation of teeth.

July 2024

Mitsuhiro Tsukiboshi, Nozomu Yamauchi, Yosuke Tsukiboshi, Taisuke Tsukiboshi

Acknowledgment

I would like to express my sincere gratitude to the mentors who provided materials for the publication of this book. As the father of modern autotransplantation of teeth, Dr. Jens Ove Andreasen (Aug,1935~Sept, 2020) pioneered many significant studies that have served as the stepping stones for so many to follow in his footsteps. I would also like to acknowledge my liberal use of his study data throughout this book and especially in Chapter 3, in which some of the figures are quoted from his research.

Dr. Yasuhiro Asai and his faculty at the Department of Endodontics at Tokyo Dental College (retired) have undertaken many important studies in transplantation and replantation. I am so fortunate to have been permitted to draw upon their valuable scientific data, which has contributed significantly to our own works and to this book.

Dr. Takeyasu Maeda of the Department of Anatomy at Niigata University School of Dentistry (retired) was kind enough to provide me with the important embryology data, for which we are also grateful.

Dr. Leif K. Bakland, Distinguished Emeritus Professor of Endodontics at Loma Linda University School of Dentistry (retired), has provided ongoing support on our transplantation journey for many years.

Finally, I would like to express my gratitude and love to all the staff, associates, and my family. To my beloved wife, Dr. Chie Tsukiboshi, for her help on many cases as a dedicated orthodontist, and more importantly as a partner for so many years.

Mitsuhiro Tsukiboshi

CONTENTS

Foreword 2

Preface 3

Acknowledgment 4

CHAPTER 1 Informed Consent on Autotransplantation of Teeth 7

CHAPTER 2 Embryology and Anatomy of Teeth and Periodontal Tissues 13

CHAPTER 3 Mechanisms of Wound Healing in Transplantation and Replantation 19

CHAPTER 4 Classification of Autotransplantation of Teeth and its Indications and Criteria 71

CHAPTER 5 Sequence and Treatment Procedures 97

CHAPTER 6 Autotransplantation of teeth in molar regions 127

CHAPTER 7 Autotransplantation of teeth in premolar regions 151

CHAPTER 8 Autotransplantation of teeth in anterior regions 173

CHAPTER 9 Autotransplantation of teeth in orthodontic treatment 187

CONTENTS

CHAPTER 10 Surgical extrusion and intentional replantation 213

CHAPTER 11 Prognosis 243

CHAPTER 12 In-house 3D replica fabrication and digital simulation using a free software 259

APPENDIX Index 269

CHAPTER 1

Informed Consent on Autotransplantation of Teeth

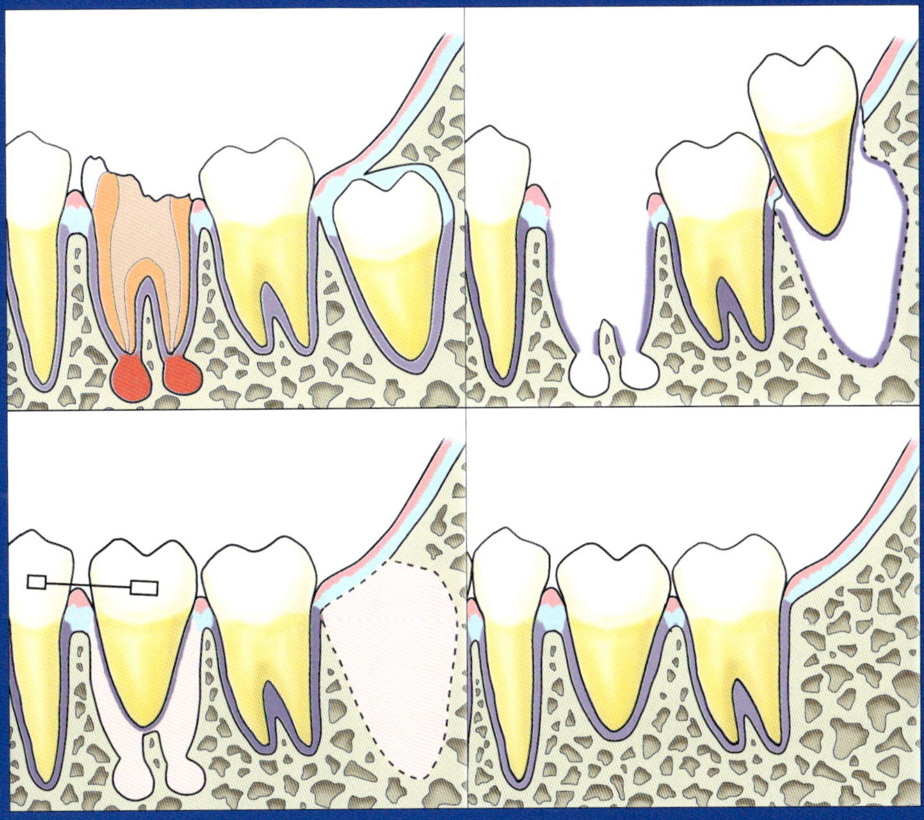

Prior to any dental examination and treatment, it is important to inform the patient about the procedure: what will be involved, the risk-benefit, cost-benefit, advantages and disadvantages, and the various expected outcomes (i.e. process-centered, disease-centered, and patient-centered outcomes) and prognosis. This chapter contains examples of typical clinical cases of autotransplantation (**Fig 1-1 to 1-3**) that may be helpful to better understand the workflow of the procedure.

Autotransplantation of Teeth and its Modalities

Autotransplantation of teeth (ATT) is a procedure that surgically moves a tooth from one position to another in the same oral cavity. For example, removing a hopeless tooth and replacing it with a healthy, nonfunctional tooth, like when an impacted third molar is transplanted into a socket/site of a deeply decay, unrestorable first molar (**Fig 1-1, 1-2**). Another example would be treatment for a congenitally missing tooth, e.g. a third molar is transplanted into the socket of a deciduous mandibular second molar where a mandibular second permanent premolar is congenitally missing (**Fig 1-3**). One of the advantages of ATT is that periodontal tissue lost due to periodontal disease can be restored (see **Chapter 6 Fig 6-7**).

In addition to conventional transplantation, there are included surgical extrusion and intentional replantation (see **Chapter 4** and **Chapter 10**), by which teeth that can hardly be treated by other methods may be preserved.

Clinical Examination and Diagnosis

Assessing and treatment planning an ATT case requires careful evaluation of the patient, including clinical and radiographic findings. It is necessary to measure and assess the donor tooth (e.g. the tooth to be removed and placed into the new site) and the recipient site (e.g. the site where the transplanted tooth will be placed) as well as the root form/shape and periodontal ligament (PDL) of the donor tooth. A preoperative Cone Beam Computed Tomography (CBCT) study is strongly advised.

Patients will need to know that it is always possible that a procedure may have to be discontinued for a variety of reasons, such as complications in extracting the donor tooth, problems with the recipient site (such as extensive bony defect), and unanticipated difficulties. The patient's compliance, as well as attitude toward having a complex and somewhat uncertain procedure performed, must be taken into account when presenting this treatment option.

Advantages and Disadvantages of Transplantation

Advantages include the following:

1. The patient can avoid a fixed bridge which helps preserve tooth structure of the adjacent teeth.
2. The patient can avoid an implant, which carries its own risks and higher costs.
3. ATT is more biocompatible than implants. If successful, the donor tooth will heal with a healthy PDL, which can induce bone formation and adapt/move naturally. It can also be orthodontically moved.

Disadvantages include the following:

1. ATT is technique-sensitive, and requires multiple steps and appointments.
2. Treatment outcomes may be difficult to predict.
3. Possible complications are root resorption, which may result in the eventual loss of the tooth.

Sequence of Treatment

In cases where the unsalvageable tooth is still in the socket (future recipient site), there are typically two approaches for ATT: The clinician can perform the transplantation immediately after extraction of the tooth in the recipient site, which is known as immediate transplantation, or within 1 and a half months after extraction of the tooth in the recipient site, known as delayed transplantation. If more than 2 months have elapsed, healing of the recipient site may progress with decrease in bone height and width, thus making the transplantation more difficult. The prognosis of immediate transplantation is thought to be better due to the PDL tissues remaining on the recipient socket wall. If there is not enough keratinized gingiva at the recipient site to achieve adequate primary closure, the immediate transplantation may have higher risks, and delayed transplantation is preferred because there will be more available keratinized gingival tissue, typically 3 to 5 weeks after tooth extraction (see **Chapter 5**). Therefore, the timing of tooth extraction of the recipient site should be carefully assessed for ATT.

The author's surgical procedures for immediate transplantation are as follows:

1. Extraction of the tooth in the recipient site.
2. Preparation of the recipient socket, ideally using a replica of the donor tooth (see **Chapter 12**).
3. Extraction of the donor tooth and placement of the donor into the recipient socket.
4. Suture and surgical dressing.
5. Irrigation with saline the next day.
6. Removal of the sutures and the dressing after 7 days. If the mobility is high, connect the transplant with the adjacent tooth with wire and resin.

Transplantation of an immature tooth to replace a hopeless first molar

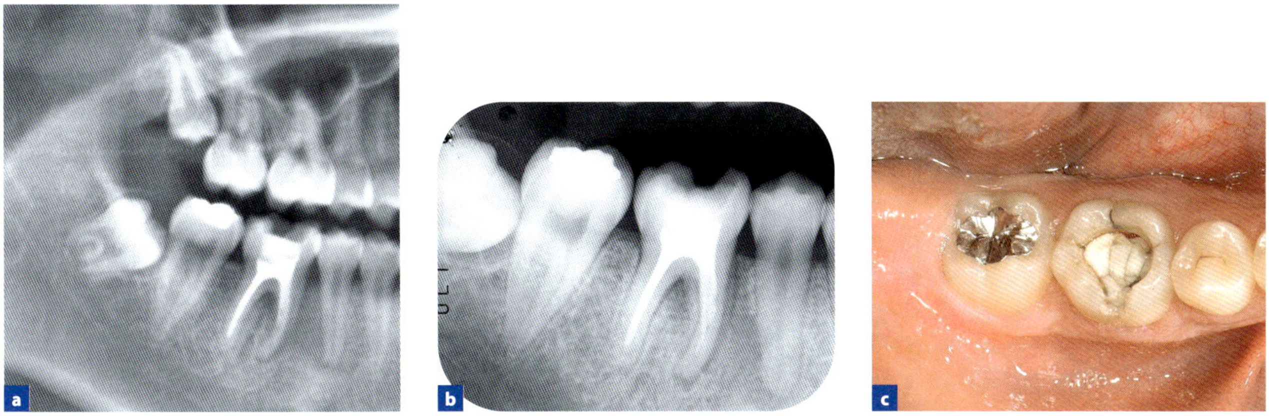

Fig 1-1a to c Preoperative views of an 18-year-old male with a vertical root fracture of the mandibular right first molar. The impacted mandibular right wisdom tooth has incomplete root formation, and is a good candidate for a donor tooth for autotransplantation.

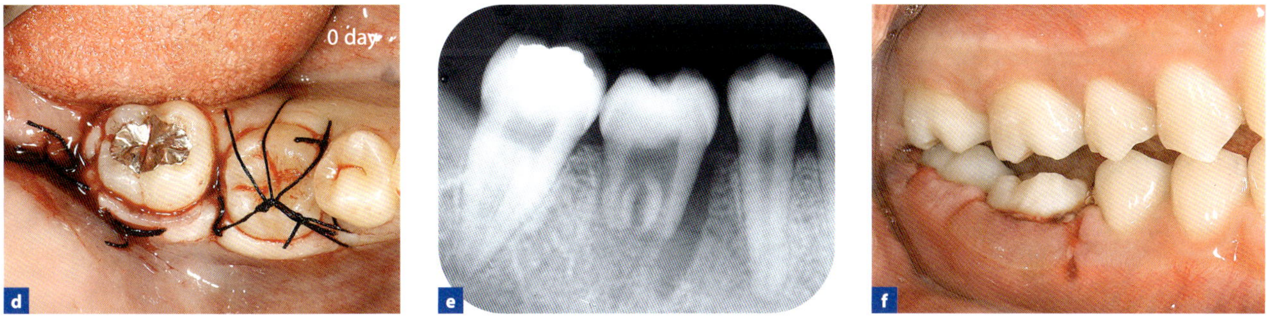

Fig 1-1d to f The day of the transplantation procedure. Interproximal and occlusal spaces are observed around the transplanted tooth.

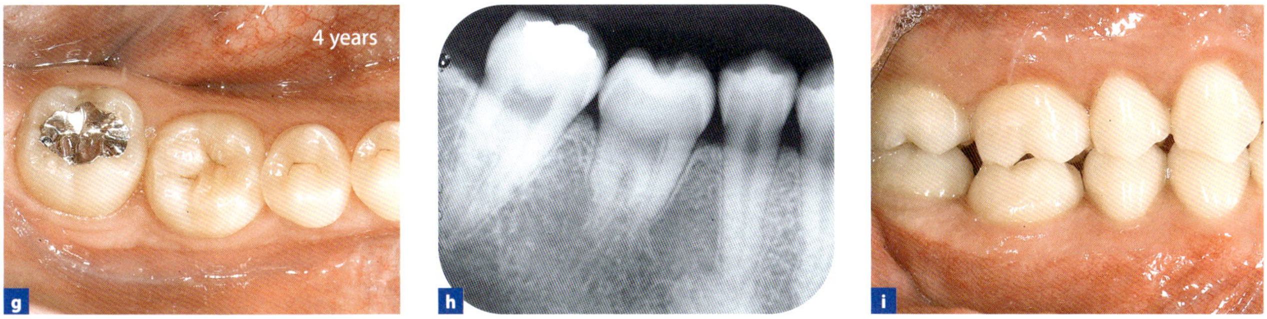

Fig 1-1g to i Four years after the procedure. Pulp canal obliteration (spontaneous healing of pulp) and root development are observed. EPT (+) response. The aforementioned spaces have spontaneously closed by the natural eruption of the transplanted tooth.

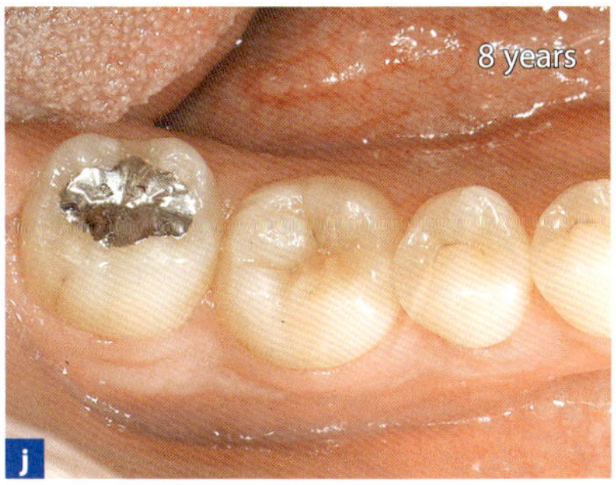

Fig 1-1j Occlusal view after 8 years.

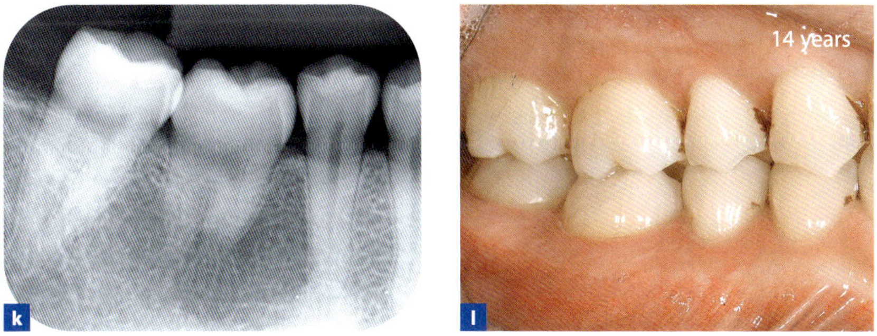

Fig 1-1k, l 14 years after the procedure. EPT (+) response. The tooth is asymptomatic, functional and the radiograph shows no apparent abnormalities such as root resorption.

Transplantation of a mature tooth to replace a hopeless first molar

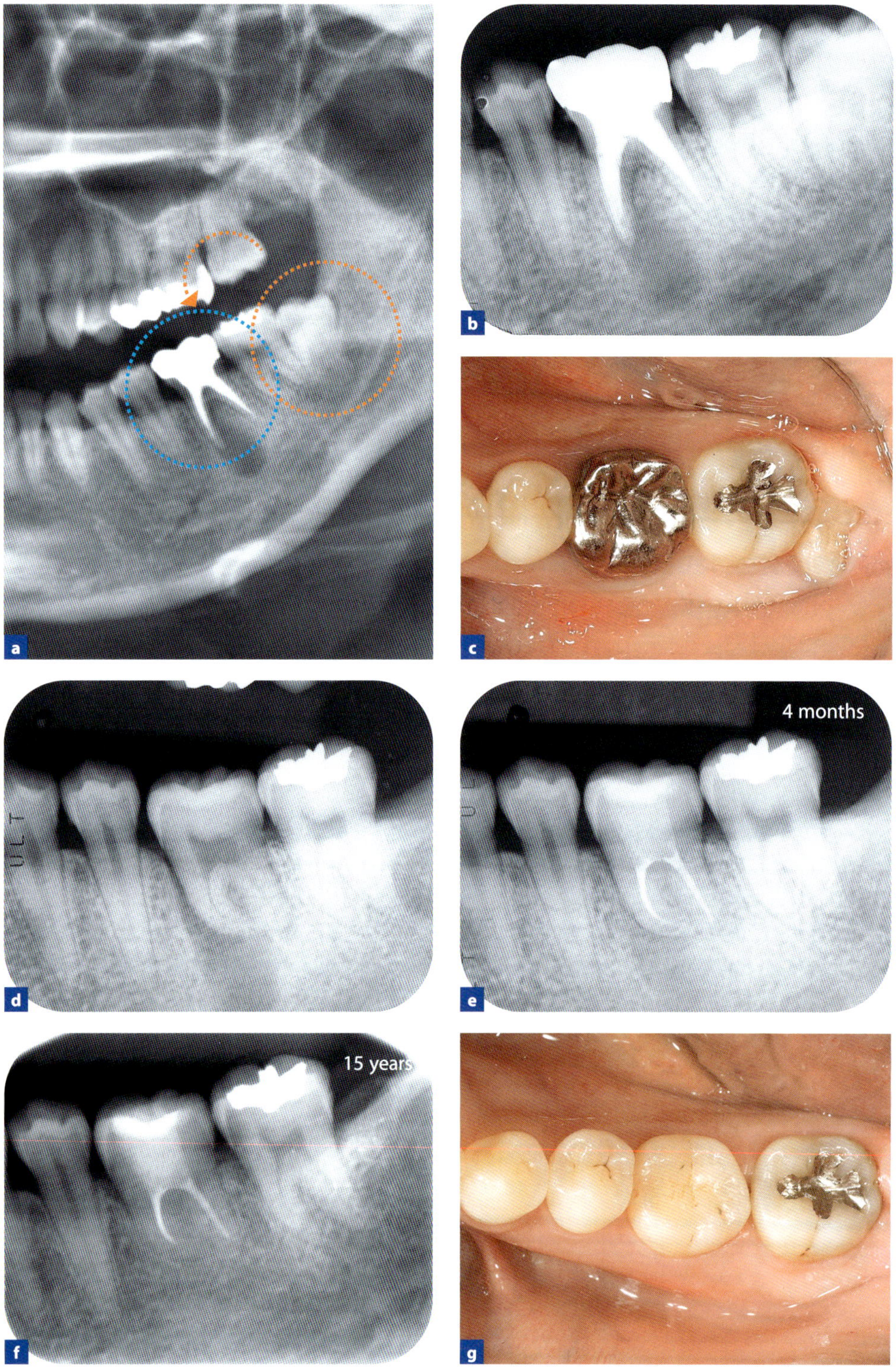

Fig 1-2a to c Preoperative views of a 27-year-old female with a vertical root fracture of the mandibular left first molar. The half-impacted mandibular left wisdom tooth is not in occlusion and can be used as a donor tooth.

Fig 1-2d Immediately after transplantation.

Fig 1-2e Four months after the procedure. Since spontaneous healing of the pulp is not expected in a tooth with mature root formation, root canal procedure should be done at the appropriate time. Usually, root canal treatment is initiated 2 weeks after transplantation, and root canal completion at 1month after transplantation.

Fig 1-2f and g 15 years postoperative. The transplanted tooth is restored using composite resin. No complications are observed.

7. Start root canal treatment (RCT) of the coronal portion after 2 weeks, place an interappointment medicament, and finish RCT around 4 weeks later. Remove the splint.
8. Restore the transplant with an appropriate method and schedule regular recalls.

In the case of ATT of immature teeth, root canal therapy is usually not necessary; if the apex is wide open, revascularization of the pulp and continuation of root development are expected (**Fig 1-1 and 1-3**).

Transplantation for a patient suffering a congenitally missing tooth

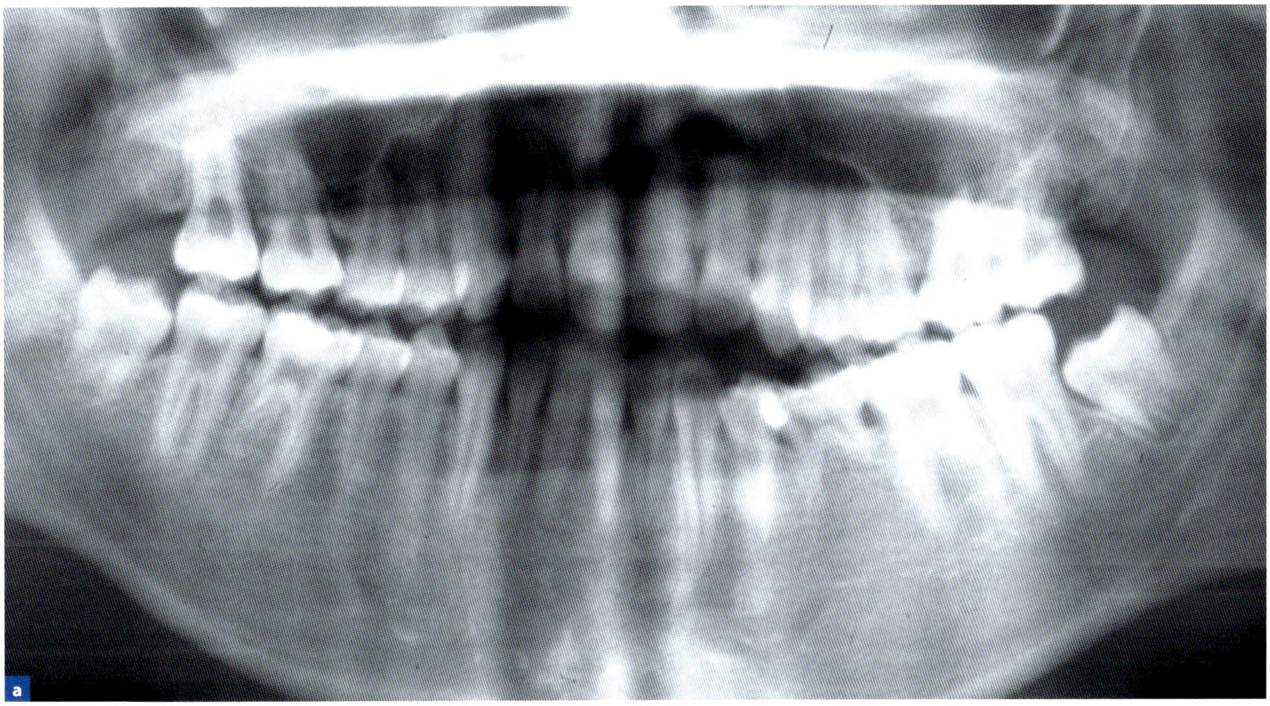

a

Fig 1-3a Panoramic radiograph of a 17-year-old female with a congenitally missing mandibular left second premolar. The mandibular wisdom teeth are at stage 4 of root development (see **Chapter 3 Fig 3-27**), indicating appropriate timing for autotransplantation.

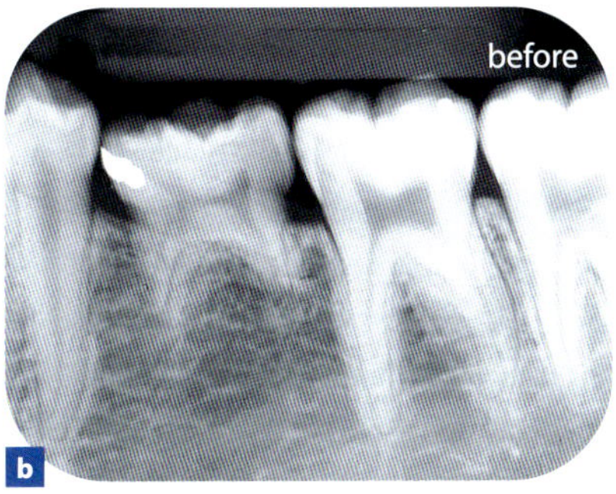

b

Fig 1-3b Preoperative radiograph. A deciduous tooth is retained in the area of the congenitally missing tooth.

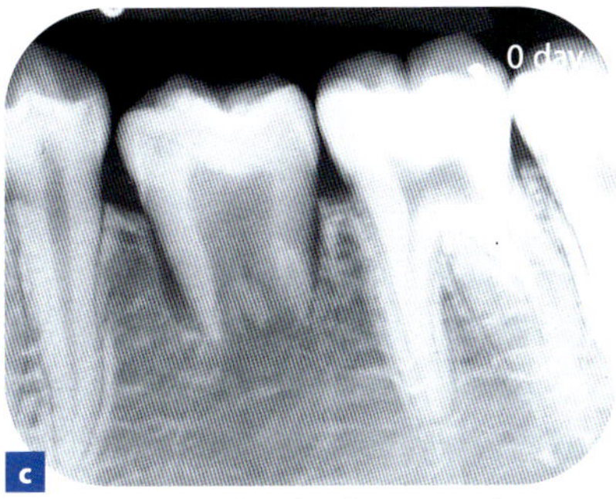

c

Fig 1-3c Immediately after transplantation. The mandibular right wisdom tooth is used as a donor tooth since it is easier to extract.

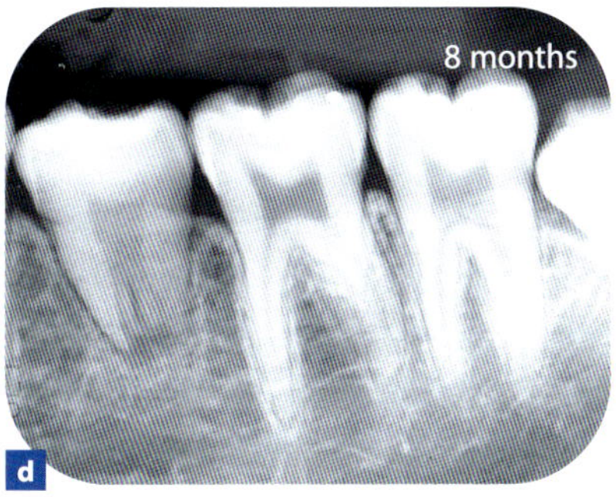

d

Fig 1-3d Eight months after the procedure. The transplanted tooth appears to be undergoing pulp canal obliteration and continued root development.

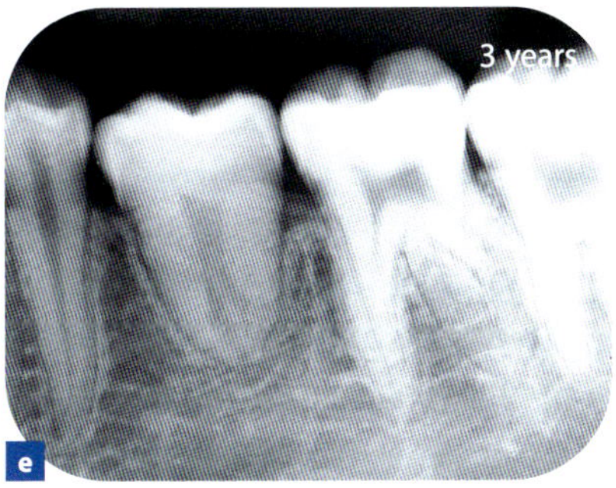

e

Fig 1-3e Three years after the procedure. Root development appears complete.

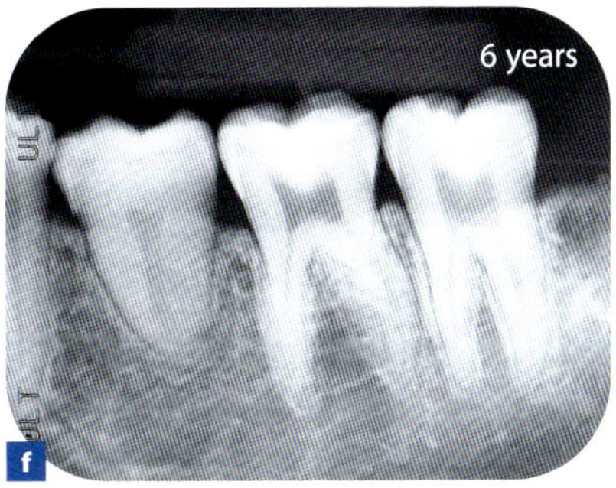

f

Fig 1-3f Six years postoperative.

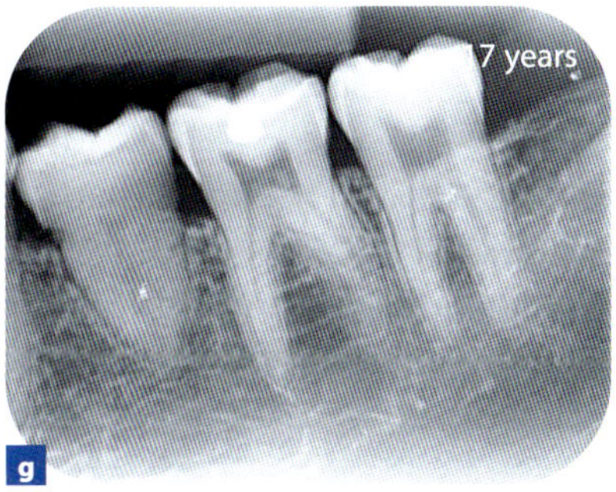

g

Fig 1-3g 17 years postoperative. Possible slight surface root resorption (not progressive) on the mesial aspect is observed. The tooth is asymptomatic, functional, and continues to respond to EPT.

CHAPTER 2

Embryology and Anatomy of Teeth and Periodontal Tissues

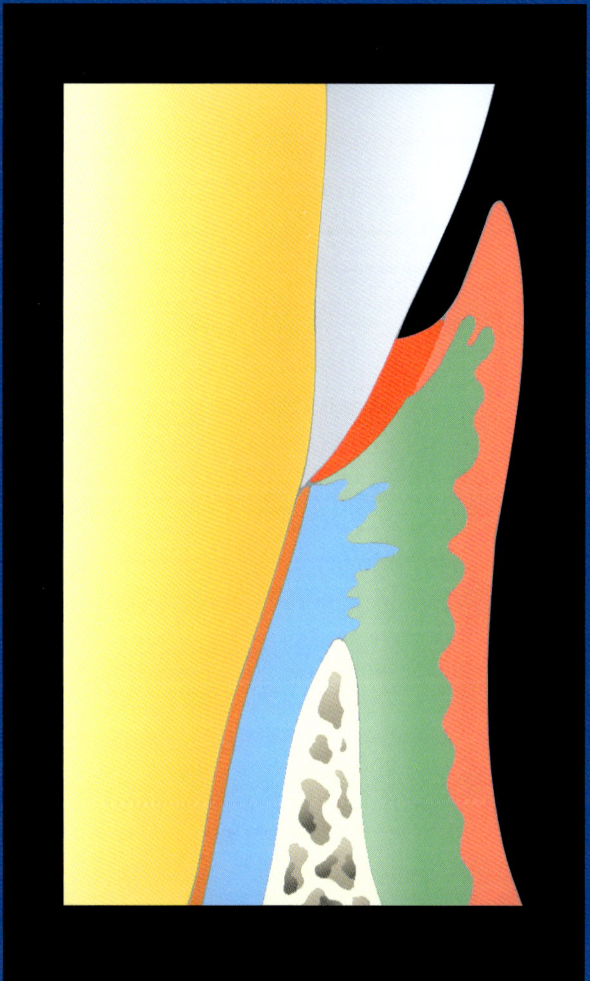

In order to understand wound healing associated with transplanted teeth, it is important to have a working knowledge of the development and anatomy of teeth and periodontal tissues. In recent years, the progress in this field, particularly the research and understanding of molecular mechanisms of tooth germ differentiation, has been remarkable. This chapter will go over the fundamentals of tooth and periodontal tissue development at the macroscopic and histological levels.

Development of Teeth and Periodontal Tissues[1–3]

Development of tooth germ

The formation of the tooth germ, composed of enamel organ, dental papilla and dental follicle begins when neural crest cells migrate to the site of the future tooth development and form the dental mesenchyme (**Fig 2-1**). The dental mesenchyme then induces epithelial cells that eventually become an enamel organ (**Fig 2-2**). The epithelial cells are then morphologically divided into inner and outer enamel epithelium. Neural crest cells reside in the dental papilla at the concavity of the inner enamel epithelium and differentiate into odontoblasts, pulpal cells, sensory neurons and other cells (**Fig 2-3**). The enamel organ and dental papilla are surrounded by fiber-rich mesenchyme (**Fig 2-3**). This saclike structure is called the dental follicle and eventually form the periodontal tissues, including cementum, periodontal ligament, and alveolar bone.

Dentin and enamel formation

The inner epithelial cells differentiate into ameloblasts (enamel-forming cells). This event sends signals to mesenchymal cells in the dental papilla and they differentiate into odontoblasts to start forming mineralized dentin. On the surface of the mineralized dentin, ameloblasts synthesize enamel matrix and form mineralized enamel. Upon completion of dentin and

Development of tooth germ

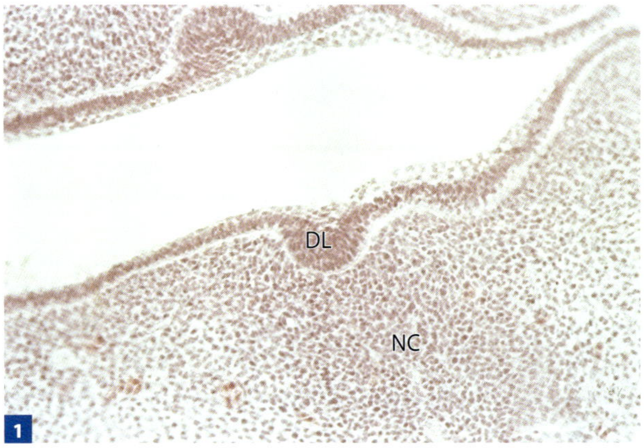

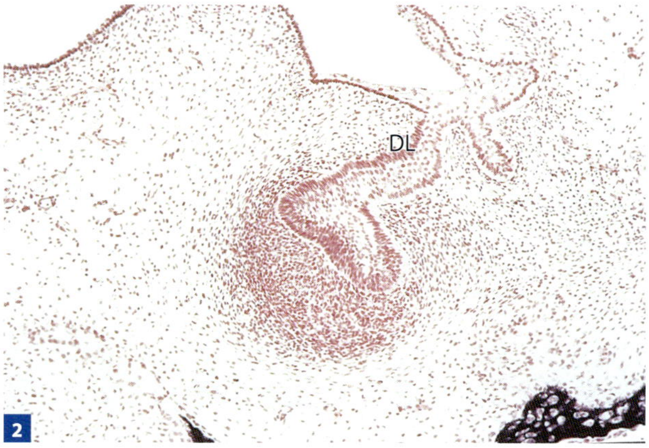

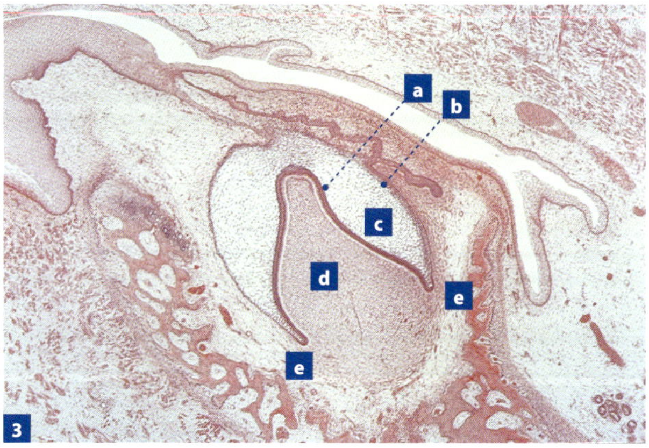

Fig 2-1 (above left) Neural crest cell migration and formation of dental ledge. Thickening of the epithelium occurs in the region of the future tooth development after migration and proliferation of mesenchymal cells derived from the neural crest (NC); then the dental ledge (DL) is formed.

Fig 2-2 (above right) Cap stage of tooth germ at 9 to 10 weeks of embryonic development. The dental ledge proliferates and differentiates, forming enamel organ.

Fig 2-3 (right) Bell stage of tooth germ at 14 week of embryonic development. Inner enamel epithelium (**a**), outer enamel epithelium (**b**), stellate reticulum (**c**), and dental papilla cells (**d**) can be distinguished, and dental germ is held in the dental follicle (**e**). The dental follicle is a sac-like structure composed of fiber-rich mesenchymal tissue.

(courtesy of Dr. Takeyasu Maeda, Niigata University School of Dentistry, Department of Oral Anatomy).

Formation of Hertwig's epithelial root sheath and root dentin

Fig 2-4 After the enamel and dentin of the tooth crown is formed, the inner and outer dental epithelia fuse together forming a bilayer of cells from the cervical curvature towards the apex. This bilayer of epithelial cells, "Hertwig's root sheath", plays a critical role in determining the shape of the tooth root and induction of odontoblast differentiation.
(courtesy of Dr. Takeyasu Maeda, Niigata University School of Dentistry).

Fig 2-5 Epithelial diaphragm. The portion of the root sheath bending toward the dental papilla.
(courtesy of Dr. Takeyasu Maeda, Niigata University School of Dentistry).

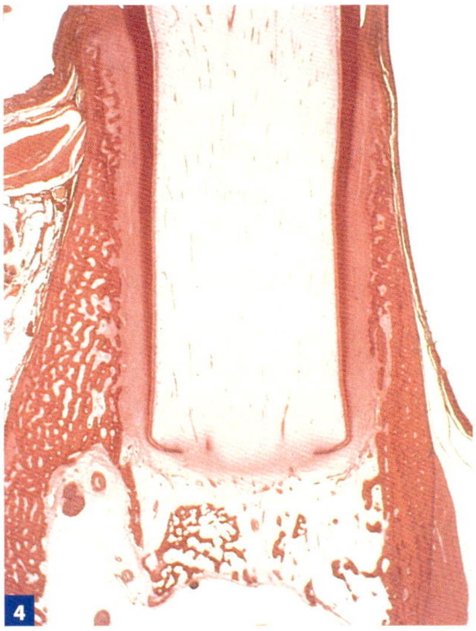
4

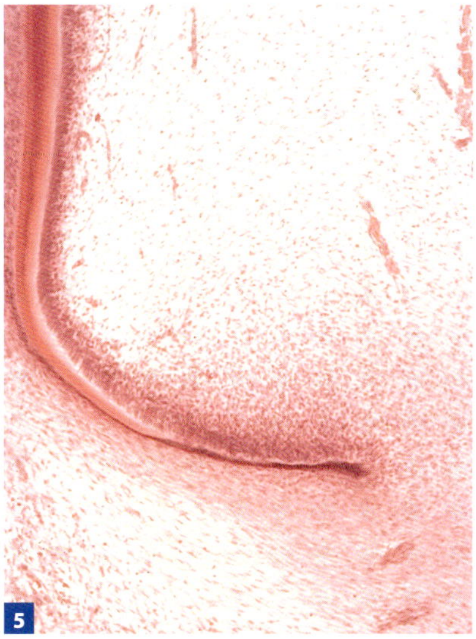
5

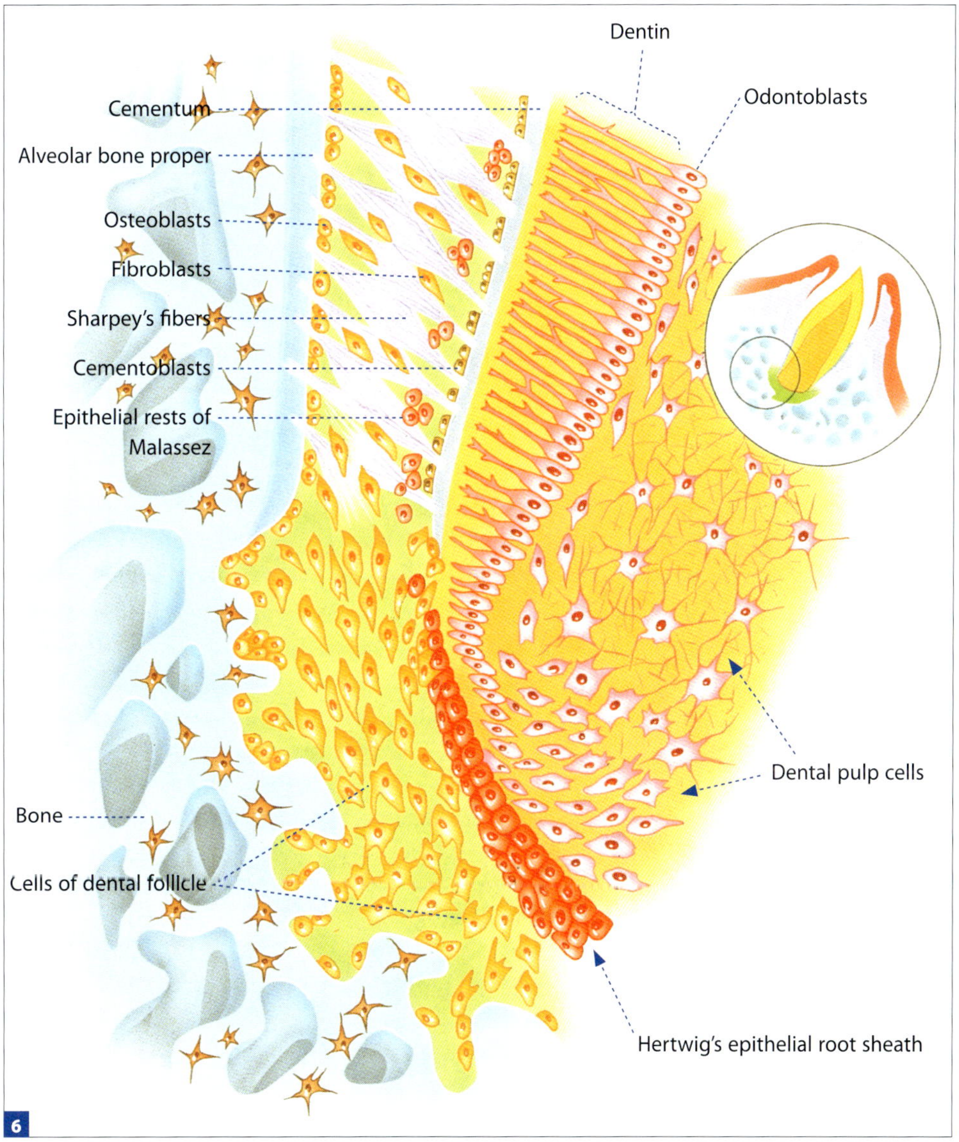

6

Fig 2-6 Illustration of apex and periodontal tissues of developing teeth.
Inside Hertwig's epithelial root sheath (epithelial diaphragm), odontoblasts differentiated from dental pulp cells form root dentin. Cementum is deposited on the surface of newly formed dentin by cementoblasts differentiated from cells of the dental follicle. Sharpey's fibers are embedded in cementum by fibroblasts derived from the dental follicle. At the same time, the alveolar bone proper is formed by osteoblasts differentiated from cells in the dental follicle and the Sharpey's fibers are embedded into this new bone.

enamel formation in the tooth crown, the inner and outer enamel epithelia fuse together forming a bilayer cell sheath and extend into the apex of the tooth from the cervical curvature. The bilayer of epithelial cells is called "Hertwig's epithelial root sheath," and it is thought to induce the differentiation of mesenchymal cells in dental papilla into odontoblasts leading to the formation and completion of the root dentin [4]. As the root dentin grows toward the apex, the "Hertwig's epithelial root sheath" separates from the enamel epithelium, moves toward the apex (**Fig 2-4** and **2-5**) and eventually disintegrates. the remnants of the Hertwig's epithelial root sheath are present in the periodontal ligament and they are called the epithelial rest of Malassez (**Fig 2-6**).

Periodontal tissues are formed by cells derived from the dental follicle cells derived from the dental follicle differentiate into cementoblasts (cementum-forming cells), fibroblasts (principal cells involved in the formation of periodontal ligament), and osteoblasts (bone-forming cells). Cementum is deposited on the root surface, while fibroblasts form the periodontal ligament. In the meantime, osteoblasts, which are differentiated from cells derived from the dental follicle, form the alveolar bone proper on the inner surface of the alveolar process. The periodontal ligament (made up primarily of collagen fibers) attach and embed into the cementum and alveolar bone, and is called Sharpey's fibers (**Fig 2-6**). Thus, Sharpey's fibers serve as attachment for the tooth root to the surrounding alveolar bone (**Fig 2-7**). By completing all of these intricate and synchronized events, healthy tooth and periodontal tissues are formed.

Histology of the periodontal ligament

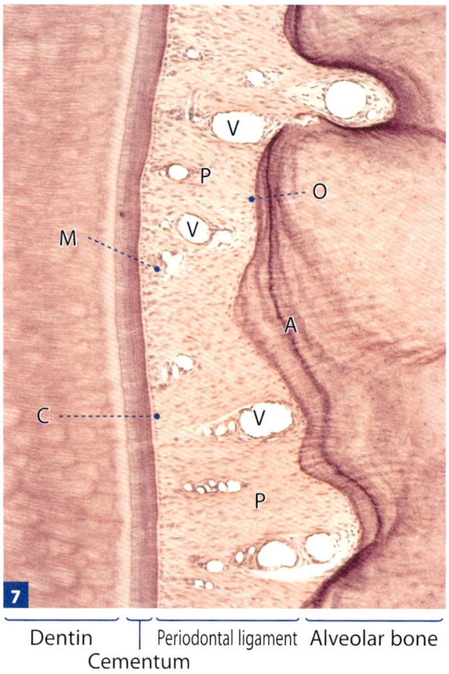

Fig 2-7 The periodontal ligament contains many blood vessels (**V**). A single layer of cementoblasts (**C**) is aligned on the surface of the cementum, and epithelial rests of Malassez (**M**) are observed near the cementum. Osteoblasts (**O**) align on the surface of the alveolar bone proper (**A**), and collagen fibers in the periodontal ligament (**P**) connect the bone and cementum (courtesy of Dr. Takeyasu Maeda, Niigata University School of Dentistry).

Anatomy of Teeth and Periodontal Tissues

Supracrestal tissue attachment (biologic width)

The anatomy of fully erupted teeth and periodontal tissues[1-3,5] is illustrated in **Fig 2-8**. In an average, healthy erupted tooth, the cementoenamel junction (CEJ) is generally located about 1 mm coronal to the crest of the alveolar bone. The junctional epithelium on average is 1 mm coronal to the CEJ, which is attached firmly to the tooth (epithelial attachment) by hemidesmosomes. The root dentin apical to the CEJ is attached to gingival connective tissue and alveolar bone through cementum and Sharpey's fibers. This type of attachment is called connective tissue attachment. A band of soft tissue attachment between the base of the gingival sulcus and the alveolar crest, which is composed of approximately 1 mm of attachment epithelium and 1 mm of connective tissue attachment, thus a total of 2mm, is referred to as biological width or supracrestal tissue attachment[6-11] (**Fig 2-8d**). A healthy biological width is thought to be important in maintaining healthy periodontal tissues, so the clinician should be aware of it in the treatment strategy of autotransplantation and replantation.

Alveolar bone, gingiva and alveolar mucosa

Alveolar bone (also called alveolar process) is composed of two parts: the basal bone including bone marrow and alveolar bone proper (lamellar bone). The alveolar bone proper is a thin, dense/compact bone deposited on the inner surface of the alveolar process by osteoblasts in the periodontal ligament. It surrounds the root and is observed as the lamina dura in radiographs (**Fig 2-8b**). Gingiva and alveolar mucosa surround the teeth and cover the alveolar bone. The alveolar mucosa is an unkeratinized and movable mucosa containing musculature. Gingival tissue is a keratinized soft connective tissue located coronal to the alveolar mucosa. It consists of attached gingiva, which is "attached" to teeth or alveolar bone, and free gingiva (or marginal gingiva), which is the gingival sulcus surrounding teeth (**Fig 2-8a** and **2-8c**).

Anatomy of teeth and periodontal tissues

Fig 2-8 Anatomy of teeth and periodontal tissues.

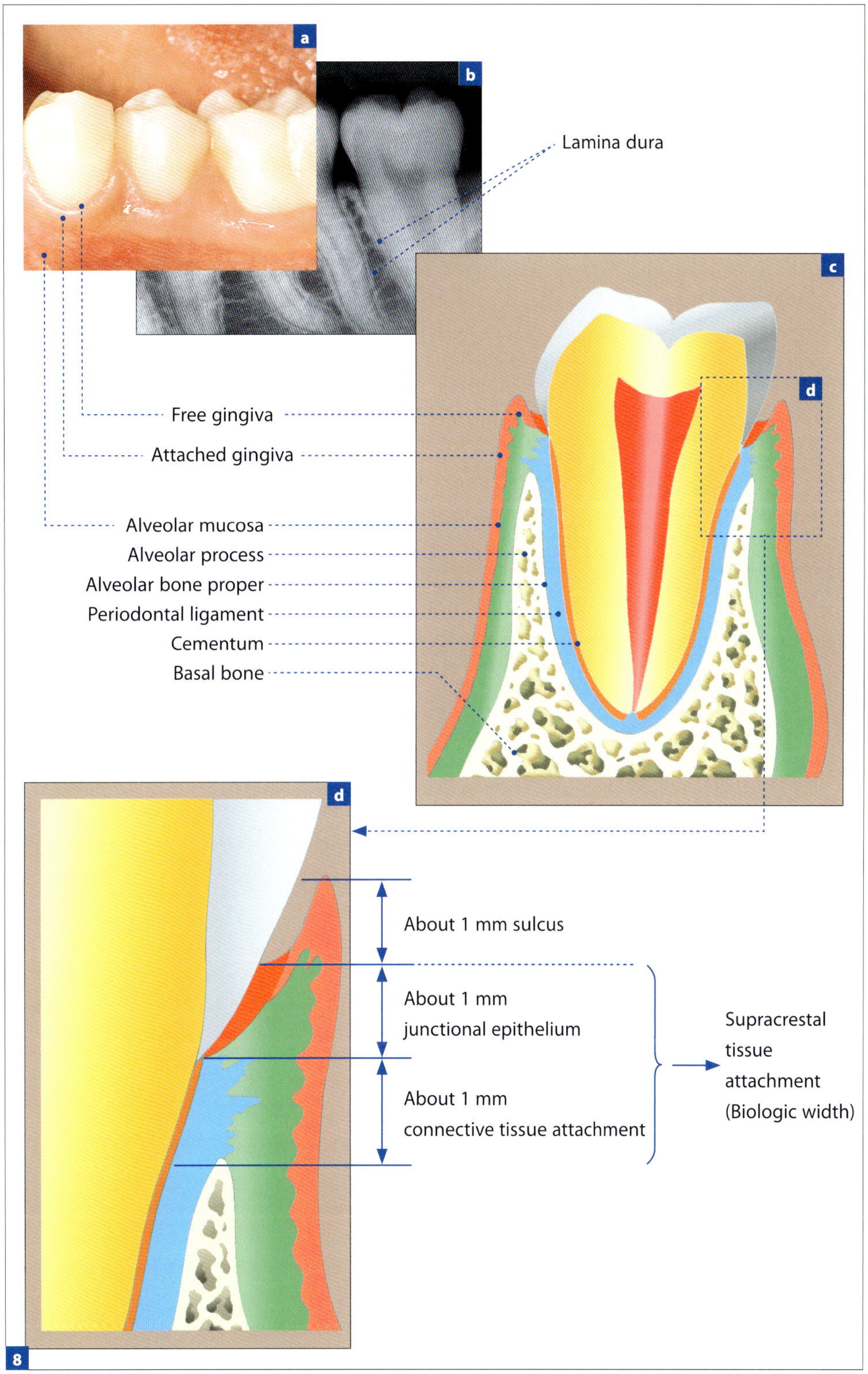

Fig 2-8a to d A fully erupted permanent tooth and its periodontal tissues shown by clinical photography (**a**), radiographic image (**b**) and illustrations (**c, d**). Alveolar bone embryologically consists of the alveolar bone proper and the alveolar process. The alveolar process is derived from the basal bone and the alveolar bone proper is derived from the periodontal ligament. The alveolar bone proper is observed as lamina dura on the radiograph. Gingiva consists of free gingiva and attached gingiva transitioning to alveolar mucosa. The CEJ is located 1 mm coronal to the crest of the alveolar bone and 1 mm of connective tissue attachment above the crest of the alveolar bone. Moreover, 1 mm of junctional epithelium and 1 mm of gingival sulcus are formed coronal to it. Because these connective tissue attachments and junctional epithelia above the crest of bone are observed on almost all tooth surfaces, they determine supracrestal tissue attachment (biological width). In healthy periodontal tissue, supracrestal tissue attachment is 3 mm after adding 1 mm of gingival sulcus.

References

1. Ten Cate AR. Oral Histology, development, structure and function, ed 3. St Louis: Mosby, 1989.
2. Bhaskar SN. Orban's oral histology and embryology, ed 10. St Louis: Mosby, 1986.
3. Lindhe J. Textbook of clinical periodontology. Copenhagen: Munksgaard, 1984.
4. Hammarström L. Enamel matrix, cementum development and regeneration. J Clin Periodontol. 1997; 24: 658-68.
5. Rateitschak KH, Wolf HF, Hassell TM. Color atlas of dental medicine. Periodontology, ed 2. New York: Thieme, 1989.
6. Maeda T, Ohshima H, Tsukiboshi M. Tooth and periodontium: development and structure [in Japanese]. the Quintessence. 1997; 16: 2051-72.
7. Gargiulo AW, Wentz FM, Orban B. Dimensions and relations of the dentogingival junction in humans. J Periodontol. 1961; 32: 261–7.
8. Maynard JG, Wilson RD. Physiologic dimensions of the periodontium significant to the restorative dentist. J Periodontol. 1979; 50(4): 170.
9. Ingber JS, Rose LF, Coslet JG. The "biologic width"-a concept in periodontics and restorative dentistry. Alpha Omegan. 1977; 70(3): 62-5.
10. Nevins M, Mellonig JT. Clinical approaches and evidence of success. Vol 1. Periodontal therapy. Chicago: Quintessence publishing, 1998.
11. Tsuji S. "Europian periodontal disease classification" revised for the first time in 20 years [in Japanese]. the Quintessence. 2018; 37(9): 55-8.

CHAPTER 3

Mechanisms of Wound Healing in Transplantation and Replantation

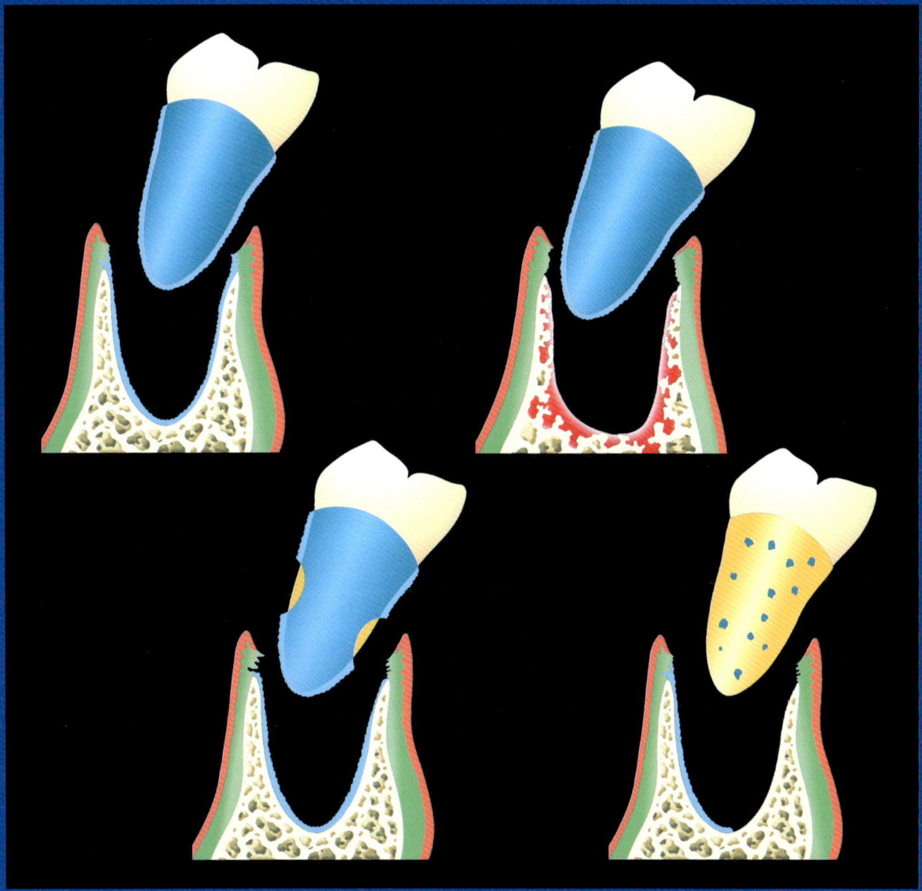

In the past 40 years, an increase in understanding of wound healing following transplantation and replantation has improved the success of these procedures significantly.

Through good understanding of the healing mechanisms, it is possible to achieve successful outcomes in different case types and also to be able to manage possible complications that may occur after transplantation. The healing mechanism of transplantation will be discussed in the following five categories: the healing of the periodontal ligament, the mechanism of root resorption, healing of the gingival tissue, healing of the pulp and continuation of root development and healing of the alveolar bone.

Healing of the Periodontal Ligament

Reattachment

Ideal healing of the periodontal ligament occurs when the extracted tooth is replanted in the original extraction socket within a short period of time (**Fig 3-1** and **3-2**). This type of healing is described as a reattachment of the periodontal ligament. Reattachment is defined as "the reunion of connective tissue and a root surface that have been separated by incision or injury"[1,2]. In transplantation and replantation, reattachment may be further defined as connective tissue (fibrous) reunion with the root surface, in which the vital periodontal ligament attaches and surrounds the root after replantation.

Reattachment in replantation

A number of studies have demonstrated that healing by reattachment occurs if an extracted tooth with adequate periodontal ligament attachment is replanted in the extraction socket within a short period of time[3–11].The periodontal ligament is usually separated in the middle. The inner layer is attached to the tooth and the rest is left in the extraction socket. The healing process of the replanted tooth in an animal study (monkey) is as follows[5]:

- Three days after replantation: fibrin and erythrocytes are scattered between the root's attached periodontal ligament and the remaining PDL left on the extraction socket walls. Hemorrhage is observed in some areas (**Fig 3-2a, b**).
- One to 2 weeks after replantation: fibroblasts and collagen fibers are visible in the torn area, which indicates the beginning of repair of the periodontal ligament (**Fig 3-2c, d**).

Healing by reattachment after replantation

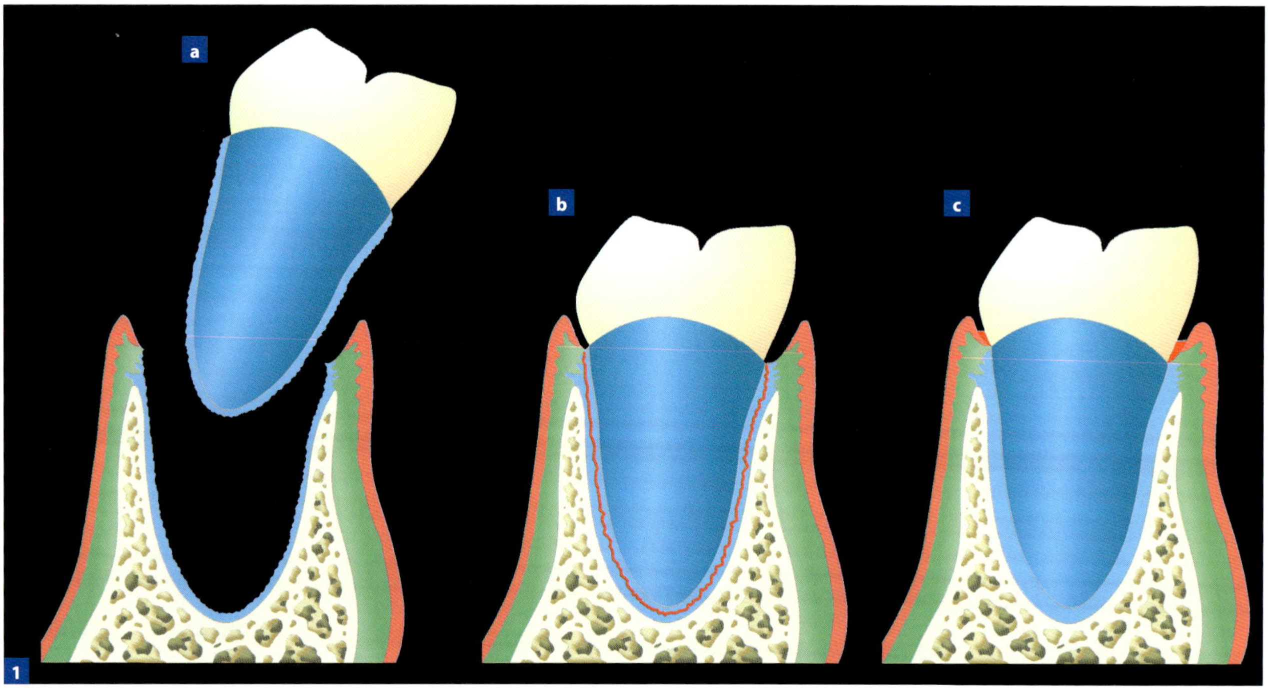

Fig 3-1a Before replantation. The extracted tooth is ready to be placed back in its alveolar socket. The periodontal ligament is intact both on the root surface and the wall of the alveolar socket.

Fig 3-1b Immediately after replantation. There is a thin blood clot in the periodontal ligament space between the root and the socket wall.

Fig 3-1c After healing (4 to 8 weeks postoperative). Reattachment of the periodontal ligament is complete.

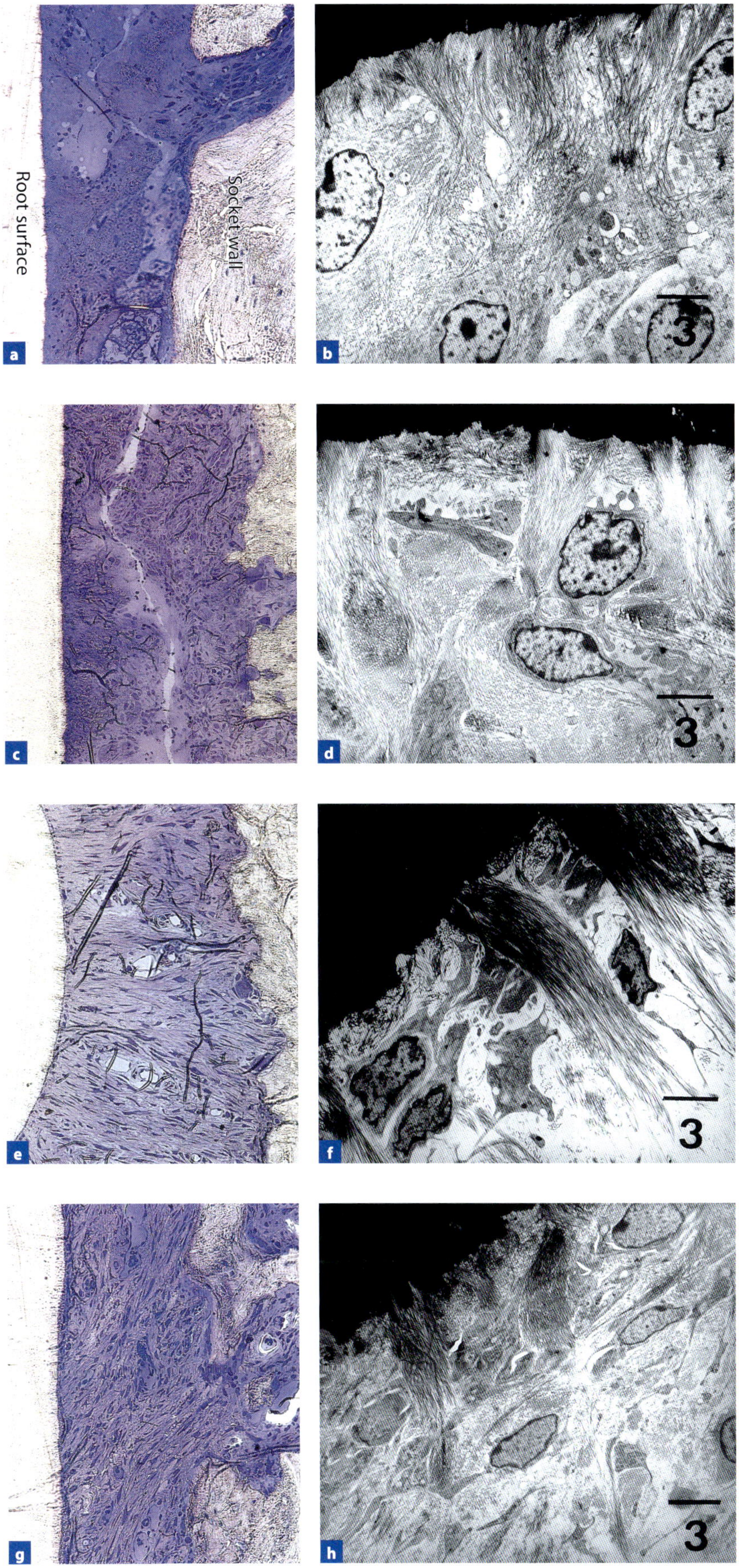

Fig 3-2 Histologic healing showing reattachment following replantation of monkey teeth (courtesy of Tokyo Dental College).

Fig 3-2a Three days after replantation. Periodontal ligament can be seen attached to both the root surface and alveolar socket wall; blood clot with fibrum reticulumis present.
Fig 3-2b Electron micrograph of root surface in **Fig 3-2a**. Collagen fibers run perpendicular to the cementum with interspersed cementoblasts and cells undergoing degeneration.

Fig 3-2c One week after replantation. Note the empty space between the periodontal ligament fibers from the root surface and the alveolus. Resorption cavities and osteoclasts are visible on the socket wall; spindle cells can be seen near the root surface.
Fig 3-2d Electron micrograph of root surface in **Fig 3-2c**. Bundles of collagen fibers are attached to the cementum with cementoblasts interspersed among the fibers.

Fig 3-2e Two weeks after replantation. Cementoblasts are present on the root surface and periodontal ligament fibers run from the root surface to the alveolar wall with fibroblasts aligned parallel to the fibers. Also note apposition of new bone on the socket wall.
Fig 3-2f Electron micrograph of root surface in **Fig 3-2e**. Note bundles of collagen fibers with high density extending at right angles from cementum. Spindle-shaped cementoblasts are parallel to the cementum.

Fig 3-2g Four weeks after replantation. Cementoblasts are aligned on the root surface and osteoblasts are aligned on the bony wall. In between these surfaces functionally arranged periodontal ligament fibers are aligned with many fibroblasts present.
Fig 3-2h Electron micrograph of root surface in **Fig 3-2g**. Bundles of collagen fibers run perpendicular to the cementum with cementoblasts interspersed. Also note fibroblasts present among the fibers.
(**a**, **c**, **e**, **g**: toluidine blue staining)

- Two to 3 weeks after replantation: proliferation of fibroblasts and regularly aligned bundles of collagen fibers are observed, which indicates that functional alignment of the periodontal ligament tissue is in progress(**Fig 3-2e, f**) .
- Four weeks after replantation: near normal periodontal ligament and alignment of collagen fiber bundles are observed (**Fig 3-2g, h**).

The timing of this process may vary from one study to another, but it is clear that reattachment healing does take place in replantation. It appears that it takes around 1 month for periodontal ligament healing to reach the initial stage (functional arrangement of fibers), and in the gingival and cervical areas of the root, reattachment occurs sooner (around 1 to 3 weeks)[10,11].

Reattachment in transplantation

Healing of the periodontal ligament in transplantation to surgically prepared (newly formed) alveolar sockets is different than that observed in replantation or the transplantation to existing (freshly extracted) sockets[12-17](**Fig 3-3** and **3-4**). The difference in healing is likely related to the absence of periodontal ligament fibers on the walls of the surgically prepared sockets (**Fig 3-5** and **3-6**).

Reattachment of gingival fibers to cervical root fibers is similar to that which is seen in replantation and transplantation to existing sockets (**Fig 3-5b**). Below the crest of bone, however, there appears to be a different healing process which occurs. During the first week after transplantation the root surface periodontal ligament is kept vital in the presence of the surrounding blood clot (see **Fig 3-5b**). During the next 2 weeks the blood clot is replaced by granulation tissue, which provides a favorable environment for the periodontal ligament, supplying nutrients and setting the stage for connective tissue reattachment. Over the next 2 to 6 months, the granulation tissue and immature bone is gradually replaced by mature bone and tooth-bone reattachment occurs (see **Fig 3-5c**). According to research at the Tokyo Dental College[12-17], it appears that transplantations to surgically prepared sockets result in less functionally aligned periodontal ligament compared with that

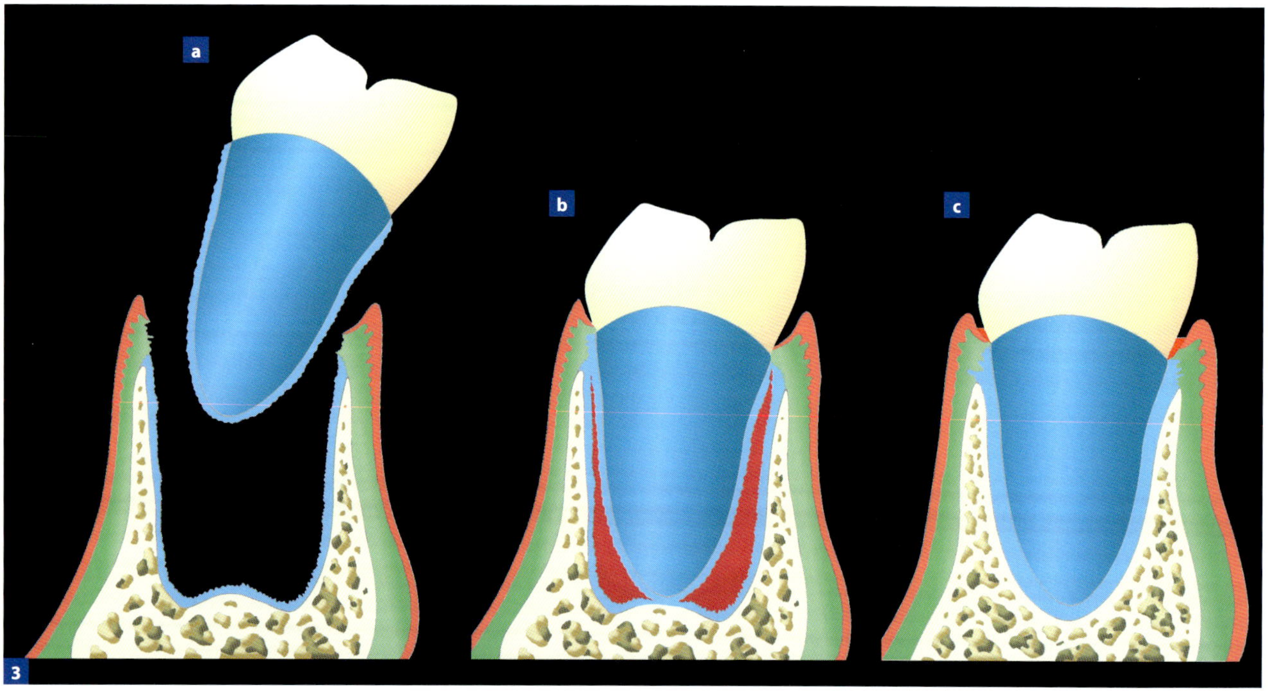

Fig 3-3 Healing by reattachment after transplantation.
Fig 3-3a Before transplantation. The empty recipient alveolar socket is ready to receive the donor tooth, which has periodontal ligament fibers attached to the root.
Fig 3-3b After transplantation. The gingival connective tissue and supra-crestal periodontal ligament tissues are closely approximated to the cervical area of the tooth. In the remainder of the socket, a blood clot forms between the tooth and the socket wall.
Fig 3-3c After healing. Reestablishment of the periodontal ligament connection between the root and the reformed alveolar socket has occurred. Early healing can be expected between the periodontal ligament of the recipient socket and the transplant tooth.

Fig 3-4 Histologic healing showing reattachment following transplantation of monkey teeth a freshly extracted socket (courtesy of Tokyo Dental College).

Fig 3-4a One week after transplantation of a donor tooth with periodontal ligament attached to the root system. Note the periodontal ligament attached to the root surface and granulation tissue present in the middle of the periodontal ligament space.
Fig 3-4b Two weeks after transplantation. There is no change involving the root surface, but new bone apposition can be seen on the socket wall. The periodontal ligament fibers are not yet continuous from the root to the bone. odontal ligament fibers between the root and bone.

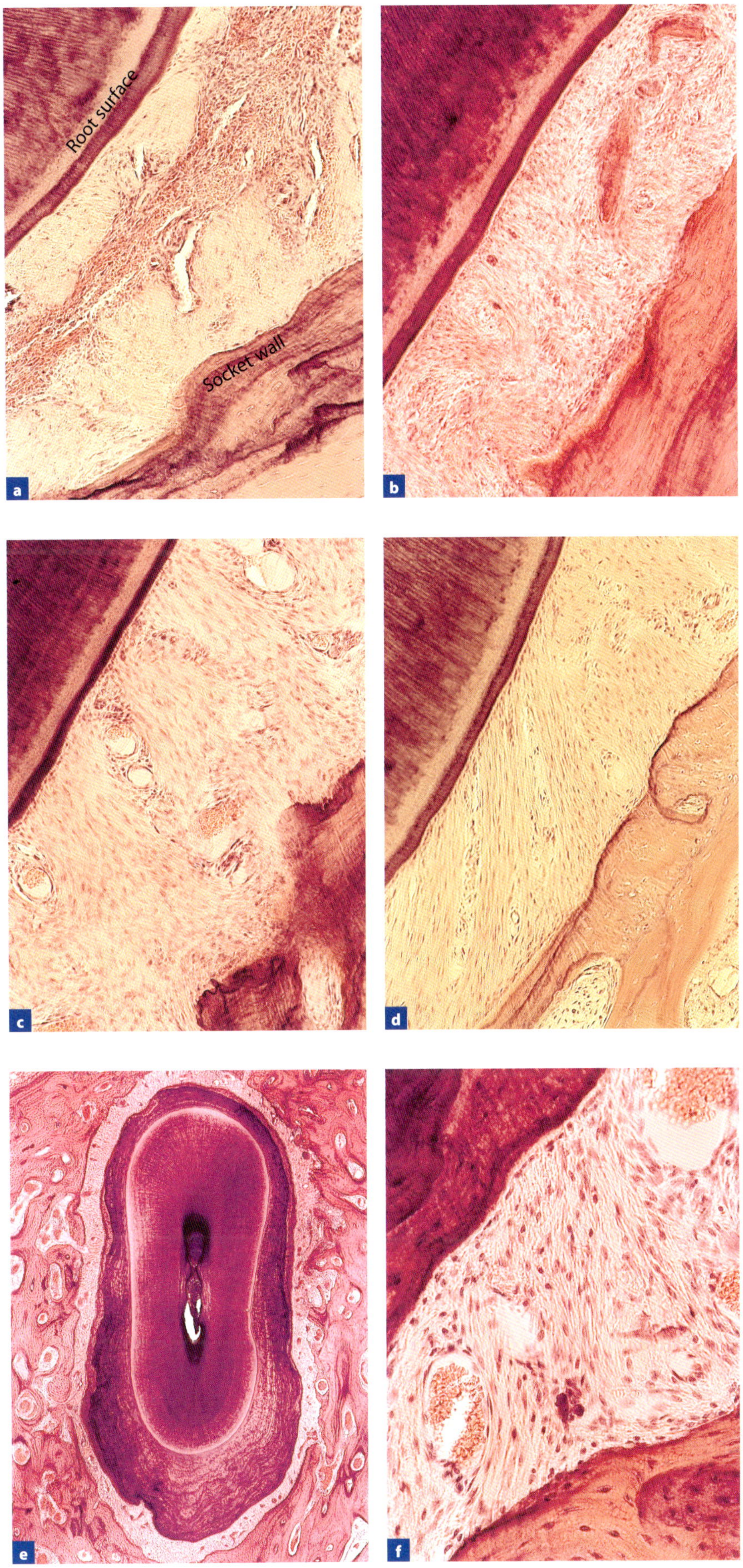

Fig 3-4c Four weeks after transplantation. The root surface is unchanged but new bone is present on the socket wall and a few thin periodontal ligament fibers can be seen running from the root to the bone.
Fig 3-4d Eight weeks after transplantation. Periodontal ligament fibers are functionally aligned between the root surface and the socket wall.

Fig 3-4e 16 weeks after transplantation. Transverse section of the root shows normal periodontal ligament space around the root with no evidence of ankylosis.
Fig 3-4f Higher magnification of the root surface in **Fig 3-4e**. Cementoblasts are aligned adjacent to the root surface and osteoblasts are aligned similarly to the socket wall. Also noticeable is the functionally aligned periodontal ligament fibers between the root and bone.
(H-E staining).

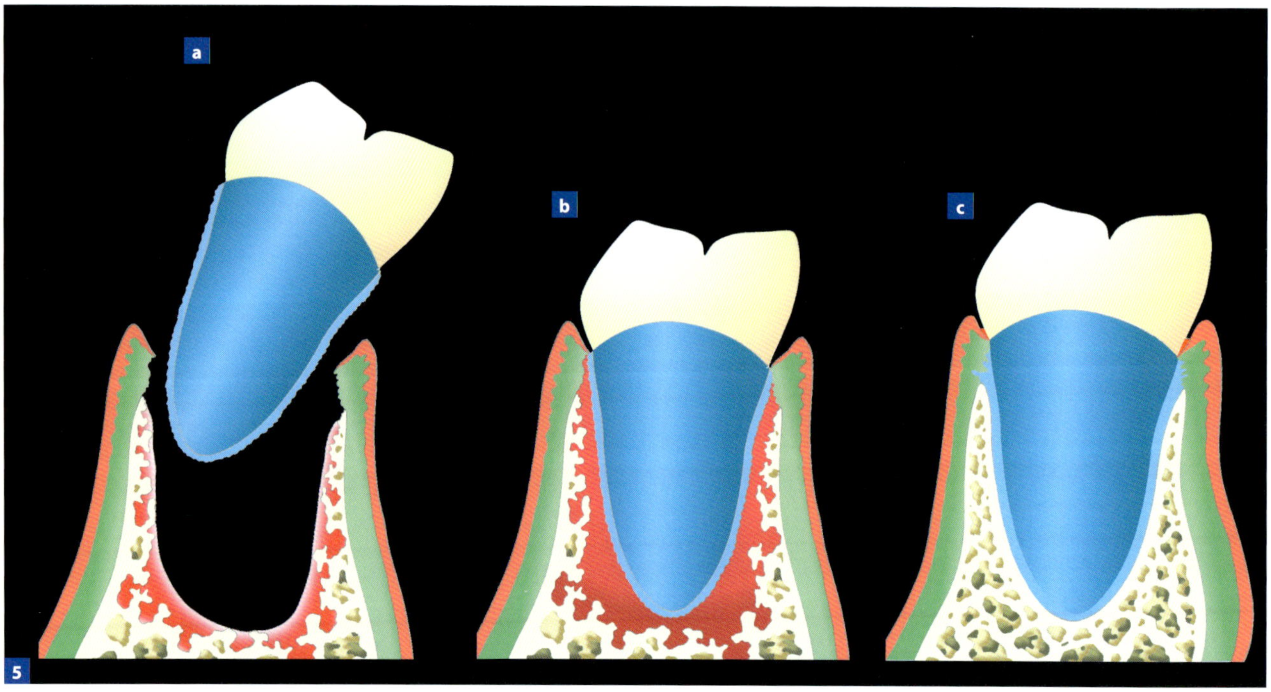

Fig 3-5 Healing by reattachment after transplantation to a newly prepared alveolar socket.

Fig 3-5a Before transplantation. Periodontal ligament fibers are present only on the root of the donor tooth. The recipient socket has been surgically prepared in the alveolus.

Fig 3-5b After transplantation. The gingival connective tissue and the tooth's cervical periodontal ligament fibers can be brought in close contact manually; a blood clot forms between the bony socket walls and the rest of the root. The blood clot is replaced by granulation tissue and immature bone in 1 to 3 weeks and mature bone is in place in 2 to 6 months.

Fig 3-5c After healing. Clinically, healing may be similar to **Fig 3-1** and **3-3**, but histologically, the healing may not be the same, and even if it is, it may require a longer period of time (see **Fig 3-6** and **3-7**).

achieved in transplantations to sockets with remaining bony wall periodontal ligament attachment, as demonstrated histologically up to 16 weeks after transplantation. As shown in **Fig 3-6** and **3-7**, the periodontal ligament aligns more parallel, rather than perpendicular, to the root surface in these transplantations. One study[17] found the width of the periodontal ligament space decreased after healing (**Fig 3-7**), which may be in part due to the decrease in the epithelial rests of Malassez in transplantations to surgically prepared sockets. Clinically, however, it appears that satisfactory healing (i.e. no root resorption, maintenance of a periodontal ligament space, and apparent normal tooth mobility) takes place in the transplantation to surgically prepared alveolar sockets.

A comparison study of transplantation and replantation by Andreasen[18] demonstrated that the prognosis in transplantations depends more so on the presence of vital periodontal ligament on the root surface, and not so much on the presence of periodontal ligament in the alveolar socket. The periodontal ligament on the alveolar socket wall lacks the ability to protect the root surface from resorption and does not induce the growth of new periodontal ligament on the root surface. Other studies have shown similar results[5,7,15]. These studies defined successful transplantation as the absence of root resorption.

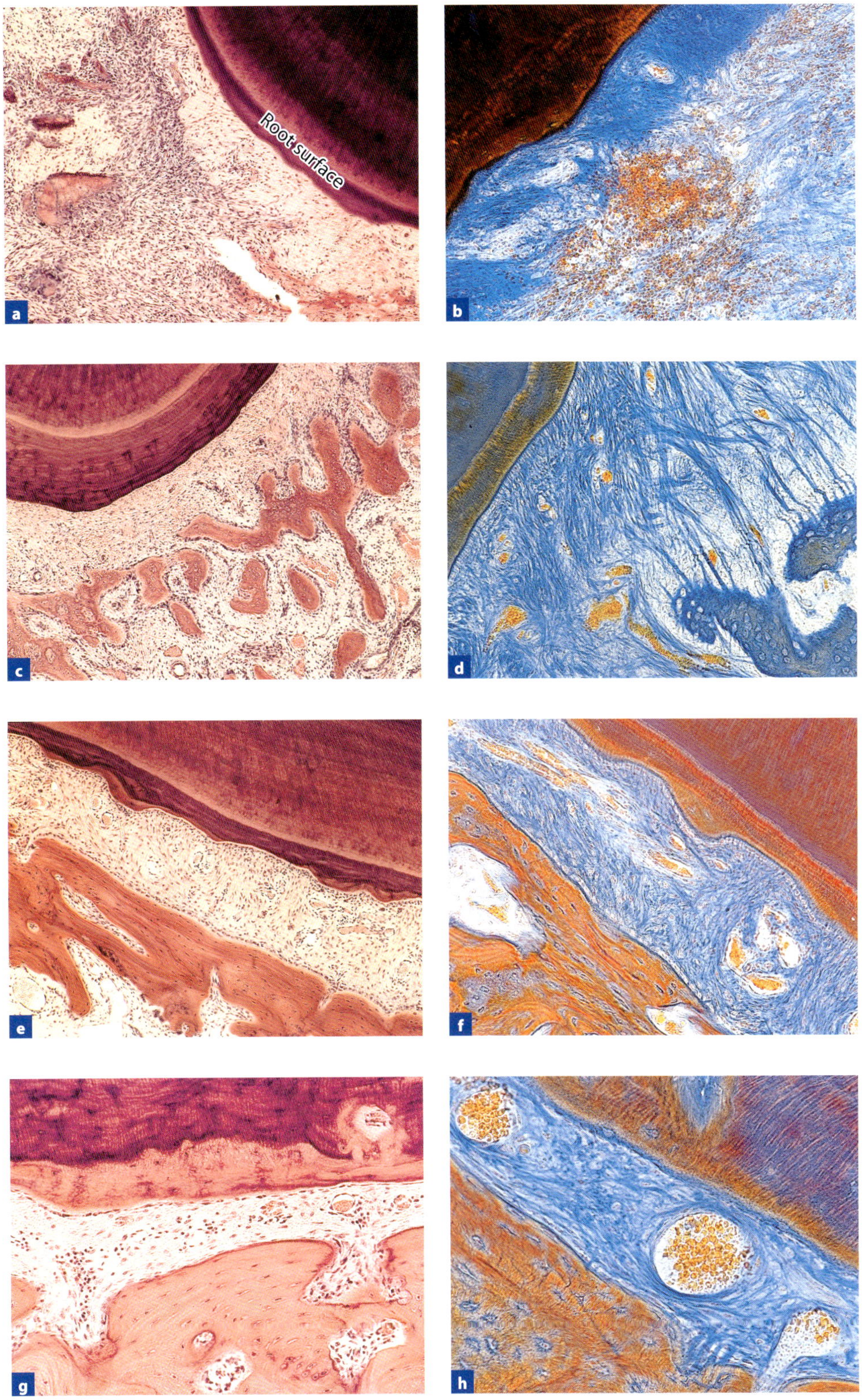

Fig 3-6 Histologic demonstration of the healing process after transplantation to surgically prepared sockets in monkeys (courtesy of Tokyo Dental College).

Fig 3-6a and 3-6b One week after transplantation of a donor tooth to a surgically prepared socket in a monkey. The donor tooth had periodontal ligament attached to the root surface; the recipient site had no ligament present. Note that periodontal ligament tissue can be seen on the root surface and that the fibers are aligned perpendicular to the cementum. Cementoblasts are present.

Fig 3-6c and 3-6d Three weeks after transplantation. Cementoblasts are aligned along the root surface, but there is no resorption or apposition of new hard tissue. It does appear that apposition of a newly formed bone crest is taking place.

Fig 3-6e and 3-6f Eight weeks after the procedure. A new layer of cementum has formed with cementoblasts appearing alongside. The alveolar socket wall appears well formed with osteoblasts along the new bone. The connective tissue fibers observed between the root and the bone do not appear to be functionally well aligned.

Fig 3-6g and 3-6h 16 weeks after the procedure. Apposition of newly formed cementum in a resorption cavity and alignment of adjacent cementoblasts are observed. The alveolar socket wall is formed at a constant distance from the donor tooth and osteoblasts are aligned adjacent to it. Although fibers between the cementum and the alveolar socket wall are observed, they are slightly misaligned.

(**a**, **c**, **e**, **g**: H-E staining; **b**, **d**, **f**, **h**: Mallory staining)

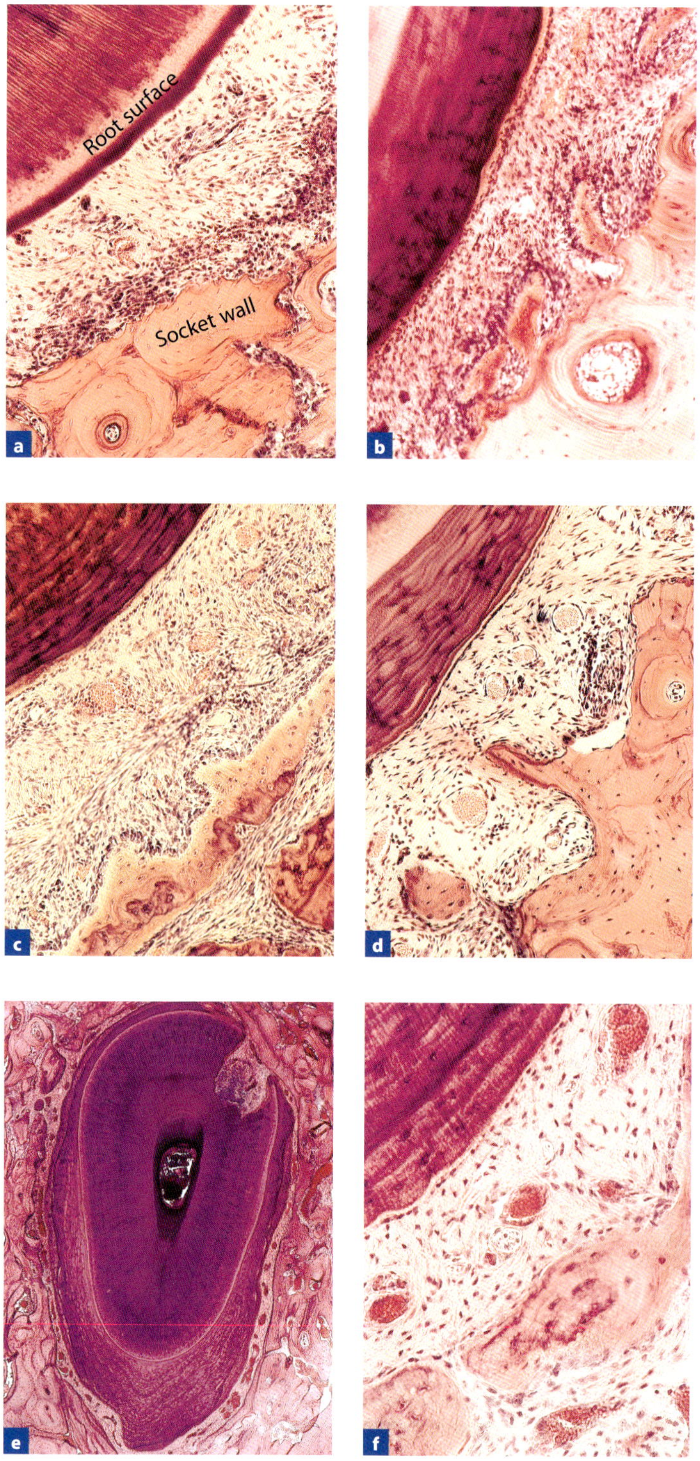

Fig 3-7 Tissue healing shown histologically following transplantations to monkey sockets in which periodontal ligament tissue was removed (courtesy of Tokyo Dental College).

Fig 3-7a One week after the procedure. Ruptured periodontal tissue is left on the root surface but not on the alveolar socket wall. Resorption of the alveolar socket wall and granulation tissue is observed along the socket wall.

Fig 3-7b Two weeks after the procedure. The periodontal ligament fibers are still left on the root surface. Resorption of the alveolar socket wall and apposition of new bone can be observed.

Fig 3-7c Four weeks after the procedure. Apposition of new bone and alignment of osteoblasts on its surface are visible on the alveolar socket wall. There is no evidence of continuity of fibers running between the root surface and the alveolar socket wall.

Fig 3-7d Eight weeks after the procedure. Cementoblasts can be seen aligned on the surface of the root, and apposition of new bone is apparent on the opposite alveolar socket wall. Fibers between them show partial functional alignment, but most of them are misaligned.

Fig 3-7e 16 weeks after the procedure. A resorption cavity can be seen on the surface of the donor tooth; ankylosis, however, is not apparent. Width of the periodontal ligament space is rather narrow.

Fig 3-7f Higher magnification of **Fig 3-7e**. Cementoblasts on the root surface and osteoblasts on the alveolar socket wall can be observed. Fibers between them are mostly misaligned. (H-E staining).

New attachment

Studies on replantation have demonstrated that deficits of the periodontal ligament on the root surface are repaired by new attachment[5-7,9-11,19-26] (**Fig 3-8**). New attachment is defined as "the reunion of connective tissue with a root surface that has been deprived of its periodontal ligament"[1]. It could also be defined as "regeneration and attachment of periodontal ligament tissue to a root surface that has lost periodontal ligament pathologically or mechanically" (**Fig 3-9**). The mechanism of new attachment is the formation of connective tissue between exposed root surface and surrounding tissue (bone or gingival connective tissue) by proliferation of the cells derived from the periodontal ligament around the exposed root surface with addition of cementum on the root and inclusion of Sharpey's fiber into the cementum[2] (Fig 3-10).

The size of the defect and deficit of periodontal ligament on the root surface and the distance from the socket wall of the recipient site to the root are likely factors that affect the likelihood of repair by new attachment. Andreasen and Kristerson[22] found that up to 2 mm of surface area of periodontal ligament loss on the root surface can be repaired by new attachment (Fig 3-11). The greater the distance between the bone and the root, the more time that may be necessary for the bone tissue to reach the root, which may lead toa wider range of repair processes of the periodontal ligament by new attachment.

On a clinical level, one can never be sure that all the peri-

New attachment

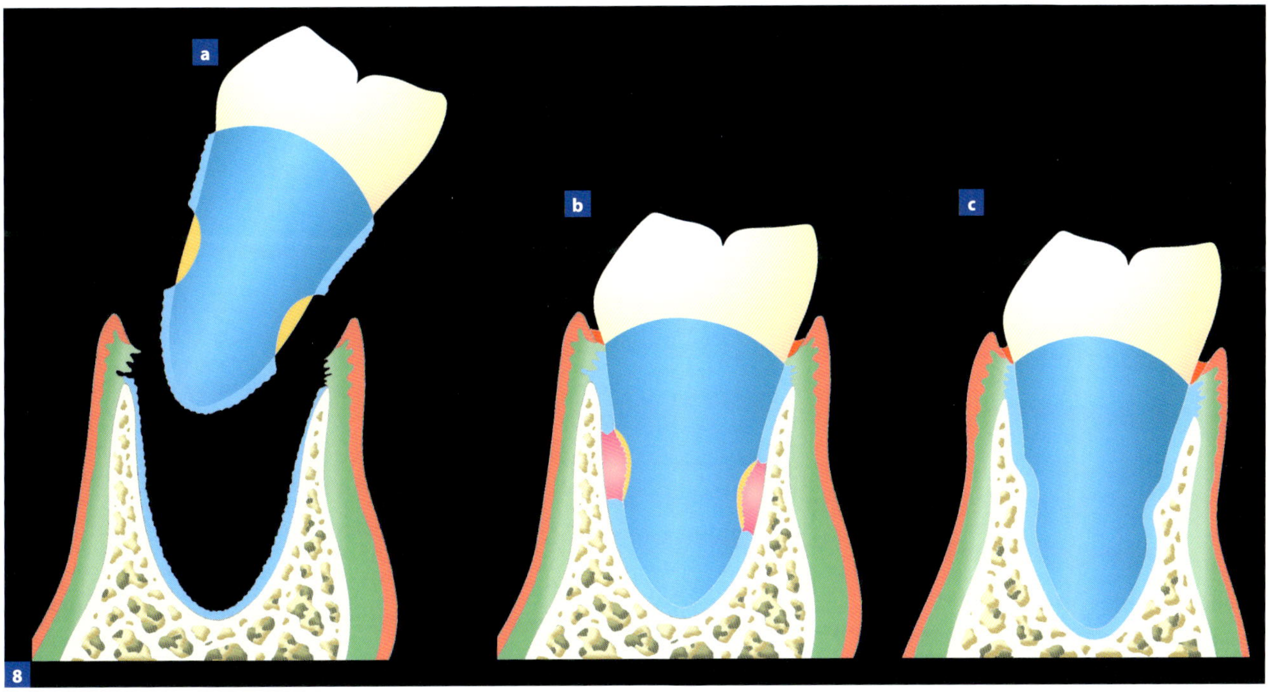

Fig 3-8 Healing by new attachment after transplantation and replantation of teeth with partially missing periodontal ligament.
Fig 3-8a Before transplantation. The donor tooth is partially missing periodontal ligament from its root surface.
Fig 3-8b After transplantation. Transient initial ankylosis and surface resorption involving the root surface without periodontal ligament are expected.
Fig 3-8c After completion of the healing process. New periodontal ligament attachment takes place in the resorbed areas with no further ankylosis.

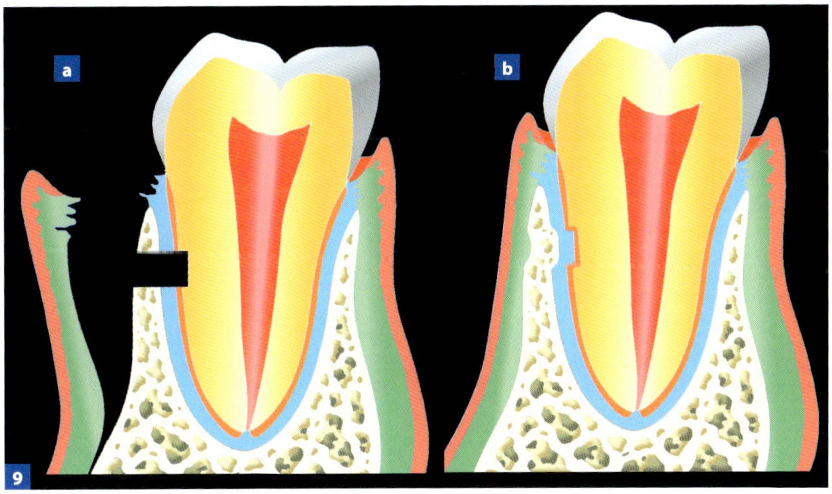

Fig 3-9 New attachment demonstrated experimentally.
Fig 3-9a After elevation of a gingival flap. A cavity is prepared through the bone, periodontal ligament, cementum, and dentin, following which the flap is replaced.
Fig 3-9b After healing. The surgically prepared cavity in dentin is restored by cementum and periodontal ligament (new attachment).

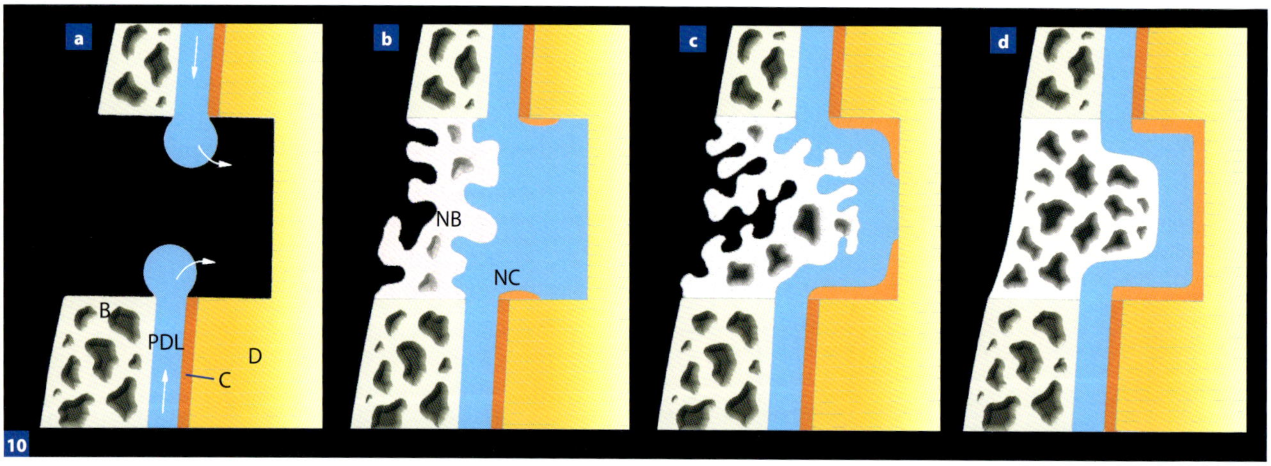

Fig 3-10 Mechanism of new attachment shown in **Fig 3-9** (modified from refs. 26, 27).

Fig 3-10a At 3 to 9 days. The periodontal ligament proliferates from the ruptured ligament tissue.

Fig 3-10b At 14 to 21 days. New periodontal ligament tissue fills the cavity, and new cementum is deposited on the dentin. The bony defect is repaired with newly formed bone at the same time.

Fig 3-10c At 28 to 42 days. Healing of bone progresses.

Fig 3-10d At 60 to 470 days. The cavity is repaired with new cementum and periodontal ligament. The proper periodontal ligament space is reestablished between the bone and the new root surface.

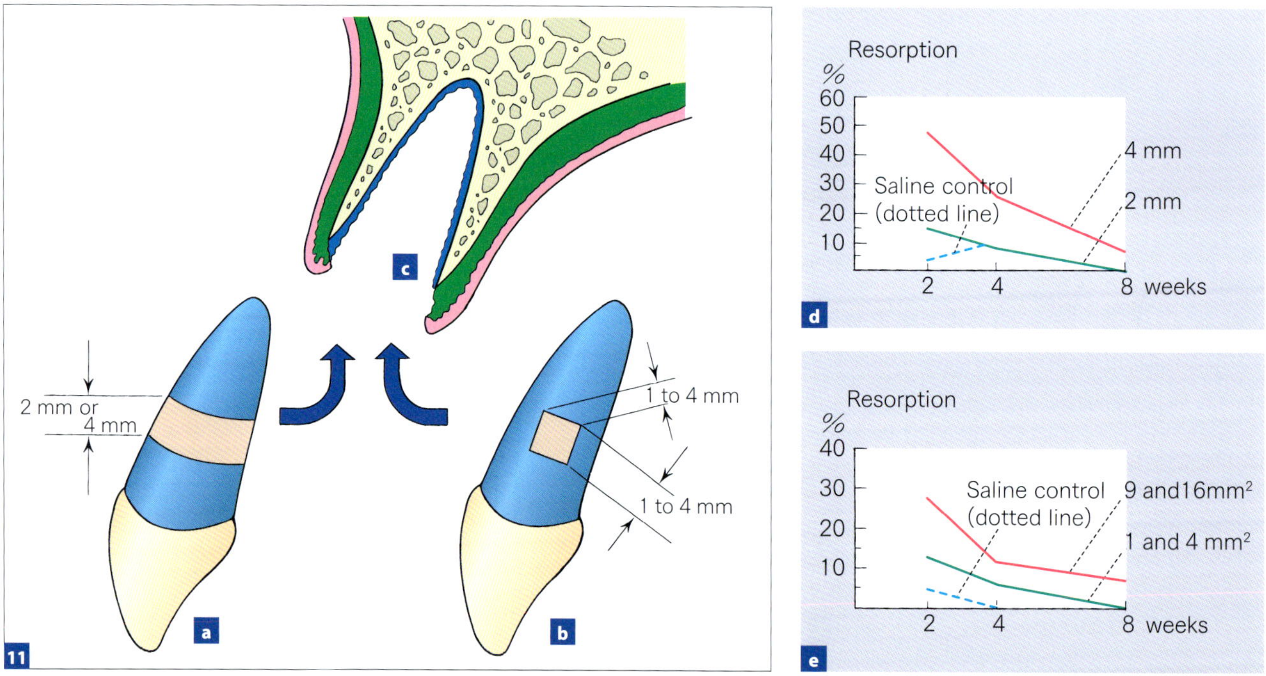

Fig 3-11 Limited drying or removal of the periodontal ligament and new attachment after replantation of mature permanent incisors in monkeys.

Methods:

Fig 3-11a Periodontal ligament of extracted teeth is either partially (2 or 4 mm of width) dried and necrotized (the periodontal ligament of other area is vital) and the teeth are replanted in the original extraction sockets (**c**).

Fig 3-11b Periodontal ligament is partially removed mechanically (1×1, 2×2, 3×3, or 4×4 mm) and the teeth are replanted in the original extraction sockets (**c**).

Results:

Fig 3-11d Graph shows that ankylosis occurs in the necrotic area of teeth with 2 mm defects at 2 weeks but is repaired by new attachment over time. However, ankylosis exists even 8 weeks after replantation with the teeth of 4 mm defects.

Fig 3-11e Graph shows that complete healing by new attachment was achieved with the teeth of 1×1 mm and 2×2 mm defects. On the other hand, ankylosis exists even 8 weeks after the replantation with the teeth of 3×3 mm and 4×4 mm defects. This result indicates that healing by new attachment can be expected to some extent, but in teeth with larger defects permanent ankylosis will result.

(Reprinted with permission from Andreasen and Kristerson[22].)

odontal ligament is vital orundamaged after extraction of the donor tooth when performing transplantation and replantation. Therefore, if there is damaged or unhealthy periodontal ligament that may not allow for healing by new attachment there will be a higher risk that the transplanted and replanted teeth will undergo root resorption. As will be discussed later, root canal therapy of teeth with inflammatory resorption enables the repair of a resorption cavity by new attachment and cessation of root resorption. Thus, healing in transplantation and replantation is achieved by either reattachment and/or development of new attachment.

Required periodontal ligament layer for transplantation and replantation

Success of transplantation and replantation depends very much on the vitality and health of the periodontal ligament attached to the donor tooth[12–16,18]. The periodontal ligament is typically severed through the middle when the donor tooth is extracted, leaving a layer of attached periodontal ligament on the root surface that contains cells (e.g. cementoblasts, fibroblasts, pericytes, epithelial cells of Malassez) that likely play important roles in the prevention of root resorption[28–38]. It is desirable to extract a tooth with as much periodontal ligament as possible attached to it, even though the cementoblast layer by itself seems to be effective in preventing root resorption.

Survival of the periodontal ligament outside the mouth

Preserving the vitality of the periodontal ligament of donor teeth outside the mouth is essential for a successful outcome. The survival rate of the periodontal ligament under various conditions has been studied[6,7,16,39–59]. The periodontal ligament is susceptible to changes in pH and osmotic pressure. Under dry conditions, most of the periodontal ligament is still vital after 18 minutes, but after 30 minutes, more than half is nonvital, and after 120 minutes most of it has become necrotic (**Table 3-1**). Most of the periodontal ligament tissue is vital up to 120 minutes in physiologic saline. In tap water, the periodontal ligament does not survive as well due to the low osmolality, with about one-third surviving after 120 minutes[9] (**Table 3-2**). Periodontal ligament cells can be kept vital for hours (up to 24 hours) in milk[45–54] or with specialized developed preservation/storage mediums[6,7,16].

Nevertheless, it is important to complete the surgical procedure carefully and efficiently, mindful of the time, because even saline solution (or whatever medium is used during the procedure) induces necrosis of the periodontal ligament cells over time.

Survival of the periodontal ligament outside the mouth

Table 3-1 Survival of the periodontal ligament in dry conditions[39].

Time(min)	Survival rate of periodontal ligament(%)
18	70.5 ± 17.3
30	28.2 ± 18.9
60	21.2 ± 13.4
90	15.2 ± 6.2
120	20.1 ± 19.7

Table 3-2 Survival of the periodontal ligament in moist conditions[39].

	Time(min)	Survival rate of periodontal ligament(%)
In saline	18	80.0 ± 13.0
	30	71.3 ± 18.2
	60	71.4 ± 14.2
	120	61.7 ± 11.4
In top water	> 120	33.2 ± 12.2

Mechanism of root resorption (courtesy of Dr. Jens O. Andreasen[63])

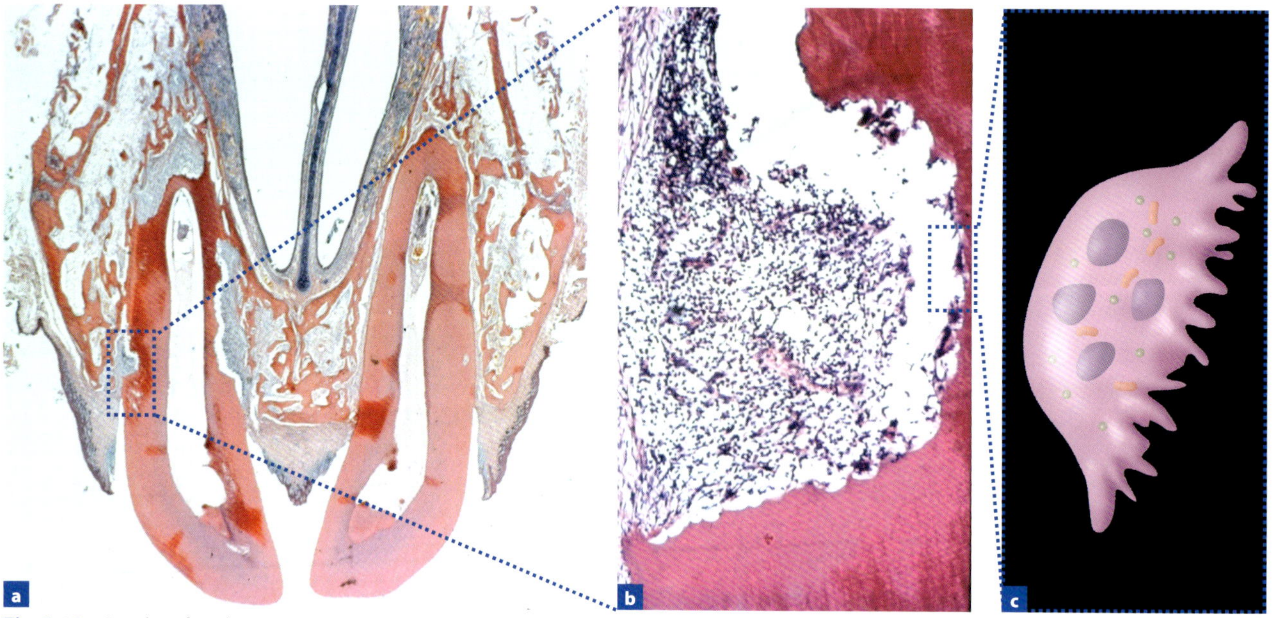

Fig 3-12a Results of replantation experiments using monkey central incisors. The maxillary right and left central incisors were extracted and replanted. The right central incisor was replanted after mechanical removal of the periodontal ligament. Three months later, tissue sections showed significant root resorption only in the root from which the periodontal ligament had been removed.

Fig 3-12b Magnified image of the resorption lacune. There are osteoclasts in the resorption lacune.

Fig 3-12c Schematic diagram of osteoclast. Osteoclasts secrete acid and lysosomal enzymes from the ruffled border to demineralize bone tissue and degrade organic matter.

Mechanism of Root Resorption

Root resorption occurs when a donor tooth with partial or total lack of viable periodontal ligament is transplanted or replanted (**Fig 3-12**). Root resorption is categorized in three groups: replacement resorption, inflammatory resorption, and surface resorption[60,61] (**Fig 3-13**). It has been demonstrated that the extent of damaged or missing periodontal ligament and pulpal status (i.e. vital or necrotic) determines which type of resorption will occur[62–64]. Others have used different terminologies for the types of root resorption, with replacement resorption being classified as "ankylosis-related resorption, inflammatory root resorption as "inflammation-related resorption, and surface root resorption as "repair-related resorption"[65]. In this book, the 1966 classification and terminology proposed by Andreasen et al. will be used.

Replacement resorption

Replacement resorption occurs when a tooth with extensive loss of vital periodontal ligament is transplanted or replanted[18,20,21,62,63] (**Fig 3-14**). Replacement resorption is the phenomenon by which the root is resorbed and replaced by bone. It results in ankylosis, in which bone and root fuse together.

Remodeling is always occurring in the bone as part of homeostasis of the body[66,67]. Bone resorption is a function of osteoclasts and bone apposition is that of osteoblasts. These cells always work together in the resorption-apposition process (the so-called "coupling phenomenon")[68-71]. The development of osteoclasts begins with the chemotaxis of monocytes (osteoclast precursors) derived from bone marrow stem cells, which disseminate out of blood vessels and become multinuclear osteoclasts through fusion, differentiation, and maturation[72] (**Fig 3-15**). When osteoblasts are activated, a bone resorption-promoting factor, called RANKL (receptor activator of nuclear factor κB ligand) is expressed on the cell surface, and binds with a signaling molecule called RANK (receptor activator of nuclear factor κB) on osteoclast precursors. Activated osteoblasts also release MCSF (macrophage colony stimulating factor), which binds to the cell surface receptors on osteoclast precursors.

Classification of root resorption

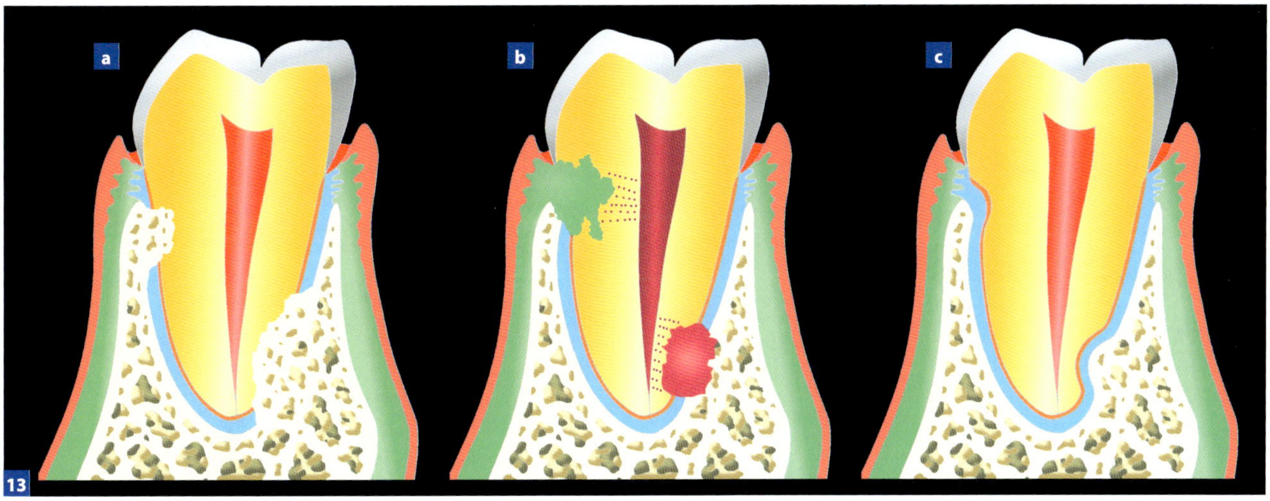

Fig 3-13a Replacement resorption. Root dentin is replaced by bone, which results in a fusing of bone to tooth (ankylosis).
Fig 3-13b Inflammatory resorption. The resorption of tooth structure is stimulated by adjacent inflammatory tissue, which is often induced by infected pulp tissue. The resorption cavity (both in the root and the adjacent bone) is filled with granulation tissue.
Fig 3-13c Surface resorption. This is a relatively minor and transient resorption in which the initial resorption has been repaired by new attachment.

This binding also causes the precursor cells to differentiate, fuse, and mature into multinucleated osteoclasts[72-80] (**Fig 3-15**). Mature osteoclasts secrete acid and lysosomal enzymes from the ruffled border to demineralize bone and degrade organic matrix components, resulting in bone resorption[81-91].

When roots with necrotic or lost periodontal ligament come in contact with bone and its osteoclasts, the hard tissues of the root (cementum and dentin) become involved in the remodeling

Mechanism of replacement resorption

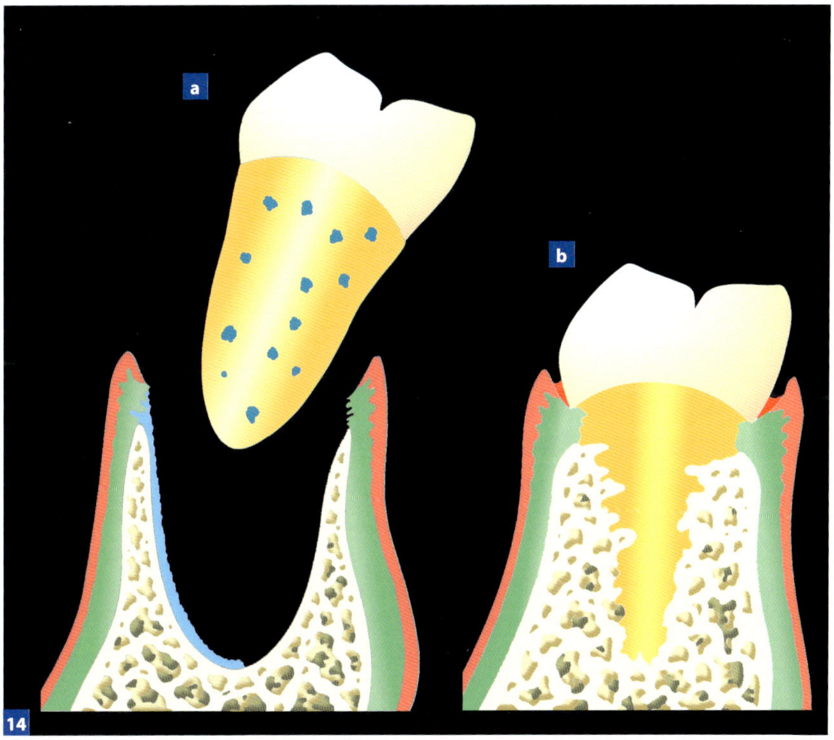

Fig 3-14a Preoperative. If a donor tooth with either missing or necrotic periodontal ligament tissue is placed in an alveolar socket, postoperative replacement resorption will occur regardless of the presence or absence of periodontal ligament tissue in the recipient site.
Fig 3-14b Postoperative. The outcome of this type of replantation or transplantation is that the root becomes part of normal bone remodeling; that is, the root is replaced with new bone. The rate of replacement resorption is related to the rate of bone remodeling in the host (i.e. faster in children, slower in adults).

Lineage of osteoclasts (modified from Kahn, et al.[72])

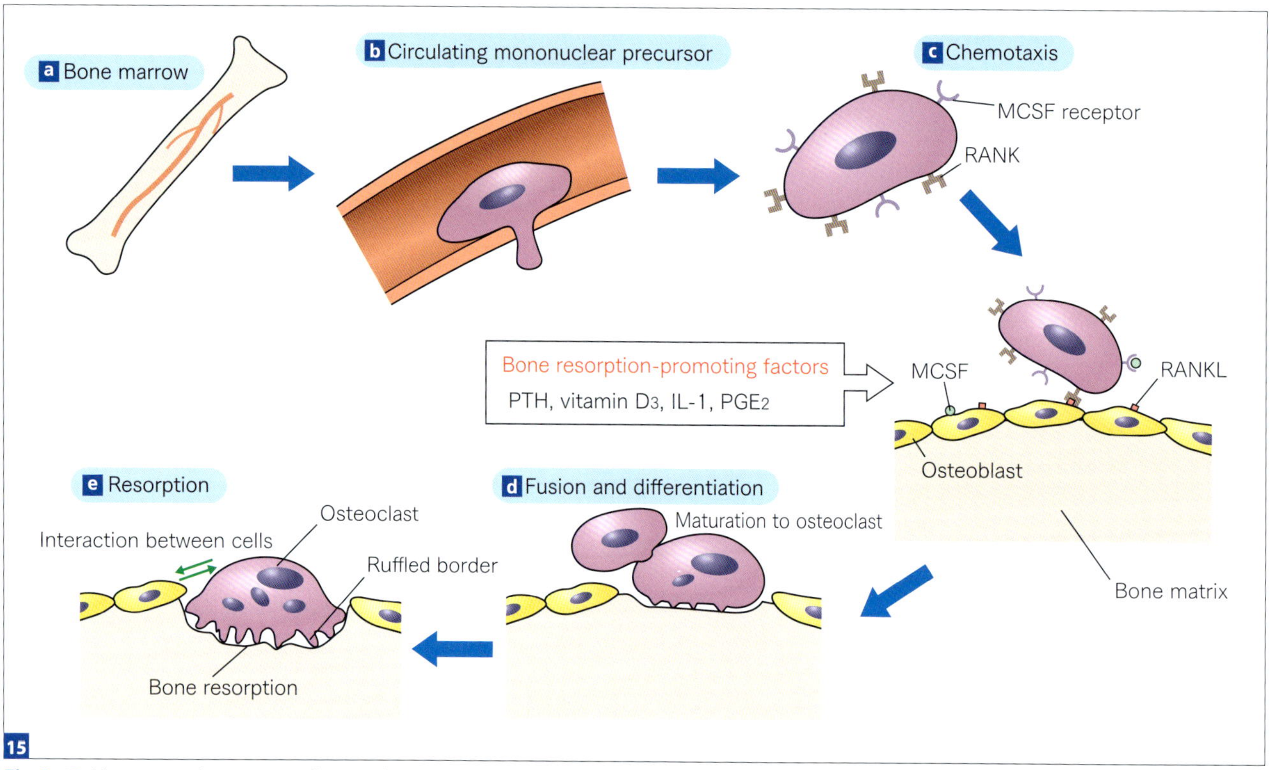

Fig 3-15 Monocytes (precursors of osteoclasts) are derived from bone marrow (**a**), migrate from vessels by chemotaxis (**b**), fuse together on bone substance, and differentiate into multi-nuclear osteoclasts. On the other hand, when osteoblasts are activated by bone resorption-promoting factors, a signal called RANKL is expressed on the surface of osteoblasts and binds to a signal receptor called RANK on osteoclast precursors (**c**). Activated osteoblasts also release macrophage colony stimulating factor (MCSF), which also binds to the signal receptor on the osteoclast precursors. This binding of MCSF and MCSF results in the fusion, differentiation, and maturation of monocytes into multinucleated osteoclasts (**d**). Mature osteoclasts secrete acid and lysosomal enzymes from the ruffled border to demineralize bone tissue and degrade organic matter, thereby causing bone resorption (**e**). Monocytes can differentiate into osteoclasts, macrophages, and all other leukocytes. Bone resorption-promoting factors include PTH (parathyroid hormone), vitamin D3, IL-1 (interleukin 1) released by macrophages, PGE_2 (prostaglandin E_2), and other cytokines.

process of bone, where root resorption and bone apposition occur simultaneously on the root surface[92-94].

A study by Ichinokawa[5] in which they investigated the replantation of teeth with the periodontal ligament totally removed mechanically in monkeys (**Fig 3-16**) demonstrated apposition of hard tissue on the root surface 1 week after replantation (**Fig 3-16c** and **3-16d**). An interesting finding of this study is that apposition of hard tissue by osteoblasts derived from periodontal ligament tissue left in the alveolar socket precedes root resorption. Partial fusion through bone apposition on the root surface and the alveolar bone was observed 4 weeks after the surgical procedure, indicating that ankylosis had already begun in this area (**Fig 3-16g** and **3-16h**). Clinically, ankylosis is detected typically between 4 months to 1 year after replantation (**Fig 3-17**). Partial ankylosis is often difficult to detect because these teeth show some mobility and respond normally to percussion tests. Long-term radiographic follow-up will show if partial ankylosis will progress to replacement resorption with complete loss of the root structure, or if it will be repaired by new attachment.

The rate at which replacement resorption occurs seems to depend on the age of the patient[44,66,92]. The rate of replacement resorption is proportional to the rate of the remodeling process of the patient —faster in children and slower in adults (in general, bone remodeling in children: 50%/year; adults: 2%/year)[66]. Therefore, if ankylosis occurs after transplantation or replantation, the tooth may function normally for a long period of time if the rate of root resorption/bone remodeling is slow (**Fig 3-17**).

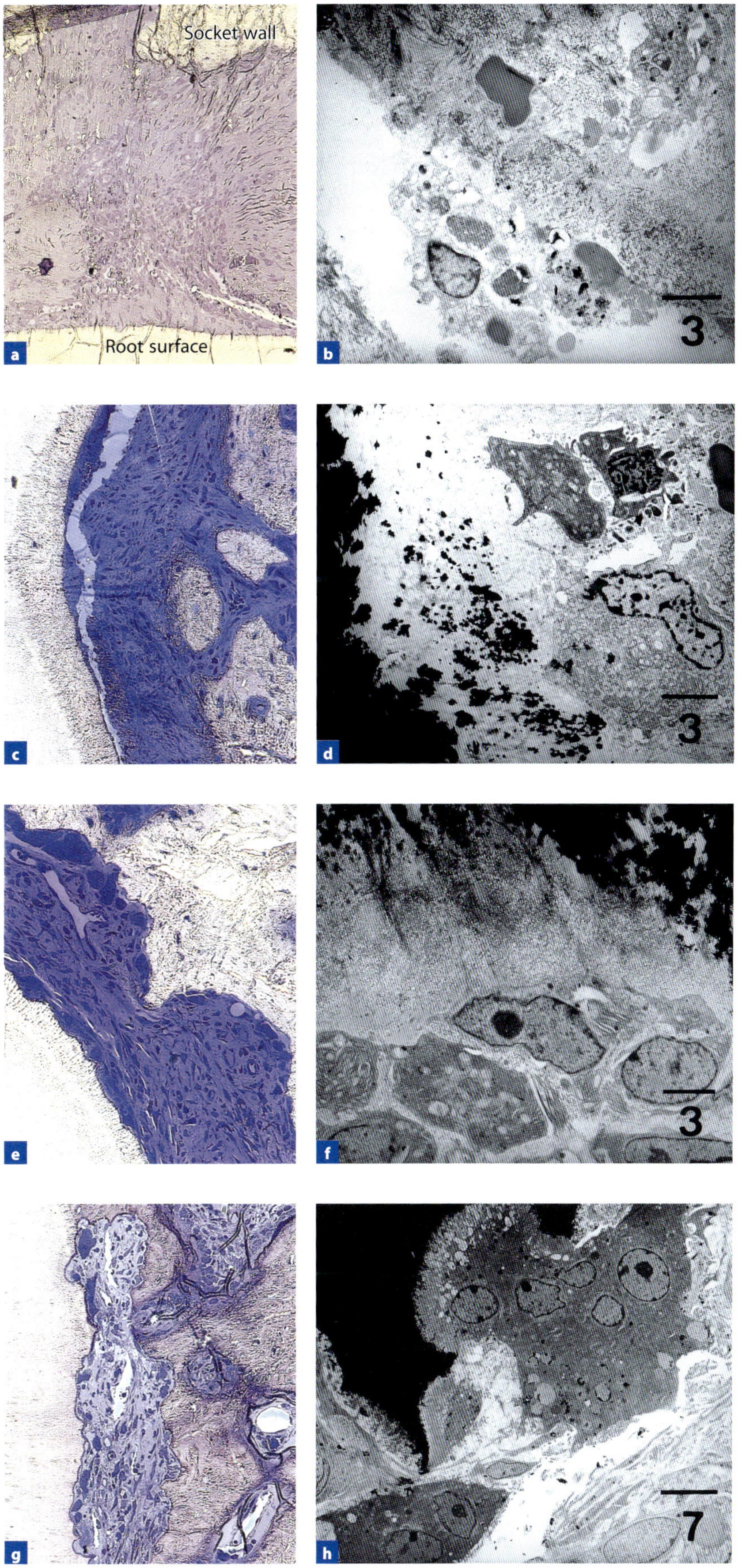

Fig 3-16 Histologic appearance of teeth in monkeys after replantation in which the periodontal ligament was removed from the roots (courtesy of Tokyo Dental College).

Fig 3-16a Three days after replantation. The periodontal ligament fibers can be seen only on the alveolar socket wall. An amorphous area can be seen along the sectioned edge of the fibers. Many spindle and ellipsoid cells are also observed.

Fig 3-16b Electron micrograph of the middle section of **Fig 3-16a**. Cells with vacuolation in cytoplasm mix with erythrocytes (cells without membrane). Irregularly aligned collagen fibers are visible in intercellular cement.

Fig 3-16c One week after the procedure. Newly formed hard tissue is observed on one part of the root surface. In the middle of the area, spindle-shaped cells or polygonal cells are irregularly aligned. Apposition of newly formed hard tissue and osteoblasts are visible.

Fig 3-16d Electron micrograph of the root side of **Fig 3-16c**. Pointed and rounded structures are scattered on the root surface and cells enriched with small intracellular organs are observed. Sparse collagen fibers and erythrocytes are observed in intercellular cement.

Fig 3-16e Two weeks after the procedure. Resorption with osteoclasts and apposition of newly formed hard tissue with osteoblasts are observed on both the root surface and the alveolar socket wall. Irregularly aligned polygonal and spindle-shaped cells are observed in the middle.

Fig 3-16f Electron micrograph of the root side of **Fig 3-16e**. Osteoid, composed of noncalcified bundles of collagen fibers, is observed on the root surface, and alignment of osteoblast-like cells, which are enriched with small intracellular organs, is seen around it.

Fig 3-16g Four weeks after replantation. Apposition of newly formed hard tissue is observed on both the root surface and the alveolar socket wall and many osteoclasts are observed in the resorption cavity.

Fig 3-16h Electron micrograph of the root side of **Fig 3-16g**. Porykaryotic (multi-nuclear) osteoclasts with clear zones or ruffled borders are observed in the severely resorbed area adjacent to the root surface.

(**a**, **c**, **e**, **g**: toluidine blue staining)

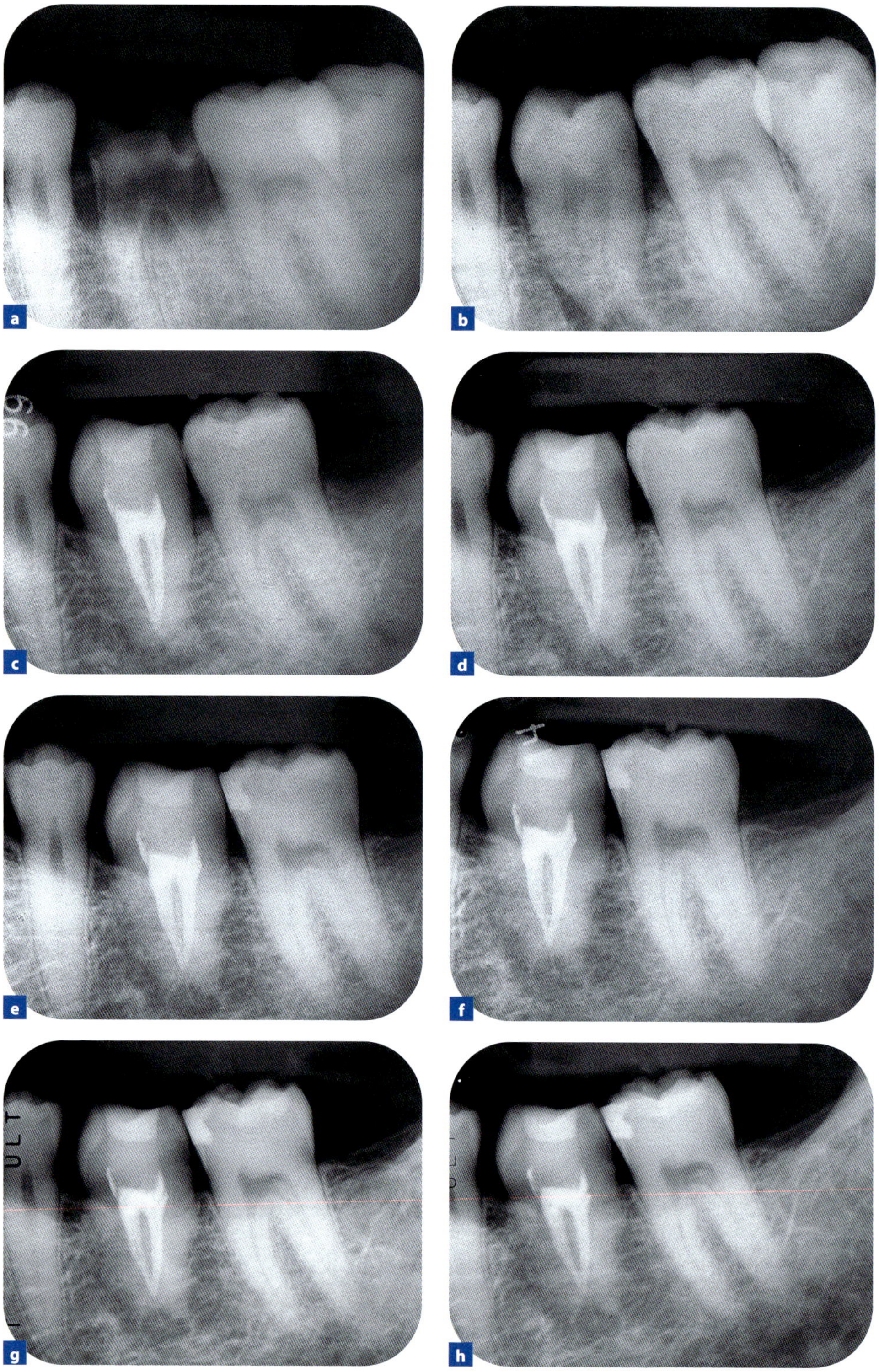

Fig 3-17 Clinical case of replacement resorption.

Fig 3-17a Preoperative radiograph of a non-preservable first mandibular molar in a 46-year-old male. The treatment plan was to transplant the patient's maxillary third molar.
Fig 3-17b After transplantation.

Fig 3-17c 10 months after transplantation. No periodontal ligament space is observed and there is no mobility.
Fig 3-17d Two years after transplantation. Obvious replacement resorption is observed.

Fig 3-17e Four years after transplantation.
Fig 3-17f Five years after transplantation. Continued resorption is observed but seems slow.

Fig 3-17g 10 years after transplantation.
Fig 3-17h 13 years after transplantation. In adults (postpubertal patients), the progression of root resorption due to ankylosis is very slow.

Inflammatory resorption

Inflammatory resorption is observed when a tooth with pupal infection and partial loss of periodontal ligament is transplanted or replanted[64, 95] (**Fig 3-18**). The process begins where surface resorption of cementum by osteoclasts has exposed the root dentin in areas where the periodontal ligament either was missing or necrotic[64]. The exposed dentin areas leave tubules that communicate with the pulp space in which infected pulp tissue is present. Bacteria and their byproducts (e.g. endotoxin) migrate through the dentin tubules to the root surface

Mechanism of inflammatory resorption

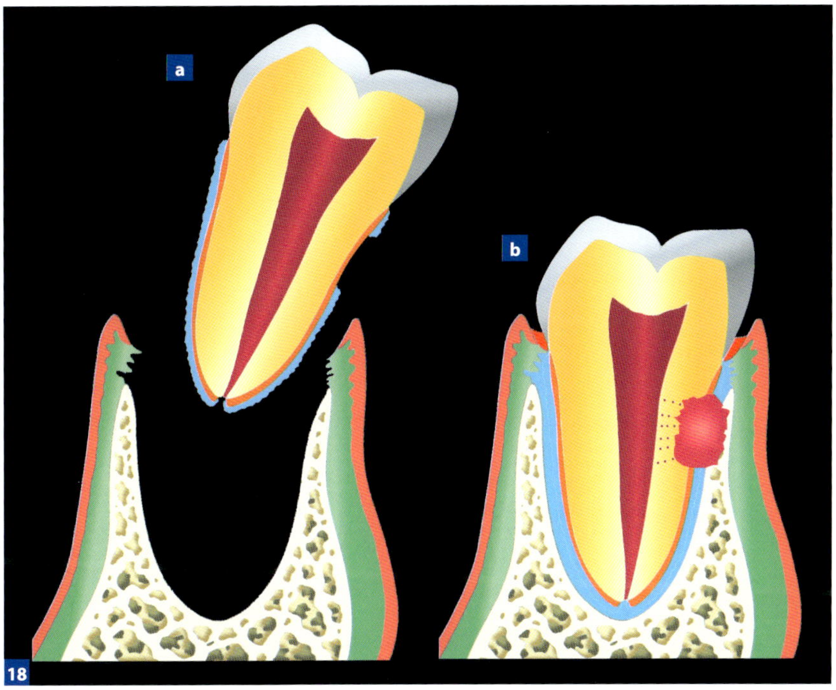

Fig 3-18a Before replantation or transplantation. The donor tooth has necrotic pulp tissue and partially missing or necrotic periodontal ligament.

Fig 3-18b Following replantation or transplantation. Initial surface resorption of cementum will expose dentinal tubules, which communicate with infected pulp tissue, allowing bacteria and endotoxin to induce additional osteoclastic activity, resulting in inflammatory resorption of both root structure and adjacent alveolar bone. The resorption cavity is filled with capillary-rich inflammatory granulation tissue which supply osteoclast as a member of defense systems and, unless the infected pulp tissue is removed, resorption will continue.

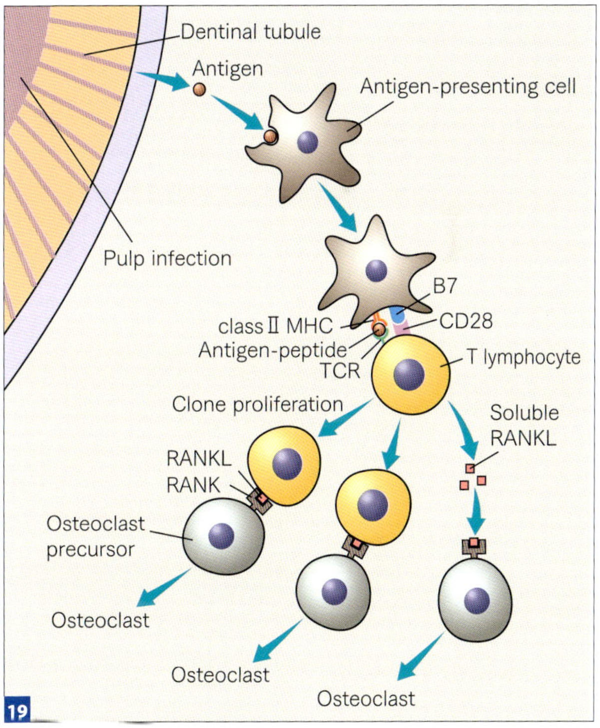

Fig 3-19 Ontogenesis of Osteoclast by activated lymphocytes (courtesy of Dr. Hiromasa Yamamoto.[96]). Antigen-presenting cells (dendritic cells, macrophages, and B lymphocytes) transmit antigen information and activation signals to T lymphocytes. Only lymphocytes that are specific for the antigen are selected for T lymphocytes. The activated T lymphocytes then produce osteoclasts by expressing RANKL on the plasma membrane. Soluble RANKL secreted by activated lymphocytes may also play a role.

Fig 3-20 A long-term follow-up result of inflammatory resorption after root canal treatment

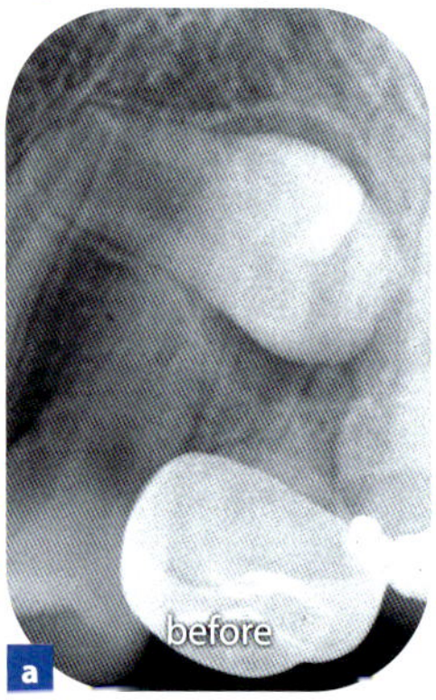

Fig 3-20a Preoperative radiograph of a 17-year-old female. The impacted second premolar is to be transplanted into the primary second molar site.

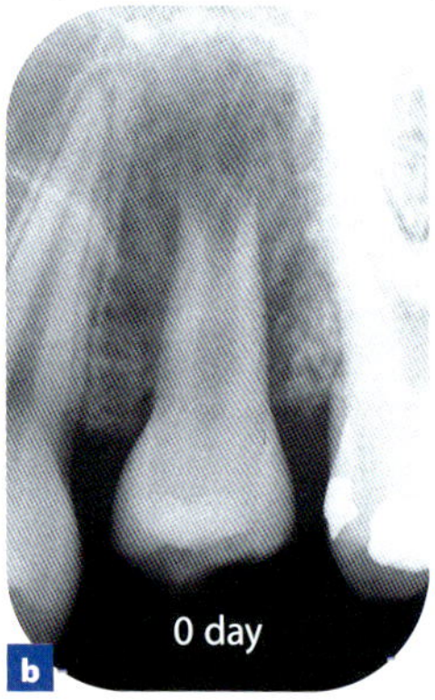

Fig 3-20b Immediately after transplantation.

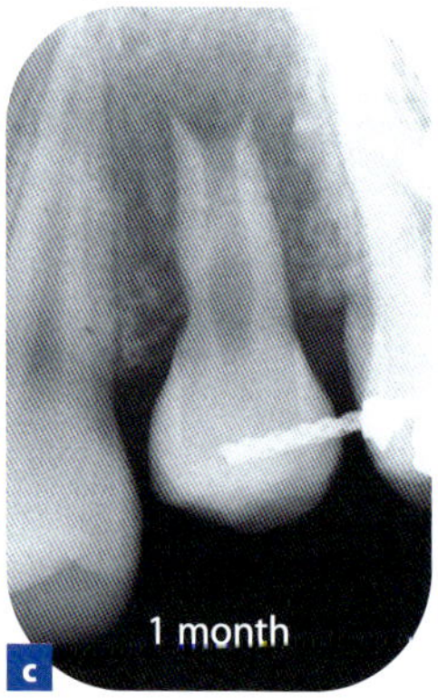

Fig 3-20c One month postop. Root resorption has begun to occur on the mesial aspect.

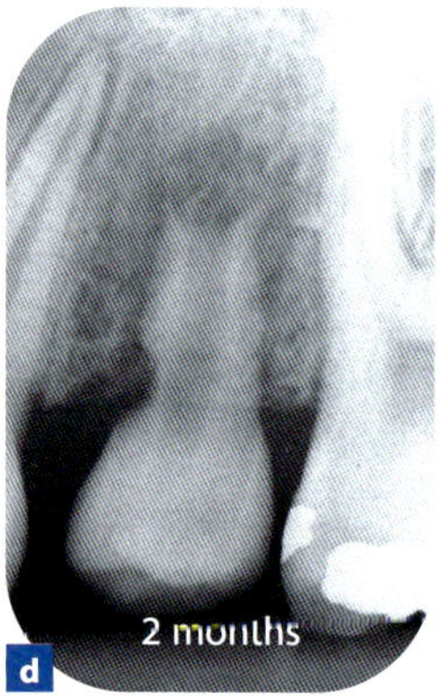

Fig 3-20d Two months postop. Inflammatory resorption is progressing rapidly.

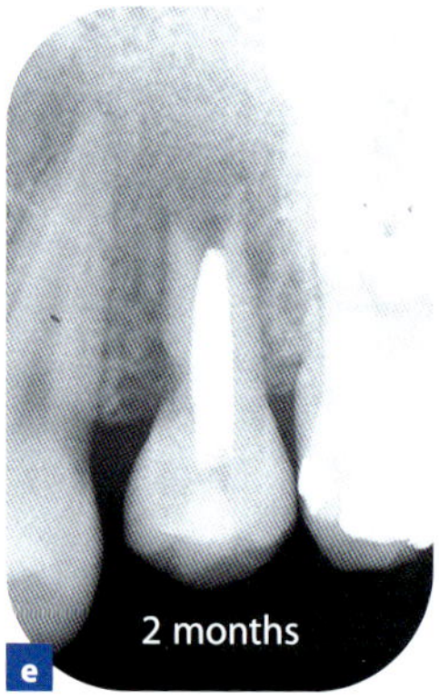

Fig 3-20e Same day as **Fig 3-20d**. Immediately after root canal treatment. The root canal was filled with a calcium hydroxide preparation, 'Vitapex' (Neo, Tokyo, Japan).

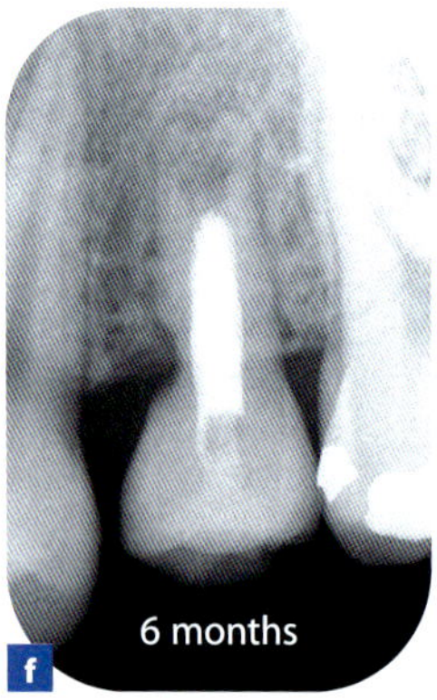

Fig 3-20f Six months postop. Root resorption seems to have completely ceased and the resorption lacuna is separated from the bone by a normal periodontal ligament space.

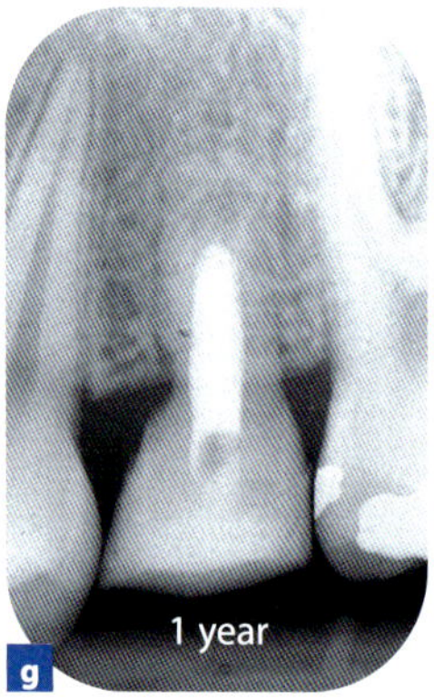

Fig 3-20g One year postop. Root resorption has not progressed. Normal periodontal ligament space is seen in the resorption cavity (lacune). A small amount of continued root growth can be seen.

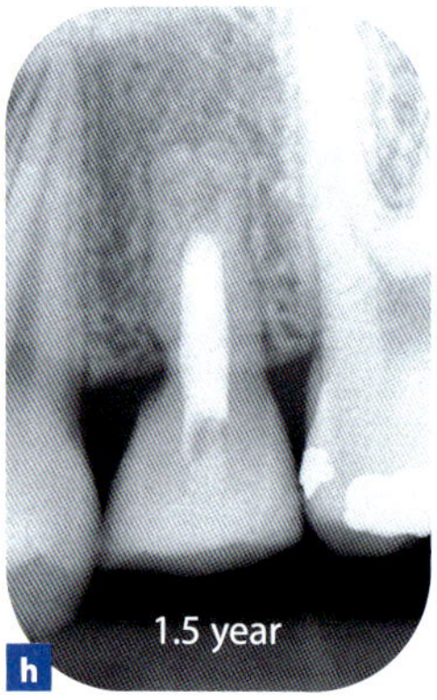

Fig 3-20h One year and 6 months postoperative.

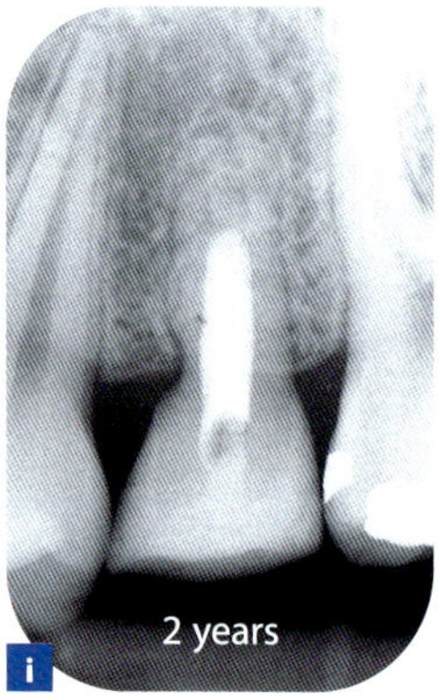

Fig 3-20i Two years postoperative.

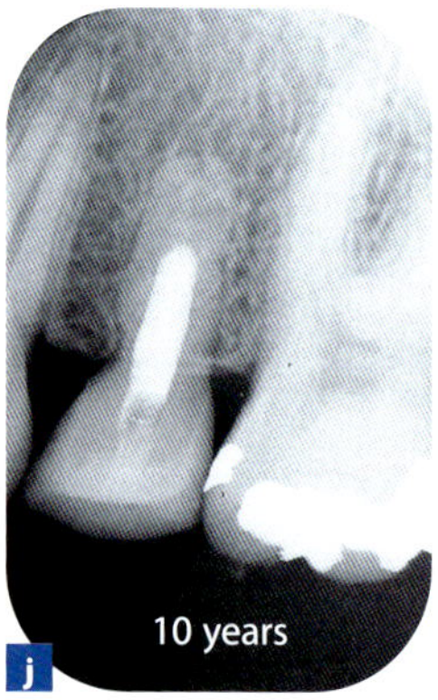

Fig 3-20j 10 years postoperative.

Fig 3-20k 17 years postoperative.
Fig 3-20l CBCT coronal image after 17 years. There is no root resorption observed on the buccal and lingual aspects.
Fig 3-20m CBCT sagittal image of the same tooth on the same day as **Fig 3-20l**, showing that the proximal resorption has been arrested and is separated from the bone by the periodontal ligament space.

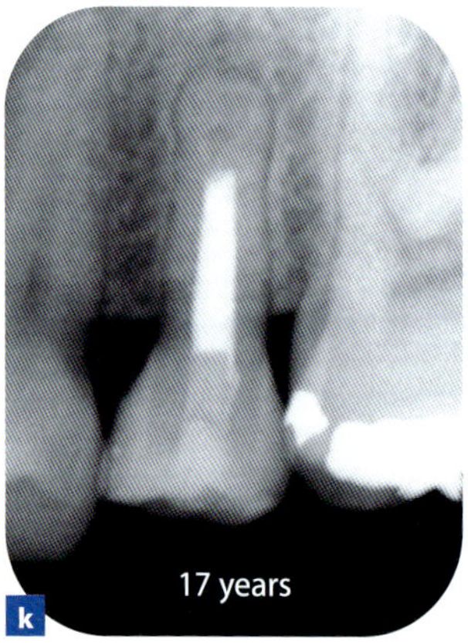

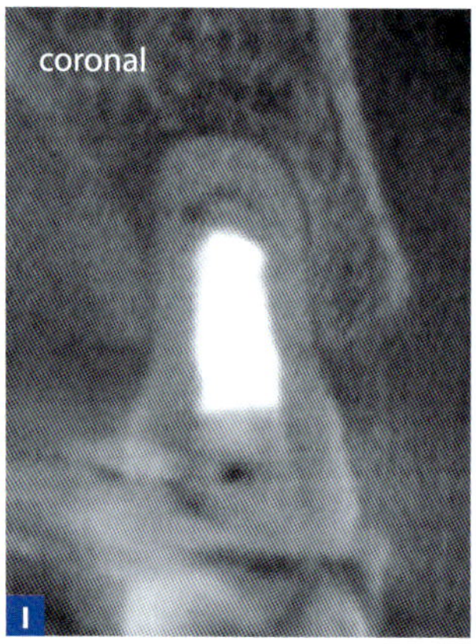

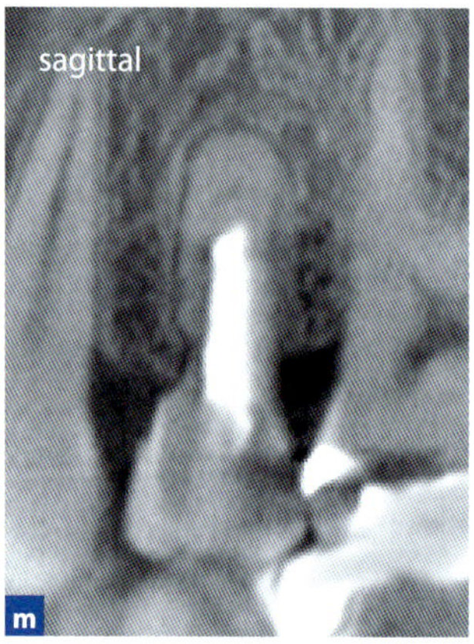

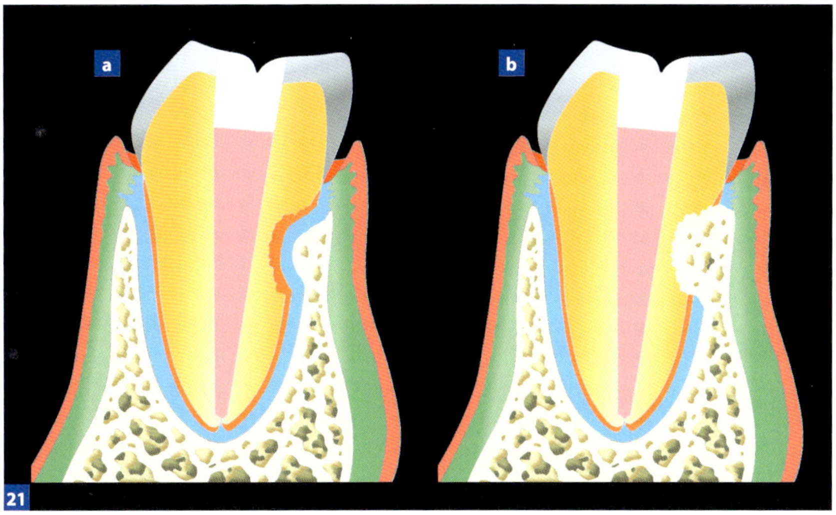

Fig 3-21 Types of healing in cases of inflammatory resorption after root canal therapy.

Fig 3-21a Repair by new attachment. Arrested resorption is followed by deposition of cementum on the resorbed dentin surface. Sharpey's fibers are attached to the new cementum and normal periodontal ligament is formed. New bone fills the resorption cavity with normal periodontal ligament space separating the root and bone.

Fig 3-21b Repair by progressive replacement resorption (ankylosis). This undesirable outcome results from failure of cementoblasts to lay down cementum before osteoclasts begin their process of hard tissue resorption as part of normal bone remodeling.

and induce an inflammatory response in the host tissue (**Fig 3-18b**). In addition to osteoblast-induced differentiation (see **Fig 3-15**), osteoclasts are also thought to disseminate from the circulating blood as a host response and contribute to the progression of the root resorption[96-98] (**Fig 3-19**).

A characteristic of inflammatory resorption is the existence of granulation tissue, which contains many capillary vessels in the resorptive cavity, which appears as a radiolucent finding radiographically[60, 61] (**Fig 3-20d**). The radiolucency from the resorption can be observed as early as 1 month after transplantation or replantation (**Fig 3-20a** to **3-20d**). Age of the host does not seem to affect the speed of inflammatory root resorption, which can develop fairly rapidly. Unlike replacement resorption, inflammatory resorption can be arrested by root canal treatment if it is done early[64]. After root canal treatment, the granulation tissue is replaced with periodontal ligament tissue and healing by new attachment occurs[19, 22-25, 64, 99] (**Fig 3-21a**). If the resorption area is large, there is a higher risk that osteoclastic activity may take place before new cementum and periodontal ligament fiber attachment occurs, resulting in replacement resorption (ankylosis)[22] (**Fig 3-21b**). In teeth which develop ankylosis, delayed inflammatory resorption may occur near the cervical area several years after transplantation (**Fig 3-22**). This change from replacement resorption to inflammatory resorption may be due to invasion of microorganisms into the pulp space and dentin tubules.

Surface resorption

Surface resorption is resorption that is limited to the surface of the cementum or dentin. Surface resorption is part of the repair mechanism in which new cementum is laid down on newly resorbed areas and periodontal ligament fibers become embedded in the new cementum (see **Fig 3-8** to **3-10**). Surface resorption likely occurs when there is limited or partial injury to the periodontal ligament[10, 19, 22, 64]. Inflammatory resorption that arrests after root canal treatment and shows evidence of healing by new attachment can also be referred to as surface resorption[64, 65].

Fig 3-22 A Clinical case of delayed inflammatory root resorption.

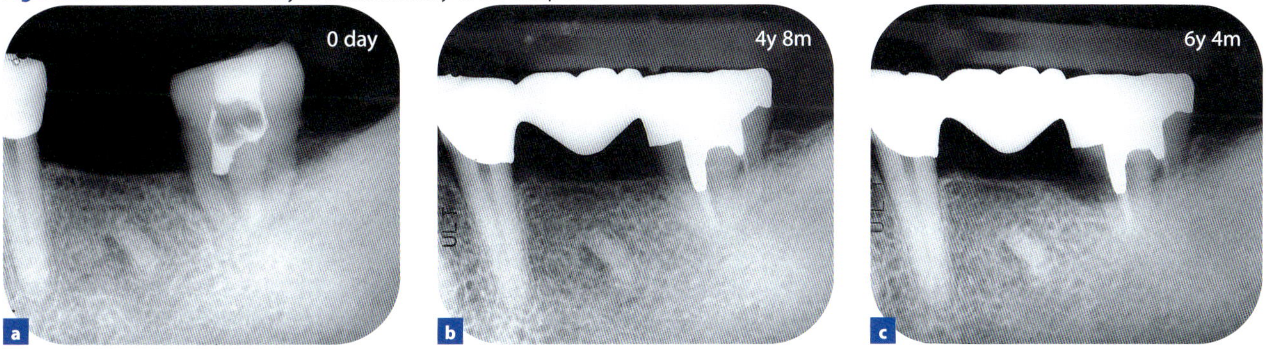

Fig 3-22a After transplantation in a 41-year-old male.

Fig 3-22b Four years and 8 months after transplantation. It looks like no ankylosis but actually ankylosis might have initiated.

Fig 3-22c Six years and 4 months after transplantation. Emergence of inflammatory resorption at mesial lingual cervical area. It is possible that the initial ankylosis may develop into inflammatory resorption due to bacteria in the dentinal tubules.

Healing of gingiva

If the concept of biologic width[100-104] is applied to transplantation, the transplanted tooth (**Fig 3-23a**) should be positioned with the CEJ and about 1 mm of periodontal ligament (PDL) exposed above the bone crest (**Fig 3-23b**). This positioning allows for proper connective tissue attachment around the cervical area. If the donor tooth is placed deeper into the recipient site, there will be apical migration of the epithelium to the level of the PDL, which leads to crestal bone resorption and re-establishment of the biologic width. This would result more likely in horizontal bone loss if the alveolar crest is thin and vertical bone loss if the crestal bone is thick (**Fig 3-23c**). If the tooth is transplanted into a position more coronally above the crest, there may be a longer connective tissue attachment that is established (**Fig 3-23d**). This long connective tissue attachment may eventually develop into alveolar bone proper, depending on the condition of the surrounding bone (this will be discussed later in the chapter on the section "healing of alveolar bone"). The junctional epithelial attachment of approximately 1 mm will be also be established naturally at the base of the gingival sulcus.

Healing of gingiva

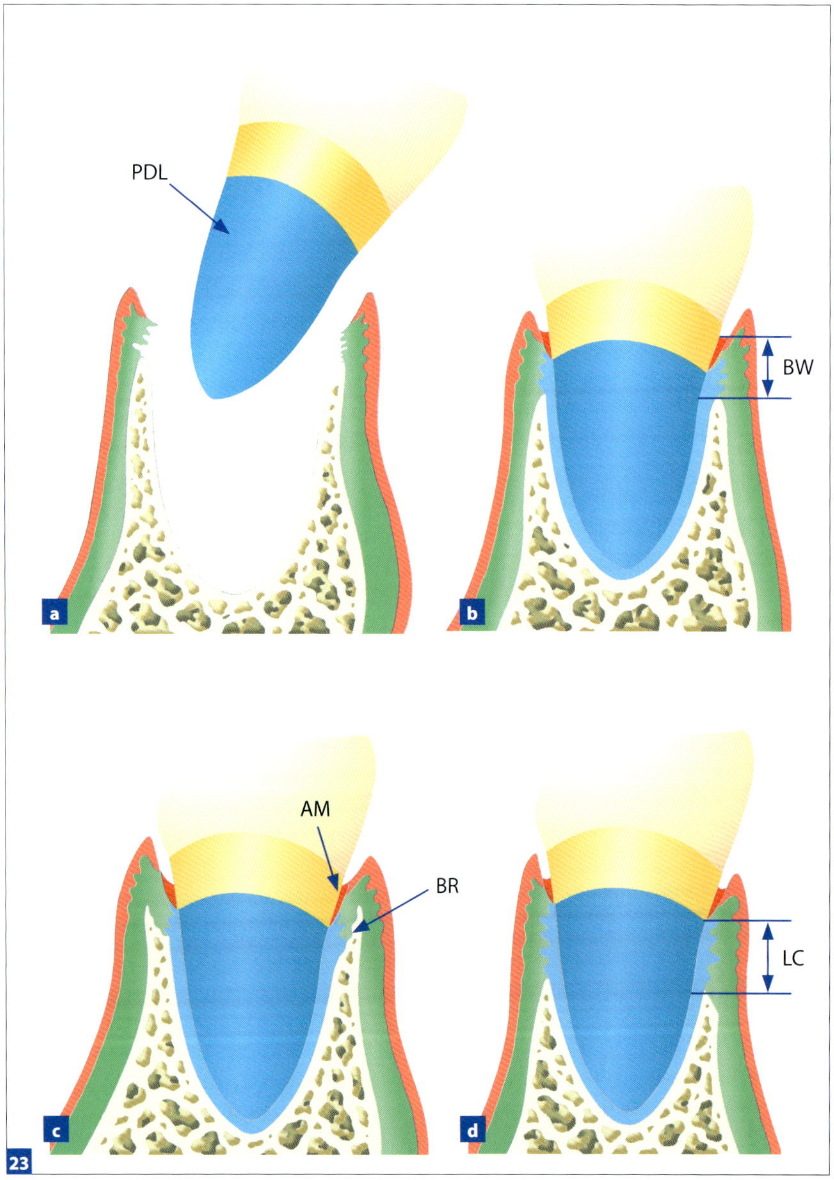

Fig 3-23 Healing of gingiva.
Fig 3-23a Before transplantation of a tooth without coronal one fifth of the periodontal ligament.
Fig 3-23b Ideal position. Ideal biologic width (BW) can be achieved by placing the donor tooth at a level so that a 1 to 2 mm width of the periodontal ligament is located above the bone crest.
Fig 3-23c Donor tooth placed too deep. Apical migration (AM) of epithelium occurs, creating vertical bone resorption (BR).
Fig 3-23d Donor tooth placed too shallow. Long connective tissue attachment (LC) may result.

From the standpoint of biologic width, the ideal positioning for the transplanted tooth is with a band of about 1 mm of periodontal ligament above the bone crest margin. In practice, however, it is recommended that the transplanted tooth be placed slightly deeper into the recipient socket to avoid too much contact with the opposing tooth (especially in the transplantation of an immature tooth). In most cases the tooth will spontaneously erupt after a few months and naturally re-establish the biological width (see **Fig 3-57**).

Pulpal healing and root development

When an immature tooth (i.e. tooth with incomplete root formation) is used as a donor, healing of the pulp and continued root development can be expected after transplantation[107-120] (**Fig 3-24** and **3-25**).

Pulpal Healing

(1) Revascularization and Pulp canal obliteration

Pulpal healing in transplantation can be explained through the phenomenon of revascularization (regeneration of capillaries into the pulp canal) and subsequent pulp canal obliteration. In immature teeth, Hertwig's epithelial sheath still remains (**Fig 3-26a**), and regeneration of capillary vessels progresses through the apical foramen surrounded by this epithelial sheath. As capillaries regenerate, pulp cells inside the epithelial sheath proliferate into the pulp canal[111-114] (**Fig 3-26b**). The rate of this proliferation is thought to be about 0.5 mm/day, and within a few months the pulp canal is filled with vital tissue months (**Fig 3-26c**). Thereafter, the pulp canal space undergoes rapid calcification and is called pulp canal obliteration (PCO)[108]. PCO is classified into two categories; total PCO in which the root canal is closed completely with calcified tissues (**Fig 3-26d** and **3-24**) and; partial PCO in which some pulp canal space remains[109] (**Fig 3-26e** and **3-25**).

In total obliteration, the root canal space is not detected radiographically (**Fig 3-24m** to **3-24o**). In partial obliteration, part of the pulp chamber and canal space can be detected radiographically (**Fig 3-25g** to **3-25i**). Even after the pulp canal undergoes obliteration, the transplanted tooth responds to electronic pulp test (EPT), but the response may diminish over time. In partial obliteration the tooth typically responds to EPT if pulp necrosis does not occur.

Pulpal healing and root development

Fig 3-24 A Clinical case of pulp healing and root development after transplantation①

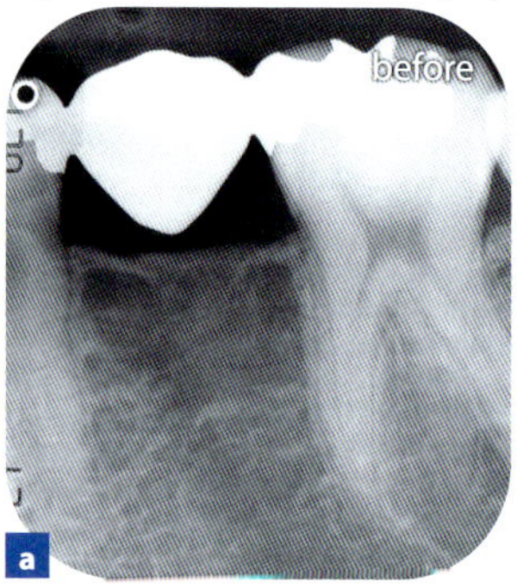

Fig 3-24a Preoperative radiograph of a 16-year-old girl with a congenital missing of #35.

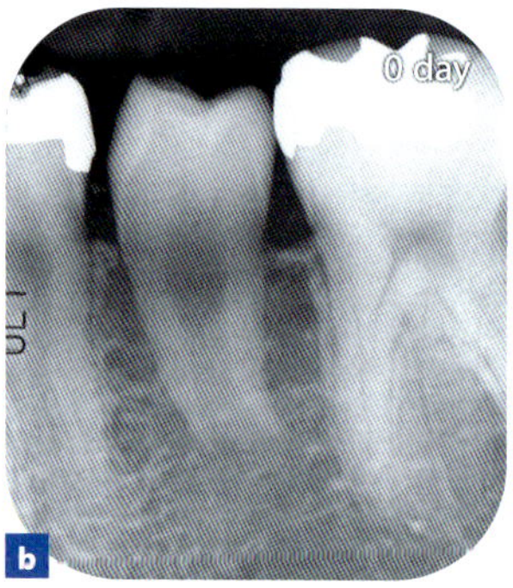

Fig 3-24b Immature #45 was transplanted to the missing site.

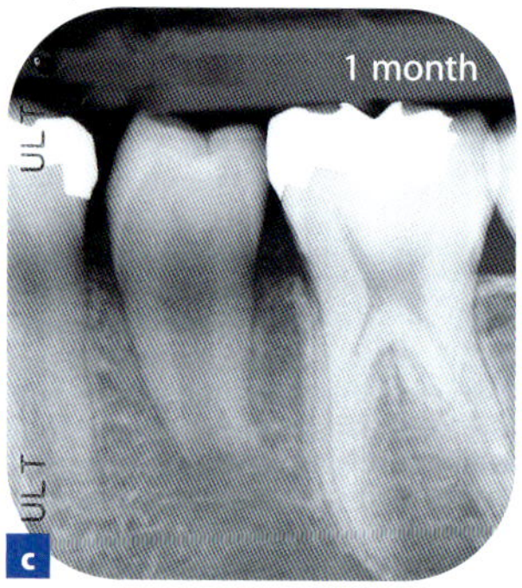

Fig 3-24c One month postoperative. No change was observed.

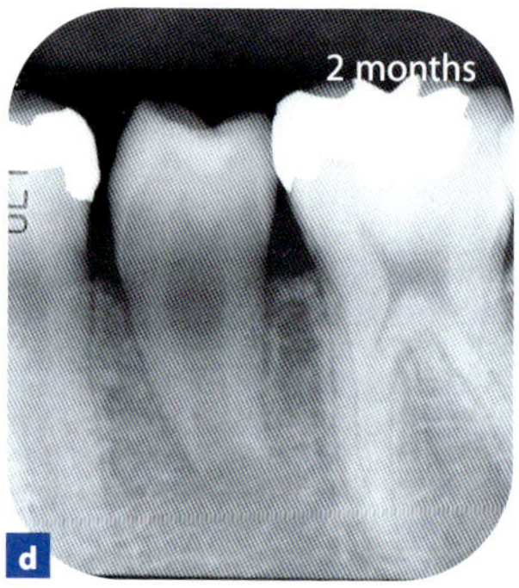

Fig 3-24d Two months postoperative. No change was observed.

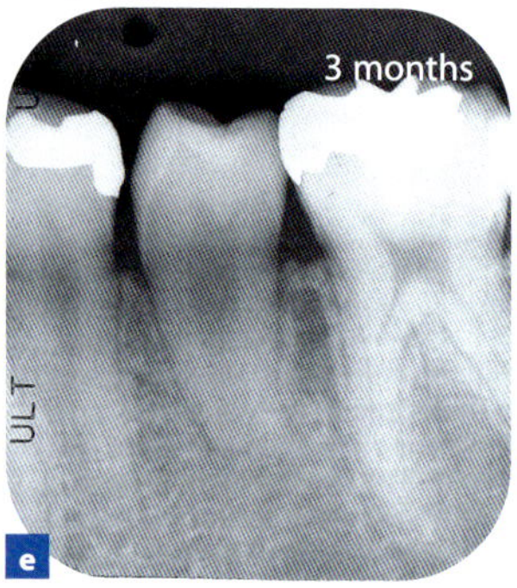

Fig 3-24e Three months postoperative. Slight calcification of the pulp canal is observed.

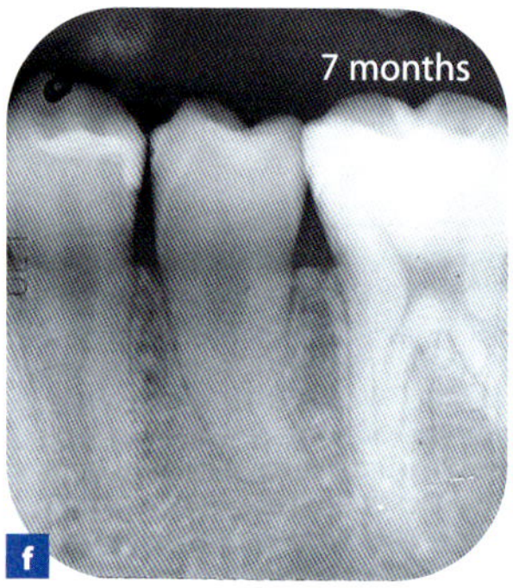

Fig 3-24f Seven months postoperative. Slight progression of the calcification. The transplant responds EPT (+).

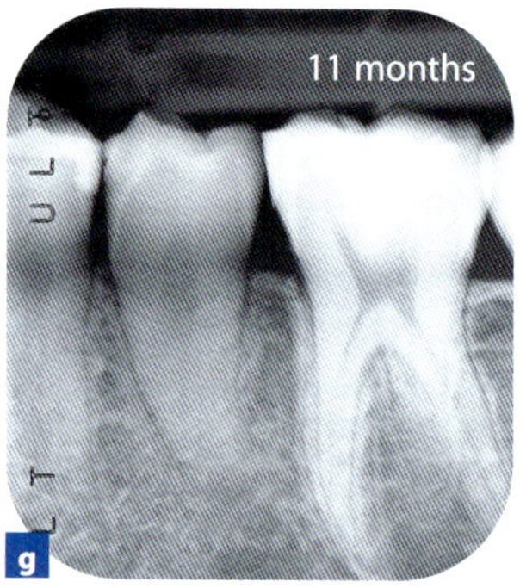

Fig 3-24g 11 months postoperative.

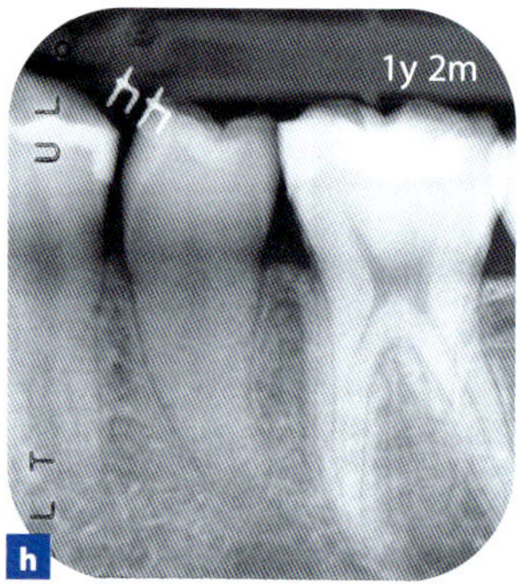

Fig 3-24h One year and 2 months postoperative. Calcification of the pulp cavity and root development are obvious.

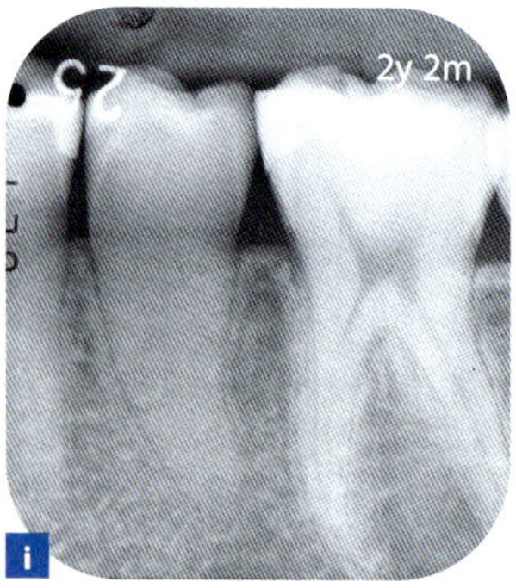

Fig 3-24i Two years and 2 months postoperative. The pulp canal obliteration is almost completed and the root development is in its final stage.

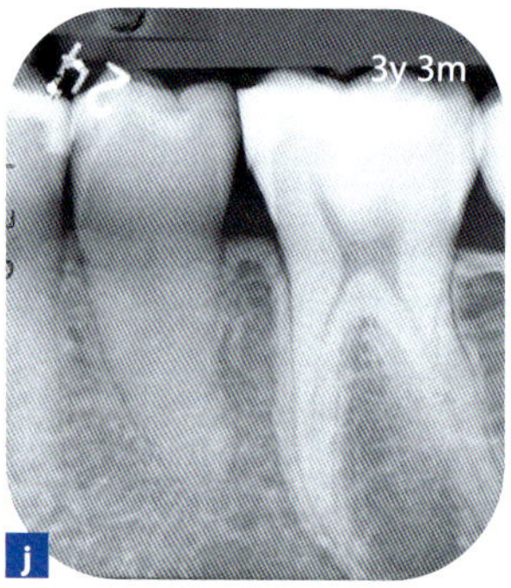

Fig 3-24j Three years and 3 months postoperative, there is little change compared to **Fig 3-24i**.

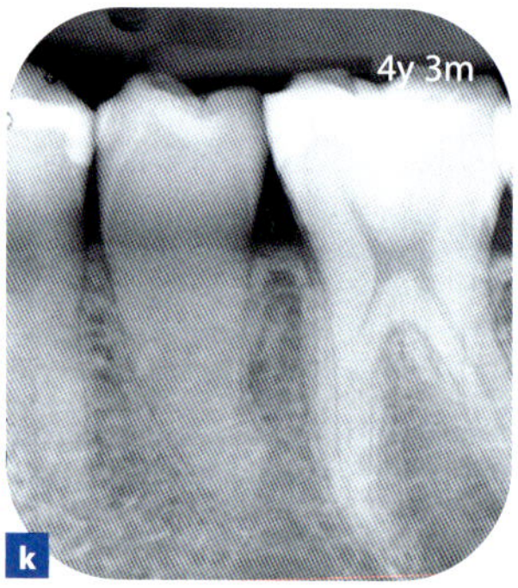

Fig 3-24k Four years and 3 months postoperative. The transplant responded EPT positive.

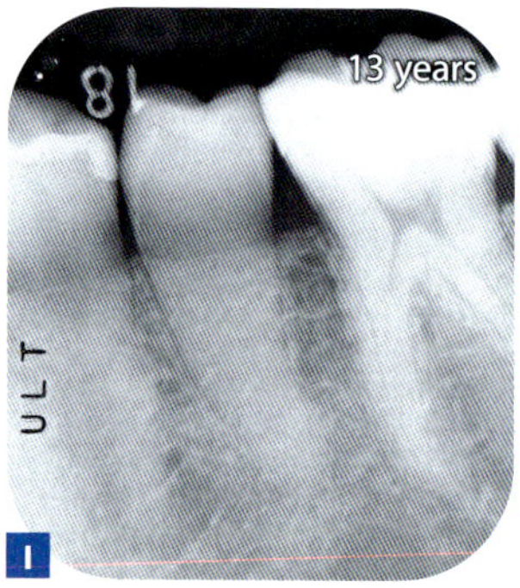

Fig 3-24l 13 years postoperative. No radiographic changes, but the response to EPT is less.

Fig 3-24m-o CBCT images after 13 years. No resorption is observed though almost the entire pulp space of the transplant is obliterated.

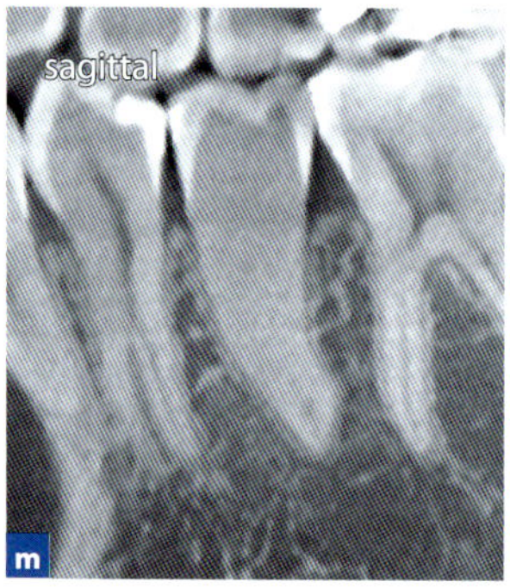

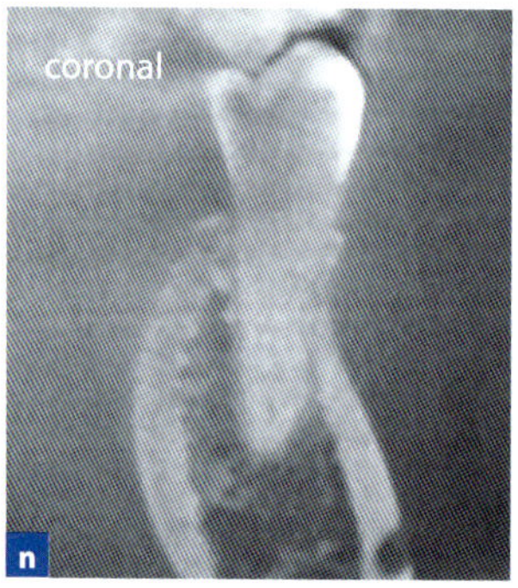

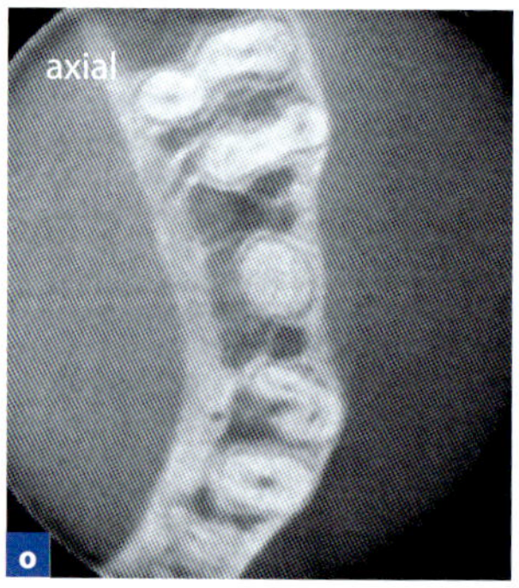

Fig 3-25 A Clinical case of pulp healing and root development after transplantation②

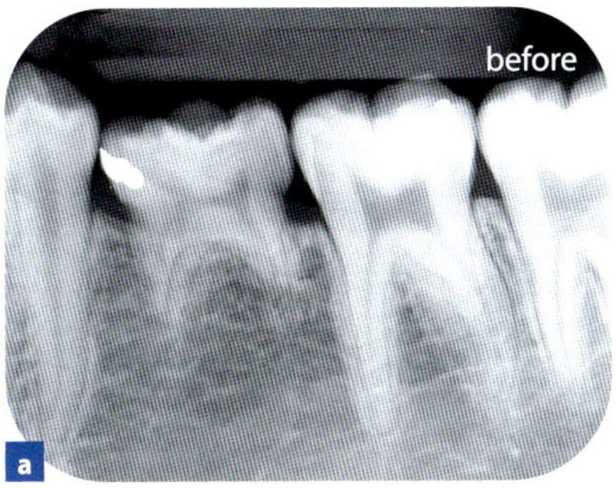

Fig 3-25a Preoperative radiograph of a 17-year-old female with a congenital missing of #35.

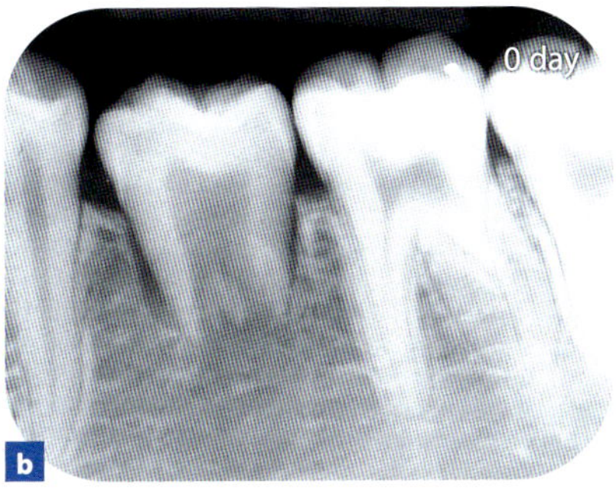

Fig 3-25b Immediately after transplantation. A partially impacted immature #48 was transplanted.

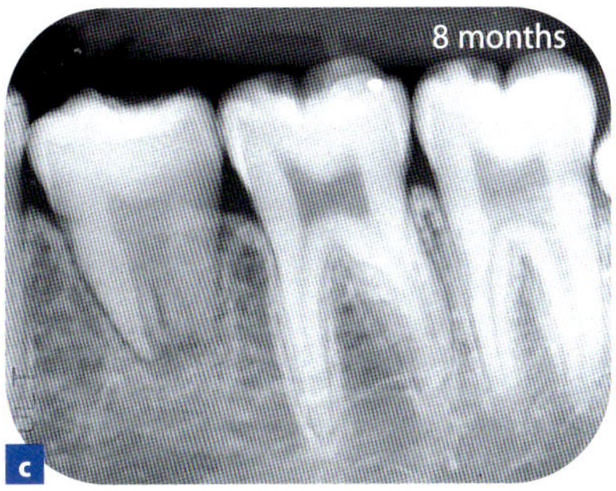

Fig 3-25c Eight months postoperative. The transplant responded EPT positive.

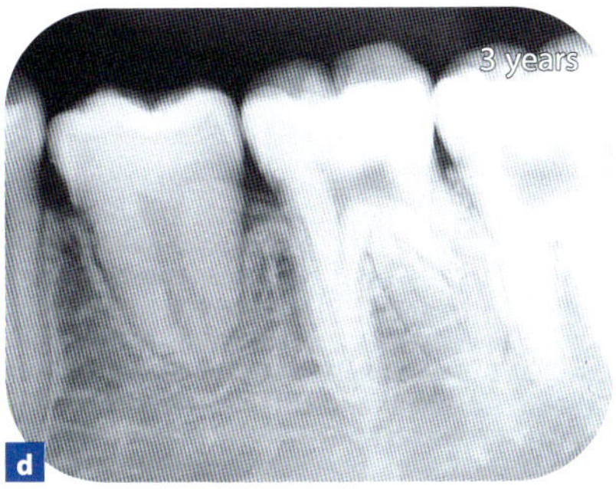

Fig 3-25d Three years postoperative. Pulp canal obliteration and root development were observed.

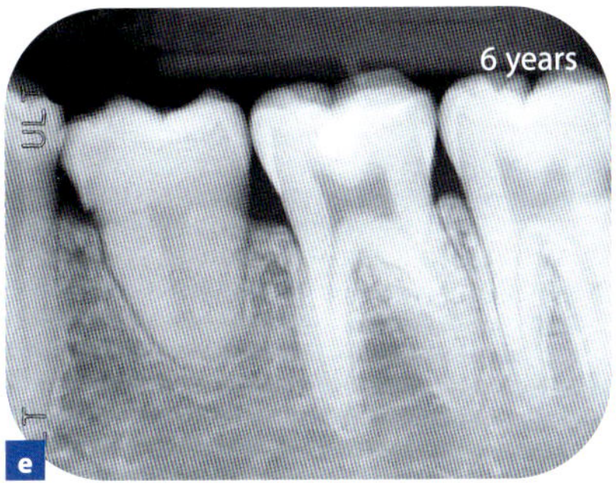

Fig 3-25e Six years postoperative.

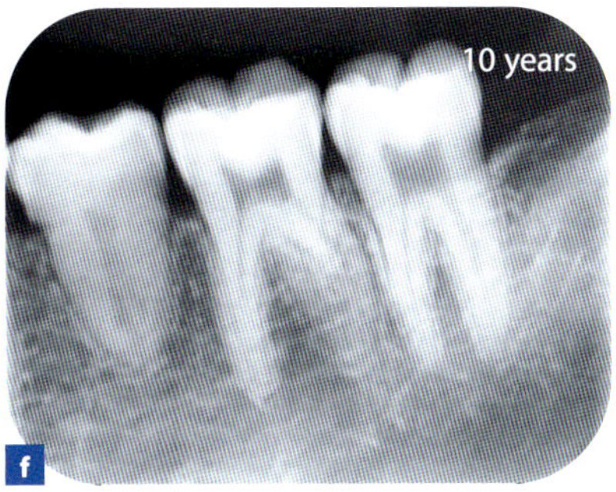

Fig 3-25f 10 years postoperative. Note the pulp cavity can be observed.

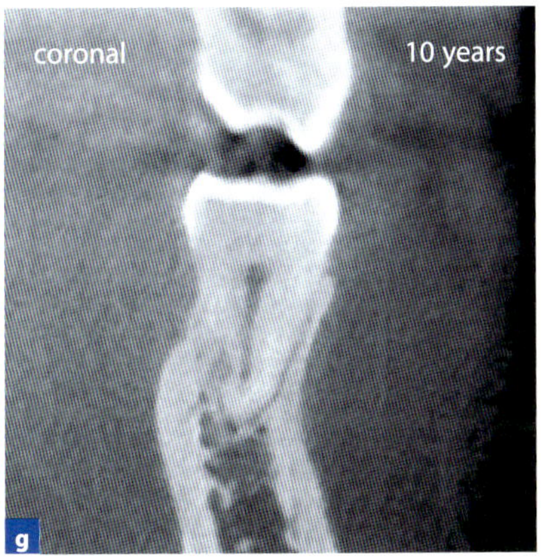

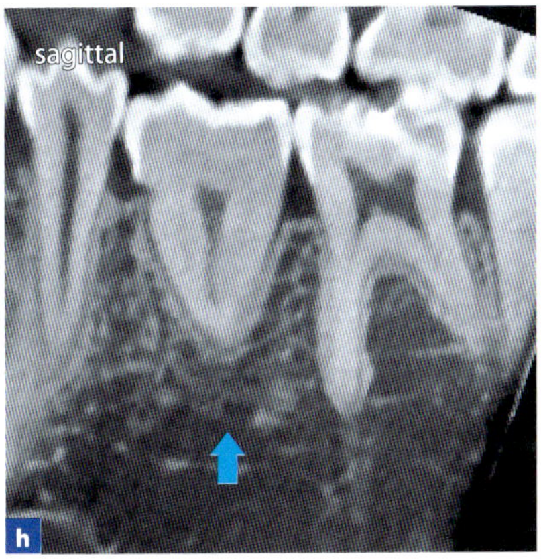

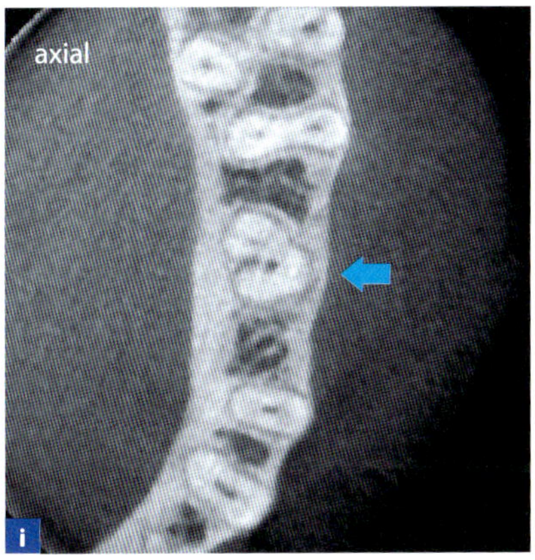

Fig 3-25g-i CBCT images 10 years after transplantation. The pulp cavity is preserved. The pulp has healed as partial obliteration. It can also be observed that the surface resorption on mesial aspect has not progressed.

Mechanism of pulp healing in transplantation of an immature tooth

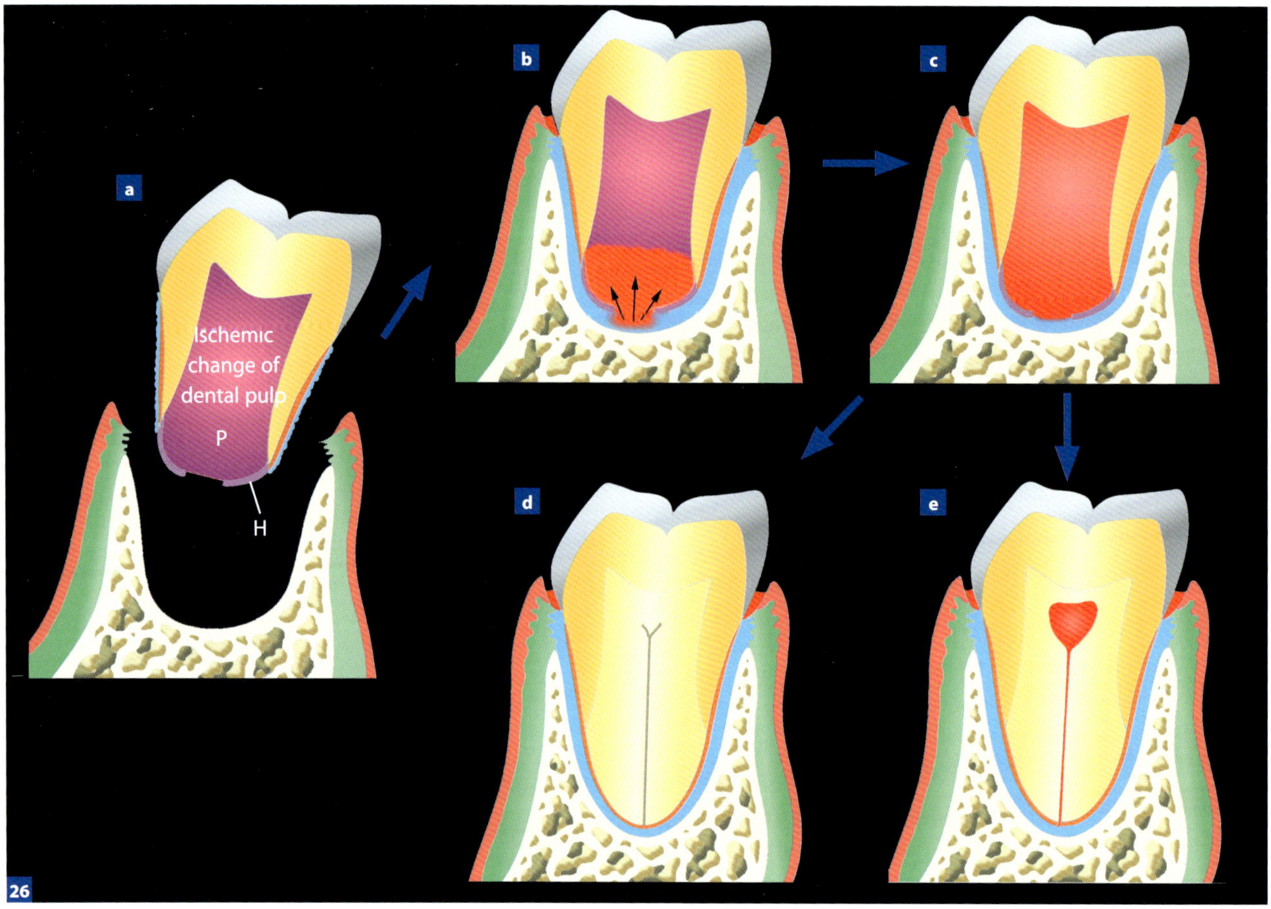

Fig 3-26a Preoperative. Transplantation of an immature tooth. The pulp (P) of the donor tooth is suffering ischemic change. Hertwig's epithelial root sheath (H) is attached to the apex.
Fig 3-26b A few days after transplantation. Capillary vessels proliferate coronally from the apical foramen and pulp cells proliferate along with them.
Fig 3-26c A few weeks after transplantation. The pulp canal is filled with vital tissue first, then rapid calcification occurs from the canal walls.
Fig 3-26d Total obliteration of the pulp canal with hard tissue.
Fig 3-26e Partial obliteration of the pulp canal with some remaining pulp tissue.

Fig 3-27 shows the stages of root development as proposed by Moorrees, et al[121]. **Fig 3-28** shows results from a study looking at the percentage of pulpal healing that occurred after transplantation of 370 premolars at various stages of root development[108]. According to this study, pulpal healing can be predictably observed in teeth up until stage 5 of root development. The study also investigated pulpal healing based on the diameter of the root's apical foramen and showed that if the

Table 3-3 Pulp healing in relation to the diameter of apical foramina of donor teeth (Reprinted with permission from Andreasen et al.[108]). The probability of pulp healing was summarized according to the diameter of the apical foramina. The data may indicate that about 94% of pulp healing can be expected with no less than 1 mm of diameter. Contrarily there is little chance with less than 1 mm.

Diameter foramen (mm)	0.1~0.9	1.0~1.9	2.0~2.9	3.0~3.9	4.0~4.9	5.0~6.9
Pulp healing	4(13%)	53(87%)	107(97%)	63(98%)	10(83%)	6(86%)
Pulp necrosis	26	8	3	1	2	1

Stage1	Beginning of root formation
Stage2	1/4 root formation
Stage3	1/2 root formation
Stage4	3/4 root formation
Stage5	Complete root formation, apical foramen is wide open
Stage6	Complete root formation, apical foramen is half closed
Stage7	Complete root formation, apical foramen is nearly closed

Fig 3-27 Developmental stages of roots (classification of Moorrees et al.[121]).

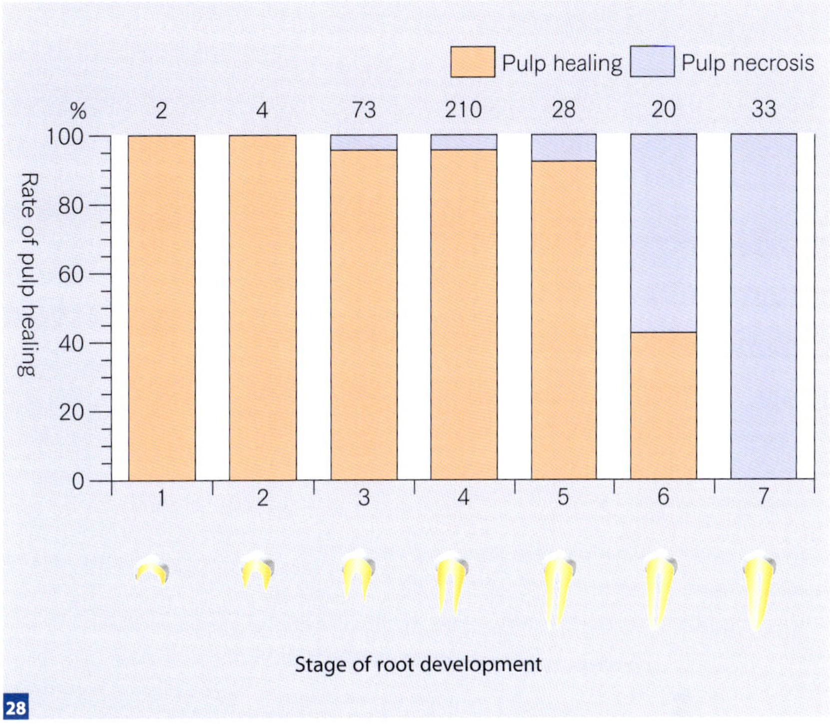

Fig 3-28 Healing of pulp in relation to stage of root development.
After 370 premolars at various stages of root development were transplanted, the data on pulp healing were collected. The results show that healing of pulp cannot be expected at stage 6 or 7. (Reprinted with permission from Andreasen et al.[108]).

Fig 3-29 A case of transplantation to determine the criteria of whether or not pulp healing will occur.

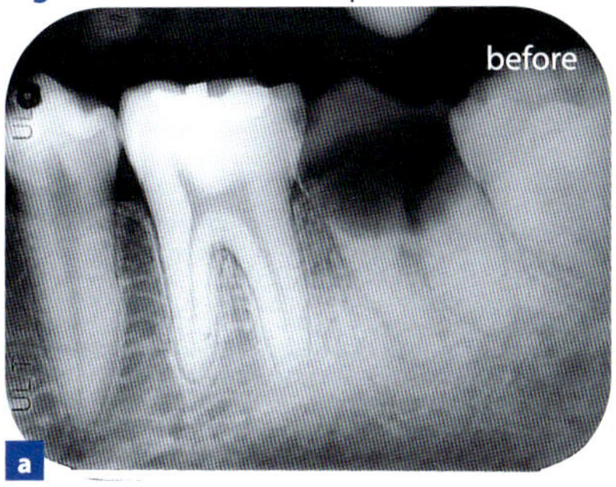

Fig 3-29a Preoperative radiograph of a 21-year-old male whose #38 was to be transplanted into the adjacent second molar site.

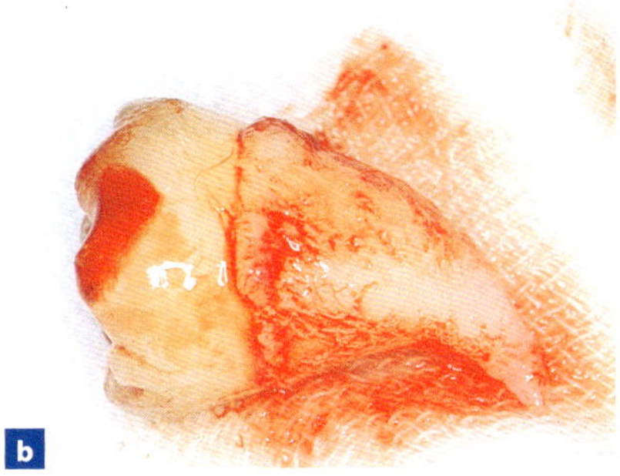

Fig 3-29b The donor tooth extracted for transplantation. Note the small amount of Hertwig's epithelial sheath attached to the root apex.

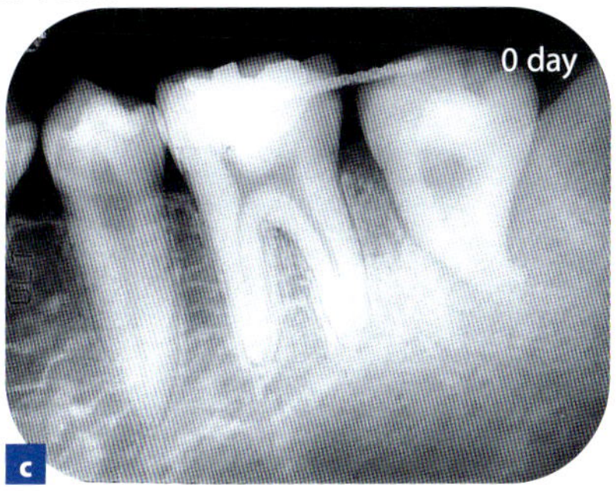

Fig 3-29c Immediately after transplantation.

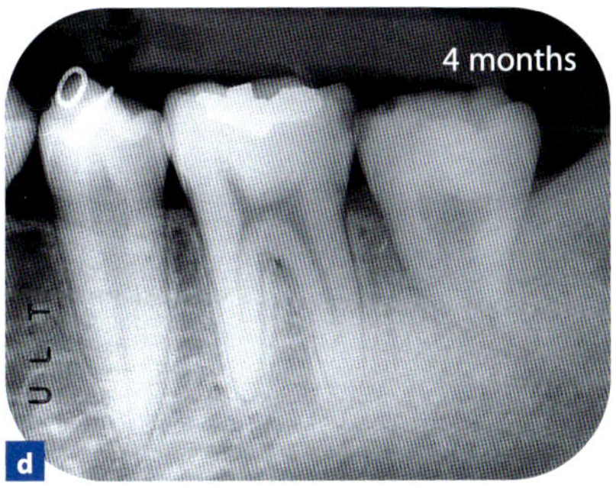

Fig 3-29d Four months after transplantation.

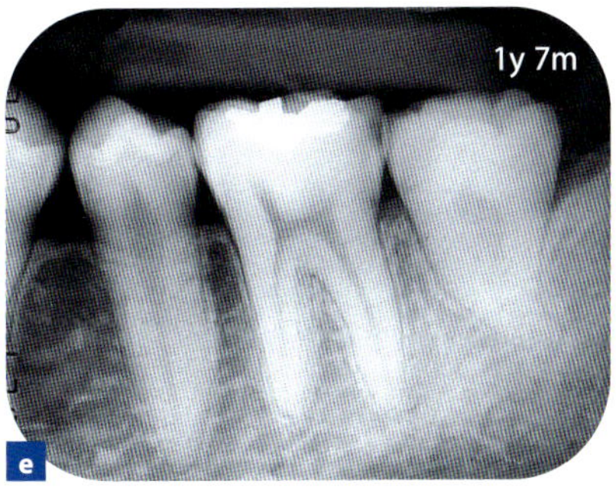

Fig 3-29e One year and 7 months after transplantation, showing the pulp healing. EPT (+).

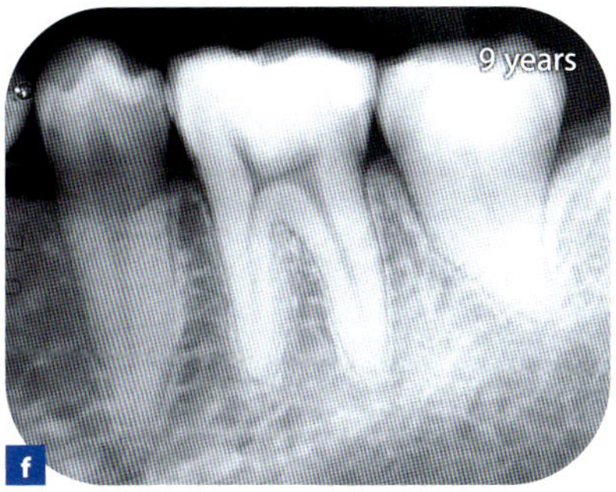

Fig 3-29f Nine years after transplantation. The presence of Hertwig's epithelial sheath at the root apex of the donor tooth at the time of transplantation may determine whether or not pulp healing can be expected.

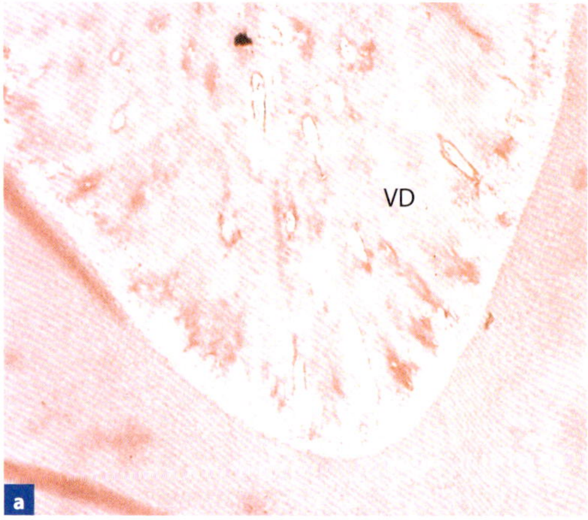

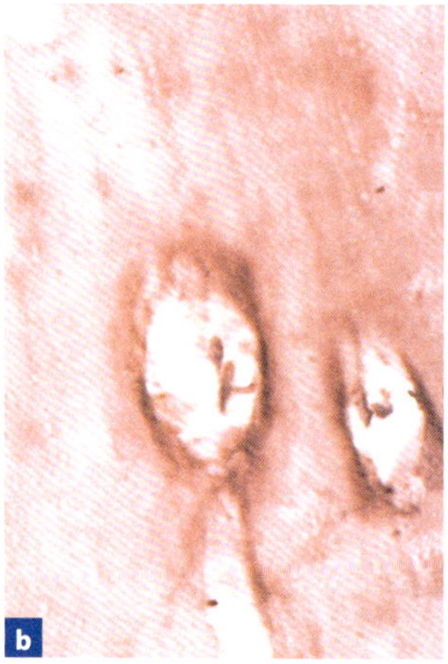

Fig 3-30 Histology of the hard tissue found in teeth with pulp canal obliteration. (Courtesy of Dr. Jens O. Andreasen)

Fig 3-30a Dentin formed after transplantation is called vascular dentin (VD) because of the presence of cavities that are the traces of vessels.

Fig 3-30b Higher magnification of **Fig 3-34a**. Hard tissue seems to consist of osteodentin.

diameter of the apical foramen was 1 mm or greater, pulpal healing was observed in 94% of cases (**Table 3-3**). Clinically the author has observed that in most cases, healing of the pulp occurs when the Hertwig's epithelial root sheath is present on the donor tooth (**Fig 3-29**).

The hard tissue formed in the root canal space after transplantation is called 'vascular dentin' or osteodentin because in the dentin-like hard tissue there are the small vascular spaces present (**Fig 3-30**). Bacterial infection into the obliterated tissue can result in periapical/periradicular infection that is difficult to treat due to the calcification (**Fig 3-31**). Therefore, in teeth that undergo pulp canal obliteration (in the transplantation of an immature tooth), it is important to avoid tooth preparation that may expose dentin and prevent dental decay[122].

Fig 3-31 A clinical case of periapical lesion developing after healing of a transplanted immature tooth.

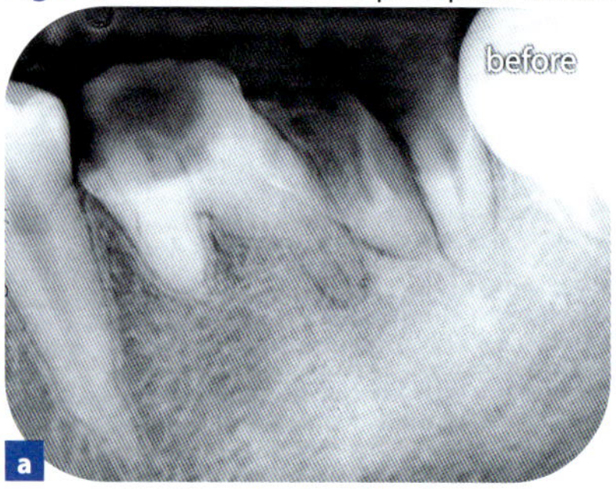

Fig 3-31a Preoperative radiograph of a 17-year-old male.

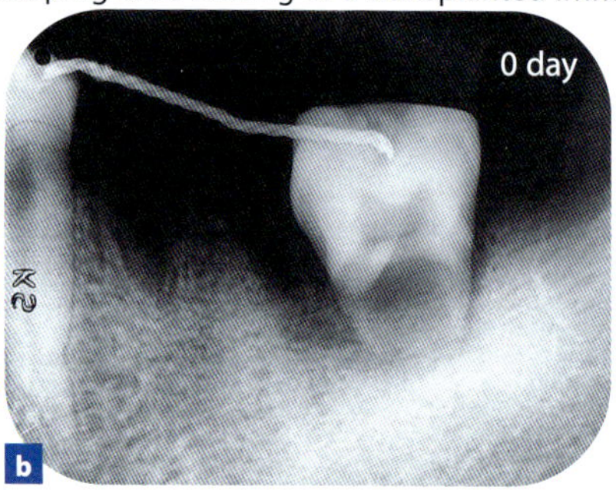

Fig 3-31b Immediately after transplantation. #36 and #37 were extracted and #38 was transplanted to #37 site.

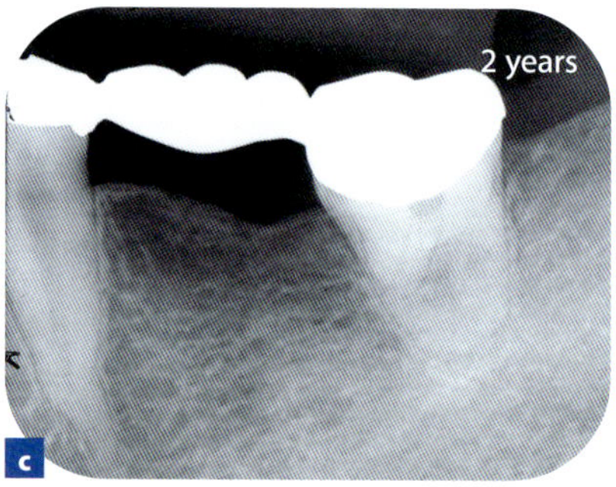

Fig 3-31c Two years after transplantation. Pulp healing and root development are observed.

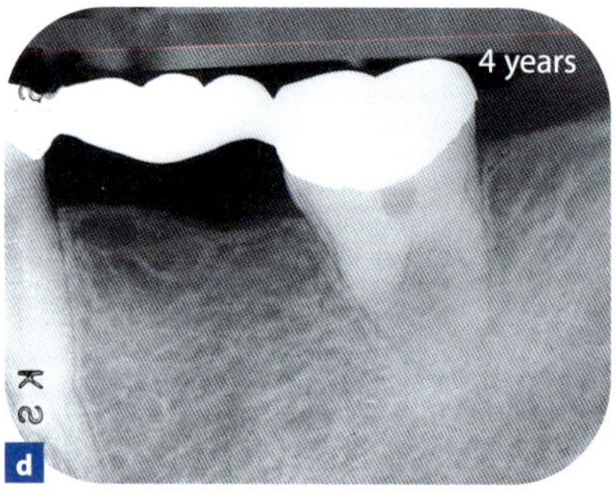

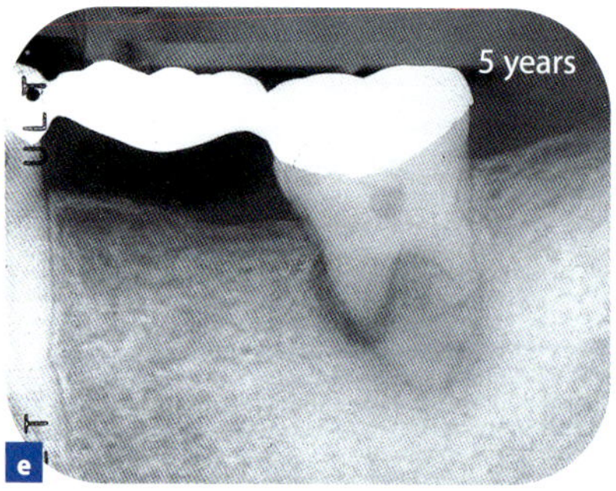

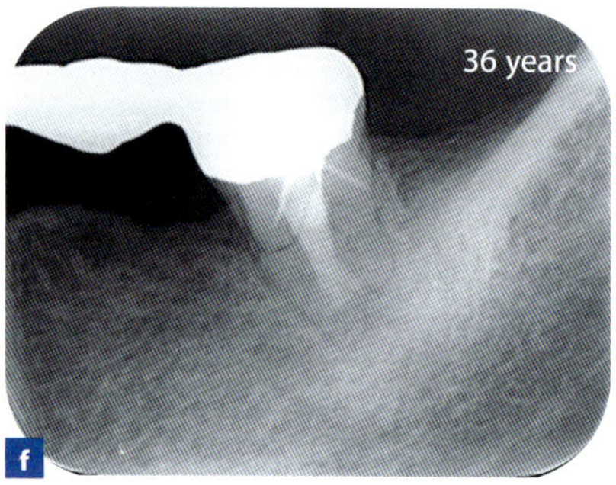

Fig 3-31d Four years after transplantation.

Fig 3-31e Five years after transplantation. A periapical lesion has developed. The cause may be that the tooth was prepared over the enamel as the abutment of a bridge. As the cement layer was washed out and secondary caries progressed, bacterial infection of the pulp cavity occurred. The canal was treated endodontically.

Fig 3-31f 36 years after transplantation. The lesion has disappeared and the transplant is maintained successfully.

Inner periodontal ligament (inner PDL)

An inner periodontal ligament may develop after transplantation or replantation of a developing tooth (Fig 3-32). This is thought to occur through the invasion and regeneration of the periodontal ligament and bone tissue into the pulp canal instead of the pulp tissue. This may be caused by necrosis, damage, or mechanical removal of Hertwig's epithelial sheath during the surgery, PDL regenerates along the inner root canal

Healing with inner periodontal ligament(inner PDL)

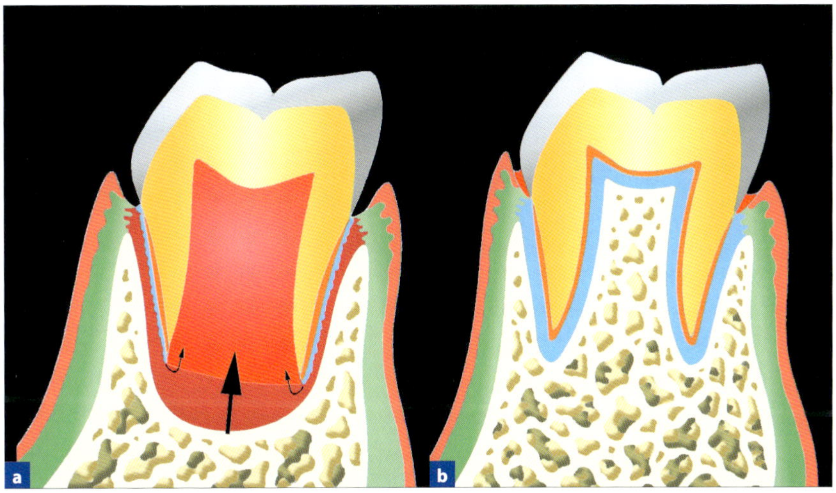

Fig 3-32a After transplantation of a donor tooth without Herwig's epithelial root sheath. Proliferation of periodontal ligament cells and bone cells into the canal may occur. The periodontal ligament proliferates coronally, depositing cementum on the inner wall of the root canal, and bone tissue grows along with it.
Fig 3-32b Healing with inner periodontal ligament. It should be noted that if alveolar bone fills the pulp space before cementum and periodontal ligament fibers attach to the inner dentin wall, replacement resorption (ankylosis) will take place.

Fig 3-33 A case of inner PDL healing.

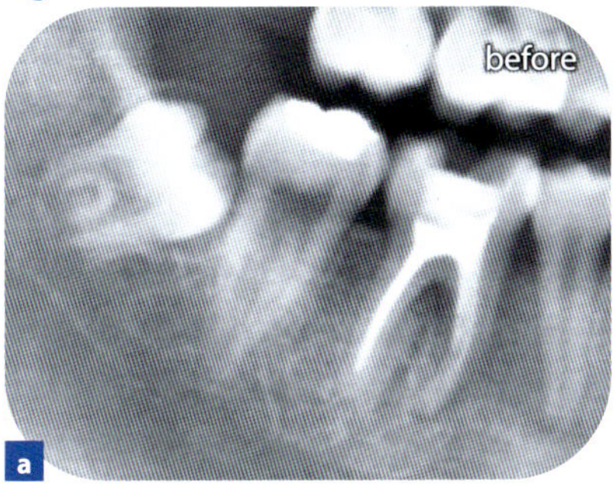

Fig 3-33a Preoperative radiograph of an 18-year-old male before transplantation of #48 into #46 which suffered crown-root fracture.

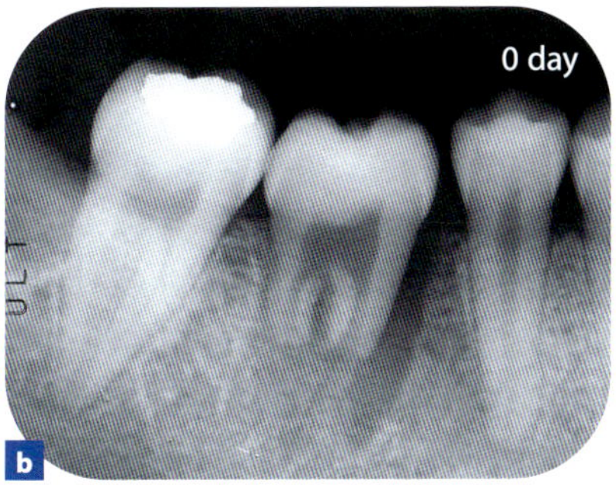

Fig 3-33b Immediately after transplantation.

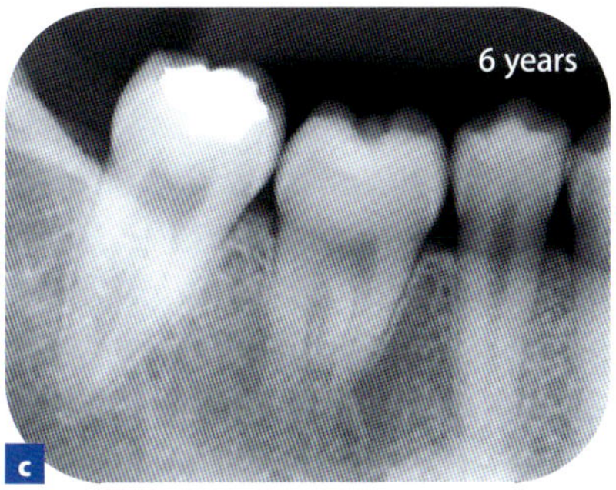

Fig 3-33c Six years after transplantation. The healing of the transplant seemed normal but inner PDL may have occurred in the mesial root though #46 responded EPT positive.

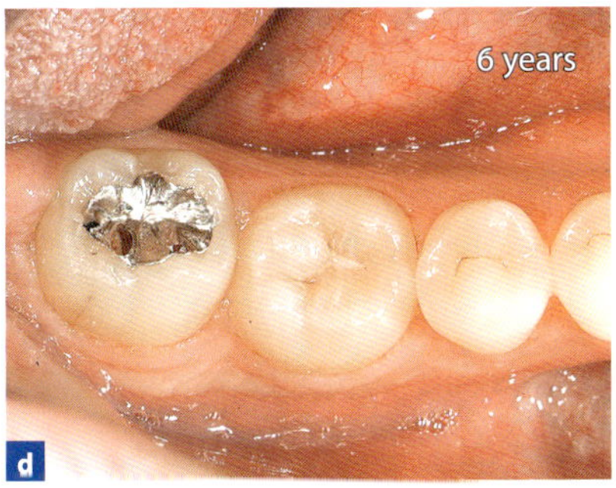

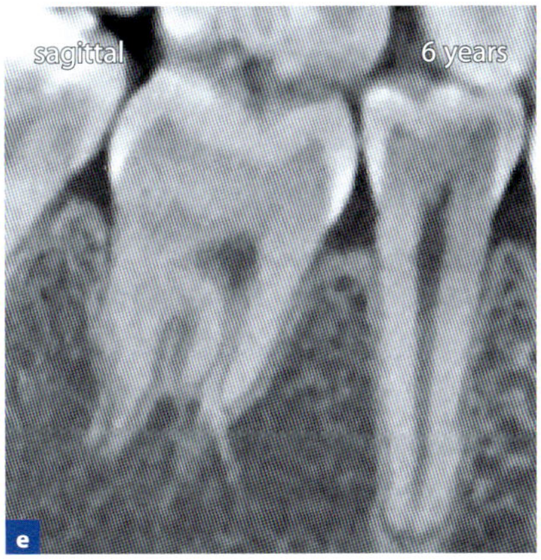

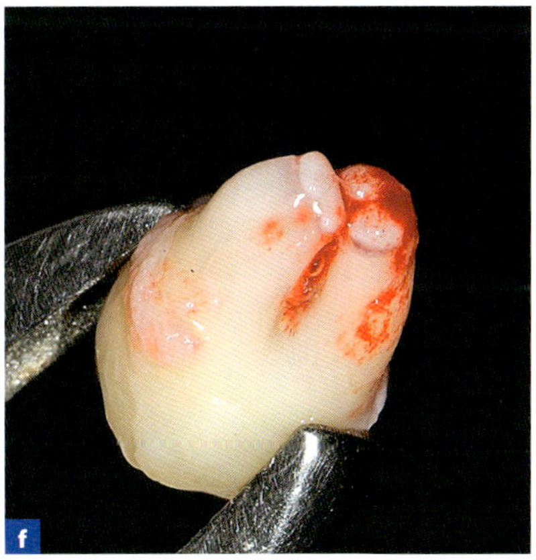

Fig 3-33d Occlusal view 6 years after transplantation.
Fig 3-33e CBCT image 6 years after transplantation, showing root development and pulp cavity closure in the distal root, whereas no root development and inner PDL were observed in the mesial root.
Fig 3-33f The donor tooth at time of transplantation. All of the apices are covered with Hertwig's epithelial sheath, but it is more likely that it was actually separated from the pulp tissue in the mesial root. It is possible that the Hertwig's epithelial sheath was removed during the surgery.

wall from the apical foramen, along with apposition of cementum and bone tissue formation in the canal space. Teeth with inner PDL are typically asymptomatic and functional and thus no treatment is necessary (**Fig 3-33**).

Root canal therapy for infected immature teeth

In cases that the pulp does not heal after transplantation of an immature tooth, root canal therapy is necessary. The reason for the failure in most cases is due to bacterial infection of the pulp tissue. If the infection extends to the periapical region and the Hertwig's epithelial sheath is necrotic, apexification is the treatment of choice[123-127] (**Fig 3-34** and **3-35**). If there is partial necrosis of the pulp and the Hertwig's epithelial sheath is healthy, apexogenesis type of treatment[128] (**Fig 3-36**) can be a performed (**Fig 3-37**). In both cases, the necrotic tissue is removed/cleaned and calcium hydroxide can be placed to aid in disinfection and healing.

Fig 3-34 Necrosis of pulp and apexification.

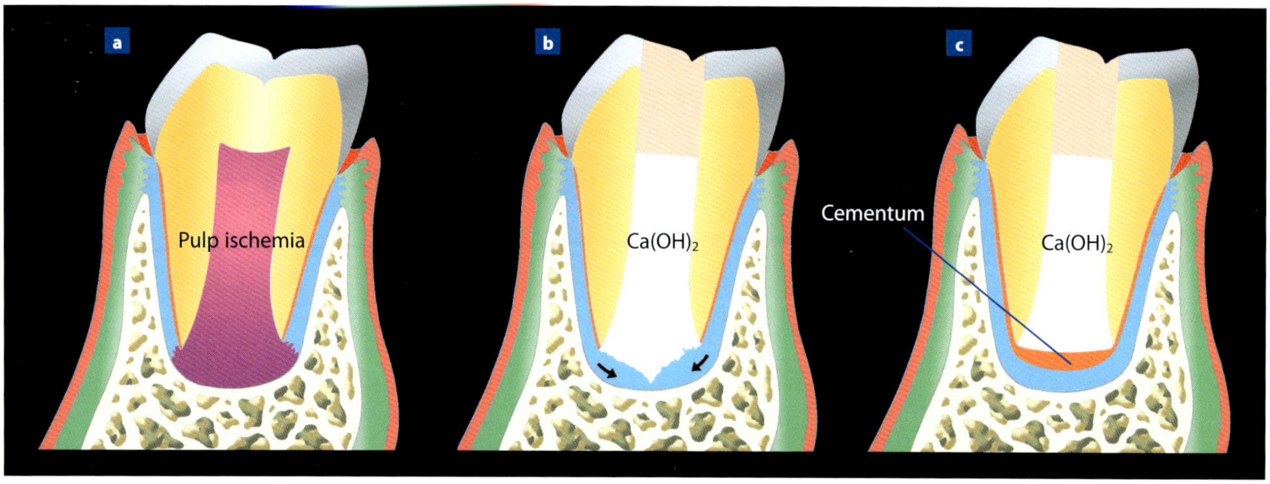

Fig 3-34a Complete necrosis of the pulp after transplantation of an immature tooth. Apexification is indicated as the endodontic option.
Fig 3-34b Apexification. Calcium hydroxide is medicated up to the apex. Cells of the periodontal ligament proliferate on the calcium hydroxide.
Fig 3-34c After healing of the apex. The apex will be closed with cementum in a few months.

Fig 3-35 A case of apexification of a transplanted immature tooth involved in pulp necrosis.

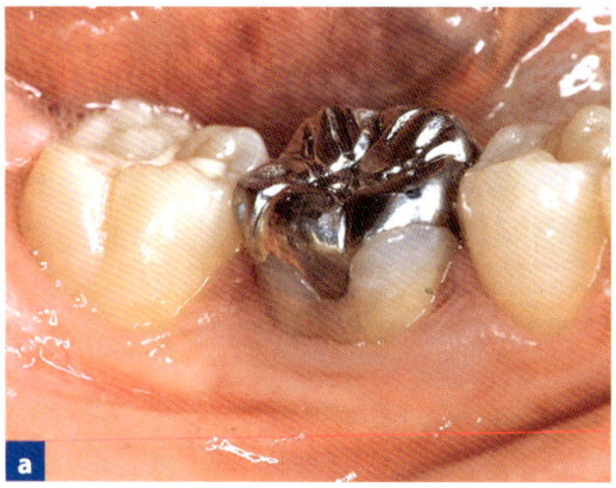

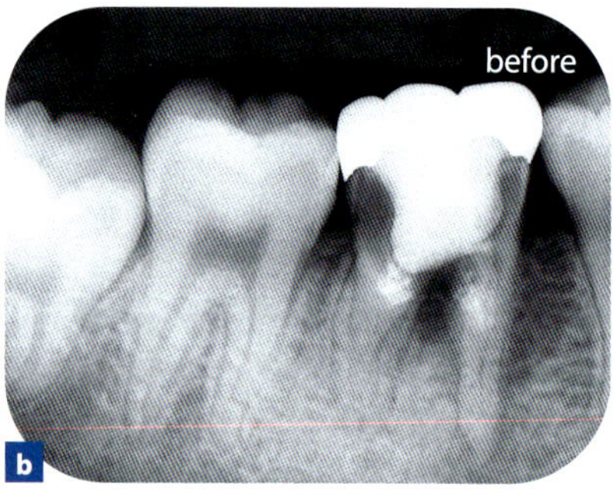

Fig 3-35a, b Preoperative view and radiograph of a 20-year-old female. #46 involved in progressive external resorption is to be replaced by #48.

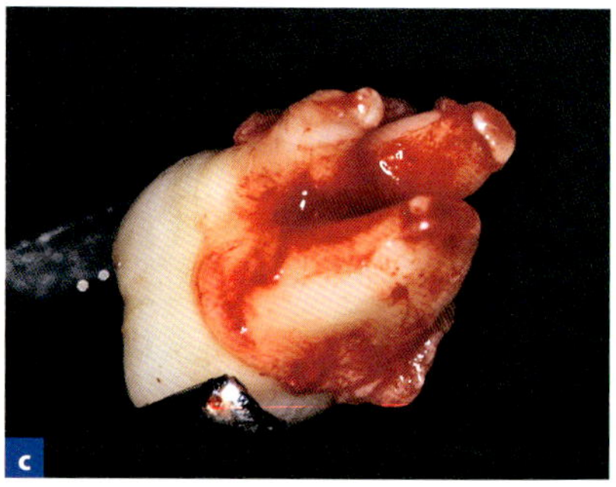

Fig 3-35c The extracted donor tooth.

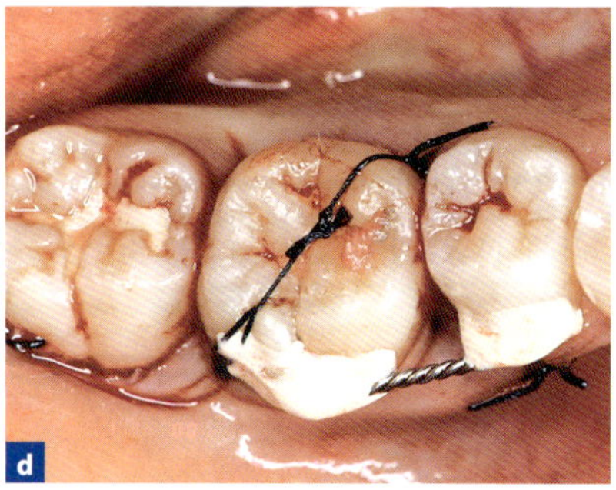

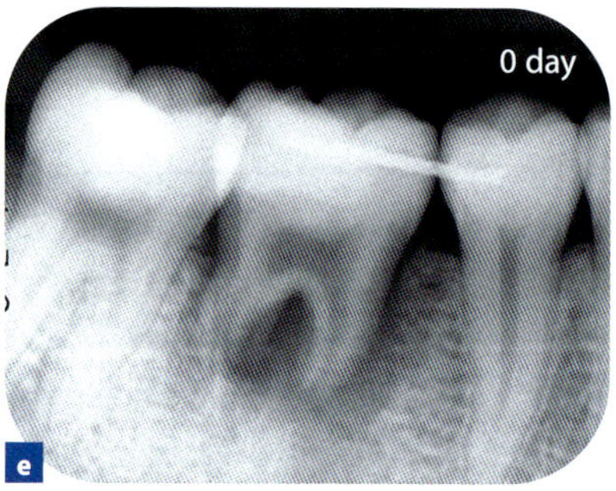

Fig 3-35d, e Immediately after transplantation.

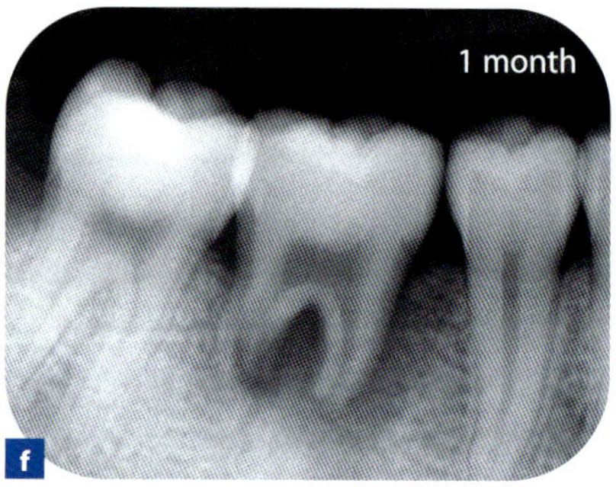

Fig 3-35f One month after transplantation. Radiolucency around the root remains.

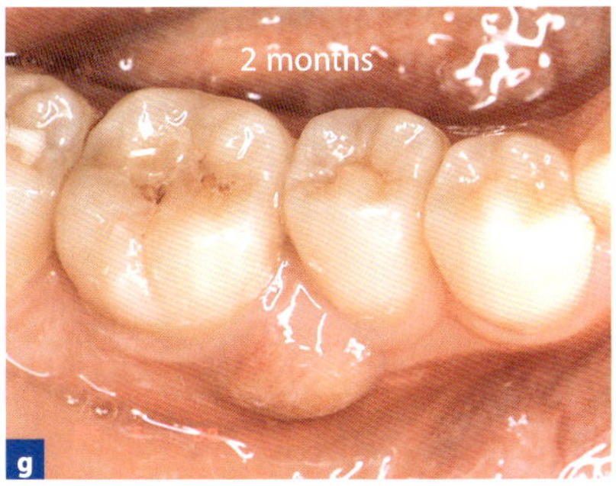

Fig 3-35g Two months after transplantation. Abscess can be observed.

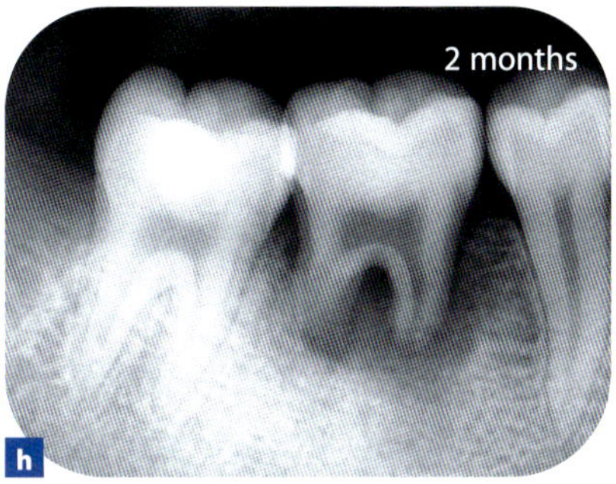

Fig 3-35h Radiograph of the same day as **Fig 3-35g**. The rarefaction has increased.

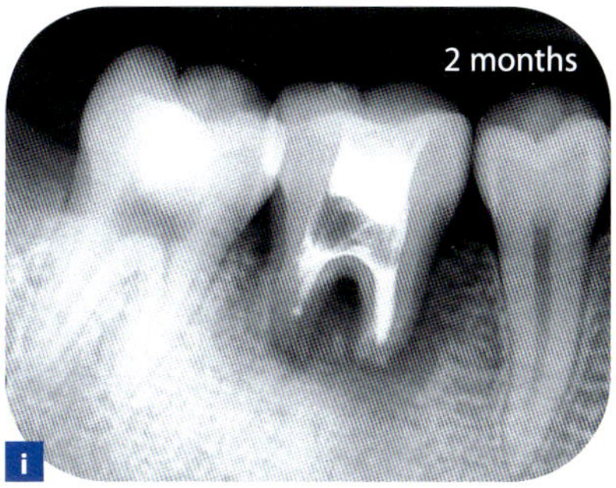

Fig 3-35i Same day as **Fig 3-35h**. Apexification was performed because of the pulp necrosis close to the apices. A calcium hydroxide preparation, "Vitapex" (Neo Dental International. Inc. Tokyo, Japan) was placed after removing necrotic tissues.

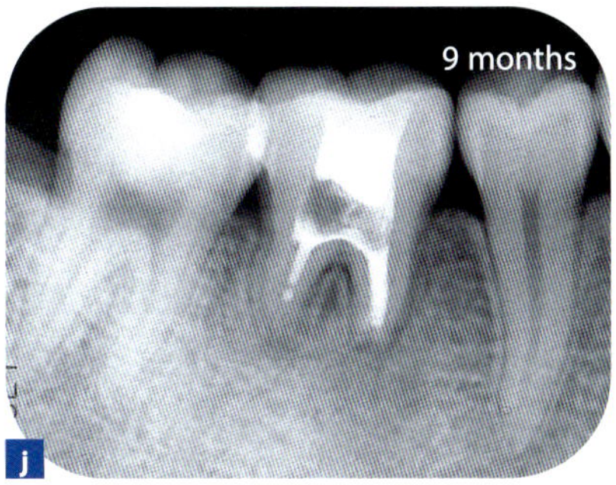

Fig 3-35j Nine months after transplantation. Radiolucency has decreased. The root apex seems to be closed by hard tissue. Then the calcium hydroxide preparation was replaced with sealer and gutta-percha .

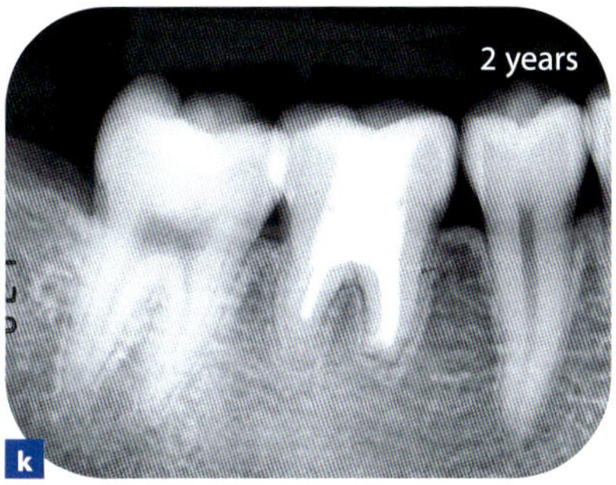

Fig 3-35k Two years after transplantation. Healing of the periodontal ligament can be observed.

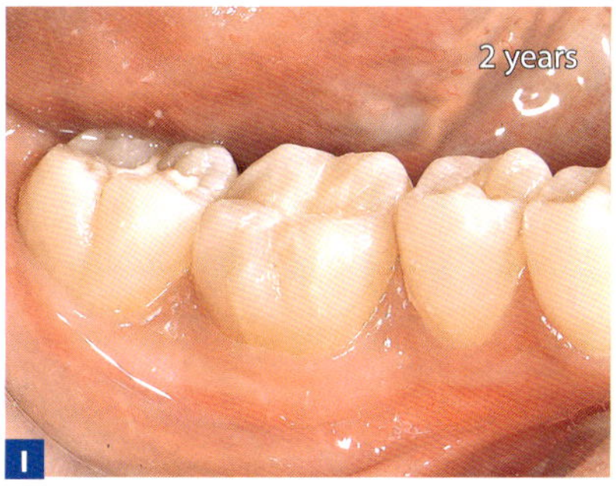

Fig 3-35l Same day as **Fig 3-35k**. The tooth is restored with CR.

Fig 3-36 Partial necrosis of pulp and apexogenesis.

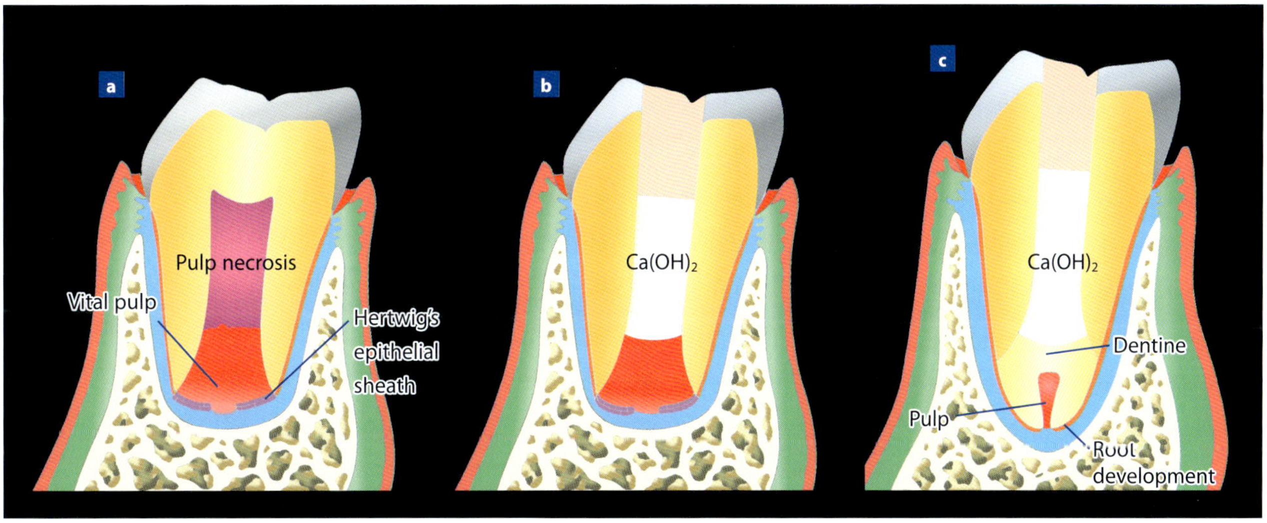

Fig 3-36a Necrosis in only the coronal part of the pulp after transplantation of an immature tooth.
Fig 3-36b Apexogenesis. Necrotic pulp tissue is removed and calcium hydroxide is placed in the canal in contact with the remaining vital pulp tissue.
Fig 3-36c After apexogenesis. Hard tissue is formed under the calcium hydroxide, and the apex develops owing to the viable Hertwig's epithelial sheath.

Fig 3-37 A case of partial necrosis of pulp and apexogenesis.

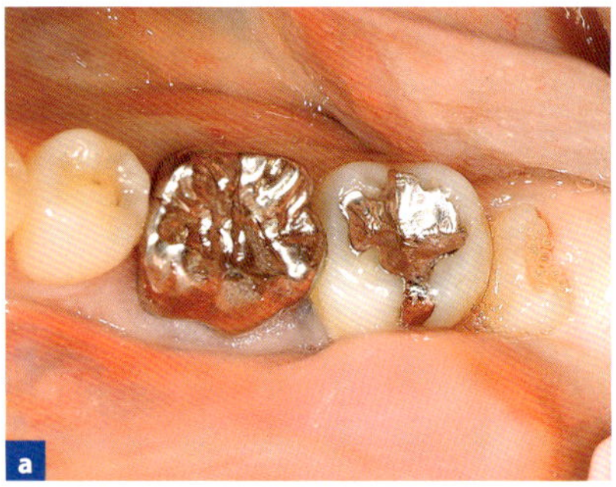

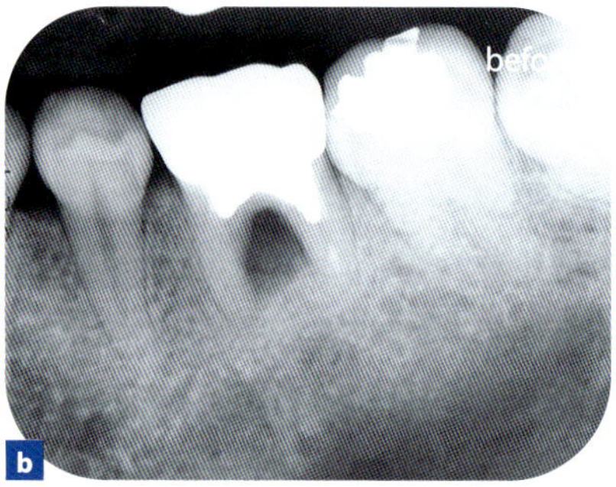

Fig 3-37a, b Preoperative view and radiograph of a 24-year-old female whose #38 was considered hopeless and transplantation was indicated using #38 as a donor.

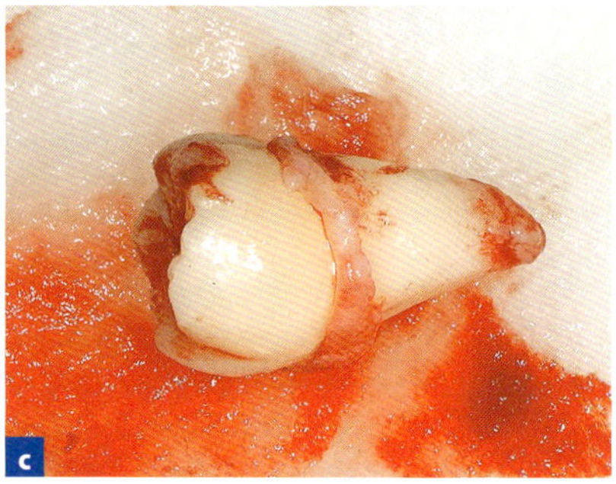

Fig 3-37c Extracted donor tooth. A small amount of Hertwig's epithelial sheath was observed around the apex.

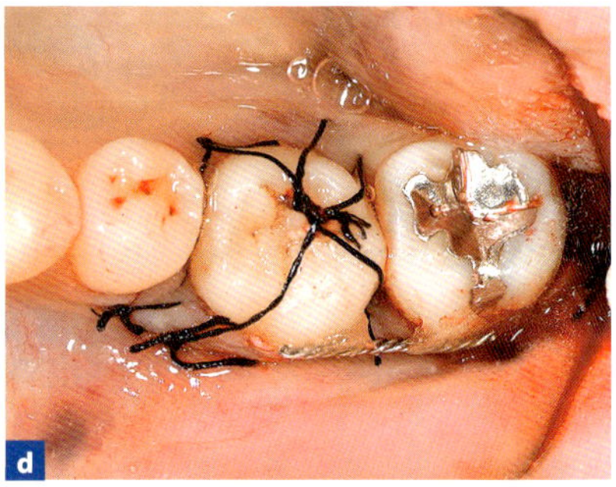

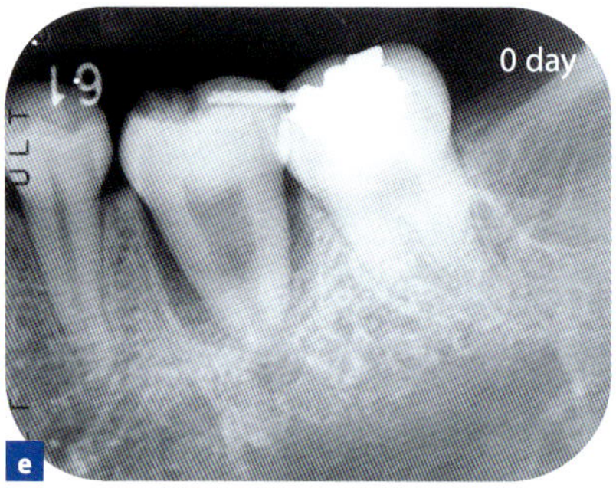

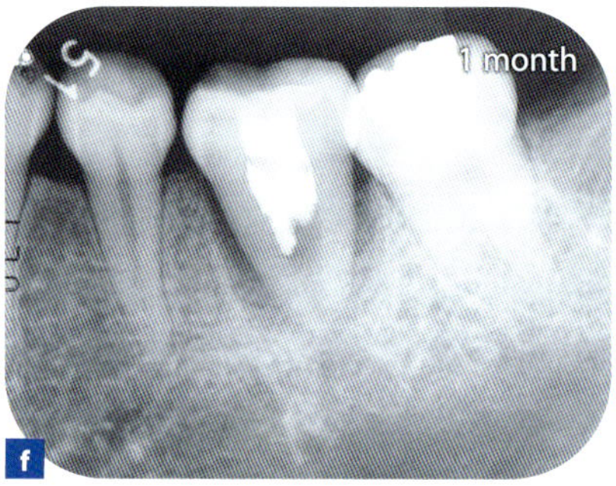

Fig 3-37d Immediately after transplantation.

Fig 3-37e Radiograph immediately after transplantation. The apex is slightly open and the pulp healing was expected.

Fig 3-37f One month after transplantation. Root canal treatment was initiated due to patient symptoms. The pulp had vital tissue starting at the mid root level and pulpotomy was performed. The necrotic pulp was removed and the space was filled with Vitapex.

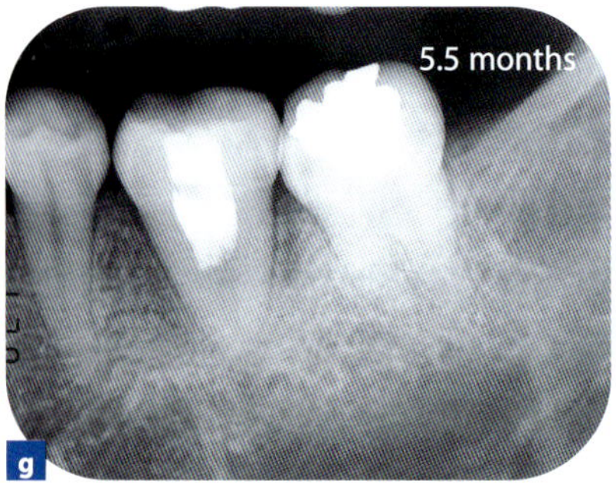

Fig 3-37g Five months and 2 weeks after transplantation. The healing of the pulp and the periodontal ligament can be observed.

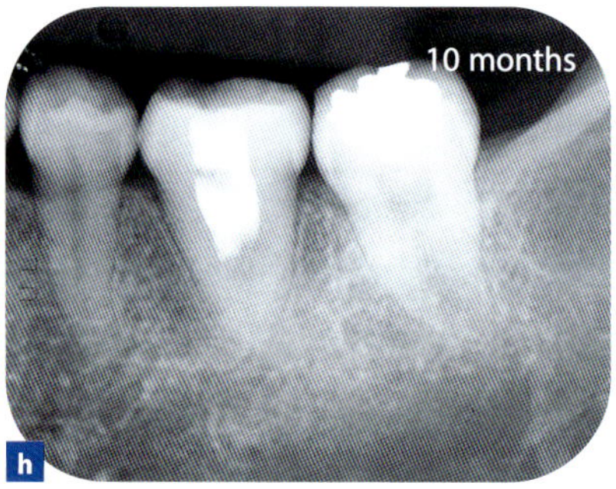

Fig 3-37h 10 months after transplantation. Immediately before replacing the calcium hydroxide preparation with MTA "PROROOT MTA" (Dentsply, USA).

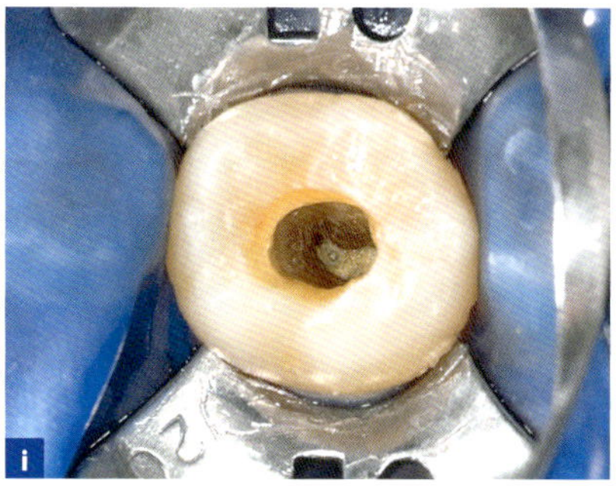

Fig 3-37i Calcified tissue can be seen on the surface of the pulpotomy after removal of the calcium hydroxide preparation. The tooth responded to EPT positively.

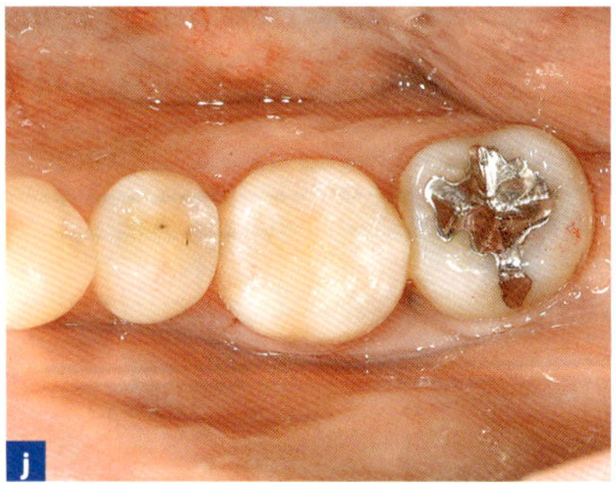

Fig 3-37j After restoration with composite.

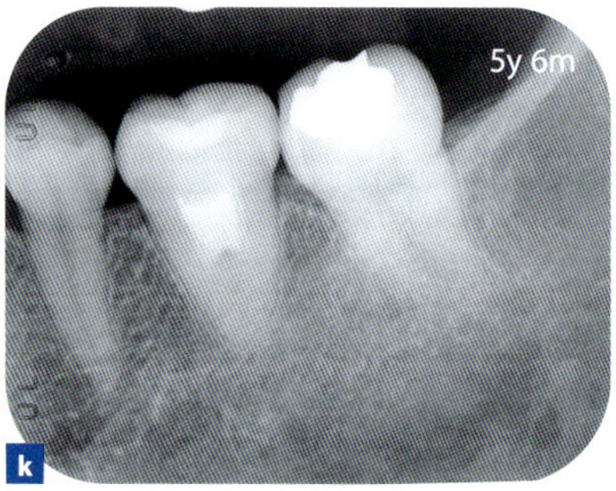

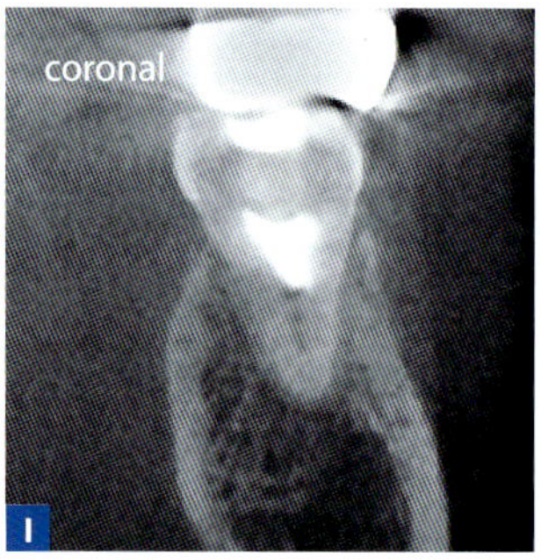

Fig 3-37k, l Five years and 6 months after transplantation. Pulp canal obliteration and slight root development were observed.

Root development

Continued development of roots is expected to occur with the healing of pulp in transplantation of immature teeth[110,117-119,129,130] (Fig 3-38). However, some cases may not have complete root development. Root development after transplantation can be classified into total arrest, which indicates no apparent development after transplantation (Fig 3-38b and 3-39); partial arrest, which indicates some development (Fig 3-38c and 3-40); and nonarrest, which indicates complete development of the roots[110] (Fig 3-38d and 3-41).

One clinical study[110] of 370 premolars that were transplanted showed root development rates of 14% total arrest, 21% nonarrest, and 65% partial arrest regardless of the developmental stage of the roots or method of surgery (Fig 3-42). Thus, if a tooth with very early stage of root development is used as a donor, it may not have a sufficient crown-to-root ratio after healing because about 80 % may result in complete arrest or partial arrest (Fig 3-39 and 3-40). Therefore, when considering root development, the root of the donor tooth should be as close to complete as possible.

From the viewpoint of pulpal healing alone, a less complete root (larger apical foramen) is better, but from the viewpoint of root length, a more developed root is better. If both pulpal healing and root development are predictably expected, the ideal timing for transplantation of an immature tooth is when the donor tooth's root is three fourths to four fifths complete (stage 4 or 5 of root development) (Fig 3-43).

Classification of root development after transplantation

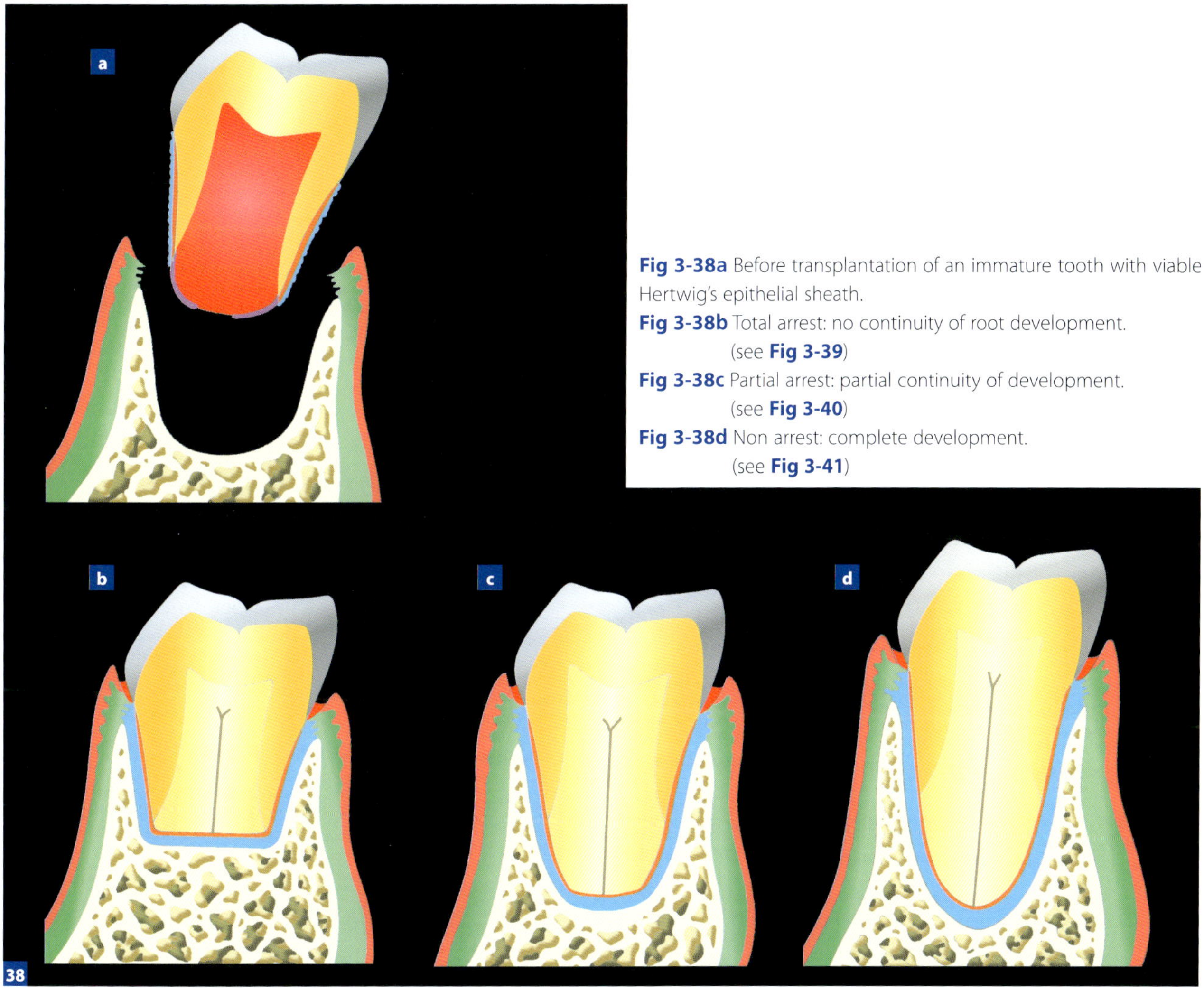

Fig 3-38a Before transplantation of an immature tooth with viable Hertwig's epithelial sheath.
Fig 3-38b Total arrest: no continuity of root development. (see Fig 3-39)
Fig 3-38c Partial arrest: partial continuity of development. (see Fig 3-40)
Fig 3-38d Non arrest: complete development. (see Fig 3-41)

Fig 3-39 A case of total arrest of root development after transplantation. (see **Fig 3-38b**)

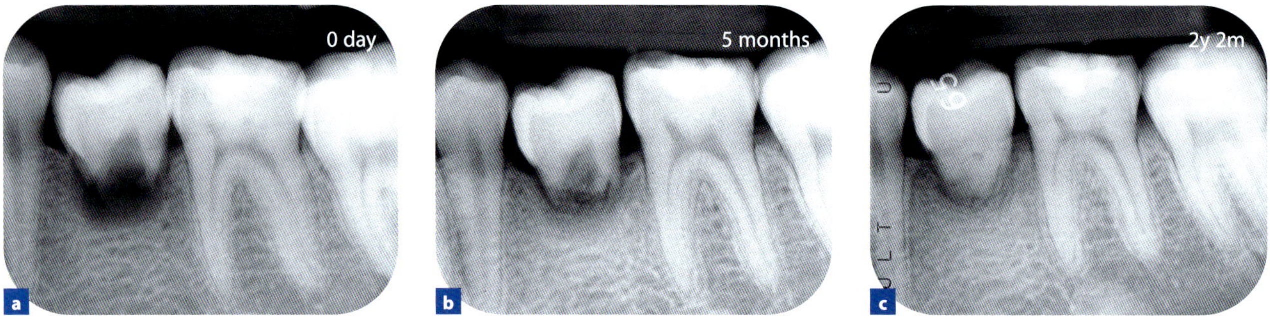

Fig 3-39a Immediately after transplantation of a 15-year-old male. #18 was transplanted into a site of a congenitally missing tooth.

Fig 3-39b Five months postoperative

Fig 3-39c Two years and 2 months postoperative. Pulp healing has progressed, but there is little root development.

Fig 3-40 A case of partial arrest of root development after transplantation. (see **Fig 3-38c**)

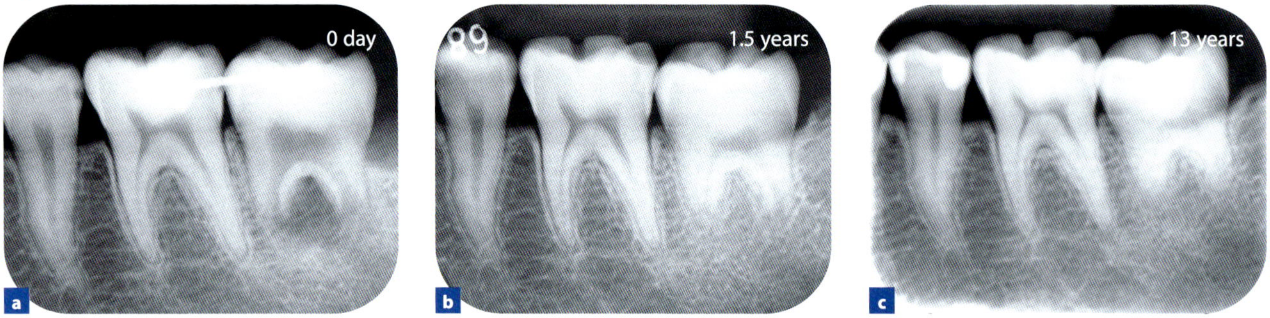

Fig 3-40a Immediately after transplantation of a 17-year-old female. # 38 was transplanted into #37 site.

Fig 3-40b One year and 6 months postoperative.

Fig 3-40c 13 years postoperative. The pulp has healed (calcified), but there is slight root development.

Fig 3-41 A case of non arrest of root development after transplantation. (see **Fig 3-38d**)

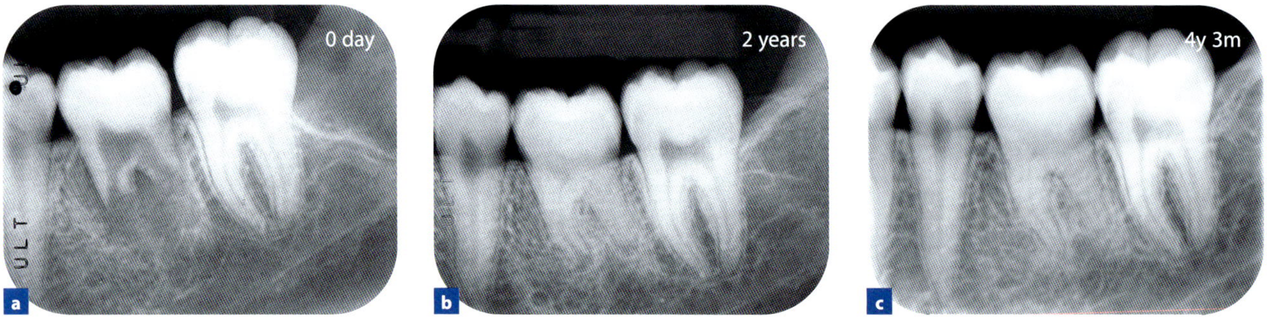

Fig 3-41a Immediately after transplantation of an18-year-old female. #38 was transplanted into #36 site.

Fig 3-41b Two years postoperative.

Fig 3-41c Four years and 3 months postoperative. The root appears to have full root development.

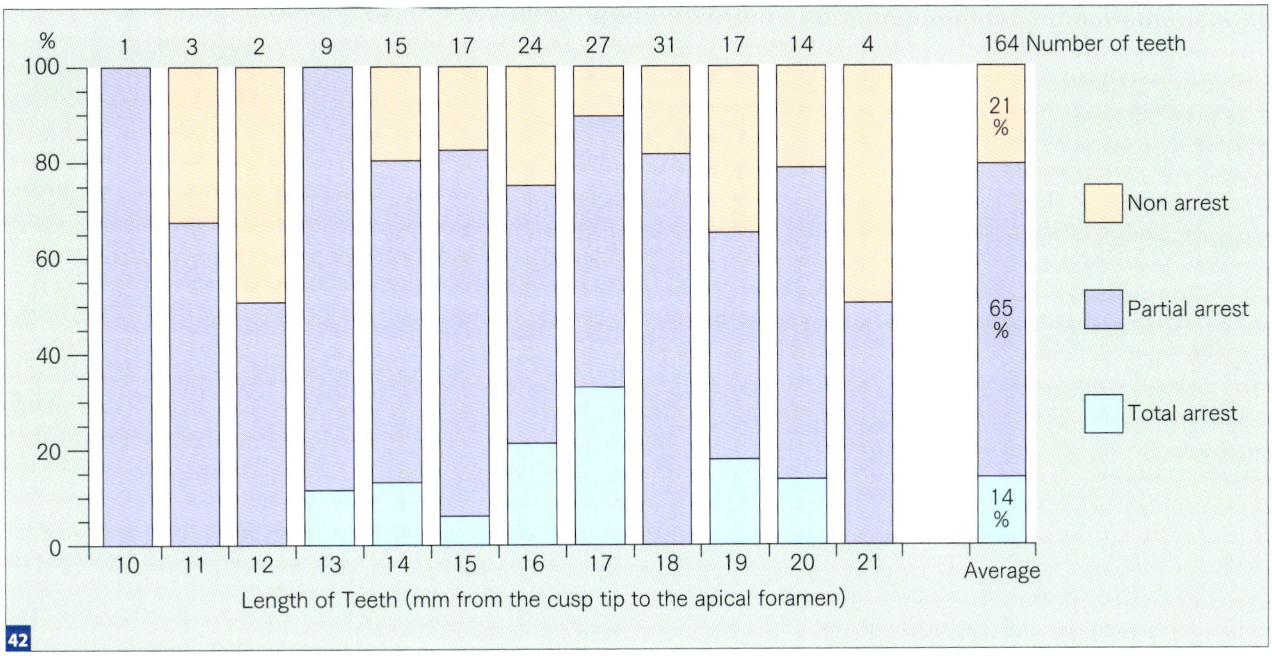

Fig 3-42 **Relationship between length of donor teeth (premolars) and continuity of root development after transplantation.**
Continuity of root development results in partial development in most cases regardless of the length of the donor teeth (65%, partial development; 14%, no development ; 21%, complete development). (Reprinted with permission from Andreasen, et al.[110]).

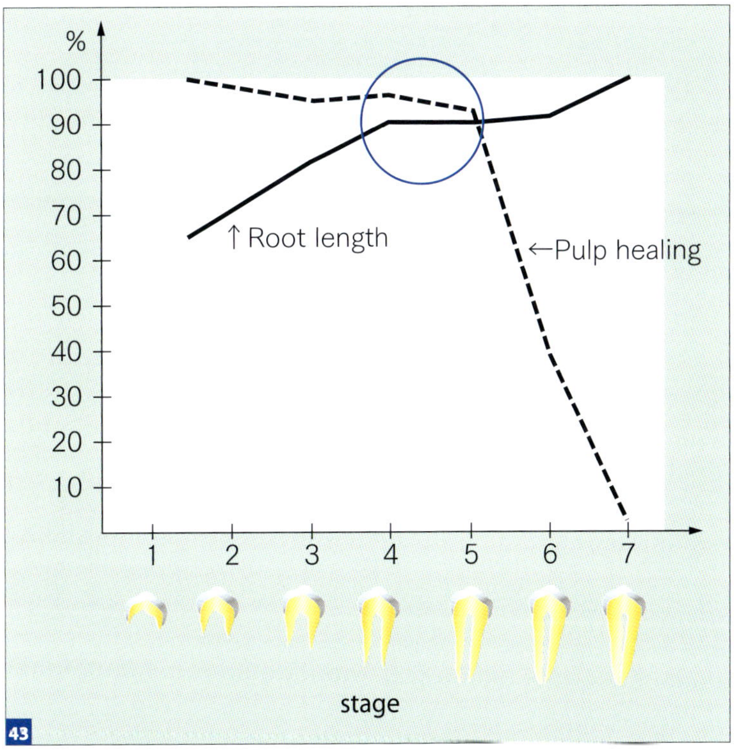

Fig 3-43 **Relationship between pulp healing and root length after transplantation of immature teeth** (Reprinted with permission from Andreasen, et al.[122]).
The line graphs show the probability of pulp healing and the expected root length for each developmental stage of the donor tooth at the time of transplantation. In healing of pulp, donor teeth in early developmental stages have better prognoses. On the other hand, donor teeth in later stages have longer roots. Thus, donor teeth at developmental stage 4 or 5 are ideal for transplantation.

Healing of Alveolar Bone

One of the advantages of transplantation is new bone formation by the periodontal ligament of the transplanted tooth. This allows periodontal tissues including the alveolar bone to develop at the recipient site where the periodontal tissues may have been lost preoperatively (**Fig 3-44** to **3-46**).

Relationship between the tooth and alveolar bone

Embryologically, the cells of the periodontal ligament are derived from the dental follicle[131-135] (**Fig 3-47**). Ameloblasts derived from the dental epithelium are responsible for the formation of dental enamel, the hardest and most mineralized tissue in the body. During differentiation and maturation, ameloblasts secrete matrix proteins such as amelogenin, enamelin, and ameloblastin, and they are thought to play important roles in mineralization. The dental papilla differentiate into odontoblasts that secrete collagen-rich matrix to form predentin, that eventually mineralize to form dentin[136-138]. As the root develops, the undifferentiated stem cells in the dental follicle differentiate into cementoblasts, fibroblasts, and osteoblasts, which form cementum, periodontal ligament, and alveolar bone proper, respectively[139-148]. During this process, a part of the collagen fibers in the periodontal ligament are embedded into the alveolar bone proper and cementum. These are called Sharpey's fibers and tightly connect the tooth root and bone. The term "periodontal ligament", as used by clinicians, refers to the collagen fiber-rich soft connective tissue between the root and alveolar bone proper. In the periodontal ligament, the principle cells are fibroblasts that actively synthesize and degrade collagen to maintain its function. Other cells in the periodontal ligament include cementoblasts, osteoblasts, and undifferentiated mesenchymal stem cells (**Fig 3-47b**), Periodontal ligament cells have the capability to reconstruct periodontal tissues including alveolar bone proper damaged by trauma or infection throughout life[149-162]. A study using monkeys[159] has shown that the periodontal ligament forms bone tissue around the roots of teeth even when transplanted under mucosa (**Fig 3-48**).

Fig 3-44 A case of alveolar bone healing after transplantation (1).

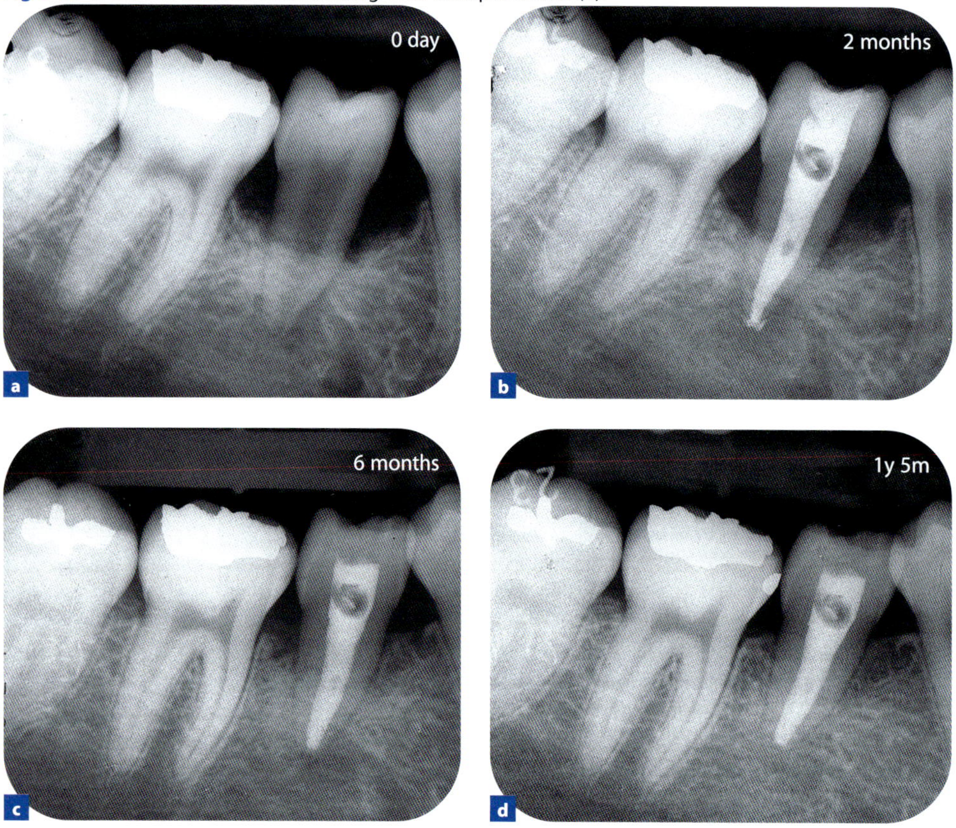

Fig 3-44a Immediately after transplantation of a 15-year-old female. Ectopically erupted #15 was transplanted into the site of congenitally missing #45.
Fig 3-44b Two months after transplantation and immediately after endodontic apexification treatment.
Fig 3-44c Six months after transplantation. There is apparent bone regeneration in the crestal and interproximal area.
Fig 3-44d One year and 5 months after transplantation. Bone regeneration is evident.

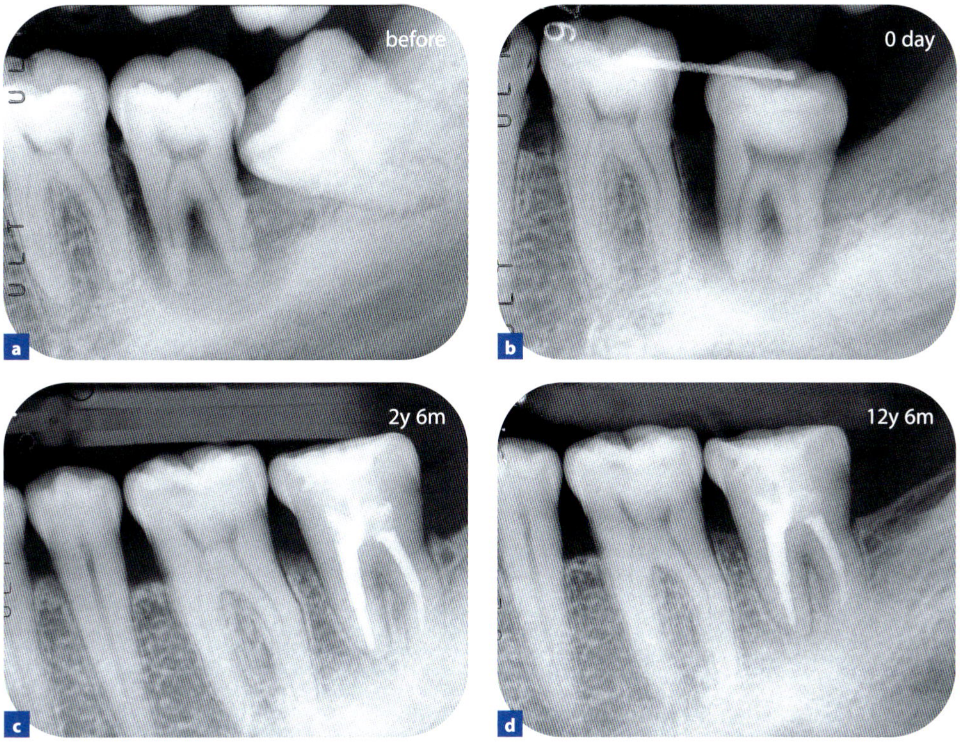

Fig 3-45 A case of Alveolar bone healing after transplantation (2).

Fig 3-45a Preoperative radiograph of a 39-year-old male. #37 hopeless due to severe periodontitis was to be replaced with the adjacent impacted #38 as a donor.
Fig 3-45b Immediately after transplantation. There is a wide bony defect seen around the transplanted tooth.
Fig 3-45c Two years and 6 months after transplantation. Natural (spontaneous) eruption of the transplant and bone regeneration has occurred.
Fig 3-45d 12 years and 6 months after transplantation. The generated bone is maintained (See **Chapter 6 Fig 6-6** for detailed treatment flow).

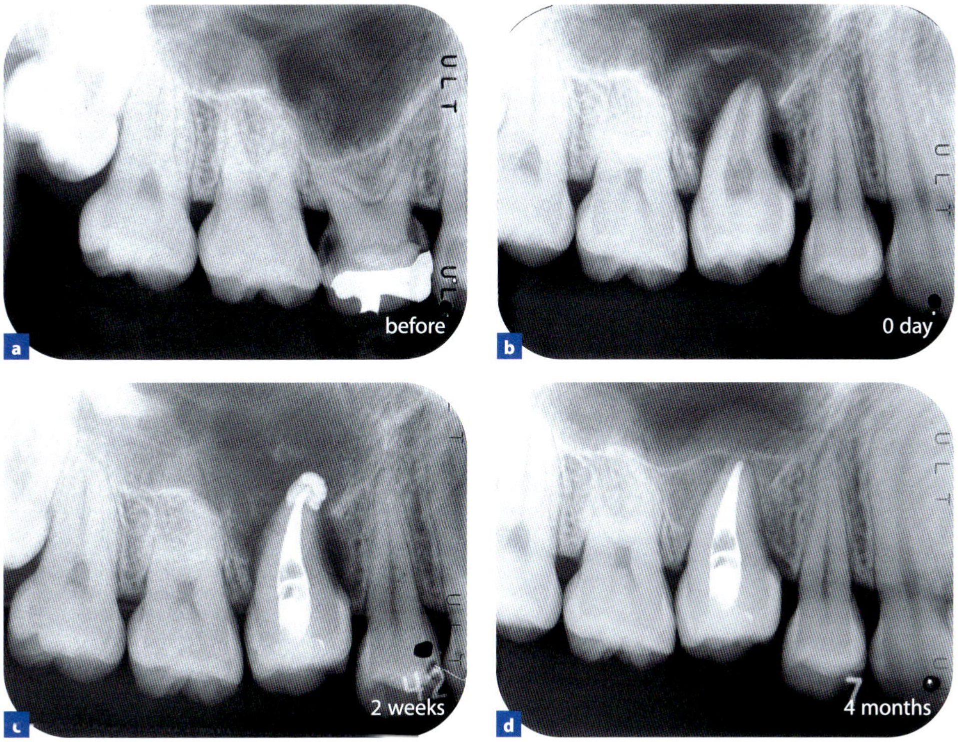

Fig 3-46 A case of Alveolar bone healing after transplantation (3).

Fig 3-46a Preoperative radiograph of a 24-year-old female, requesting transplantation of #28 to #15 site where the permanent tooth was congenitally missing.
Fig 3-46b Immediately after transplantation. The transplantation was performed in conjunction with maxillary sinus floor elevation.
Fig 3-46c Two weeks postoperative. Just after endodontic treatment of the transplant.
Fig 3-46d Four months postoperative. Bone healing around the transplant is apparent with repair of the sinus floor membrane.

Ontogenesis of periodontal tissues

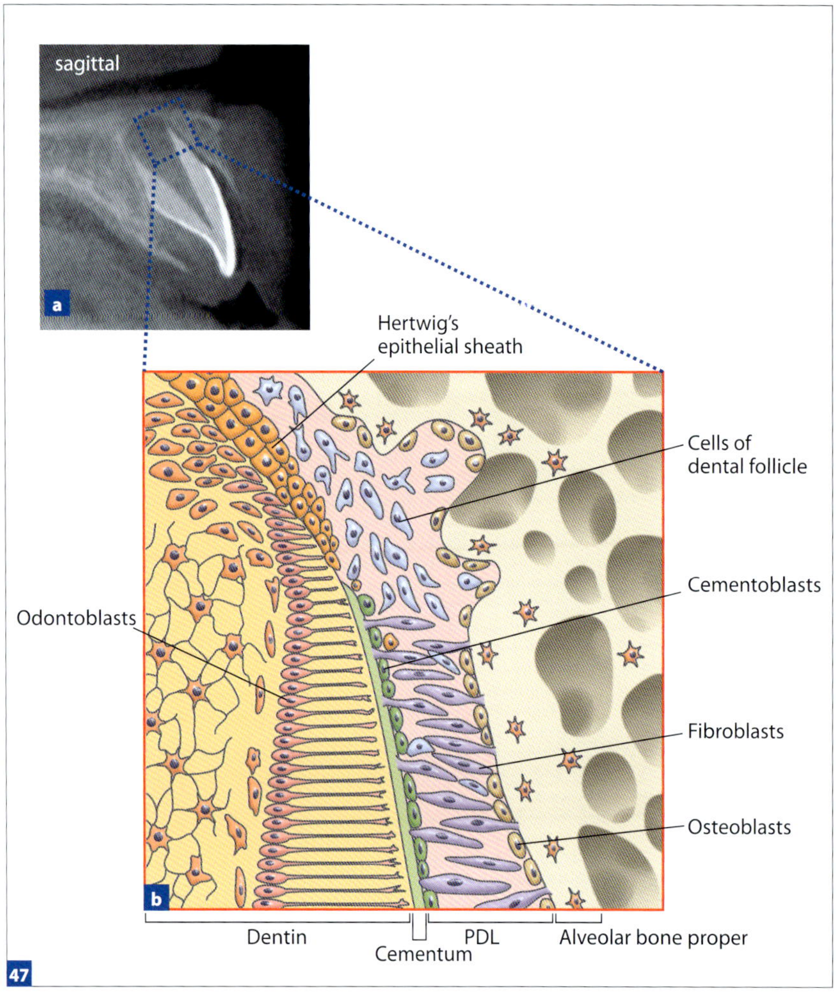

Fig 3-47a CBCT image of a maxillary immature central incisor at age 5-6 years.

Fig 3-47b Illustration of apex and periodontal tissues of developing teeth.

Inside Hertwig's epithelial root sheath (epithelial diaphragm), odontoblasts differentiated from dental pulp cells form root dentin. Cementum is deposited on the surface of newly formed dentin by cementoblasts differentiated from cells of the dental follicle. Sharpey's fibers are embedded in cementum by fibroblasts derived from the dental follicle. At the same time, the alveolar bone proper is formed by osteoblasts differentiated from cells in the dental follicle and the Sharpey's fibers are embedded into this new bone.

The periodontal ligament (PDL) is the connective tissue-rich tissue containing cementoblasts, fibroblasts, osteoblasts, or their progenitor cells, and is a layer of soft tissue that is between the cementum and the alveolar bone proper. PDL seems to have the ability to form alveolar bone proper throughout life.

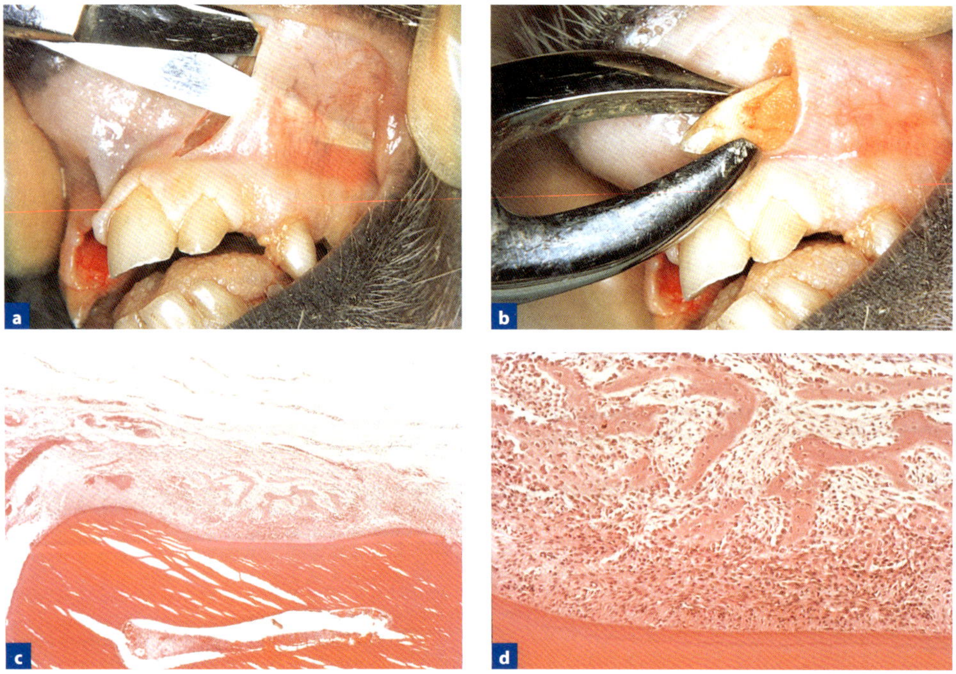

Fig 3-48 Animal experiment to demonstrate osteoinductive ability of periodontal ligament of a transplanted tooth (courtesy by Dr. Jens O. Andreasen[159]).

Fig 3-48a and **3-48b** Transplantation of a maxillary anterior tooth to the submucosa of the vestibule in a monkey.

Fig 3-48c Three weeks after transplantation. Formation of bone tissue between the periodontal ligament of the donor tooth and mucosa can be observed.

Fig 3-48d Higher magnification of **Fig 3-48c**. The periodontal ligament has the ability to form bone.

Fig 3-49 is a graph showing vertical and horizontal alveolar bone growth associated with tooth eruption in girl[163]. This data indicates that the growth (height) of alveolar bone is closely related to tooth eruption. **Fig 3-50** shows sagittal images from CBCT studies of the maxillary central incisors of different ages. The data shows that the height of the alveolar ridge increases with the eruption of teeth; the width of labial alveolar bone is thick up to around the age of 9 to 10 ; but starts to become thin, leaving the cortical plate (lamina dura/alveolar bone proper) that remains for life in most healthy individuals. The palatal side has thick cortical bone with evident cancellous bone adjacent to it, regardless of age. So, post puberty, the alveolar bone on the labial aspect of the anterior teeth is made up of cortical bone derived from the periodontal ligament (alveolar bone proper). This means that if the viable periodontal ligament is lost, the alveolar bone on the labial aspect will also be lost. Findings from delayed replantation cases have shown this to occur.

Fig 3-51 shows a case of delayed replantation which was treated by another dental office. The root resorption of tooth #11 progressed 3 years and 8 months after delayed replantation (**Fig 3-51c** and **3-51d**). The CBCT images show only the alveolar bone on the labial side is resorbed (**Fig 3-51e** to **3-51g**). Transplanting a tooth with viable periodontal ligament can lead to the development of the labial cortical bone (alveolar bone proper) (**Fig 3-52**).

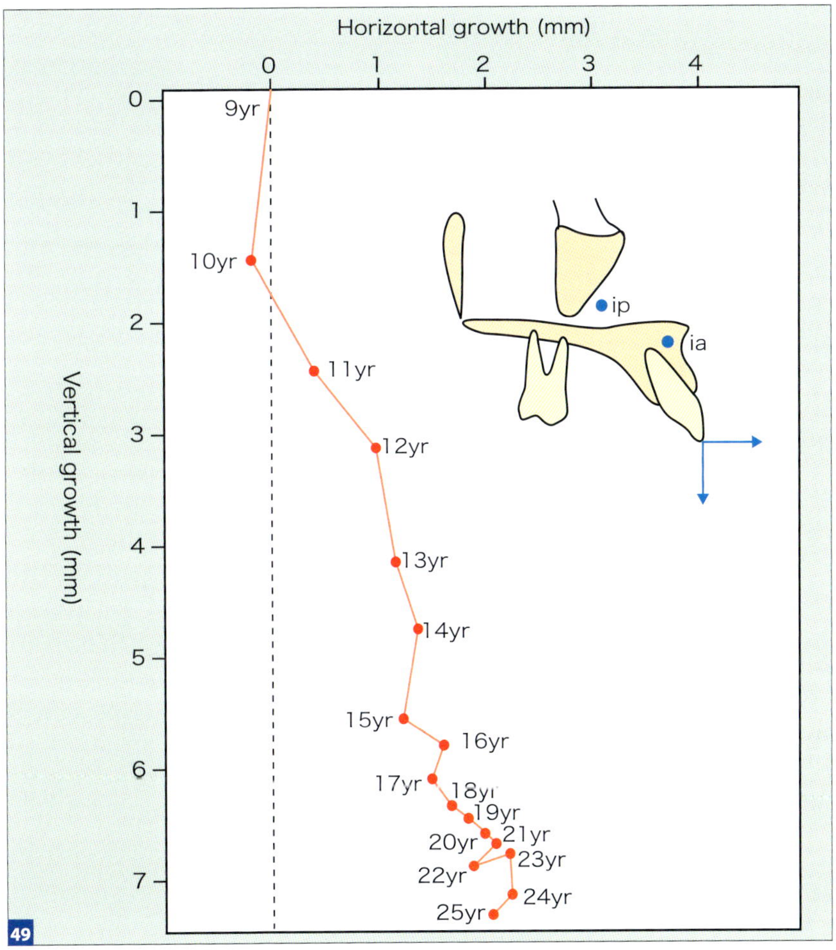

Fig 3-49 Relationship between vertical and horizontal alveolar bone growth with tooth eruption (modified from Iseri & Solow[163]).
Data from observation of 14 girls between the ages of 9 and 25 years. Transition of vertical and horizontal amount of eruption (growth of alveolar bone) of the maxillary central incisor. Alveolar bone grows mostly vertical but some horizontally as the teeth erupt.

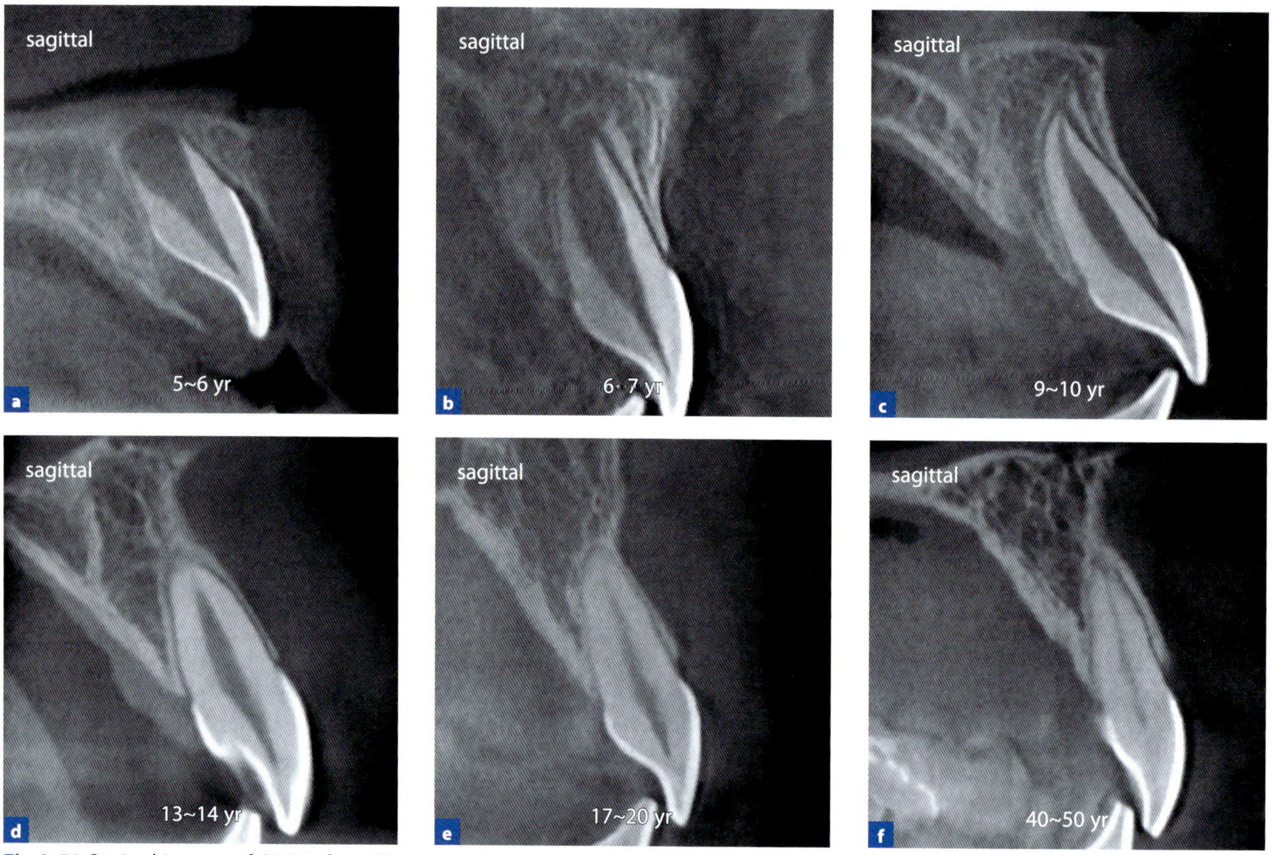

Fig 3-50 Sagittal images of CBCT of maxillary central incisors at different ages.
The data have indicated; the height of alveolar bone increases with the eruption of teeth; the width of labial alveolar bones is thick with bone marrow up to around the age of 9 to 10 years, but from the end of puberty there is typically thin cortical bone (lamina dura / alveolar bone proper) which lasts for the duration of life. The palatal side typically has thick basal bone with bone marrow cavity regardless of age. However, the above observations do not always apply when teeth have been moved orthodontically.

Summerizing the results of the discussion from **Fig 3-44** to **Fig 3-52** above, the following can be expected from autotransplantation of teeth.

1. The periodontal ligament of transplanted teeth can regenerate alveolar bone proper (basal bone is not regenerated).
2.Transplanted teeth can repair surrounding bony defects in a relatively short period of time.

Fig 3-51 Bone resorption in delayed replantation.

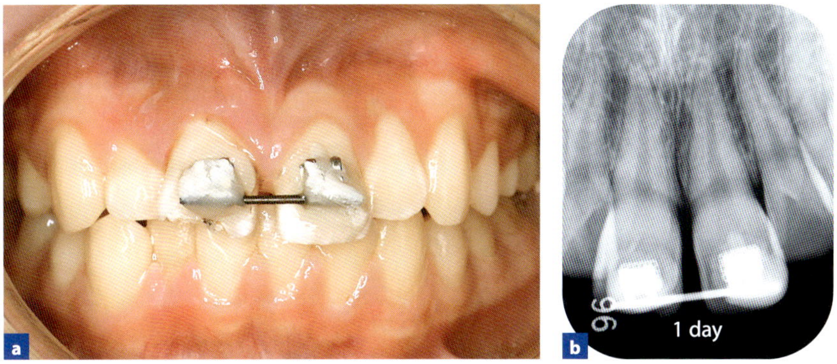

Fig 3-51a, b Preoperative view and radiograph of a 12-year 9-month-old male who underwent delayed replantation at another clinic 1 day before.

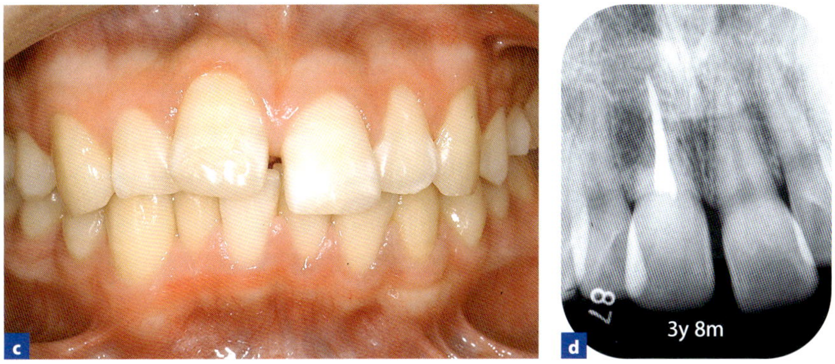

Fig 3-51c Clinical view after 3 years and 8 months. The replanted tooth is involved in infra-occlusion.

Fig 3-51d Radiograph after 3 years and 8 months. Root resorption (replacement resorption) has progressed.

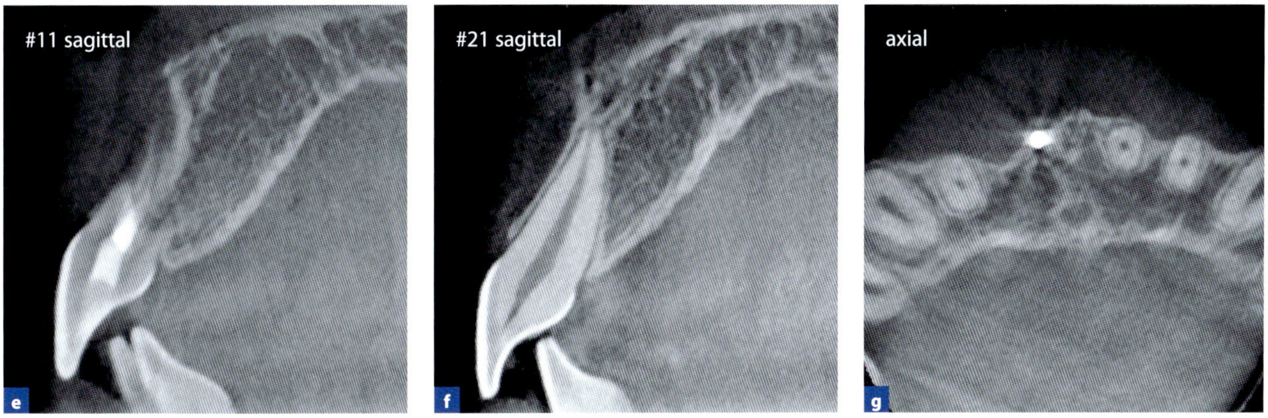

Fig 3-51e-g CBCT images after 3 years and 8 months.

Careful comparison of #11 (**e**) and the normal (untraumatized) #21 (**f**) reveals that bone resorption is seen only on the labial aspect of #11 and that the resorption has progressed up to the pulp canal. Similar findings can be seen in the axial image (**g**).

This finding suggests that the labial cortical bone (alveolar bone proper) is derived from the periodontal ligament and that the bone morphology of the labial aspect is likely controlled by the tooth with a viable periodontal ligament.

Fig 3-52 Bone regeneration by a transplanted tooth.

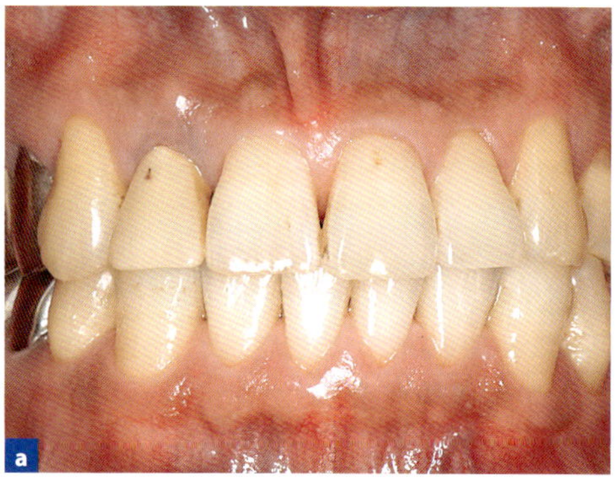
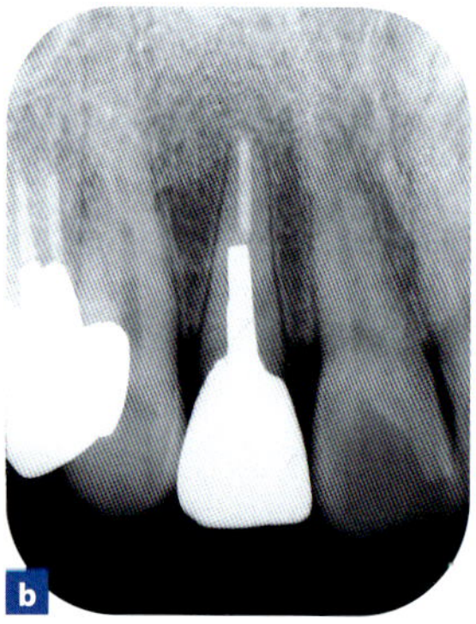

Fig 3-52a, b Preoperative view and radiograph of a 50-year-old male. #12 was involved in vertical root fracture with abscess and a deep probing depth on the labial aspect.

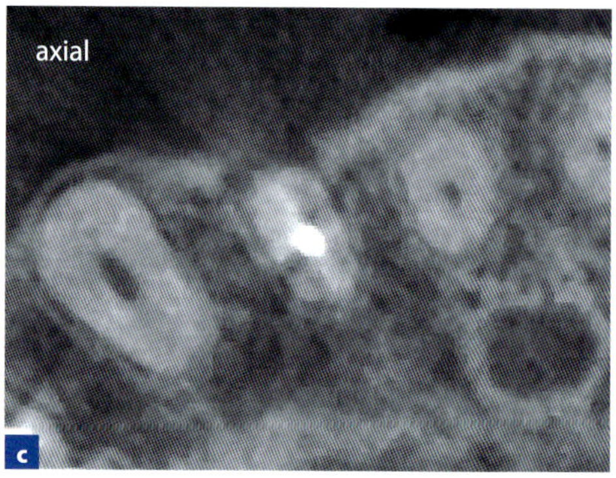

Fig 3-52c CBCT axial image before treatment, showing loss of labial cortical bone.

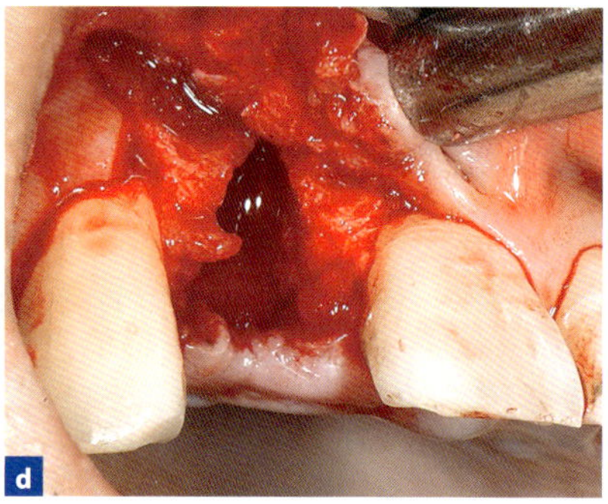

Fig 3-52d During surgery. The labial cortical bone has disappeared close to the root apex.

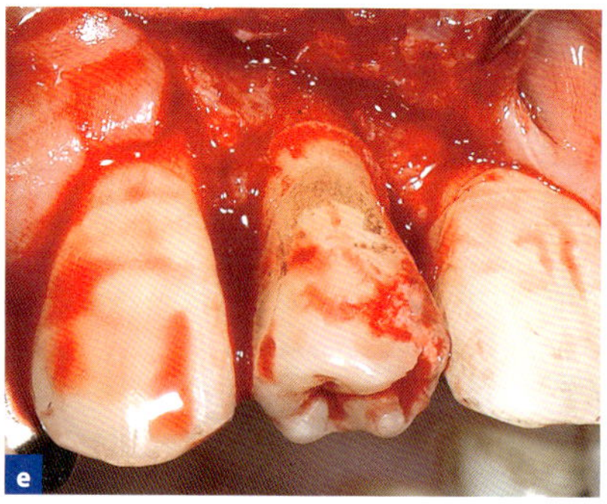

Fig 3-52e After placing the donor tooth, #35 had been displaced and was tilted.

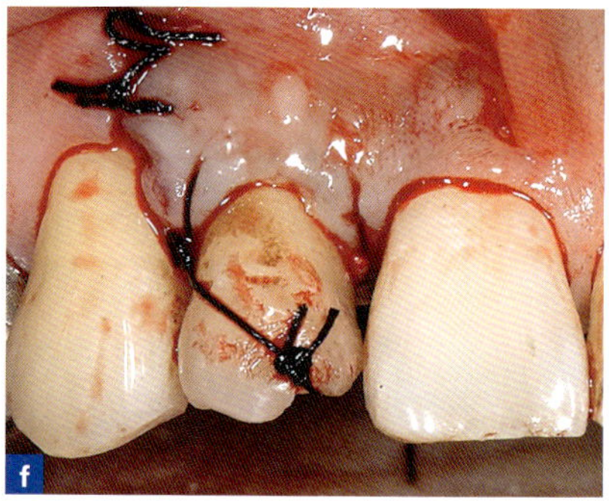

Fig 3-52f Immediately after surgery.

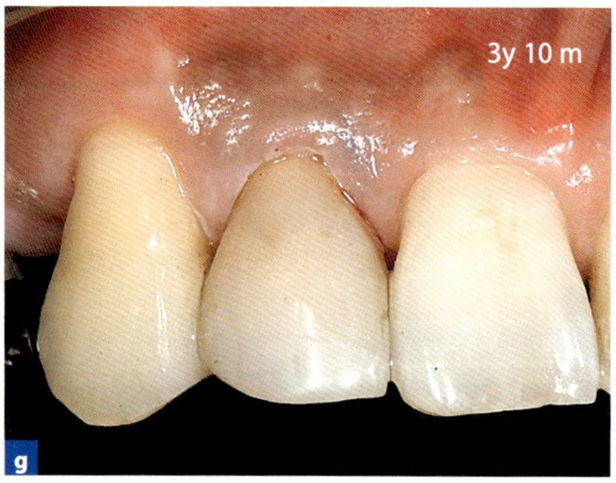

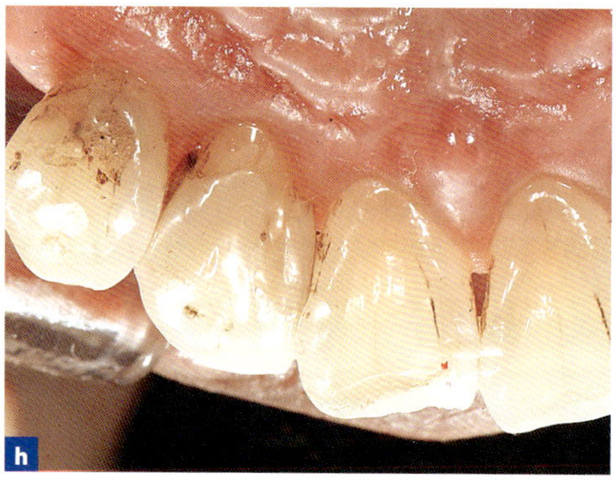
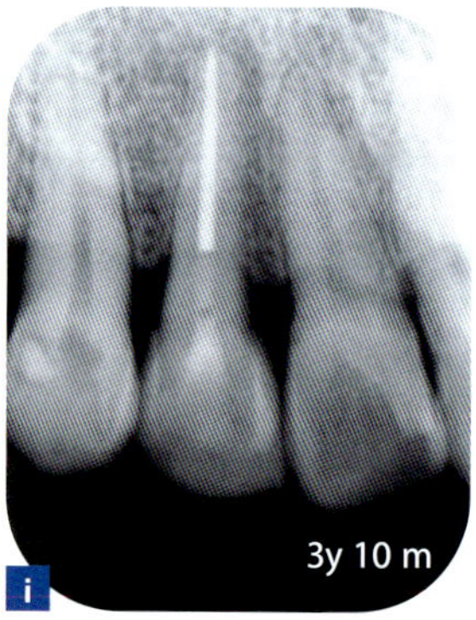

Fig 3-52g-i Three years and 10 months postoperative. No clinical or radiographic abnormality is observed.

Fig 3-52j CBCT sagittal image before treatment. Note the labial cortical bone has been lost.
Fig 3-52k Three years and 10 months after transplantation. The labial aspect of the transplanted tooth is covered by newly formed cortical bone.

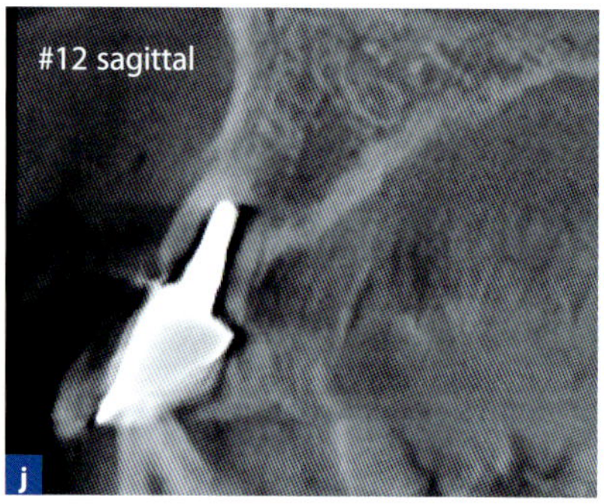

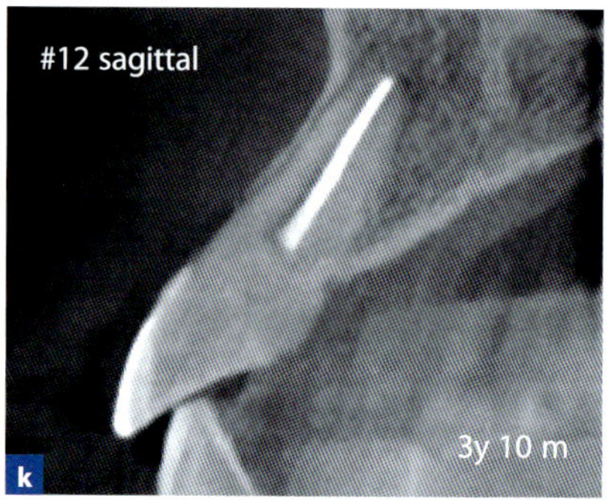

Three-dimensional analysis of alveolar bone formation after transplantation

Based on the findings discussed above, it would seem that the periodontal ligament of a transplanted tooth can induce bone formation anywhere and at any time. However, looking back at the author's clinical data over the years, it has shown that although the periodontal ligament and alveolar bone have a close interrelationship, the periodontal ligament of the transplanted tooth alone cannot predictably control bone formation.

For example, if a transplanted tooth with viable periodontal ligament is transplanted into a recipient site with sufficient bone width and height, the transplanted tooth will be predictably covered by bone, even if there is a large bony dehiscence or defect at the recipient socket (Fig 3-53). However, when a tooth is transplanted with the root exposed with a larger dehiscence of the recipient site, it is not clear whether the tooth will be completely covered by bone (formation of alveolar bone proper) (Fig 3-54 and 3-55). From the authors' experience, alve-

Three-dimensional bone regeneration around a transplanted tooth (1)

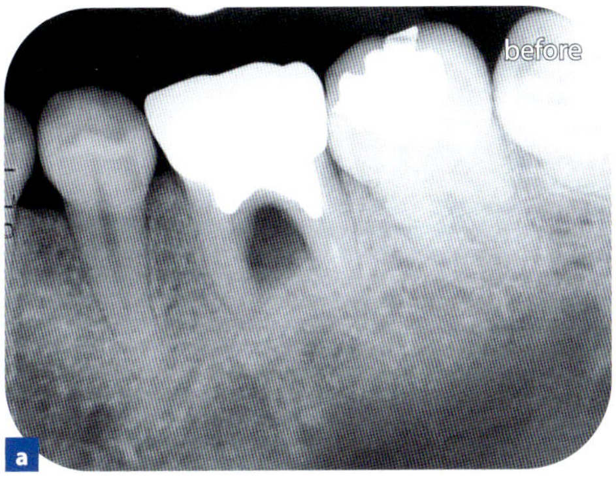

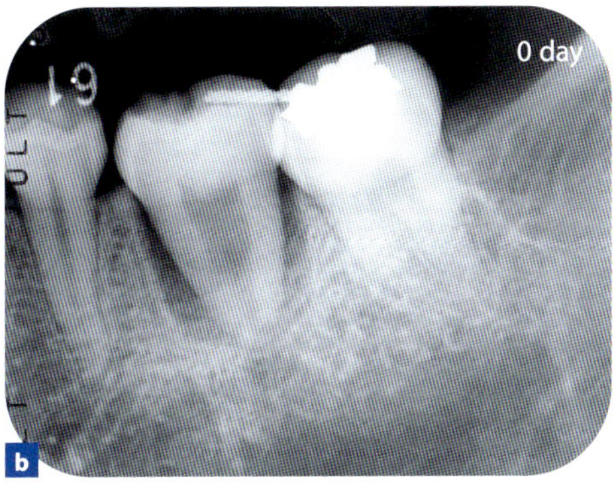

Fig 3-53a Preoperative radiograph of a 24-year-old female. #36 appears hopeless.
Fig 3-53b Immediately after transplantation. #38 was transplanted to the extracted #36 site.

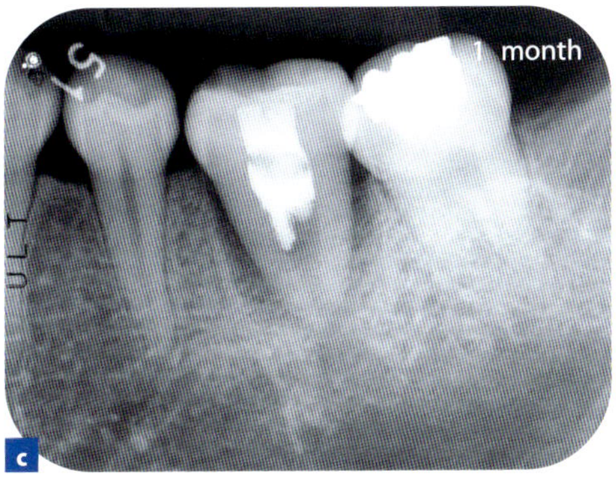

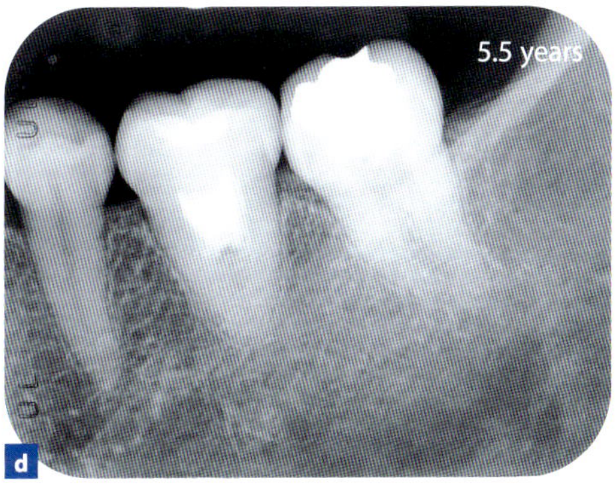

Fig 3-53c One month postoperative. The root canal treatment was started since the patient complained of slight percussion pain, but there was pulp tissue evident around the mid root level (see "Pulp healing" on page 39 and **Fig 3-37**).
Fig 3-53d Five and a half years postoperative. Note the bone healing occurred and maintained around the transplanted tooth.

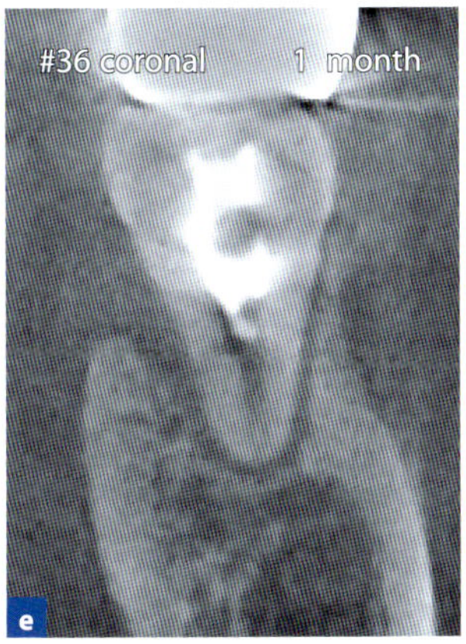

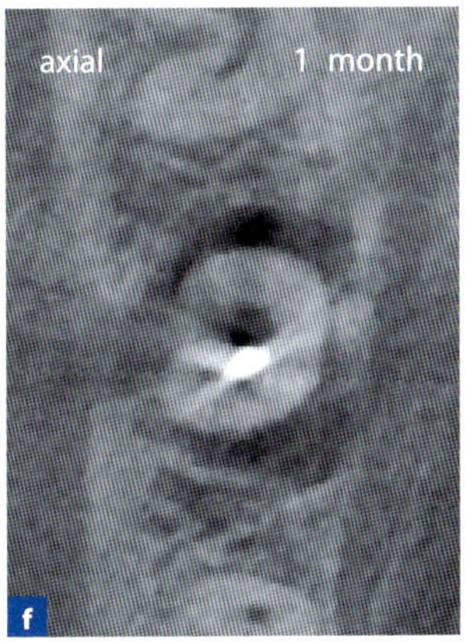

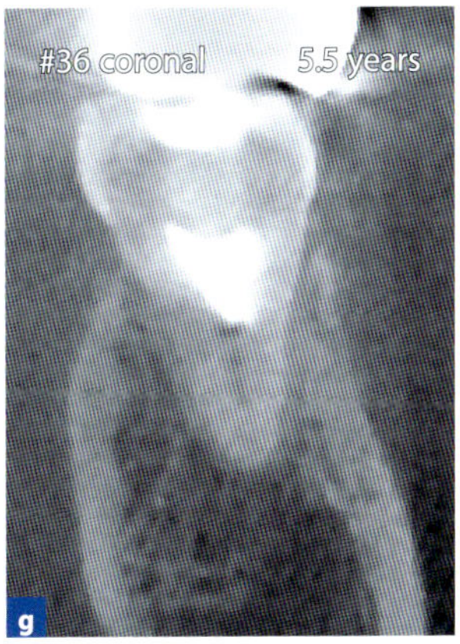

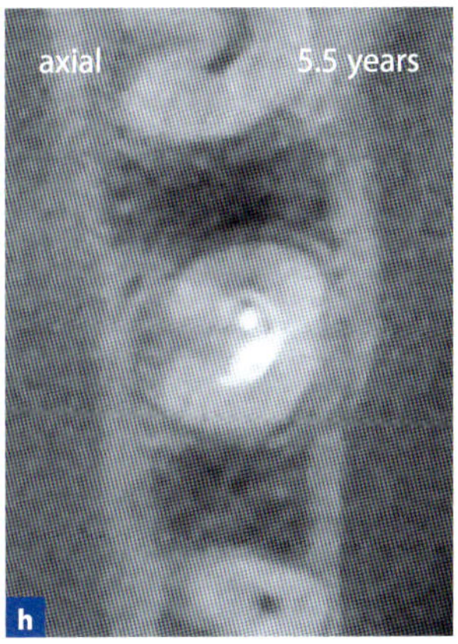

Fig 3-53e, f CBCT images 1 month after transplantation. There were large vertical and horizontal bony defects around the transplanted tooth but the root was accommodated within the bone housing.

Fig 3-53g, h CBCT images 5 and a half years postoperative. The bony defects have disappeared by the bone regenerated vertically and horizontally.

Fig 3-54 Three-dimensional bone regeneration around a transplanted tooth (2)

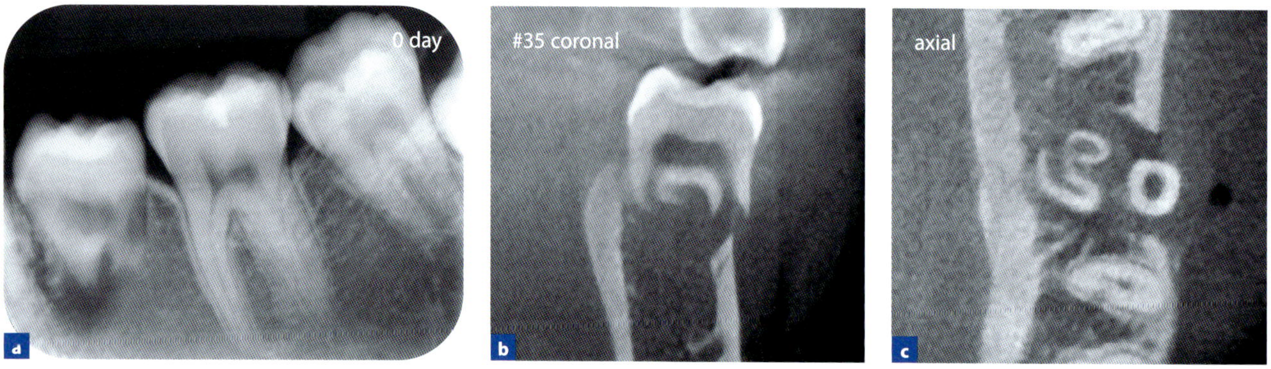

Fig 3-54a-c Immediately after transplantation of #28 into the congenital missing #35 site of a 19-year-old female (**a**). Because the width of the donor tooth was larger than that of the recipient site, the donor tooth was placed with the root completely exposed on the buccal aspect as seen (**b**) and (**c**).

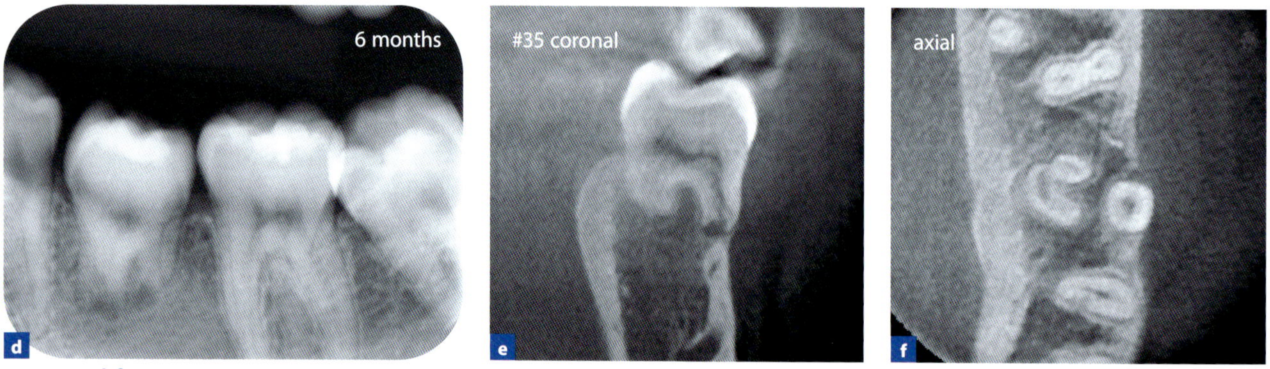

Figs 3-54d-f Six months postoperative. Natural eruption of the tooth can be seen. The bony defect around the transplant seen just after the surgery has disappeared but the exposed root surface is not completely covered by bone.

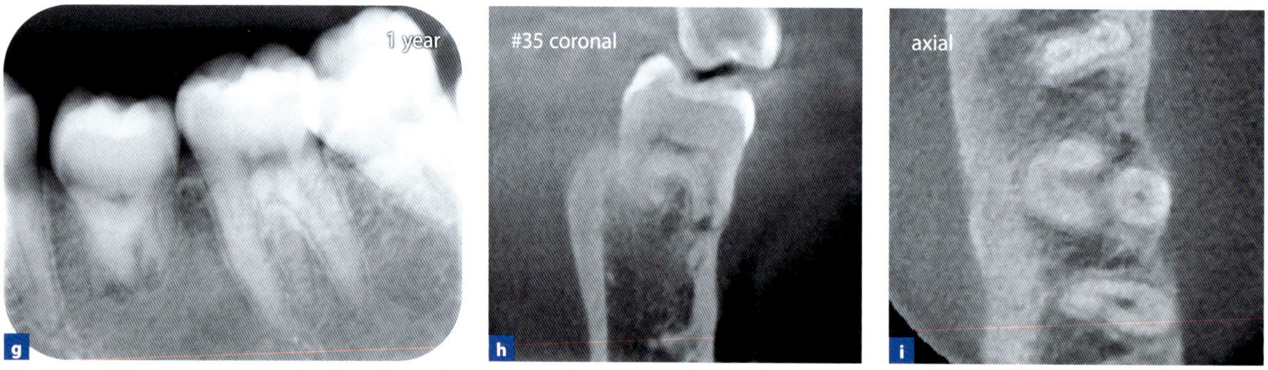

Fig 3-54g-i One year postoperative. Bone formation appears to have occurred around the exposed root.

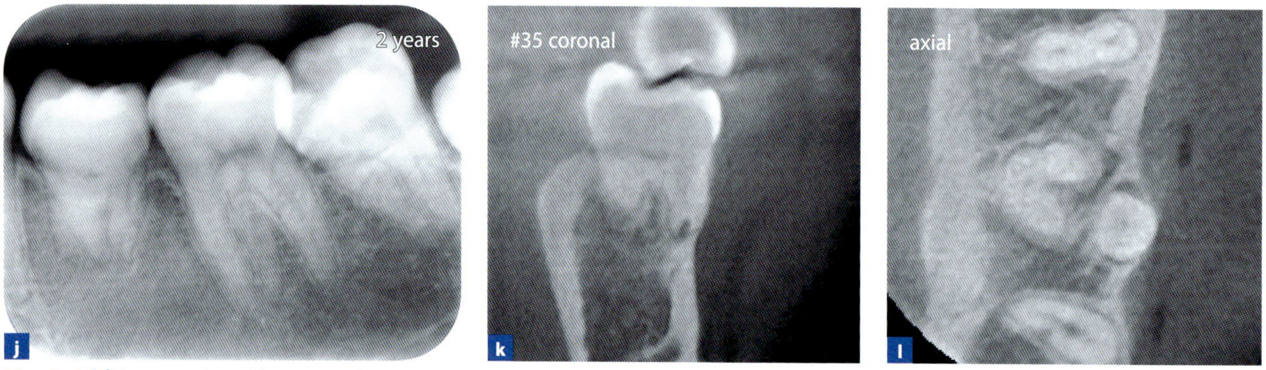

Figs 3-54j-l Two years later. The root surface around the cervical and apical area shows the formation of new bone, but it is difficult to determine whether or not bone has regenerated in the central area of the root which mostly protruded out of the socket.

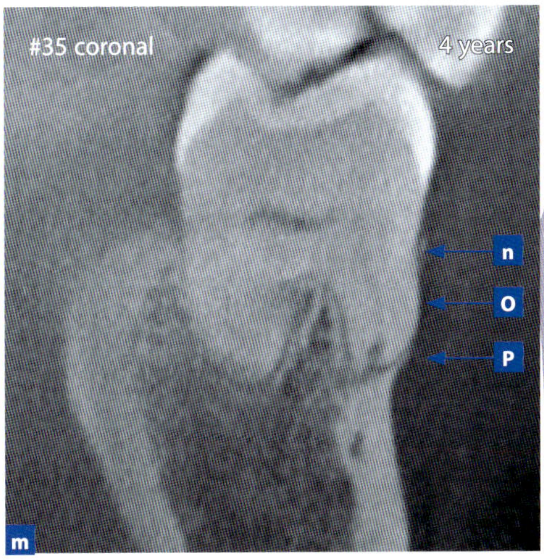

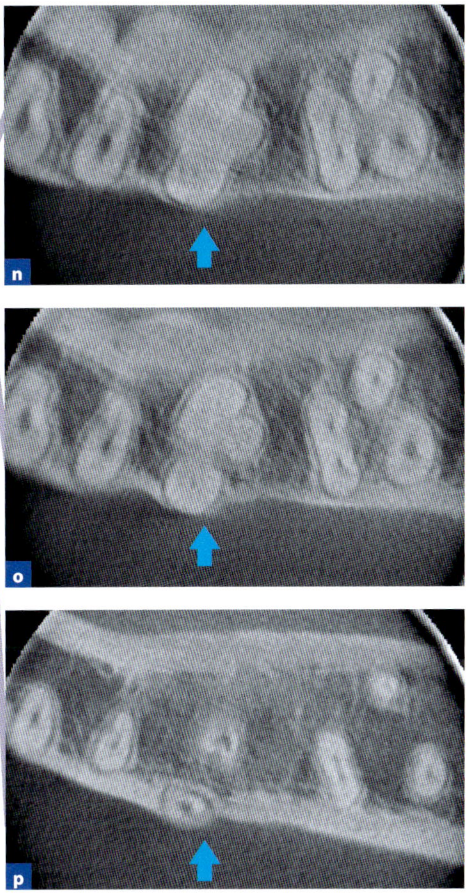

Fig 3-54m-p CBCT images after 4 years. The root appears to be covered with cortical bone at the cervical level (**n**) and near the apical level (**p**), but no clear bone regeneration can be seen in the mid root level of the root (**o**).

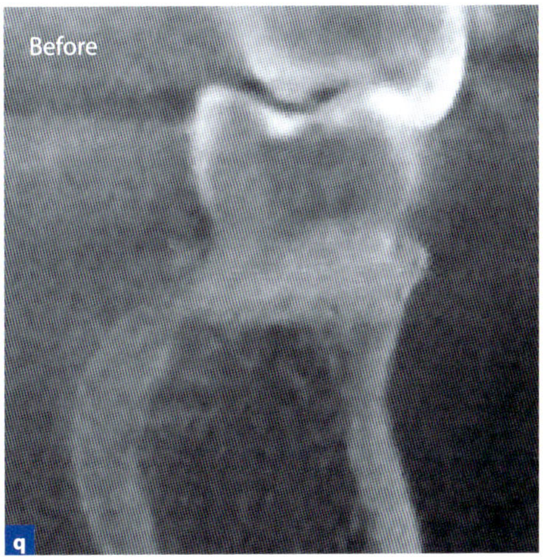

Fig 3-54q Preoperative CBCT image around the remaining deciduous tooth. Comparing **Fig 3-54m** and **Fig 3-54q**, it can be assumed that if the transplanted root protrudes too much out of the original bony housing, clear bone addition to the root surface is unlikely to occur, even if the PDL is viable.

olar bone proper is formed if the transplanted tooth is within the socket (Fig 3-54), but if the transplanted tooth is placed too far outside the original bony housing (i.e. over 2 mm), it is unlikely that alveolar bone proper will form (Fig 3-55). This means that the periodontal ligament is not always able to form and maintain alveolar bone proper but it is unclear why. It is possible that the gingival connective tissues nearby may have some inhibitory effect[38]. **Fig 3-54** shows how new bone was formed on the buccal aspect when the root was exposed outside of the original socket space.

In summary:

(1) When the transplanted root is within the bony housing or when the root exposure outside the housing is minimal, the root will likely be covered by new bone (Fig 3-56a, b).

(2)If the root is exposed too far outside the bony housing, part of the exposed root may not be covered by bone (Fig 3-56c, d).

(3) It is not clear whether bone formation can be expected on the exposed root surface by placing bone graft material around the transplanted tooth (Fig 3-56e, f).

In order to maximize the probability of new bone formation around the transplanted tooth, it would be better to place the donor tooth as deep as possible into the recipient bony tissue, especially in cases in which the width of the bone on the recipient site is not sufficient (Fig 3-57 and 3-58). Then, the teeth will either spontaneously erupt (Fig 3-57) or can be orthodontically extruded (Fig 3-58). In this way, bone regeneration around the transplanted tooth can be expected[164-166].

Fig 3-55 Three-dimensional bone regeneration around a transplanted tooth (3)

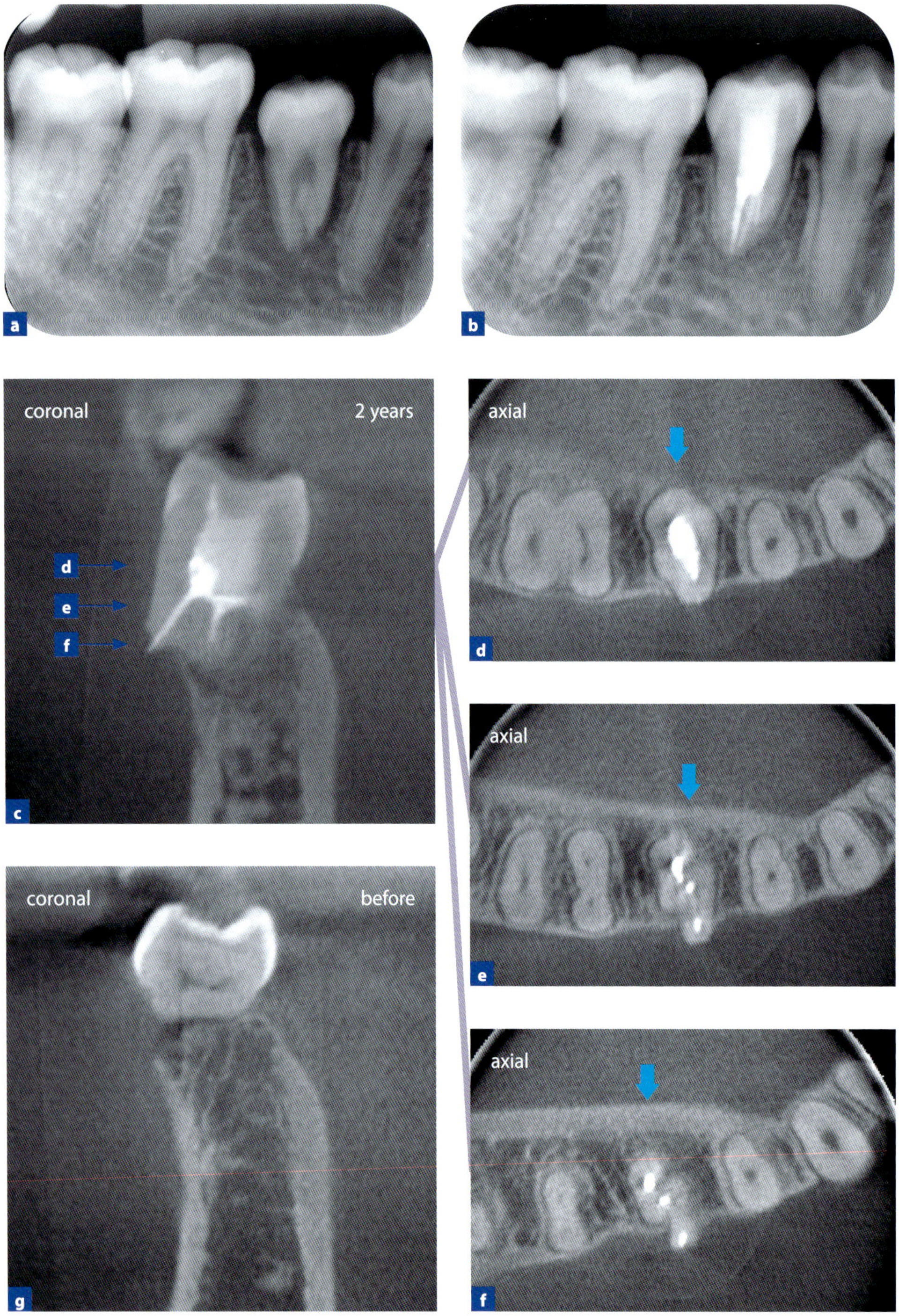

Fig 3-55a Radiograph immediately after transplantation of a 24-year-old female. #18 was transplanted into a congenitally missing #45 site.

Fig 3-55b Two years after transplantation. The patient had completed orthodontic treatment at another clinic.

Fig 3-55c-f CBCT images 2 years after transplantation. The transplanted tooth has been exposed out of the bone on the buccal aspect. There is no evidence of bone formation over the buccal aspect at the cervical (**d**), mid root (**e**), and apical (**f**) levels of the tooth root.

Fig 3-55g CBCT image before the surgery. Comparing **Fig 3-55c** and **Fig 3-55g**, one could infer that when the transplanted root is exposed too much out of the bony housing, the cortical bone (alveolar bone proper) cannot be regenerated. To prevent this situation, the teeth could have been transplanted by rotating it 45° or 90°.

Fig 3-56 Relationship between periodontal ligament of the donor tooth and horizontal bone regeneration.

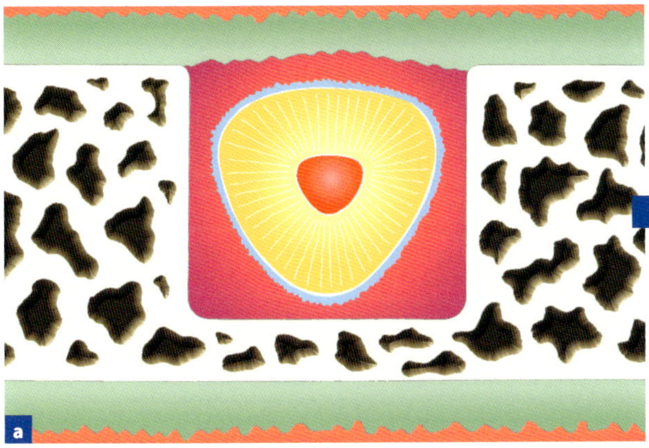

Fig 3-56a After transplantation of a tooth to a recipient site with a buccal or lingual defect.

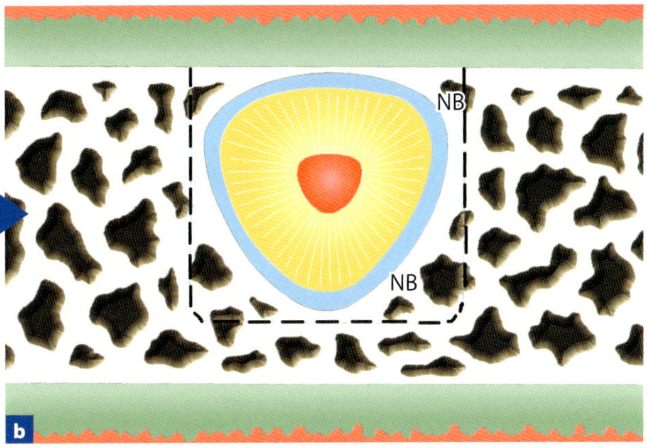

Fig 3-56b After healing. Despite defect, the donor tooth will be covered with newly formed bone (NB), which is regenerated by the periodontal ligament as long as the donor tooth with periodontal ligament is placed within the bony housing.

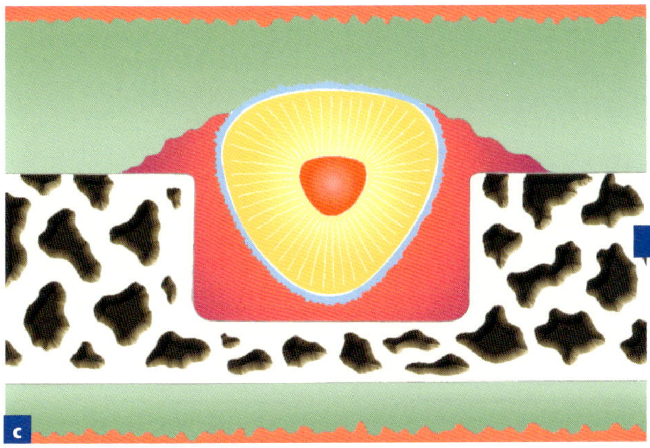

Fig 3-56c After transplantation of a tooth partially out of the bony housing, either buccally or lingually.

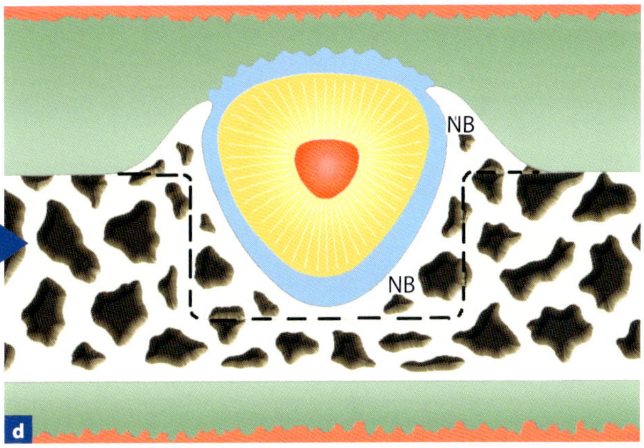

Fig 3-56d After healing. Defect with lack of buccal bone may remain if the donor tooth is placed too far outside the bony housing, despite the presence of the periodontal ligament.

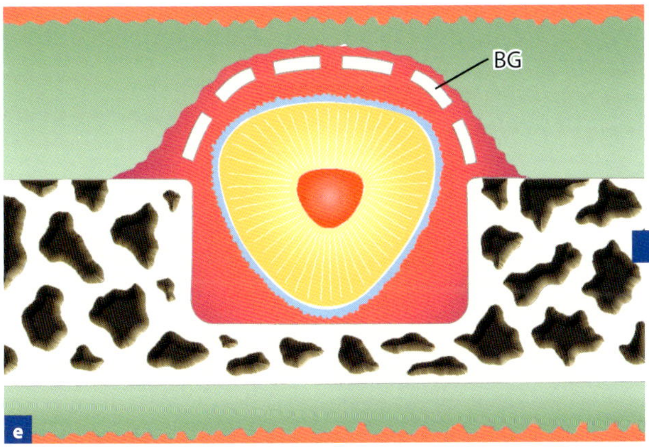

Fig 3-56e Use of bone graft material (BG). The donor tooth is placed partially outside of the bony housing but covered with bone graft materal.

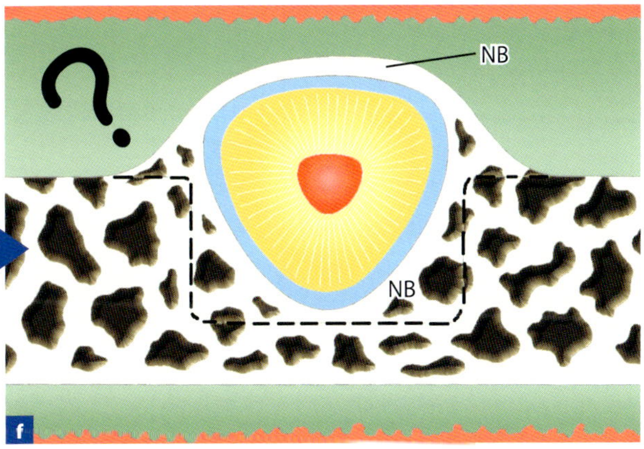

Fig 3-56f After healing. Bone graft material may or may not help the regeneration of the bone (NB) around the donor tooth.

Fig 3-57 Bone regeneration around the transplanted tooth with spontaneous eruption.

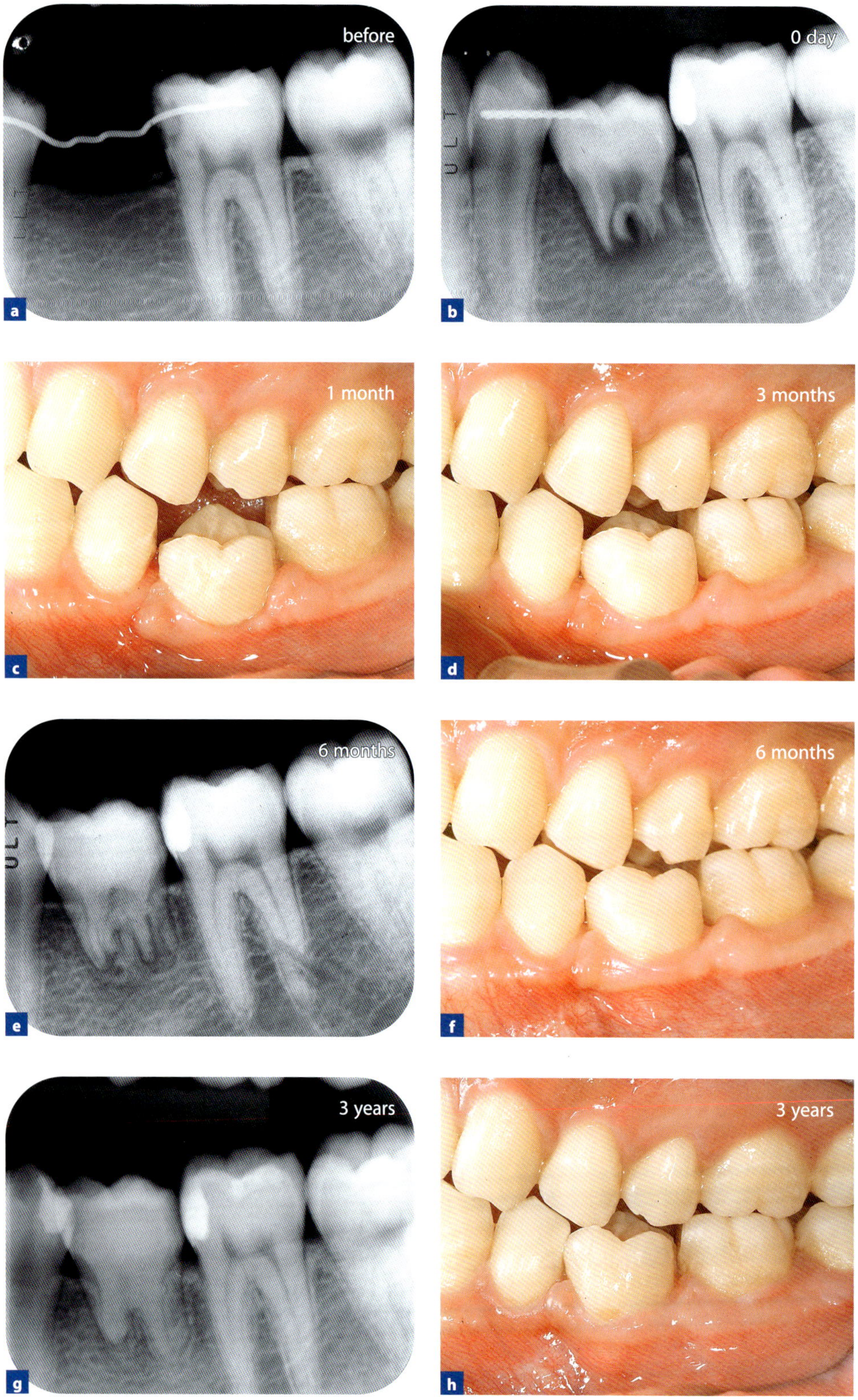

Fig 3-57a Radiograph before transplantation of a 20-year-old male. #28 was to be transplanted into congenitally missing #35 site.

Fig 3-57b Immediately after transplantation.

Fig 3-57c Lateral view 1 month after transplantation. The transplant was placed into the recipient site tilting buccally at a 20° because the ridge was too narrow to accommodate the donor in normal direction.

Fig 3-57d Three months postoperative. Spontaneous eruption of the transplant is occurring.

Fig 3-57e Six months postoperative. The healing of the pulp, periodontal ligament, and root development seem to be progressing.

Fig 3-57f Six months postoperative. Spontaneous eruption of the transplant has almost completed.

Fig 3-57g, h Three years postoperative. Healing apppears complete.

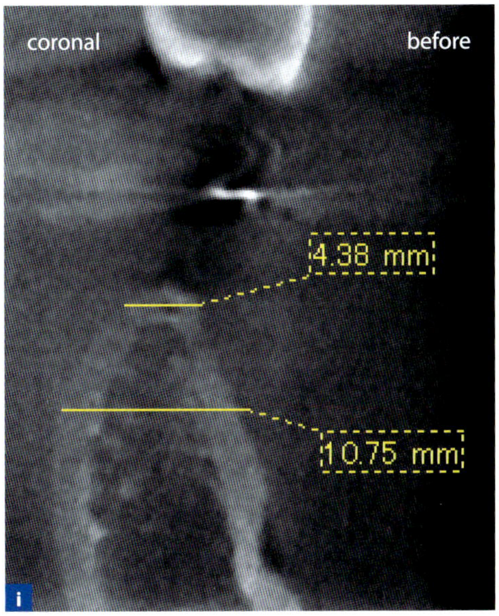

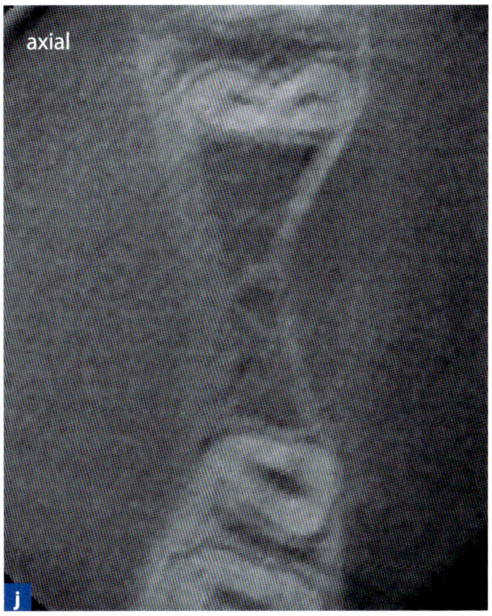

Fig 3-57i, j CBCT images before the surgery. The width of the alveolar ridge of the recipient site is narrow.

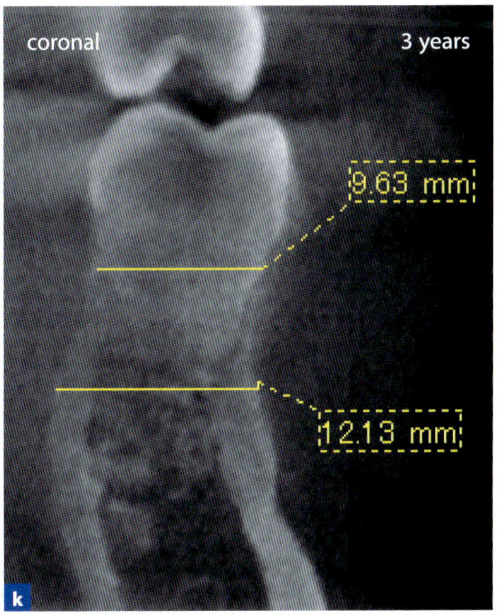

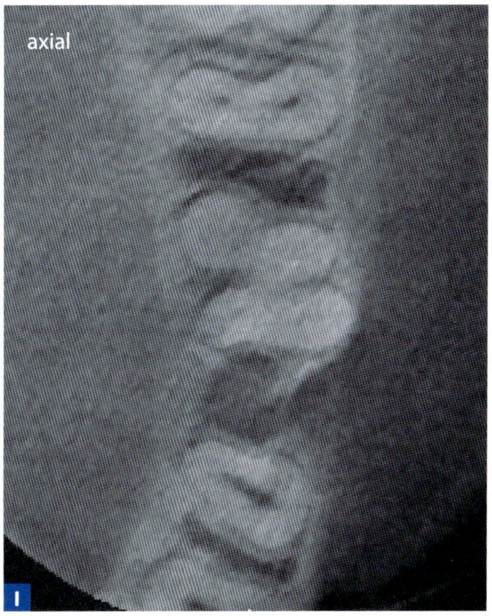

Fig 3-57k, l CBCT images 3 years after transplantation. The root of the transplant is completely covered with bone resulting in the increased ridge width. This case may indicate that if the ridge of the recipient site is narrow, it is recommended that the donor tooth is placed obliquely/tilted and deeply, and then allow for natural or orthodontic eruption.

Fig 3-58 Bone regeneration around the transplanted tooth with orthodontic eruption.

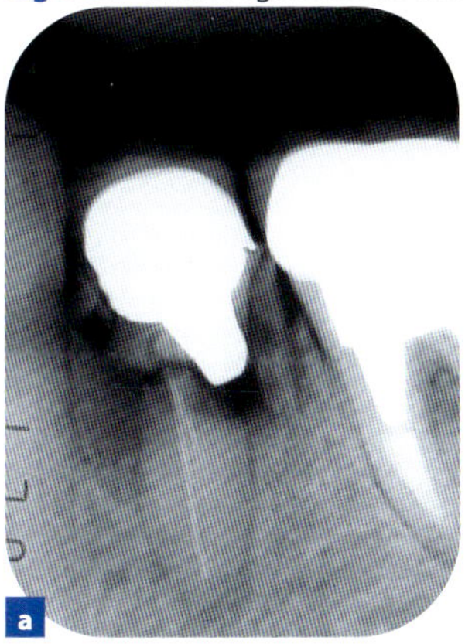

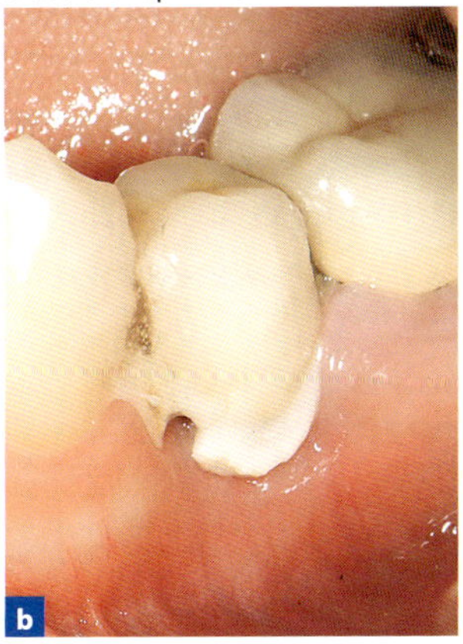

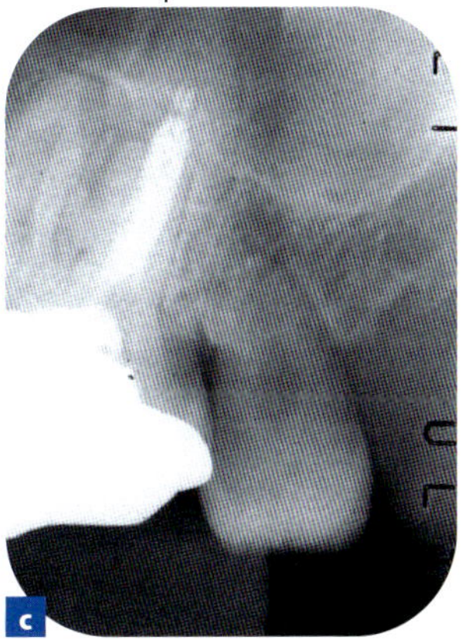

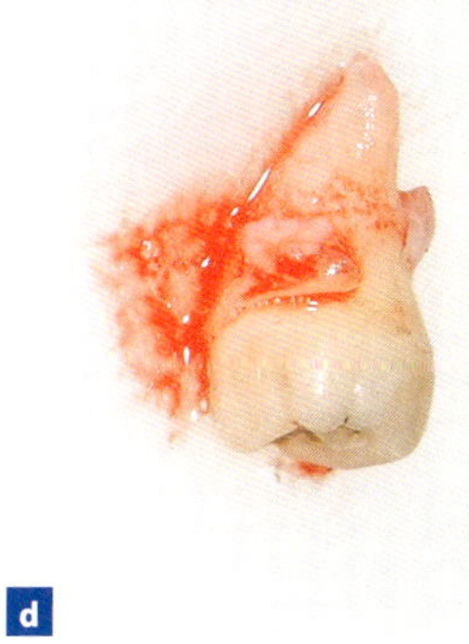

Fig 3-58a, b Radiograph and oral view before treatment of a 27-year-old female. #35 was hopeless and was to be replaced with very small #28.

Fig 3-58c Radiograph of the donor tooth, #28,

Fig 3-58d The extracted donor tooth showing a very small root preserving with two-thirds of the amount of periodontal ligament.

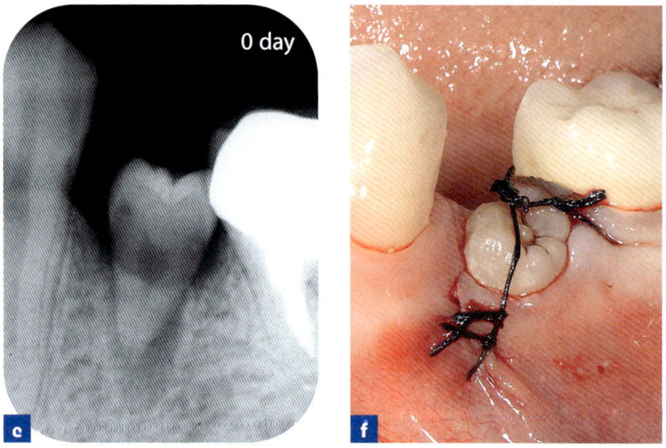

Fig 3-58e, f Immediately after transplantation.

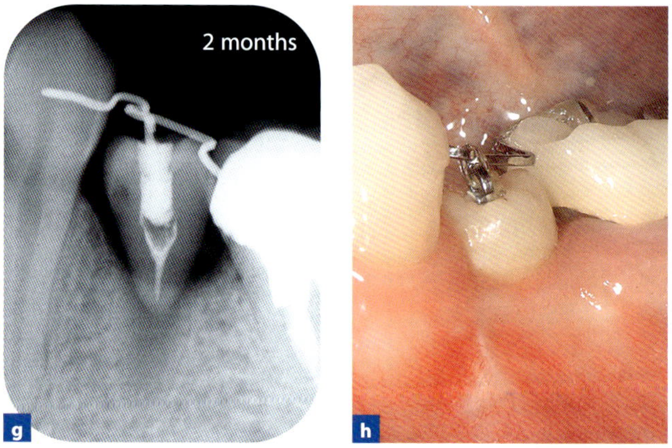

Fig 3-58g, h Two months after transplantation. One month after transplantation, orthodontic eruption was started to recover the esthetics and bone. The transplant has erupted to the goal already but looks as if it has been extruded out of the socket.

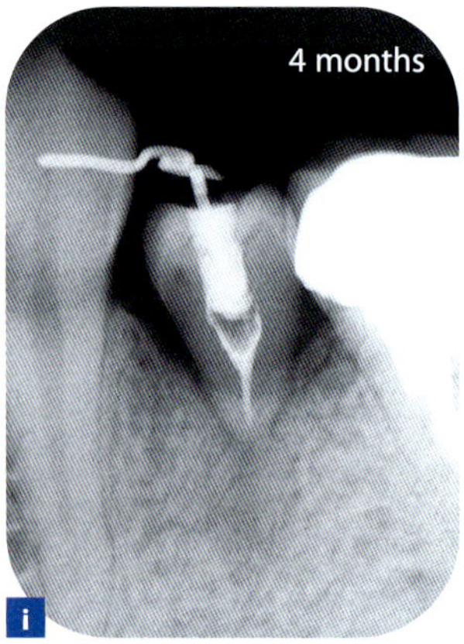

Fig 3-58i Four months after transplantation. Bone regeneration was observed around the transplant.

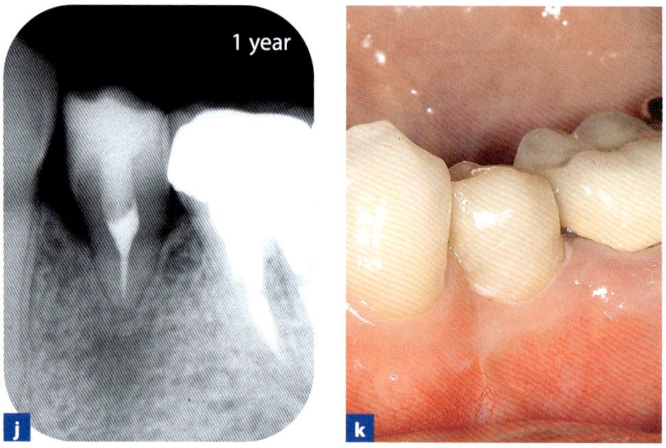

Fig 3-58j, k One year postoperative. Bone regeneration has occurred up to the level where the periodontal ligament was preserved. The transplant is restored with CR.

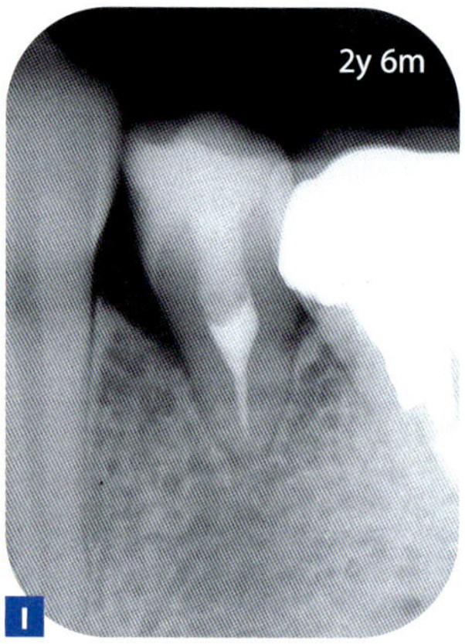

Fig 3-58l Two years and 6 months later.

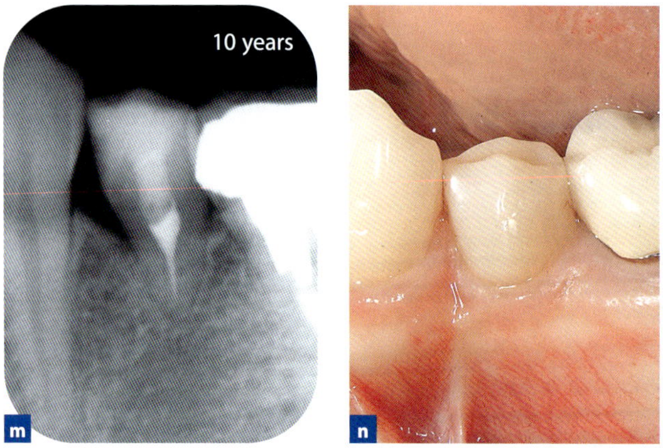

Fig 3-58m, n 10 years postoperative. The regenerated bone appears to be maintained.

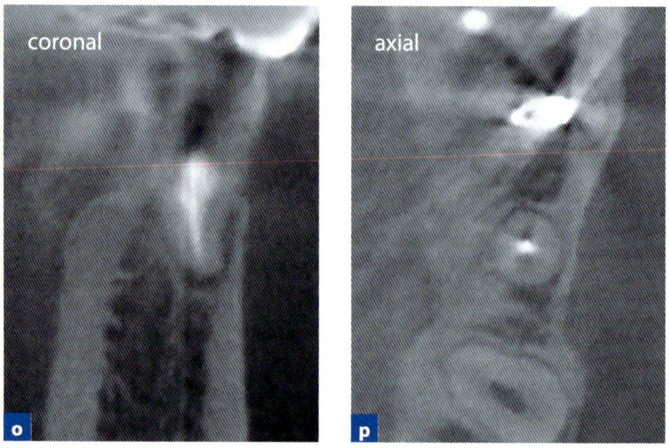

Fig 3-58o, p CBCT images 10 years after transplantation. The transplanted tooth is covered with bone up to the level where the periodontal ligament had been preserved.

References

1. Kalkwarf KI. Periodontal new attachment without the placement of osseous potentiating grafts. Periodontal Abstracts. 1974; 2 : 53-62.
2. American Academy of Periodontology: Glossary of Periodontal Terms. J Periodontal. 1986; Nov (11).
3. Tobe O. Histological studies on periodontal tissue reactions following intentional replantation of incisors in monkeys: With special reference to computer-aided three dimensional reconstruction of replanted teeth [in Japanese]. Jpn J Conserv Dent. 1990; 33: 772-802.
4. Fukuro K. Bone morphometrical studies of intentional replantation in monkeys' teeth [in Japanese]. Jpn J Conserv Dent. 1991; 34: 957-85.
5. Ichinokawa H. Ultrastructural studies on periodontal tissue reactions following intentional tooth replantation in adult monkeys [in Japanese]. Jpn J Conserv Dent. 1995; 38: 63-87.
6. Ohyama K. The effect of storage media on periodontal healing after intentional replantation of teeth in monkeys. A histopathological and morphometrical study [in Japanese]. Jpn J Conserv Dent. 1996; 39: 685-706.
7. Isono T. Effect of storage media upon periodontal healing after replantation of teeth in adult monkeys [in Japanese]. J Jpn Soc Oral Implantol. 1998; 11: 375-85.
8. Loe H, Waerhaug J. Experimental replantation of teeth in dogs and monkeys. Arch Oral Biol. 1961; 3 : 176-84.
9. Najleti CE, Caffesse RG, Castelli WA, Hoke JA. Healing after tooth reimplantation in monkeys. A radioautographic study. Oral Surg. 1975; 39: 361-75.
10. Andreasen JO. A time-related study of periodontal healing and root resorption activity after replantation of mature permanent incisors in monkeys. Swed Dent J. 1980; 4 : 101-10.
11. Proye MP, Polson AM. Repair in different zones of the periodontium after tooth reimplantation. J Periodontal. 1982; 53: 379-89.
12. Ichinokawa H, et al. The pathological analysis in the experiments on autotransplantation of teeth [in Japanese]. Jpn J Conserv Dent. 1998; 41: 38.
13. Ichinokawa H, et al. The pathological analysis in the experiments on autotransplantation of teeth: Part 2. The microstructural changes in the healing process [in Japanese]. Jpn J Conserv Dent. 1998; 41: 91.
14. Kurisaki H. The pathological analysis in the experiments on autotransplantation of teeth: Part 2 [in Japanese]. J Jpn Soc Oral Implantol. 1998; 11: 270-1.
15. Ichinokawa H, et al. The pathological analysis in the experiments on autotransplantation of teeth: Part 4. The microstructural changes in the healing process [in Japanese]. J Jpn Soc Oral Implantol. 1999; 12: 131.
16. Asai Y, Nakagawa K. PDL preservation in transplantation and replantation of teeth. Part 1. The experimental and clinical approach [in Japanese]. J Jpn Dent Assoc. 1997; 50: 6 -16.
17. Shimada T. Effect of periodontal ligament curetted in alveolar socket for autotransplantation of tooth in adult monkeys [in Japanese]. J Jpn Soc Oral Implantol. 1998; 11: 492-500.
18. Andreasen JO. Periodontal healing after replantation and autotransplantation of incisors in monkeys. Int J Oral Surg. 1981; 10: 54-61.
19. Andreasen JO. Analysis of topography of surface and inflammatory root resorption after replantation of mature permanent incisors in monkeys. Swed Dent J. 1980; 4 : 135-44.
20. Andreasen JO. Analysis of pathogenesis and topography of replacement resorption (ankylosis) after replantation of mature permanent incisors in monkeys. Swed Dent J. 1980; 4 : 231-40.
21. Andreasen JO. Relationship between cell damage in the periodontal ligament after replantation and subsequent development of root resorption. Acta Odontol Scand. 1981; 39: 15-25.
22. Andreasen JO, Kristerson L. The effect of limited drying or removal of the periodontal ligament. Periodontal healing after replantation of mature incisors in monkeys. Acta Odontol Scand. 1981; 39: 1 -13.
23. Andreasen JO, Skougaard MR. Reversibility of surgically induced dental ankylosis in rats. Int J Oral Surg. 1972; 1 : 98-102.
24. Andreasen JO. Histometric study of healing of periodontal tissues in rats after surgical injury. I. Design of a standardized surgical procedure. Odontol Revy. 1976; 27: 115-30.
25. Andreasen JO. Histometric study of healing of periodontal tissues in rats after a surgical injury. II. Healing events of alveolar bone, periodontal ligaments and cementum. Odontol Revy. 1976; 27: 131-44.
26. Yoshida M. An experimental study on regeneration of cementum, periodontal ligament and alveolar bone in the intradentinal cavities in dogs [in Japanese]. The Shikwa Gakuho. 1976; 76: 1179-222.
27. Yamamura T, et al. Pathology and Healing [in Japanese]. Tokyo: Ishiyaku, 1988.
28. Andreasen JO. Review of root resorption systems and models. Etiology of root resorption and the homeostatic mechanisms of the periodontal ligament. In: The Biological Mechanisms of Tooth Eruption and Root Resorption. Birmingham, Alabama: EBSCO Media, 1988: 9 -21.
29. Atrizadeh F, Kennedy J, Zander H. Ankylosis of teeth following thermal injury. J Periodontal Res. 1971; 6 : 159-67.
30. Cvek M, Lindvall A. External root resorption following bleaching of pulpless teeth with oxygen peroxide. Endod Dent Traumatol. 1985; 1 : 56-60.
31. Rygh P. Orthodontic root resorption studied by electron microscopy. Angle Orthod 1977; 47: 1 -16.
32. Wesselink P, Beertsen W. Initiating factors in dental root resorption. In: The Biological Mechanisms of Tooth Eruption and Root Resorption. Birmingham, Alabama: EBSCO Media, 1988: 329-34.
33. Soder PO, Otteskog P, Andreasen JO, Modeer T. The effect of drying on the viability of the periodontal membrane. Scand J Dent Res. 1977: 85: 164-8.
34. Wesselink PR, Beertsen W, Everts V. Resorption of the mouse incisor after the application of cold to the periodontal attachment apparatus. Calcif Tissue Int. 1986; 39: 11-21.
35. Hammarström L, Piece A, Blomlöf L, Feiglin B, Lindskog S. Tooth avulsion and replantation. A review. Endod Dent Traumatol. 1986; 2 : 1 -8.
36. Lindskog S, Blomlöf L, Hammarström L. Repair of periodontal tissue in vivo and vitro. J Clin Periodontal. 1983; 10: 188-205.
37. Lindskog S, Hammarström L. Evidence in favor of an anti-invasion factor in cementum or periodontal membrane of human teeth. Scand J Dent Res. 1980; 88: 161-3.
38. Melcher AH. Cells from soft connective tissue depress osteogenesis in vitro. In: The Biological Mechanisms of Tooth Eruption and Root Resorption. Birmingham, Alabama: EBSCO Media, 1988; 87-91.
39. Andreasen JO. Effect of extra-alveolar period and storage media upon periodontal and pulpal healing after replantation of mature permanent incisors in monkeys. Int J Oral Surg. 1981; 1 : 43-53.
40. Takizawa H. Studies on the teeth preservation for replantation and transplantation: viability of the POL cells [in Japanese]. J Jpn Soc Prosthodont. 1991; 35: 723-37.
41. Andreasen JO, Borum MK, Jacobsen HL, Andreasen FM. Replantation of 400 avulsed permanent incisors. 4. Factors related to periodontal ligament healing. Endod Dent Traumatol. 1995; 11: 76-89.
42. Patil S, Dumsha TC, Sykdiskis RJ. Determining periodontal ligament (PDL) cell vitality from exarticulated teeth stored in saline or milk using fluorescein diacetate. Int Endod J. 1994; 27: 1 -5.
43. Lindskog S, Blomlöf L. Influence of osmolality and composition of some storage media on human periodontal ligament cells. Acta Odontol Scand. 1982; 40: 435-41.
44. Andersson L, Bodin I, Sorensen S. Progression of root resorption following replantation of human teeth after extended extraoral storage. Endod Dent Traumatol. 1989; 5 : 38-47.
45. Courts FJ, Mueller WA, Tabeling HJ. Milk as an interim storage medium for avulsed teeth. Pediatr Dent. 1983; 5 : 183-6.
46. Blomlöf L, Otteskog P. Viability of human periodontal ligament cells after storage in milk or saliva. Scand J Dent Res. 1980; 88: 436-40.
47. Blomlöf L, Lindskog S, Andersson S, Hedström KG, Hammarström L. Storage of experimentally avulsed teeth in milk prior to replantation. J Dent Res. 1983; 62: 912-6.
48. Blomlöf L, Lindskog S, Hammarström L. Periodontal healing of exarticulated monkey teeth stored in milk or saliva. Scand J Dent Res. 1981; 89: 251-9.
49. Blomlöf L. Milk and saliva as possible storage media for traumatically exarticulated teeth prior to replantation. Swed Dent J. 1981; 8 (suppl): 1 -26.
50. Blomlöf L, Lindskog S, Hedström KG, Hammarström L. Vitality of periodontal ligament cells after storage of monkey teeth in milk or saliva. Scand J Dent Res. 1980; 88: 441-5.
51. Andersson L, Blomlöf L, Lindskog S, Feiglin B, Hammarström L. Tooth ankylosis. Clinical, radiographic and histological assessments. Int J Oral Surg. 1984; 13: 423-31.
52. Krasner P, Rankow HJ. New philosophy for the treatment of avulsed teeth. Oral Surg Oral Med Oral Pathol. 1995; 79: 616-23.

53. Trope M, Friedman S. Periodontal healing of replanted dog teeth stored in Viaspan, milk and Hank's balanced salt solution. Endod Dent Traumatol. 1992; 8 : 183-8.

54. Hiltz J, Trope M. Vitality of human lip fibroblasts in milk, Hank's balanced salt solution and Viaspan storage media. Endod Dent Traumatol. 1991; 7 : 69-72.

55. Oswald RJ, Harrington GW, Van Hassel HJ. A postreplantation evaluation of air-dried and saliva-stored avulsed teeth. J Endod. 1980; 6 : 546-51.

56. Andreasen JO, Reinholdt J, Riis I, Dybdahl R, Söder PO, Otteskog P. Periodontal and pulpal healing of monkey incisors preserved in tissue culture before replantation. Int J Oral Surg. 1978; 7 : 104-12.

57. Söder PO, Lundquist G. Autotransplantation of teeth with use of cell cultivation technique. Int Dent J. 1972; 22: 327-40.

58. Reinholdt J, Andreasen JO, Söder PÖ, Otteskog P, Dybdahl R, Riis I. Cultivation of periodontal ligament fibroblasts on extracted monkey incisors. Int J Oral Surg. 1977; 7 : 215-25.

59. Imai T. Fundamental studies on tooth transplantation: The study on preserving teeth of dogs experimentally (Part 2) [in Japanese]. J Jpn Assoc Oral Surg. 1961; 7 : 176.

60. Andreasen JO, Hjørting-Hansen E. Replantation of teeth. I. Radiographic and clinical study of 110 human teeth replanted after accidental loss. Acta Odontol Scand. 1966; 24: 263-86.

61. Andreasen JO, Hjørting-Hansen E. Replantation of teeth. II. Histological study of 22 replanted anterior teeth in humans. Acta Odontol Scand. 1966; 24: 287-306.

62. Andersson L, Jonsson BG, Hammarström L, Blomlöf L, Andreasen JO, Lindskog S. Evaluation of statistics and desirable experimental design of a histomorphometrical method for studies of root resorption. Endod Dent Traumatol. 1987; 3 : 288-95.

63. Andreasen JO. Experimental dental traumatology: development of a model for external root resorption. Endod Dent Traumatol. 1987; 3 : 269-87.

64. Andreasen JO. Relationship between surface and inflammatory resorption and changes in the pulp after replantation of permanent incisors in monkeys. J Endod. 1981; 7 : 294-301.

65. Andreasen JO, Bakland LK. Chapter 37 Pathologic tooth resorption. In: Ingle JI, Bakland LK, Baumgartner JC (eds). Ingle's ENDODONTICS. Shelton: PMPH, 2008.

66. Frost HM. Tetracycline-based histological analysis of bone remodeling. Calcif Tissue Res 1969; 3 : 221-37.

67. Suda T, et al. Biology of Bone [in Japanese]. Tokyo: Ishiyaku, 1990.

68. Martin TJ, Sims NA. Osteoclast-derived activity in the coupling of bone formation to resorption. Trends Mol Med. 2005 ; 11(2): 76-81.

69. Sims NA, Gooi JH. Bone remodeling. Multiple cellular interactions required for coupling of bone formation and resorption. Semin Cell Dev Biol. 2008 ; 19(5): 444-51.

70. Martin T, Gooi JH, Sims NA. Molecular mechanisms in coupling of bone formation to resorption. Crit Rev Eukaryot Gene Expr. 2009; 19(1): 73-88.

71. Sims NA, Martin TJ. Coupling the activities of bone formation and resorption. A multitude of signals within the basic multicellular unit. Bonekey Rep. 2014; 3 : 481.

72. Kahn A, Malone JD. Lineage of bone resorbing cells. Status and prospects of future research. The biological mechanisms of tooth eruption and root resorption. Birmingham: EBSCO Media, 1988: 313-9.

73. Yasuda H, et al. Osteoclast Differentiation factor is a ligand for osteoprotegerin/osteoclastogenesis-inhibitory factor and is identical to TRANS/RANKL. Proc Natl Acad Sci USA. 1998; 95: 3597.

74. Yasuda H, et al. Identity of osteoclastogenesis-inhibitory factor(OCIF)and osteoprotegerin(OPG): a mechanism by which OPG/OCIF inhibits osteoclastogenesis in vitro. Endocrinology. 1998; 139: 1329.

75. Hakeda Y, et al. Osteoclastogenesis inhibitory factor(OCIF)derectly inhibits bone-resorbing activity of isolated mature osteoclasts. Biochem Biophys Res Commun. 1998; 251: 796.

76. Takahashi N, et al. A new member of tumor necrosis factor ligand family, ODF/OPGL/TRANCE/RANKL, regulates osteoclast Differentiation and function. Biochem Biophys Res Commun. 1999; 256: 449.

77. Khosla S. Minireview. The OPG/RANKL/RANK System. Endocrinology. 2001; 142: 5050.

78. Simonet WS, et al. Osteoprotegerin. a novel secreted protein involved in the regulation of bone density. Cell. 1997; 89: 309.

79. Lacey DL, et al. Osteoprotegerin ligand is a cytokine that regulates osteoclast Differentiation and activation. Cell. 1998; 93: 165.

80. Kong YY, et al. OPGL is a key regulator of osteoclastogenesis, lymphocyte development, lymph node organogenesis. Nature. 1999; 397: 315.

81. Mundy GR, Roodman GD. Osteoclast ontogeny and function. In: Peck WA(ed). Bone and Mineral Research. Vol. 5. New York: Elsevier, 1987; 209.

82. Nijweide PJ, et al. Cells of bone. proliferation, Differentiation, and horumonal regulation. Physiol Rev. 1986; 66: 855.

83. Nesbitt S, et al. Biochemical characterization of human osteoclast integrins. J Biol Chem 1993; 268: 16737.

84. Aubin JE. Osteoclast adhesion and resorption. The role of podosomes. J Bone Miner Res. 1992; 7 (4): 365-8.

85. Lakkakorpi P, et al. Organization of osteoclast microfilaments during the attachment to bone surface in vitro. J Bone Miner Res. 1989; 4 : 817.

86. Teti A, Zambonin-Zallone A. Osteoclast cytoskeleton and attachment proteins. In: Rifkin BR , Gay CV(ed). Biology and physiology of the osteoclast. London: CRC Press, 1992; 245.

87. Domon T, Wakita M. A three-dimensional reconstruction of the ruffled border of osteoclast. J Bone Miner Res. 1989; 52: 1.

88. Baron R, et al. Cellular and molecular biology of the osteoclast. In: Noda M(ed). Cellular and molecular biology of bone. New York : Academic Press, 1993; 445.

89. Roodman GD. Cell biology of the osteoclast. Exp Hematol. 1999; 27: 1229.

90. Zaidi M, et al. Cellular biology of bone resorption. Biol Rev Camb Philos Soc. 1993; 68: 197.

91. Baron R, et al. Biology of osteoclast. In: Mundy GR, et al(ed). Physiology and phyamacology of bone. New York: Springer, 1993; 111.

92. Andreasen JO. External root resorption. Its implication in dental traumatology, paedodontics, periodontics, orthodontics and endodontics. Int Endod J. 1985; 18: 109-18.

93. Boyde A, Ali NN, Jones SJ. Resorption of dentine by isolated osteoclasts. in vitro. Br Dent J. 1984; 156: 216-20.

94. Jone SJ, Boyde A. The resorption of dentine and cementum. in vivo and vitro, The biological mechanisms of tooth eruption and root resorption. Birmingham: EBSCO Media, 1988; 335-54.

95. Andreasen JO. The effect of pulp extirpation or root canal treatment on periodontal healing after replantation of permanent incisors in monkeys. J Endod. 1982; 7 : 245-52, 1981; 8 : 426-7.

96. Yamamoto H. Periodontology illustrate by drawing. Tokyo: Quintessence Publishing, 2002; 161-2.

97. Kong YY, Feige U, Sarosi I, Bolon B, Tafuri A, Morony S, Capparelli C, Li J, Elliott R, McCabe S, Wong T, Campagnuolo G, Moran E, Bogoch ER, Van G, Nguyen LT, Ohashi PS, Lacey DL, Fish E, Boyle WJ, Penninger JM. Activated T cells regulate bone loss and joint destruction in adjuvant arthritis through osteoprotegerin ligand. Nature. 1999; 402(6759): 304-9.

98. Teng YT, Nguyen H, Gao X, Kong YY, Gorczynski RM, Singh B, Ellen RP, Penninger JM. Functional human T-cell immunity and osteoprotegerin ligand control alveolar bone destruction in periodontal infection. J Clin Invest. 2000; 106(6): R59-67.

99. Melcher AH. On the repair potential of periodontal tissues. J Periodontol. 1976; 47: 256-60.

100. Ingber JS, et al. The "biologic width" A concept in periodontics and restorative dentistry. Alpha Omegan. Scientific Issue, 1977 Dec; 70(3): 62-5.

101. Gargiulo AW, et al. Dimensions and relations of the dentogingival junction in humans. J Periodontol. 1961; 32: 261.

102. Maynard JG, Wilson RD. Physiologic dimensions of the perio-dontium significant to the restorative dentist. J Periodontol. 1979; 50: 170.

103. Wilson RD, Maynard JG. Intracrevicular restorative dentistry. Int J Periodontics Restorative Dent. 1981; 4 : 34.

104. Nevins M, Ono Y, Sato N. Clinical Guidance for GTR. Tokyo: Editorial House AKI, 1993; 9 - 21.

105. Caton J, Zander HA. Osseous repair of an infrabony pocket without new attachment of connective tissue. J Clin Periodontol. 1976; 3 : 54-8.

106. Caton J, Nyman S, Zander H. Histometric evaluation of perio-dontal surgery. Ⅱ. Connective tissue attachment levels after four regenerative procedures. J Clin Periodontol. 1980; 7 : 224-31.

107. Andreasen JO, Paulsen HU, Yu Z, Ahlquist R, Bayer T, Schwartz O. A long term study of 370 autotransplanted premolars. Part Ⅰ. Surgical procedure and standardized techniques for monitoring healing. Eur J Orthod. 1990; 12: 3 -13.

108. Andreasen JO, Paulsen HU, Yu Z, Bayer T, Schwartz O. A long term study of 370 autotransplanted premolars. Part Ⅱ. Tooth survival and pulp healing subsequent to transplantation. Eur J Orthod. 1990; 12: 14-24.

109. Andreasen JO, Paulsen HU, Yu Z, Schwartz O. A long term study of 370 autotransplanted premolars. Part Ⅲ. Periodontal healing subsequent to transplantation. Eur J Orthod. 1990; 12: 25-37.

110. Andreasen JO, Paulsen HU, Yu Z, Bayer T. A long term study of 370 autotransplanted premolars. Part Ⅳ. Root development subsequent to transplantation. Eur J Orthod. 1990; 12: 38-50.

111. Anderson AW, Sharav Y, Massler M. Reparative dentine formation and pulp morphology. Oral Surg Oral Med Oral Pathol. 1968; 26: 837-47.

112. Skoglund A, Hasselgren G, Tronstad L. Oxidoreductase activity in the pulp of replanted and autotransplanted teeth in young dogs. Oral Surg. 1981; 52: 205-9.

113. Kvinnsland I, Heyeraas KJ. Cell renewal and ground substance formation in replanted cat teeth. Acta Odontol Scand. 1990; 48: 203-15.

114. Skoglund A, Tronstad L, Wallenius K. A microangiographic study of vascular changes in replanted and autotransplanted teeth of young dogs. Oral Surg. 1978; 45: 17-27.

115. Schendel KU, Schwartz O, Andreasen JO, Hoffmeister B. Reinnervation of autotransplanted teeth. A histological investigation in monkeys. Int J Oral Maxillofac Surg. 1990; 19: 247-9.

116. Andreasen JO. Traumatic injuries of the teeth. 2 nd ed. Copenhagen: Munksgaard, 1981.

117. Kristerson L, Andreasen JO. Influence of root development on periodontal and pulpal healing after replantation of incisors in monkeys. Int J Oral Surg. 1984; 13: 313-23.

118. Kristerson L, Andreasen JO. Autotransplantation and replantation of tooth germs in monkeys. Effect of damage to the dental follicle and position of transplant in the alveolus. Int J Oral Surg. 1984; 13: 324-33.

119. Andreasen JO, Kristerson L, Andreasen FM. Damage of the Hertwig's epithelial root sheath. Effect upon root growth after autotransplantation of teeth in monkeys. Endod Dent Traumatol. 1988; 4 : 145-51.

120. Andreasen JO, Andreasen FM. Textbook and color atlas of traumatic injuries to the teeth. 3 rd ed. Copenhagen: Munksgaard, 1994.

121. Moorrees CFA, Fanning EA, Hunt EE Jr. Age variation of formation stages for 10 permanent teeth. J Dent Res. 1963; 42: 1490-502.

122. Andreasen JO. Atlas of replantation and transplantation of teeth. Philadelphia: WB Saunders, 1992.

123. Frank AL. Therapy for the divergent pulpless tooth by continued apical formation. J Am Dent Assoc. 1966; 72: 87-93.

124. Steiner JC, Van Hassel HJ. Experimental root apexification in primates. Oral Surg. 1971; 31: 409-15.

125. Cvek M. Treatment of non-vital permanent incisors with calcium hydroxide. I. Follow-up of periapical repair and apical closure of immature roots. Odontol Revy. 1972; 23: 27-44.

126. Dannenberg JL. Pedodontic Endodontics. Dent Clin North Am. 1974; 18: 367-77.

127. Tronstad L, Andreasen JO, Hasselgren G, Kristerson L, Riis I. Changes in dental tissues after root canal filling with calcium hydroxide. J Endod. 1981; 7 : 17-22.

128. Tenca JI, Tsamtsouris A. Continued root end development. Apexogenesis and Apexification. J Pedod 1978; 2 : 144-57.

129. Slagsvold O, Bjercke B. Autotransplantation of premolars with partly formed roots. A radiographic study of root growth. Am J Orthod. 1974; 66: 355-66.

130. Kristerson L. Autotransplantation of human premolars. A clinical and radiographic study of 100 teeth. Int J Oral Surg. 1985; 14: 200-13.

131. Cho MI, Garant PR. Development and general structure of the periodontium. Periodontology 2000. 2000; 24: 9.

132. Ten Cate AR. The development of the periodontium-a largely ectomesenchymally derived unit. Periodontology 2000. 1997; 13: 9 -19.

133. Moxham BJ, Grant DA. Development of the periodontal ligament. In: Berkovitz, BKB, et al(eds). The periodontal ligament in health and disease. London: Mosby-Wolfe, 1995; 161.

134. Schroeder HE. Gingiva. In: Handbook of microscopic anatomy, vol. 5, The periodontium. Heidelberg: Springer-Verlag, 1986; 12.

135. Bartold PK, Narayanan AS. Developmental aspects of the periodontium. In: Biology of the periodontal connective tissue. Chicago: Quintessence Publishing, 1998; 151.

136. Ruch JV. Facts and hypothesis concerning the control of odontoblast Differentiation. Differentiation. 1982; 21: 7.

137. Ruch JV. Odontoblast Differentiation and the formation of the odontoblast layer. J Dent Res. 1985; 64: 489.

138. Thomas HF, Kollar EJ. Differentiation of odontoblasts in grafted recombinations of murine epithelial root sheath and dental mesenchyme. Arch Oral Biol. 1989; 34: 27-35.

139. Thomas HF. Root formation. Int J Dev Biol 1995; 39: 231-7.

140. Diamond M, Applebaum E. The epithelial sheath. histogenesis and function. J Dent Res. 1942; 21: 303.

141. Cho MI, Garant PR. Ultrastructural evidence of directed cell migration during initial cementoblast Differentiation in root formation. J Periodontal Res. 1988; 23: 268-76.

142. Freeman E, et al. Development of a gomphosis by tooth germ implants in the parietal bone of the mouse. Arch Oral Biol. 1975; 20: 139-40.

143. Hoffman RL. Formation of periodontal tissues around subcutaneously transplanted hamster molars. J Dent Res. 1960; 39: 781-98.

144. Palmer RM, Lumsden AS. Development of periodontal ligament and alveolar bone in homografted recombinations of enamel organs and papillary, pulpal and follicular mesenchyme in the mouse. Arch Oral Biol. 1987; 32: 281-9.

145. Ten Cate AR, et al. The development of the periodontium. A transplantation and autoradiographic study. Anat Rec. 1971; 170: 365-79.

146. Ten Cate AR. Cell division and periodontal ligament formation in the mouse. Arch Oral Biol. 1972; 17: 1781-4.

147. Ten Cate AR, et al. The development of the periodontium. the origin of alveolar bone. Anat Rec. 1972; 173: 69-77.

148. Yoshikawa DK, Kollar EJ. Recombination experiments on the odontogenic roles of mouse dental papilla and dental sac tissues in ocular grafts. Arch Oral Biol. 1981; 26: 303-7.

149. Karring T, et al. Development of the biological concept of guided tissue regeneration-animal and human studies. Periodontology 2000. 1993; 1 : 26-35.

150. Caton JG, et al. Histometric evaluation of periodontal surgery. Ⅱ. Connective tissue attachment levels after four regenerative procedures. J Clin Periodontol. 1980; 7 : 224-31.

151. Karring T, et al. New attachment formation on teeth with a reduced but healthy periodontal ligament. J Clin Periodontol. 1981; 12: 51-60.

152. Becker W. Guided tissue regeneration for periodontal defects. In: Polson A M. Periodontal regeneration. Current status and directions. Chicago: Quintessence Publishing, 1994: 137.

153. Gottlow J, et al. New attachment formation at the result of controlled tissue regeneration. J Clin Periodontol. 1984; 11: 494-503.

154. Melcher AH. Periodontal ligament. In: Bhaskar SN(ed). "Orban's Oral Histology and Embryology", (10th ed). St Louis: CV Mosby, 1986: 198-231.

155. Yamamura T, Shimono M, et al. Differentiation and induction of undifferentiated mesenchymal cells in tooth and periodontal tissue during wound healing and regeneration. Bull Tokyo Dent Coll. 1980; 21: 181-222.

156. Inoue T, Shimono M, Yamamura T. Osteogenic activity of perio-dontal ligament of rat incisor. in vivo and in vitro. J Dent Res. 1988; 67: 401.

157. Inoue T, Chen SH, Shimono M. Induction of cartilage and bone formation by cells from explants of various oral tissues in vitro. Bull Tokyo Dent Coll. 1989; 68: 416.

158. Andreasen JO. Interrelation between alveolar bone and periodontal ligament repair after replantation of mature permanent incisors in monkeys. J Periodontal Res. 1981; 16: 228-35.

159. Andreasen JO. Delayed replantation after submucosal storage in order to prevent root resorption after replantation. An experimental study in monkeys. Int J Oral Surg. 1980; 9 : 394-403.

160. Houston F, Sarhed G, Nyman S, Lindhe J, Karring T. Healing after root reimplantation in the monkey. J Clin Periodontol. 1985; 12: 716-27.

161. Gottlow J, Nyman S, Lindhe J, Karring T, Wennstrom J. New attachment formation in the human periodontium by guided tissue regeneration. Case Report. J Clin Periodontol. 1986; 13: 604-16.

162. Bowers G, Chadroff B, Carnevale R, Mellonig J, Corio R, Emerson J, Stevens M, Romberg E. Histologic evaluation of new attachment apparatus formation in humans. Part Ⅲ. J Periodontol. 1989; 60: 683-93.

163. Iseri H, Solow B. Continued eruption of maxillary incisors and first molars in girls from 9 to 25 years, studied by the implant method. Eur J Orthod. 1996 Jun; 18(3): 245-56.

164. Ingber JS. Forced eruption. I. A method of treating isolated one and two wall infrabony osseous defects-Rationale and case report. J Periodontol. 1974; 45: 199-206.

165. Langer B, Wagenberg BD. Method of altering crestal levels. J Periodontol. 1979; 50: 520-31.

166. Brown IS. The effect of orthodontic therapy on certain type of periodontal defects. I. Clinical findings. J Periodontol. 1973; 44: 742-56.

CHAPTER 4

Classification of Autotransplantation of Teeth and its Indications and Criteria

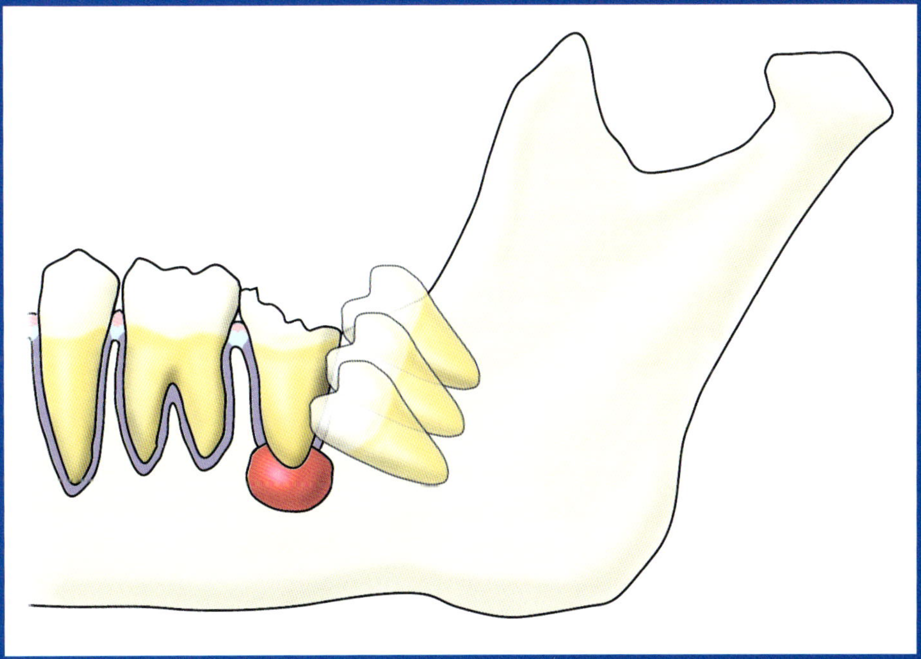

Classification of autotransplantation of teeth

Autotransplantation of teeth (ATT) is defined as "a procedure to surgically move teeth from one site to another in the same individual"[1] (**Fig 4-1**). "Surgical up-righting" (**Fig 4-2**) and surgical extrusion[2,3] (**Fig 4-3**) in which the extracted tooth is replanted into its original alveolar socket in a different and more optimal position can be considered to be a category of ATT because the healing process is essentially the same. These procedures can also be referred to as intra-alveolar transplantation[3,4,5,6,20]. Intentional replantation, which involves extract-

Classification of Autotransplantation of Teeth

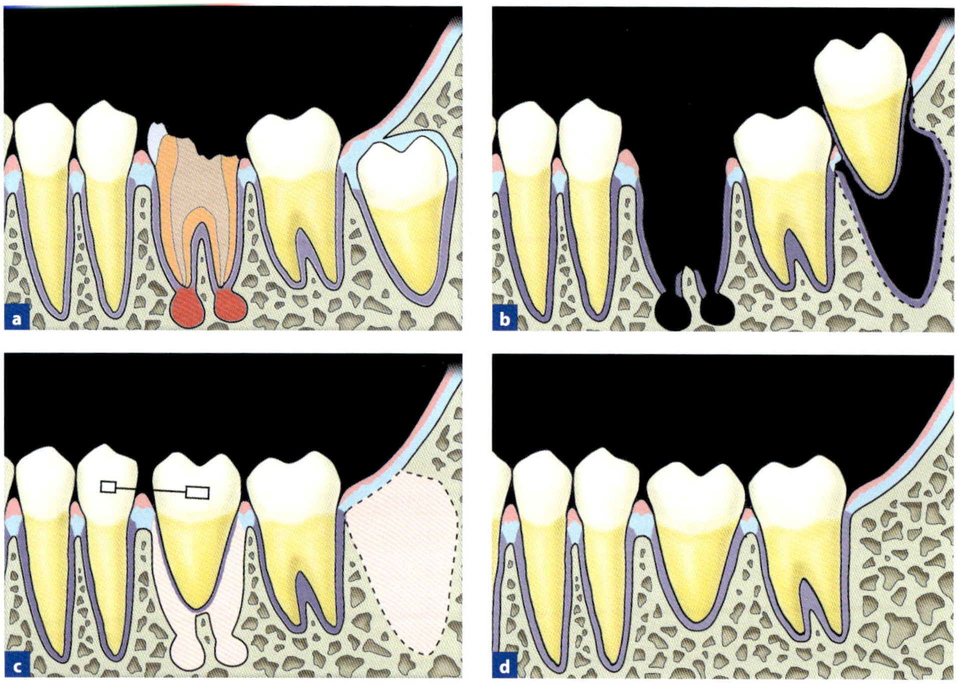

Illustration of conventional transplantation

Fig 4-1a Preoperative condition. Transplantation of a non-functional third molar to a hopeless first molar.
Fig 4-1b Recipient and donor tooth are both extracted.
Fig 4-1c Immediately after surgery. The donor tooth was placed into the extraction socket of the recipient site.
Fig 4-1d After healing.

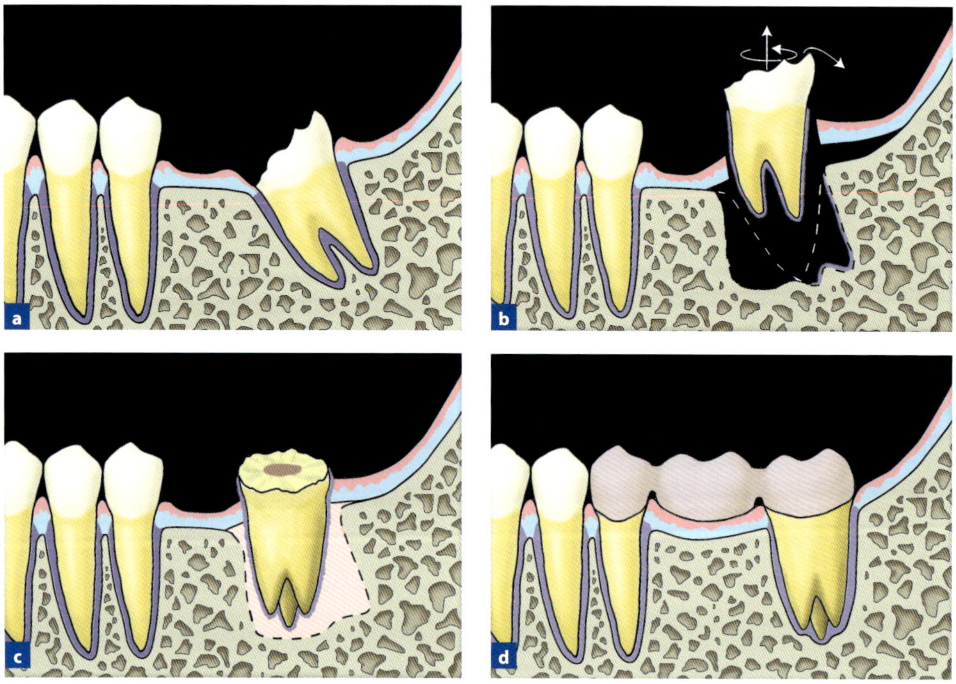

Illustration of intra-alveolar transplantation (surgical up-righting)
1. Surgical up-righting

Fig 4-2a Preoperative condition. A tooth is involved in inclination and deep caries.
Fig 4-2b After luxation of the tooth, a cavity preparation is formed within the extracted socket.
Fig 4-2c Immediately after surgical up-righting.
Fig 4-2d After healing and restoration.

ing teeth, performing extraoral procedures, and then replanting them back in the original alveolar socket[7,8] (**Fig 4-4**) may also be regarded as another category of ATT procedures. Therefore, ATT is classified into three categories: (1) conventional transplantation, (2) intra-alveolar transplantation (surgical extrusion and surgical up-righting), and (3) intentional replantation. Indications and criteria shall be discussed according to each category, along with case examples which highlight how these procedures involve a multi-disciplinary approach.

Illustration of intra-alveolar transplantation (surgical extrusion)
2. Surgical extrusion

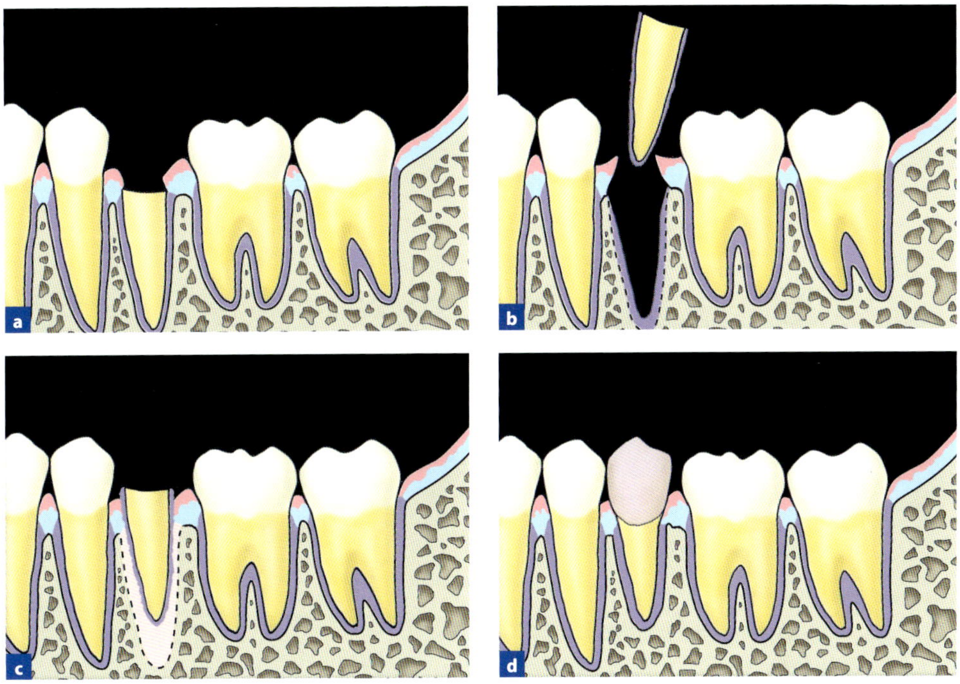

Fig 4-3a Preoperative condition. A deeply decayed tooth that can be saved by re-establishing biologic width and ferrule.
Fig 4-3b Luxation of the affected tooth.
Fig 4-3c Immediately after surgery. The tooth is placed more coronally in the extraction socket.
Fig 4-3d After healing and restoration.

Illustration of intentional replantation

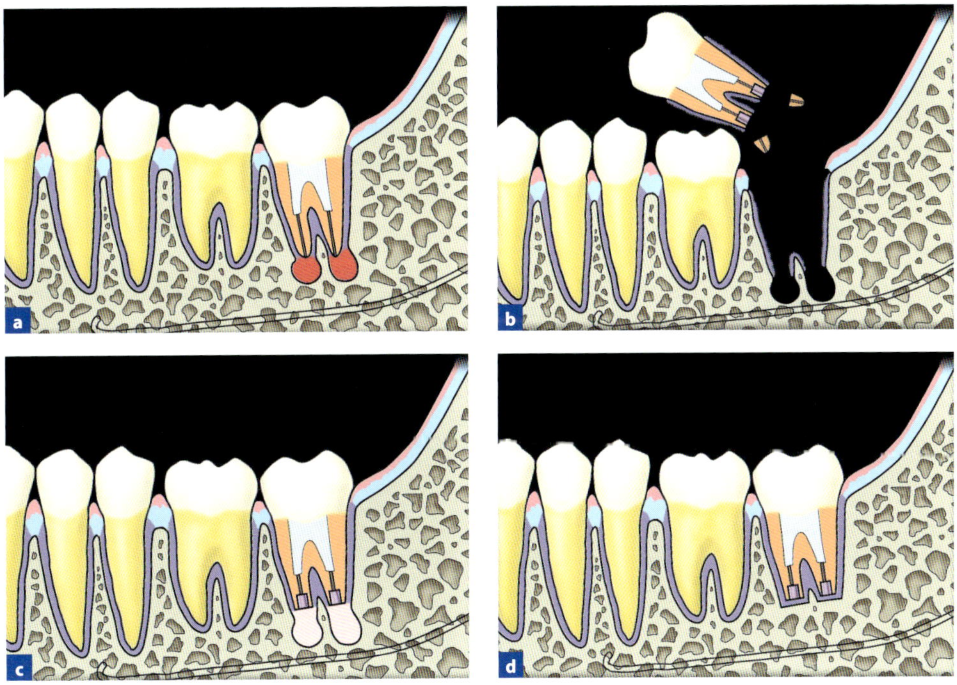

Fig 4-4a Preoperative condition. A second molar that has a symptomatic periapical lesion that cannot be treated by conventional endodontic treatment.
Fig 4-4b After luxation of the affected tooth, apicoectomy and retro-filling are performed extra-orally.
Fig 4-4c Immediately after surgery. The tooth is placed back into its original position.
Fig 4-4d After healing.

Indications and criteria for conventional transplantation

The indications and criteria for conventional transplantation will be discussed in regards to benefits over other treatments, patient factors, donor teeth, and recipient sites.

Benefits over other treatments

When considering the indications for transplantation, the advantages (functionality, time, cost, predictability, biological superiority) of transplantation over other treatments (implants, dentures, bridges, orthodontics, etc.) should be considered[9, 20, 24, 25]. In general, if there are teeth that cannot be preserved in the oral cavity and at the same time there are teeth that are not in function, such as wisdom teeth and displaced teeth, ATT can be a possible treatment option. Many of the indications for ATT are cases in which wisdom teeth (third molars) are transplanted into extraction sockets of molars which can't be preserved (**Fig 4-5** to **4-7**). If the wisdom tooth size is appropriate, it can be transplanted in a premolar regions (see **Chapter 7 Fig 7-1, 7-2,** and **7-5**) or in the anterior (see **Chapter 8 Fig 8-3**). Donor teeth are not limited to third molars. Displaced or impacted premolars may serve as donors (**Fig 4-8**). If there are no donor teeth available and the patient wants a fixed prosthesis, implant supported treatment can be a favorable option (**Fig 4-9**).

Patient factors

Because transplantation is a surgical procedure, the patient should not have major systemic problems. It is necessary to obtain informed consent, and the patient must have good compliance throughout the treatment process. In terms of predictability, treatment success appears more favorable in younger individuals (detailed in **Chapter 11**), and for those who do not have metabolic or immune disorders such as diabetes, as well as non-smokers.

Donor teeth

Suitable donor teeth are ones that are not in function and have appropriate root morphology. In terms of the stage of root development, it has been suggested that teeth with incomplete roots are more predictable than teeth with completed roots[30-33] (see **Chapter 11**), possibly due to the ease of extraction as well as higher healing potential of the periodontal ligament (PDL). It is recommended to choose donor teeth in stage 4 or 5 of root development[30-33]. If the root development stage is lower than this, root development may not occur sufficiently after transplantation, and if it is higher than this, healing of the pulp will less predictable (see **Chapter 3**). The ideal root morphology is a slightly tapered, conical, single-rooted tooth with few irregularities (**Fig 4-10a** to **4-10d**). Teeth with widely spread roots (**Fig 4-10h**), and teeth with very curved roots (**Fig 4-10e**) will have higher risks of damage to the PDL during extraction and difficulty fitting into the recipient site. Teeth with shorter root trunks used for ATT may have higher risk of furcation involvement. Sometimes multi-rooted teeth which have enamel projections (**Fig 4-10f**) and teeth with periodontal attachment loss of more than one-third of the root due are also not a favorable donor tooth (**Fig 4-10g**). If there are two or more donor teeth available in the oral cavity, the tooth with the better crown shape and fit should be used (see **Chapter 6 Fig 6-2**). Typically, maxillary third molars (as donors) are morphologically more similar to the other maxillary molars (as recipients) than the mandibular third molars, and it's easier to reshape or restore them if needed. However, if the crown morphology is very similar, choosing a root with a simpler morphology (single-root, conical type) will likely lead to a simpler surgical procedure and thus a better prognosis (see **Chapter 7 Fig 7-1**).

Recipient sites

In terms of morphology, the ideal alveolar ridge has a width and height that allows the accommodation of the donor. It appears that there is better healing potential if the recipient socket has PDL still attached when the donor tooth is transplanted[10-12](**Fig 4-5** and see **Chapter 3**). In the maxilla, a sinus lift procedure can be performed to allow for accommodation of the donor tooth[50-52] (see **Chapter 5 Fig 5-5** and **Chapter 6 Fig 6-5**). Enlarging and manipulating the recipient site can be challenging, so having a that site large enough to accommodate the donor tooth minimizes risks. It is preferred to perform the transplantation on the same day of extraction or within 1 month of the extraction of the hopeless tooth (**Fig 4-5**).

Indications and criteria for conventional transplantation

Transplantation of a mature tooth

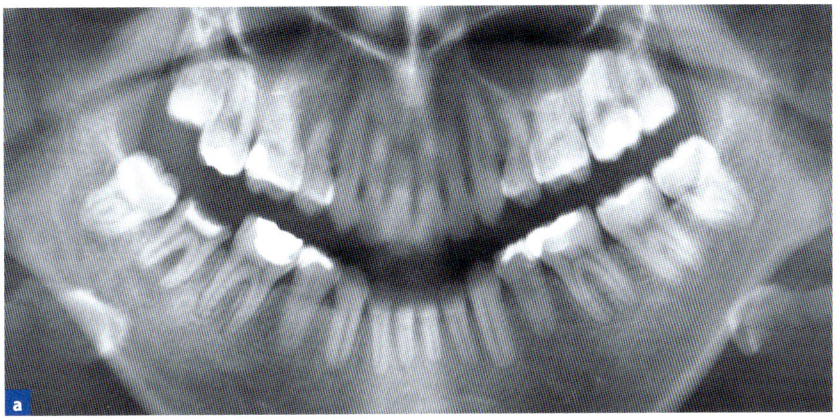

Fig 4-5a Preoperative panoramic radiograph of a 24-year-old female. The patient was referred from another clinic. Orthodontic treatment had been completed, and #47 had a previously initiated root canal treatment with an unfavorable prognosis.

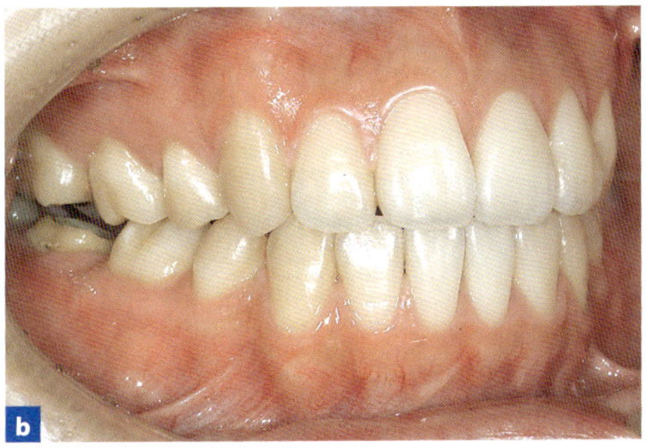

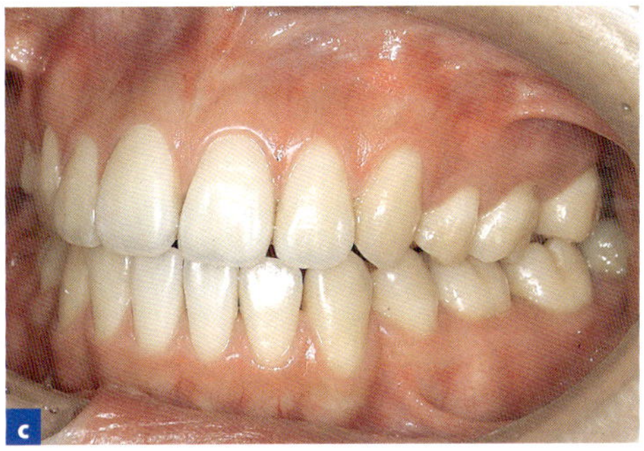

Fig 4-5b, c Preoperative lateral views of the mouth.

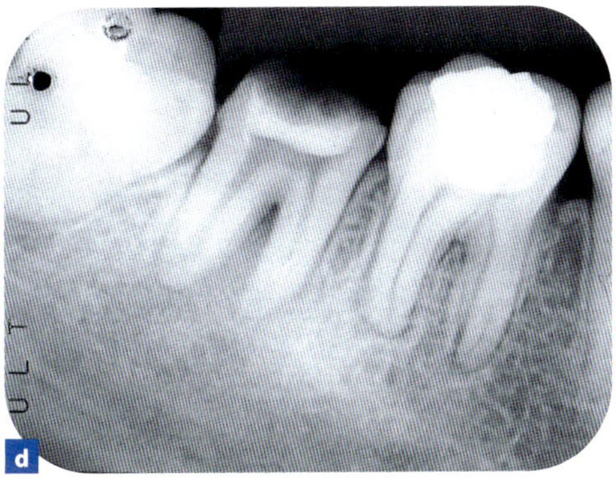

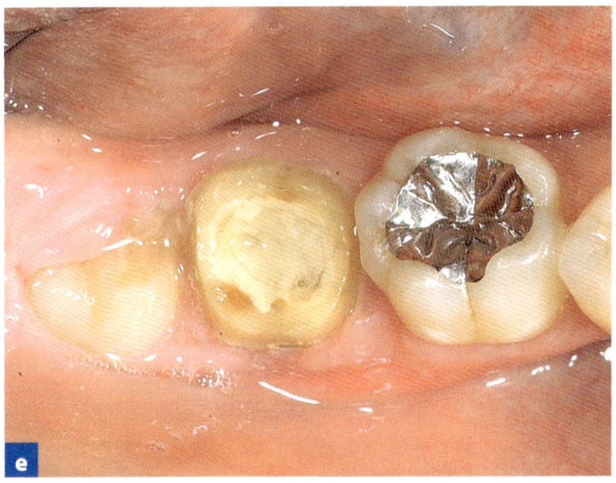

Fig 4-5d Preoperative radiograph.
Fig 4-5e Preoperative occlusal view.

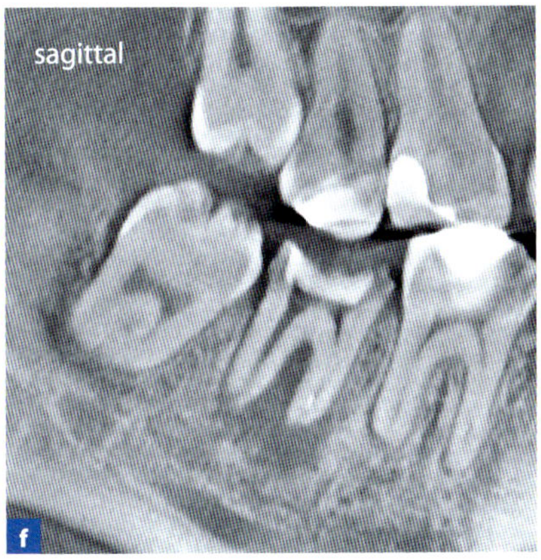

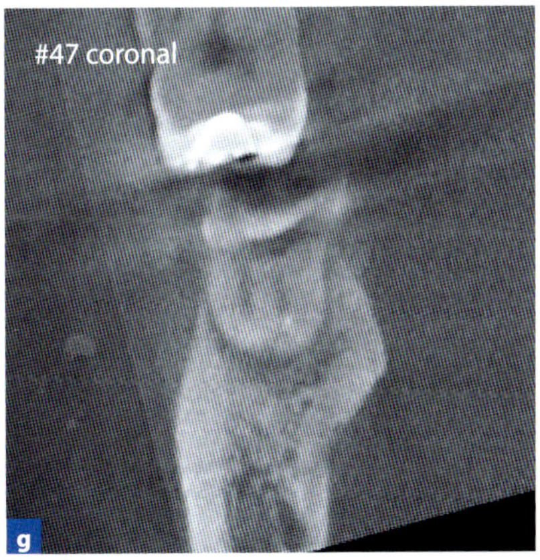

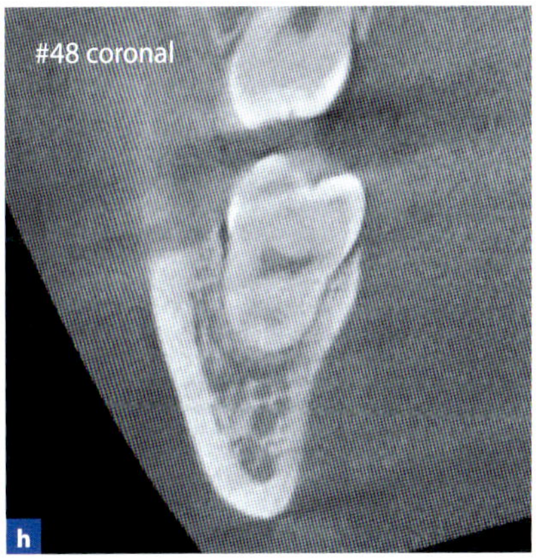

Fig 4-5f, g, h Preoperative CBCT images. #47 may be treated but the long-term outcome would be guarded due to structural compromise. When considering the morphology of the donor tooth (#48), that of the recipient (#47), the age of the patient, and the predictability, ATT was the treatment of choice. The patient did not want the option of orthodontic tooth movement of #48 because it would require a longer period of treatment time.

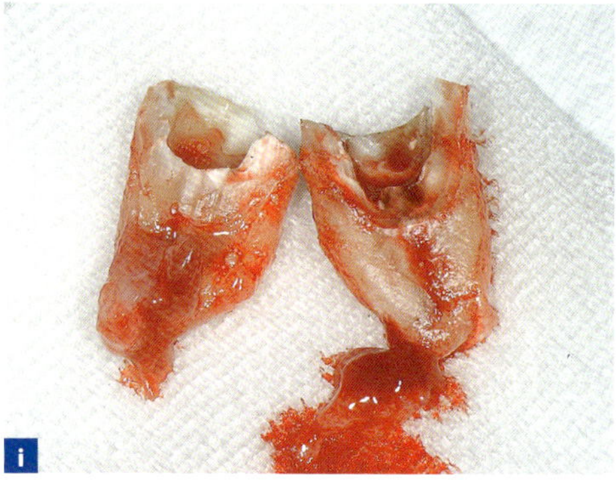

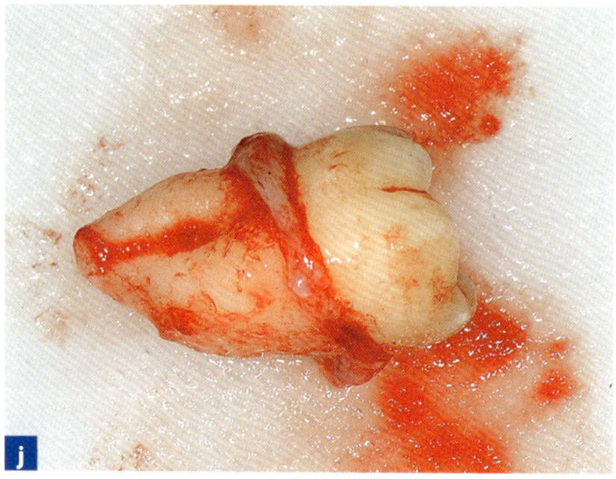

Fig 4-5i Extraction of tooth #47.
Fig 4-5j The extracted donor tooth #48.

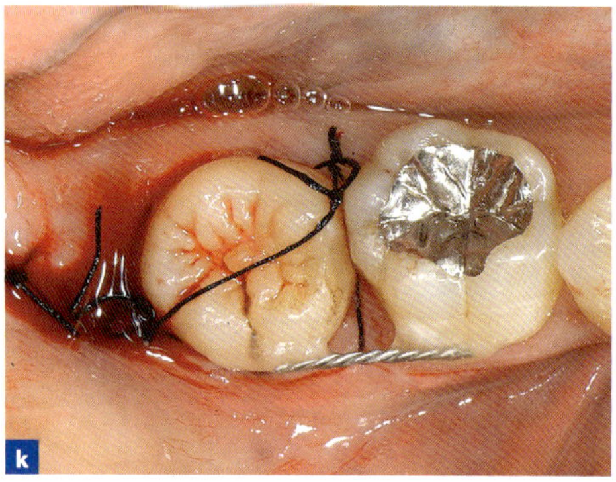

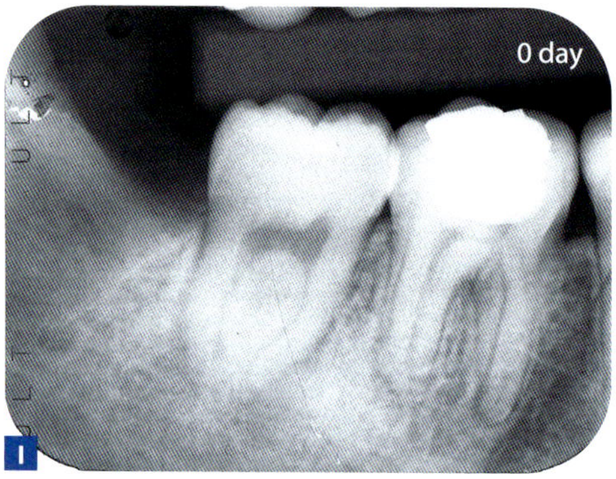

Fig 4-5k Occlusal view immediately after transplantation. The extraction of the recipient site and the transplantation of the adjacent third molar were performed on the same day (immediate transplantation).
Fig 4-5l Radiograph taken immediately after transplantation.

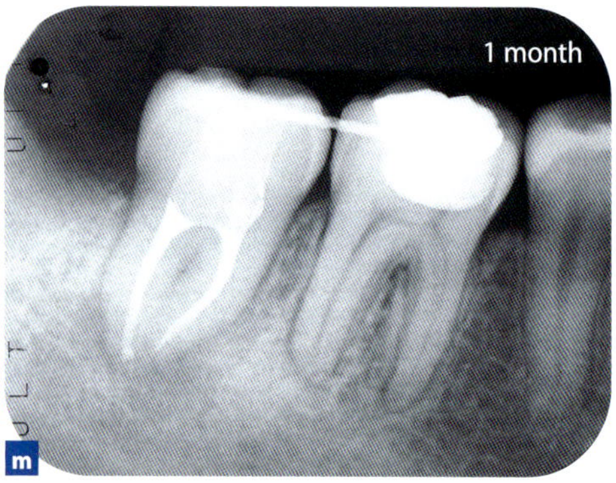

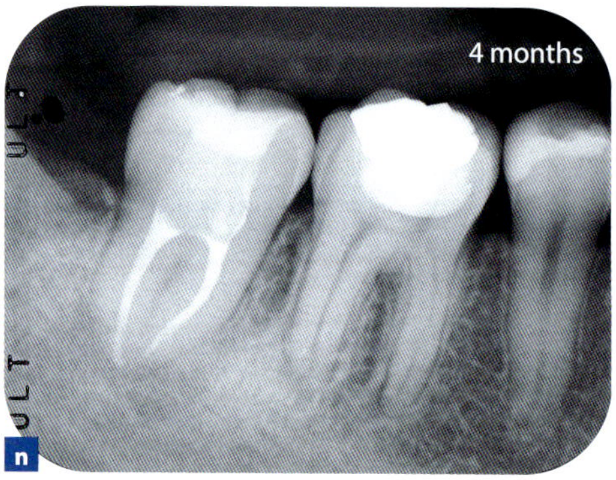

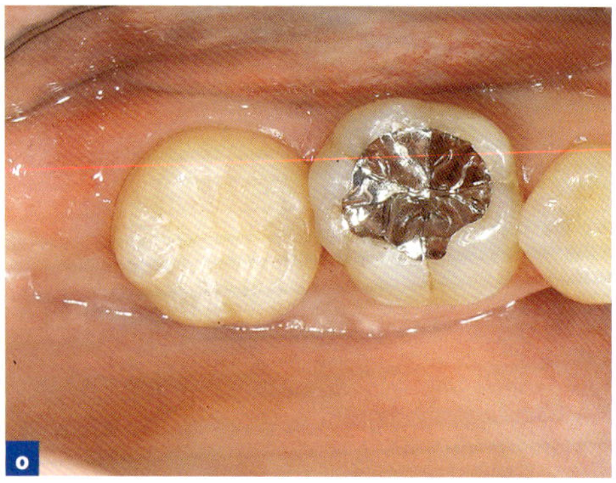

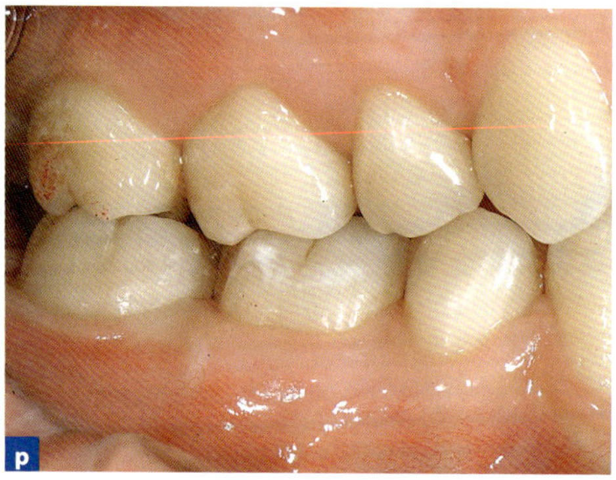

Fig 4-5m One month after the surgery and immediately after root canal filling of the transplanted tooth. The wire splinting was removed on the same day.
Fig 4-5n Four months postoperative. Findings suggestive of healing.
Fig 4-5o Clinical photograph on the same day as **Fig 4-5n**. Immediately after restoration of the transplanted tooth with composite resin (CR). Restoration with CR can preserve tooth structure and result in good esthetics and function. In addition, the time and cost required for prosthetics (indirect restoration) can be avoided.
Fig 4-5p Same day as **Fig 4-5n**. An adequate occlusal relationship was obtained.

Transplantation of an immature tooth

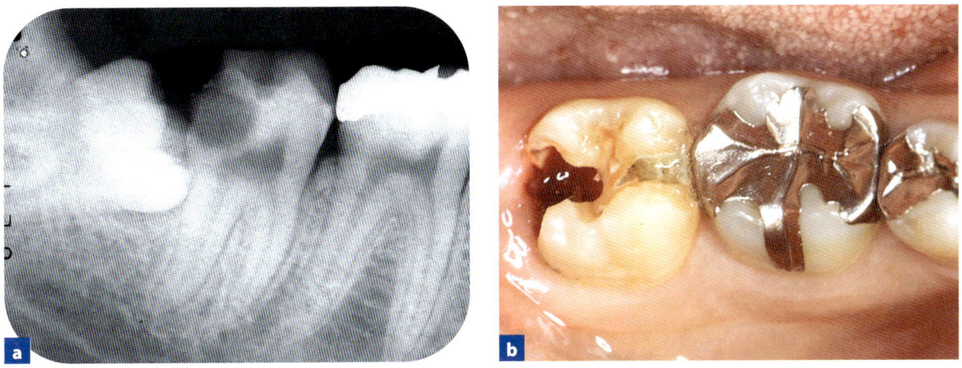

Fig 4-6a, b Preoperative radiograph and occlusal view of a 19-year-old male who visited our clinic with symptoms of pulpitis. It was thought that there were more advantages in transplantation using the adjacent third molar than to try and preserve the deeply decoyed molar.

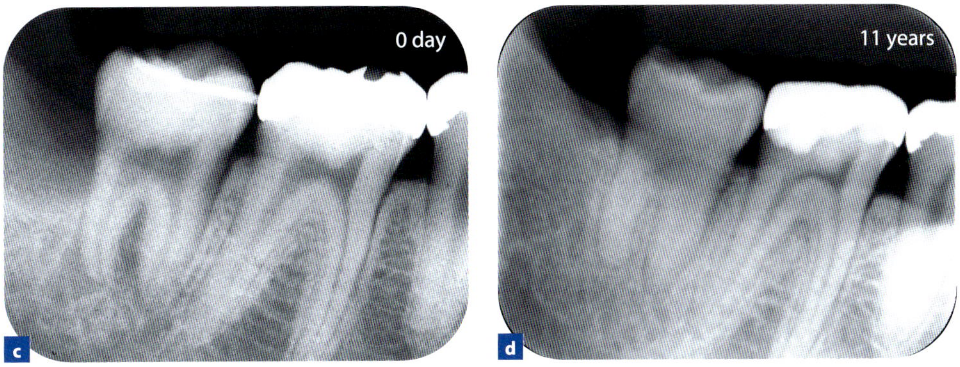

Fig 4-6c Immediately after transplantation. Although the root of the transplanted tooth was almost complete, healing of the dental pulp could be expected because Hertwig's epithelial sheath was present at the time of transplantation.

Fig 4-6d 11 years postoperative. There is positive response to EPT.

Two transplantations in the same mouth

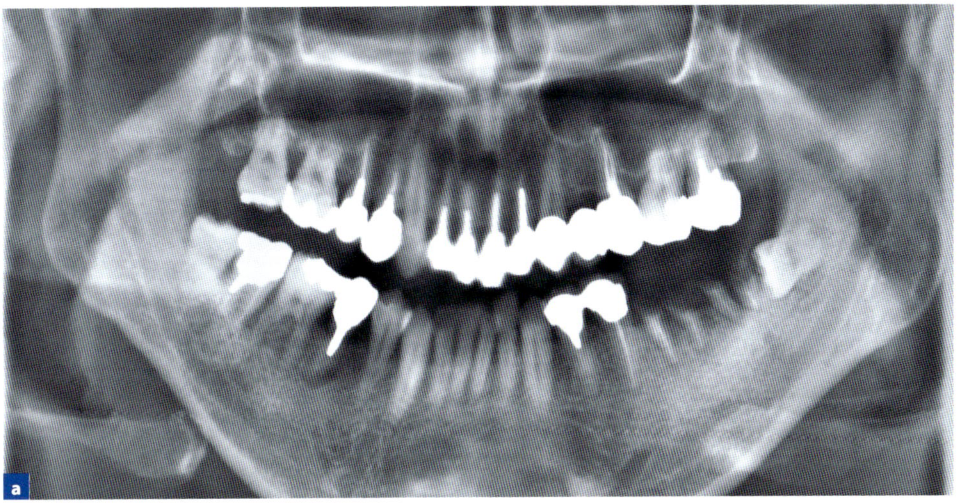

Fig 4-7a Preoperative panoramic radiograph of a 35-year-old male. He visited our clinic with the chief complaint of deep dental caries in the molar region. The patient accepted the treatment plan of transplantation of the left and right mandibular third molars into #36 and #37 sites.

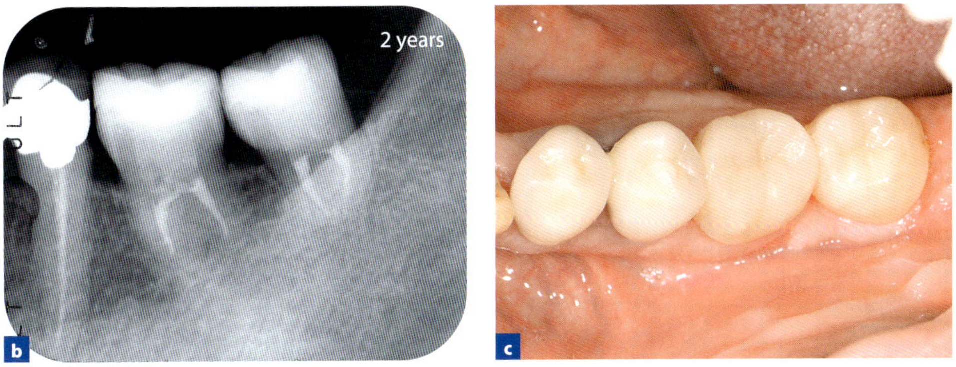

Fig 4-7b, c Two years after transplantation. The crowns are restored with CR.

Transplantation using a tilted and displaced premolar

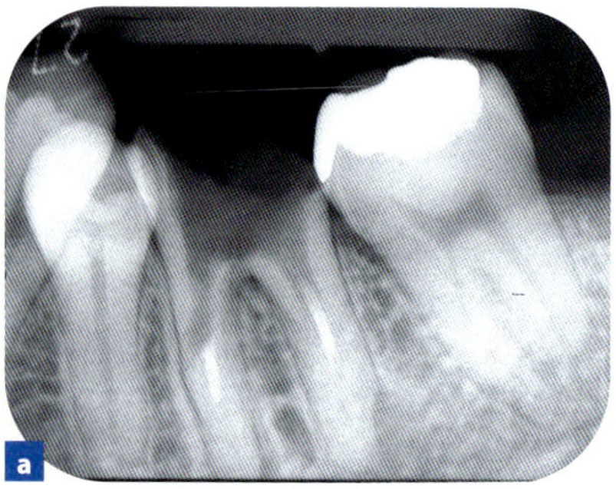

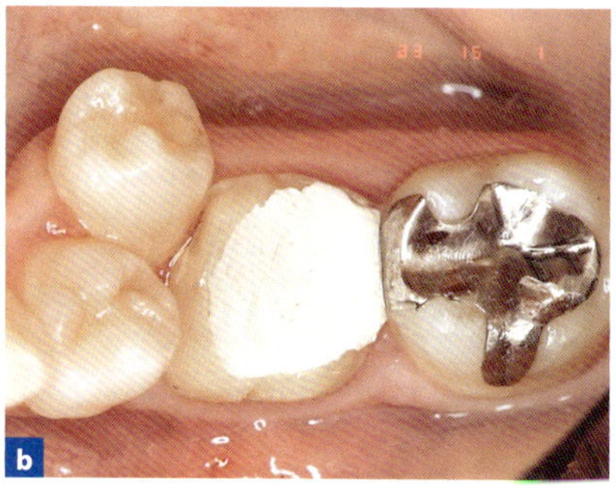

Fig 4-8a, b Preoperative radiograph and occlusal view of a 26-year-old female that presented with the chief complaint of a lost restoration on #36. It was considered that the prognosis would be unfavorable so the patient chose to have ATT of #35 that was displaced into the #36 site.

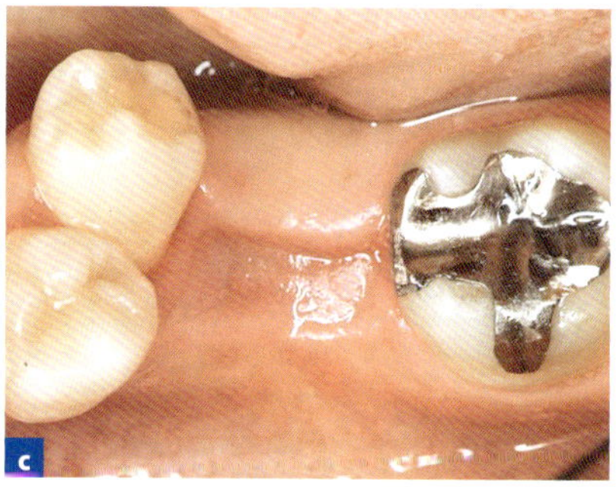

Fig 4-8c One month after tooth extraction of #36 and just before transplantation. Sufficient keratinized gingiva is formed 3 to 4 weeks after extraction, which will make it easier to close flap around the transplant.

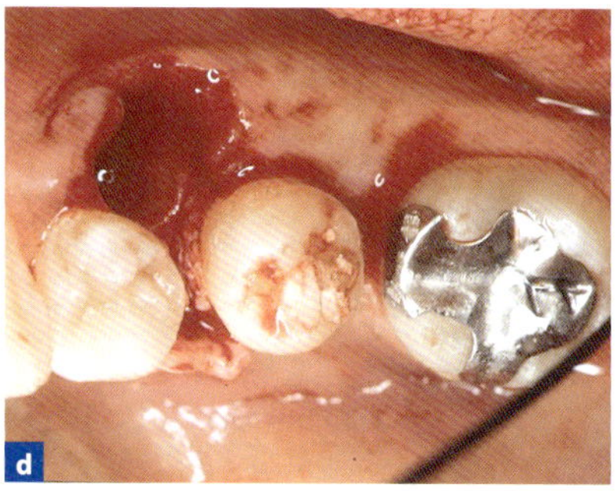

Fig 4-8d Immediately after transplantation.

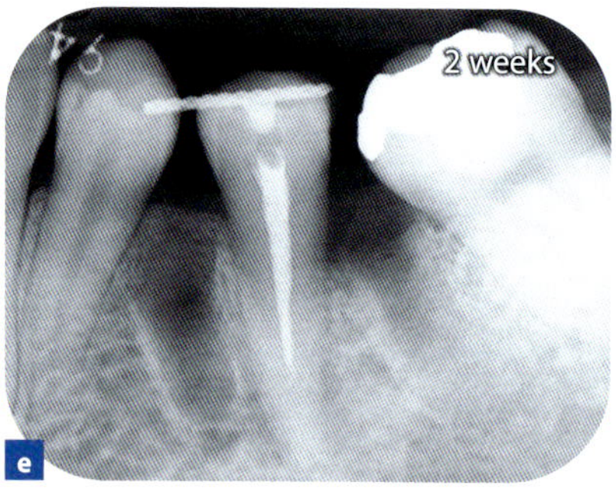

Fig 4-8e Two weeks after surgery. The root canal treatment of the transplant was initiated.

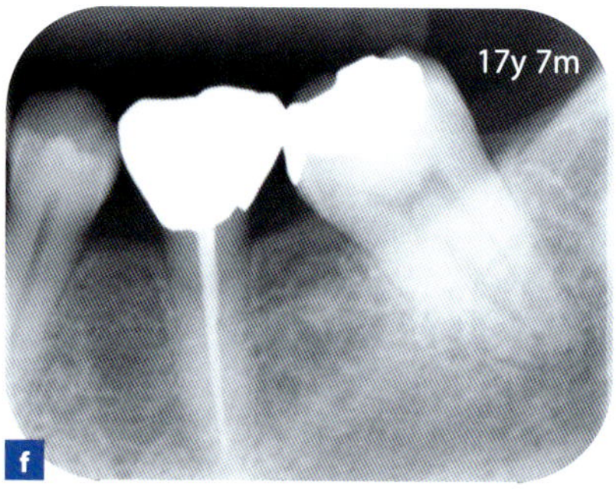

Fig 4-8f 17 years and 7 months postoperative. No problem was observed with the transplant, and the patient was content with the treatment and outcome.

A case of implant therapy

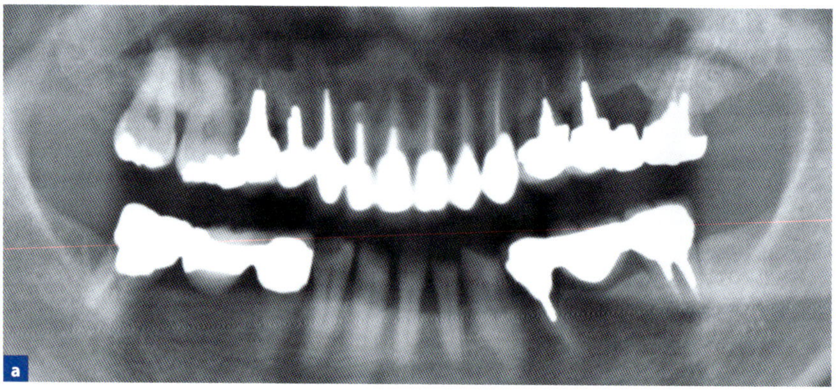

Fig 4-9a Preoperative panoramic radiograph of a 58-year-old female. The chief complaint was pain around #47. There was a diagnosis of root fracture and because there was no donor tooth, implant supported treatment was a good treatment alternative.

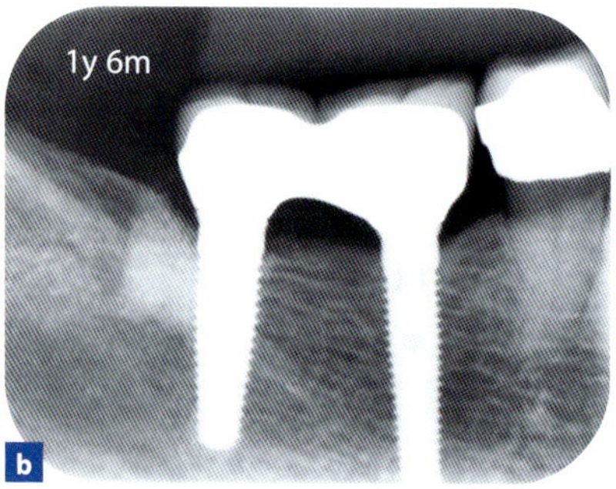

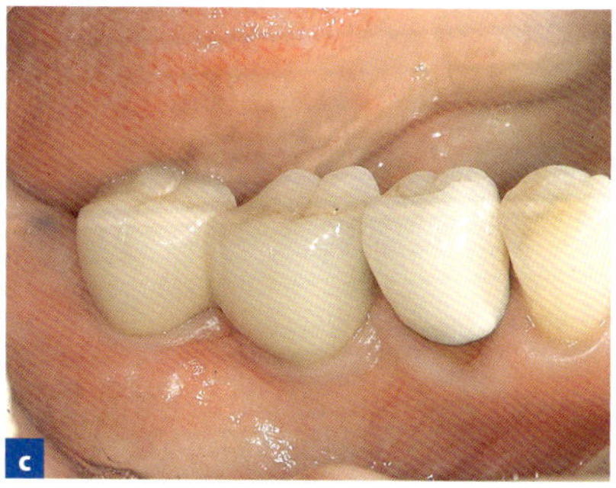

Fig 4-9b, c One year and 6 months after surgery. The patient is content with the treatment results.

Root morphology of donor teeth

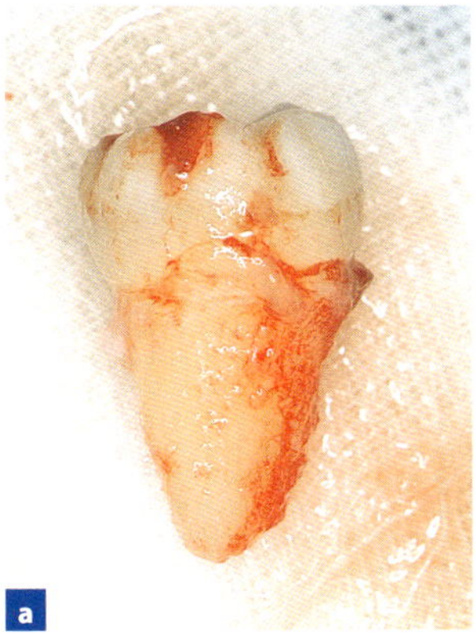

a

Fig 4-10a Ideal root morphology as a donor.

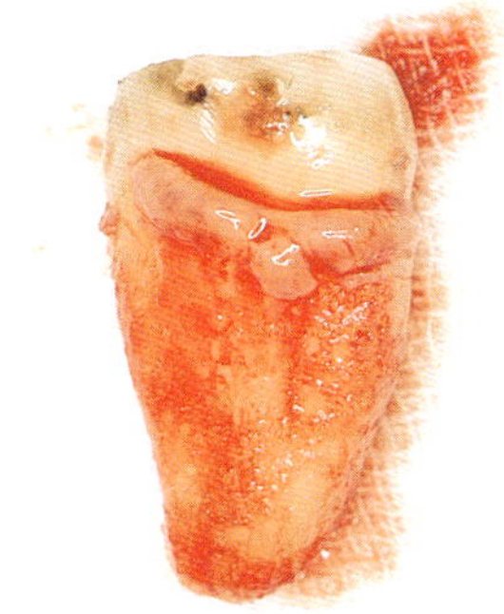

b

Fig 4-10b Wider root form but still close to ideal.

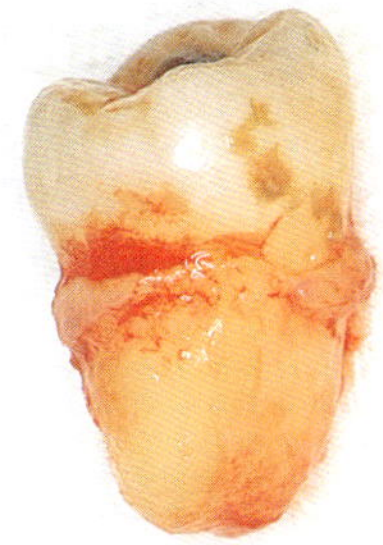

c

Fig 4-10c Root length is short, but the shape is still favorable.

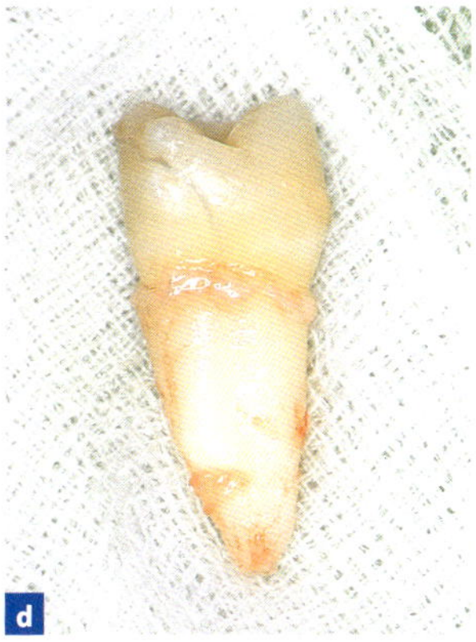

d

Fig 4-10d Premolar with a favorable morphology as a donor.

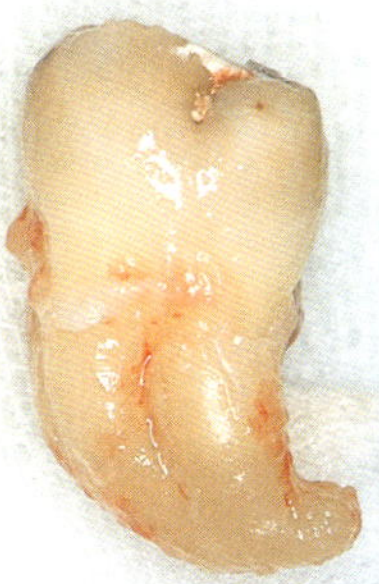

e

Fig 4-10e Tooth with higher root curvature may not be a favorable donor.

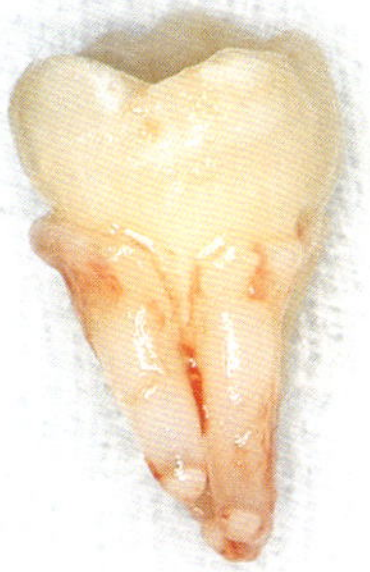

f

Fig 4-10f Tooth with enamel projection typically is not a good donor tooth.

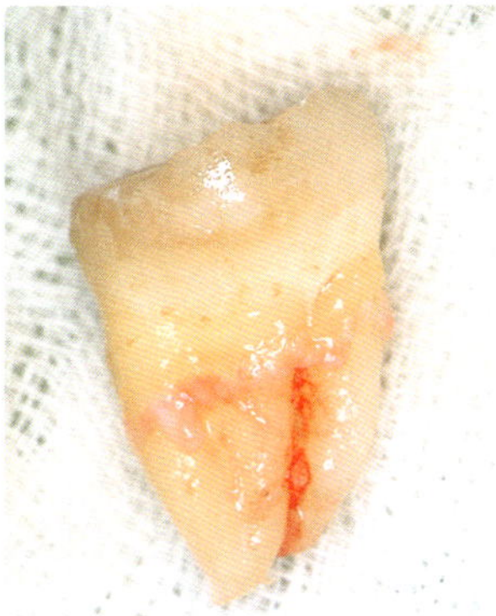

g

Fig 4-10g Tooth with visible loss of PDL attachment may not have favorable healing.

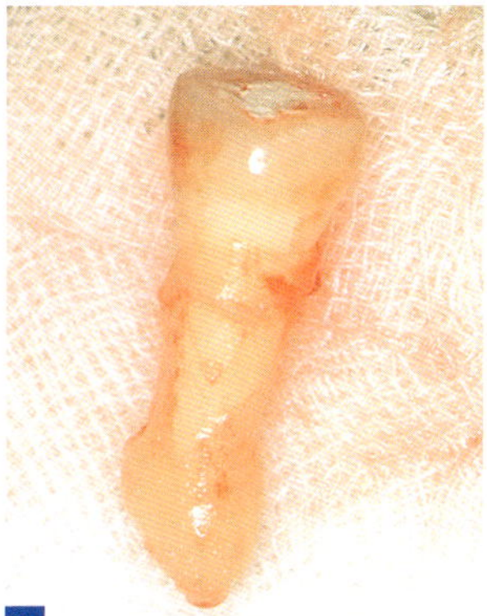

h

Fig 4-10h Tooth with bulbous root may not be a favorable donor tooth.

Mandibular horizontally impacted third molars

In many cases, horizontally impacted third molars can be transplanted into adjacent site of the hopeless second molar. The prognosis of transplantation in these cases appears to be affected by the position (depth) of the third molar (**Fig 4-11**) and the pre-existing bone loss and bony defect left after the extractions have taken place. The deeper the impaction the more difficult it is to extract the donor tooth, and the higher the risk to mechanically damage the periodontal ligament during extraction. When the horizontally impacted third molar is located more coronal, it becomes more difficult to close the gingival flap on the distal surface of the transplanted tooth, and this may lead to higher risks that the gingival reattachment fails, and deeper pockets are likely to form in this area. However, even if there are pockets on the distal aspect, the tooth can still be asymptomatic and functional long-term but good hygiene and maintenance is important. Therefore, it is better for the horizontally impacted tooth to be positioned more apically. The procedure for transplanting the mandibular horizontal impacted tooth to the adjacent second molar is further explained in **Chapter 5 Fig 5-6**.

Maxillary impacted third molars

When a young patient presents with a maxillary second molar that has poor prognosis and has an adjacent third molar that has not yet erupted, it can be expected that the third molars will spontaneously erupt into the same area after the extraction of the second molar (**Fig 4-12** and **4-13**). Therefore, when caries has progressed to the where the tooth may be questionable and mid to long-term prognosis is not favorable, it may be more beneficial for such patients to think about extracting the second molar and wait for natural eruption of third. This does not seem to happen with impacted third molars in the mandible.

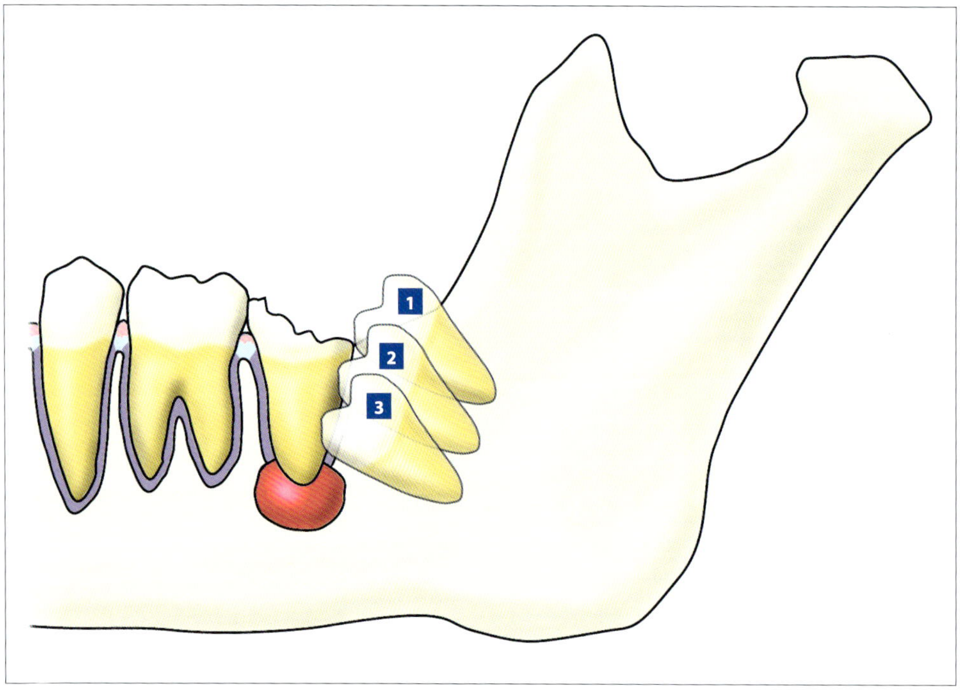

Considerations for transplantation of Horizontally impacted mandibular third molars.

Fig 4-11 When a horizontally impacted third molar is transplanted to the adjacent second molar site, the closer the impacted tooth is to the apex of the recipient side, the more difficult it is to extract the tooth, the larger the bony defect, and the more likely it is to damage the PDL of the donor tooth (position 3). When the crown of the third molar is located coronally and has erupted from the gingiva, it is more difficult to achieve closure at the distal aspect of the transplanted tooth and may decrease the prognosis of healing of the PDL (position 1). Therefore, it is ideal for the horizontally impacted molar to be positioned near the coronal third of the root of the second molar (position 2).

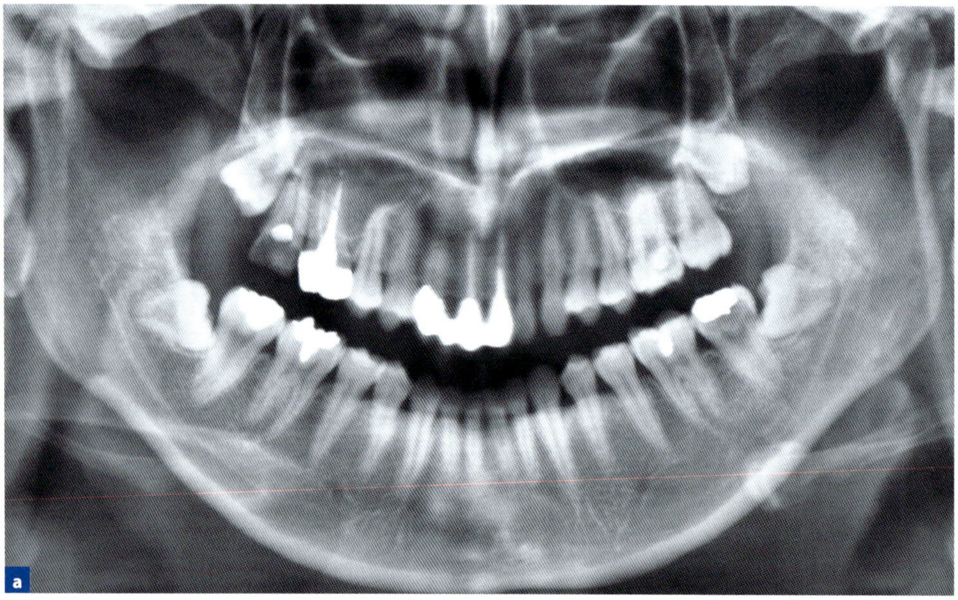

a

Maxillary impacted third molar with natural eruption and migration (1)

Fig 4-12a Preoperative panoramic radiograph of a 21-year-old female. The chief complaint was deep caries of #17 which was had an unfavorable prognosis. It was thought that the adjacent impacted third molar could erupt and migrate naturally to the extraction site of #17.

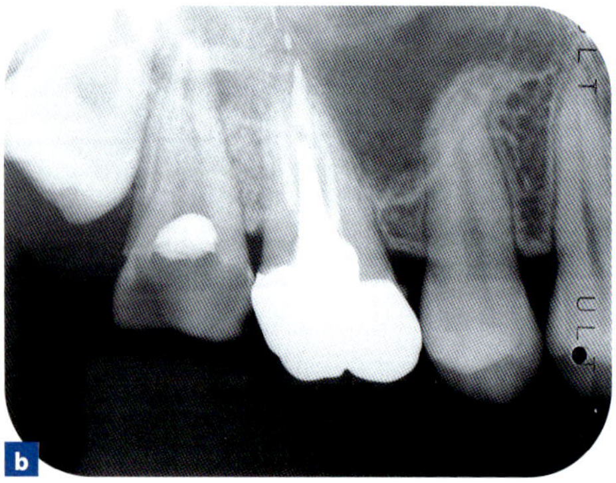

b

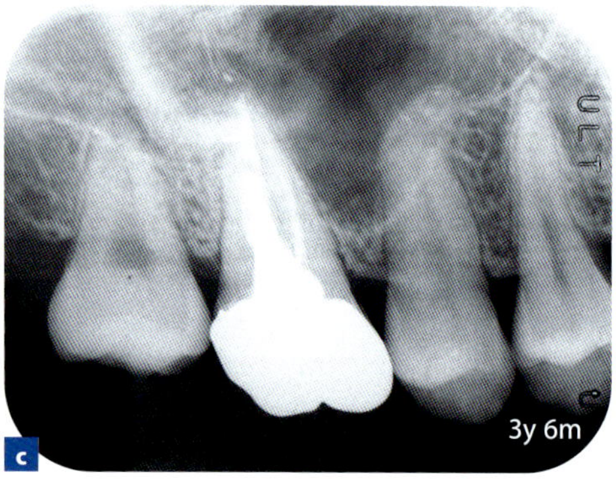

c

Fig 4-12b Preoperative radiograph.

Fig 4-12c Radiograph after 3 years and 6 months. The third molar has erupted and migrated to the position of #17.

Maxillary impacted third molar with natural eruption and migration (2)

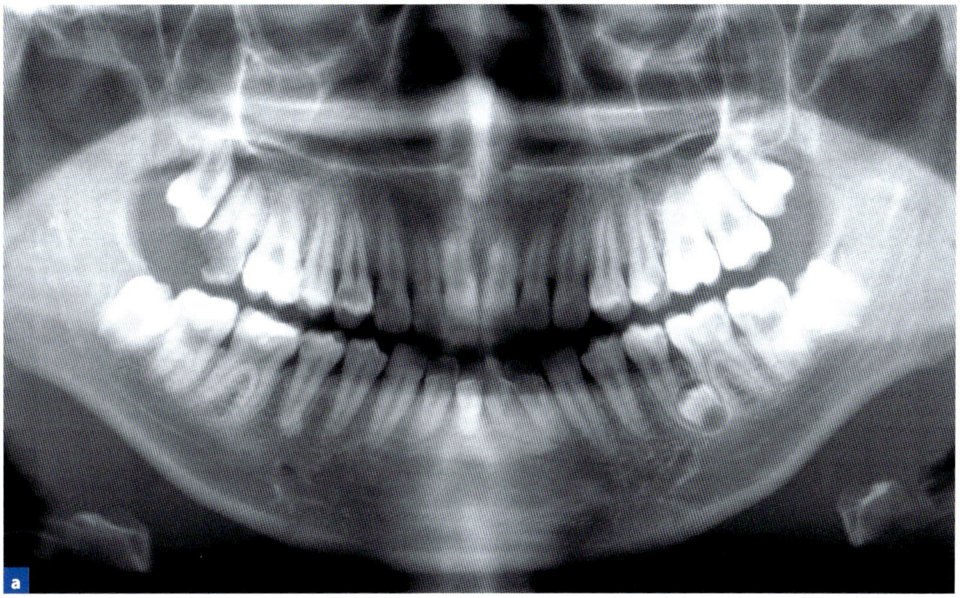

Fig 4-13a Preoperative panoramic radiograph of a 17-year-old female. The chief complaint was caries of #17 which had an unfavorable prognosis. #17 was extracted and #18 was expected to erupt and migrate naturally to the #17 position.

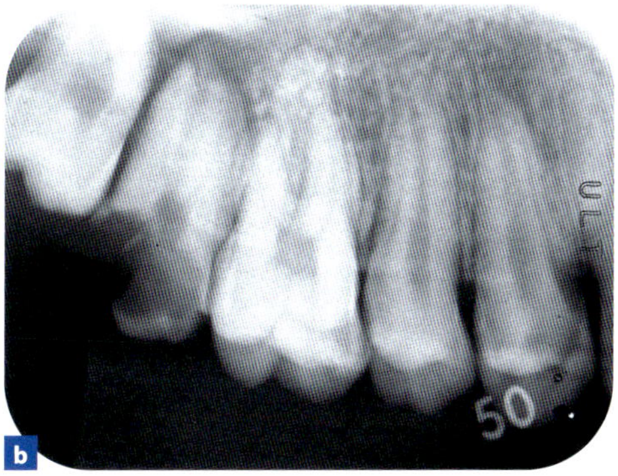

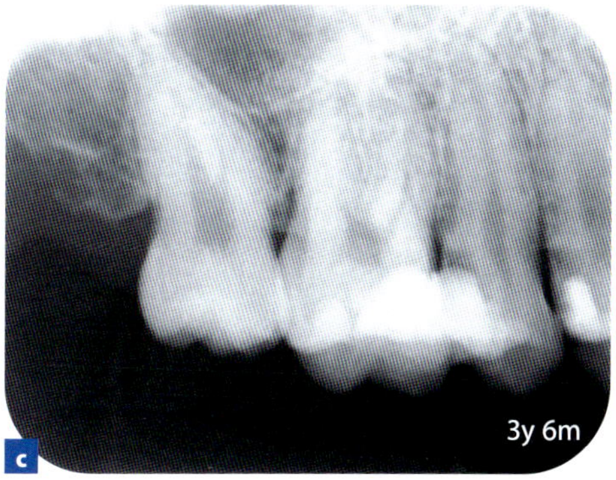

Fig 4-13b Preoperative radiograph.
Fig 4-13c Radiograph after 3 years and 6 months. The third molar has erupted and migrated nicely to #17 position.

Indications and criteria for intra-alveolar transplantation

If it is difficult to restore or preserve the tooth due to deep caries or fracture due to trauma, surgical extrusion or up-righting may be indicated, where the extracted tooth is replanted into the original socket changing the vertical position or inclination to create a better outcome[2-6].

The indications and risk-benefit for intra-alveolar transplantation must be compared to limited orthodontic treatment (LOT) [13-19]. In general, both methods are highly predictable, but LOT may have reduced risk of root surface damage but generally takes longer and possibly more costs. The following are indications for surgical extrusion and up-righting.

Appropriate root morphology

Selecting teeth that have less risk of damage to the periodontal ligament will lead to more predictable outcomes. Teeth that are single-rooted teeth, and have a conical shape, are indications for surgical extrusion and up-righting (**Fig 4-14** and **4-15**). Conversely, teeth with concave root surface, multi-rooted tooth with spread out roots, curved root, or bulbous root form is difficult to extract so these carry higher risks.

Indications for "Intra-alveolar transplantation"

1. Surgical up-righting

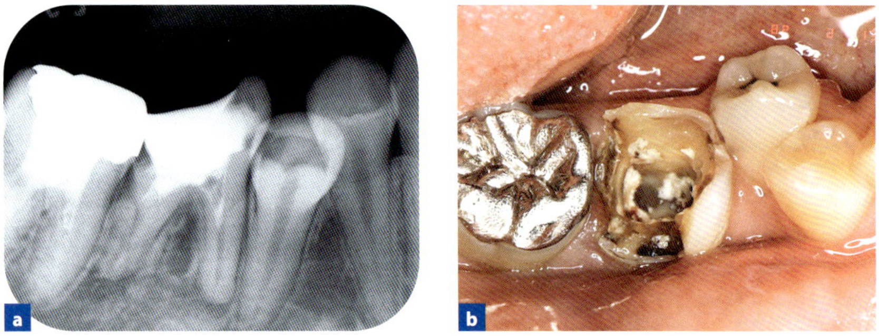

Fig 4-14a, b Preoperative radiograph and occlusal view of an 18-year-old female. #46 is involved in deep caries that leaves little remaining tooth structure. Extraction of #46 and surgical up-righting of #45 and fabricating a bridge are considered better option.

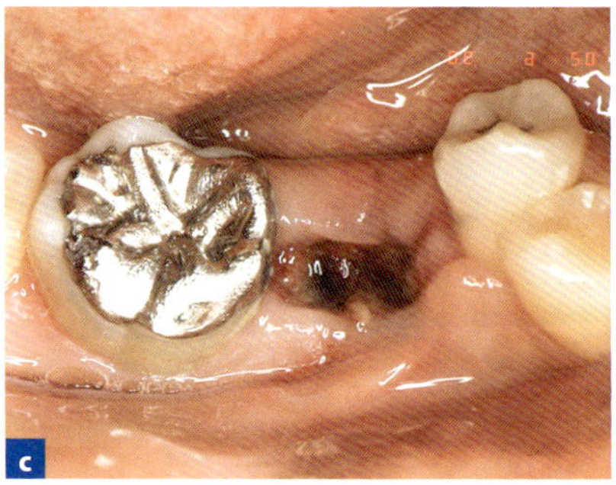

Fig 4-14c After extraction of #46.

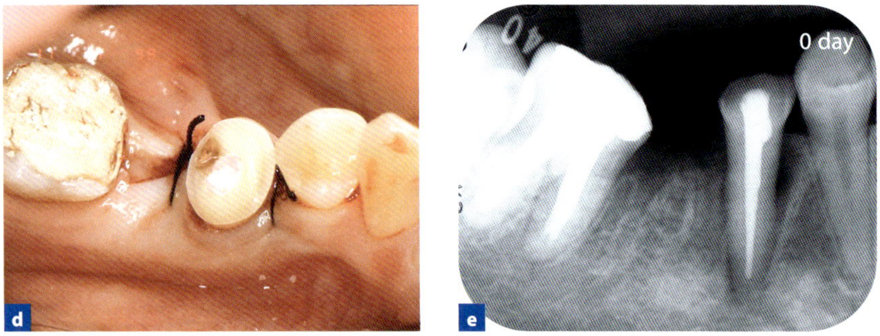

Fig 4-14d, e Immediately after surgical up-righting of #45. The root canal treatment of #45 was completed prior to surgery.

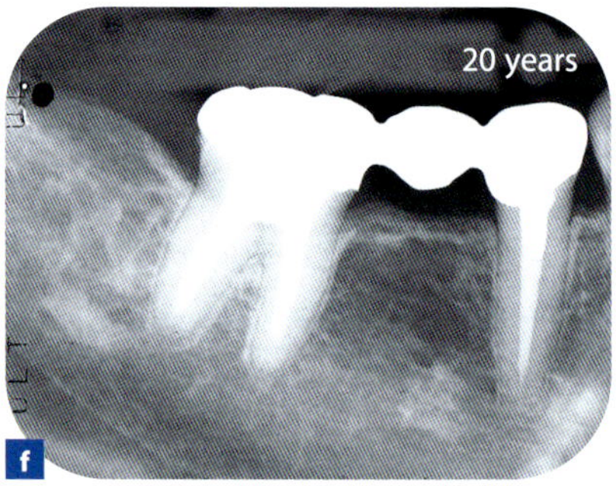

Fig 4-14f 20 years after the surgery. Tooth is asymptomatic, functional and the radiograph shows no apparent abnormalities.

Difficulty with orthodontic appliances

Surgical extrusion and up-righting may be better indicated if the orthodontic appliance cannot be properly attached due to lack of interocclusal space or isolated teeth (**Fig 4-15**).

Obliquely impacted second molars may be corrected by surgical reposition

(**Fig 4-16**)

However, this procedure ruptures the blood vessels (blood supply) to the pulp at the apex, and thus may lead to pulp necrosis and need for endodontic treatment. Although revascularization can be expected in immature teeth, pulpal healing typically results in pulp canal obliteration (**Fig 4-16**). Thus in vital teeth, LOT may be have more benefit and less risks but will take more time.

Extrusion with rotation of the tooth

For cases with deeper oblique fracture due to trauma or caries located deeply on the mesiodistal or palatal aspect, surgical extrusion may be advantageous. When trying to secure an appropriate amount of healthy tooth structure above the crest with minimal extrusion, the most damaged root surface should be brought to the buccal side to improve restorability (see **Fig 4-19** described later). Thus, surgical extrusion with rotation can be more advantageous over LOT[44].

Time and cost-benefit

In general, surgical extrusion takes less time than orthodontic extrusion. The coronal restoration (if needed) is possible to perform 3 to 5 weeks after surgical extrusion. In orthodontic treatment, if the retention period is not long enough, relapse is likely to occur[18] and can take more time to complete the restoration (**Fig 4-18** described later). Surgical extrusion may save on costs because it does not require as much orthodontic appliances and equipment.

2. Surgical extrusion

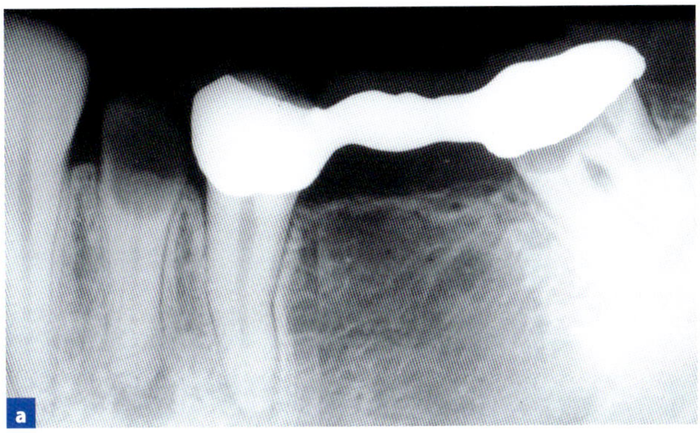

Fig 4-15a Preoperative radiograph of a 24-year-old female. #34 and #37 have deep caries. Because of the difficulty of performing orthodontic extrusion, surgical extrusion was chosen to reestablish the biological width and ferrule before the restorative procedure.

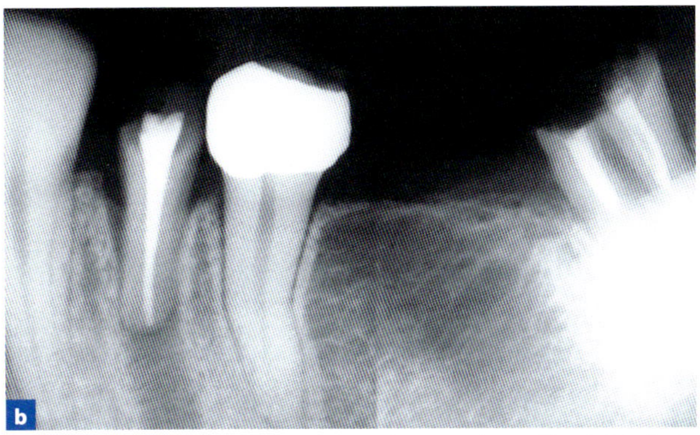

Fig 4-15b After surgical extrusion of #34 and #37. The RCT of #37 was completed after the surgery and #34 was completed before the surgery.

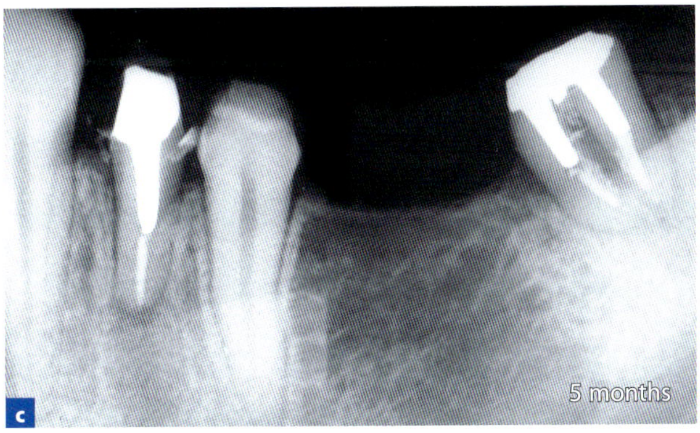

Fig 4-15c Five months after surgery.

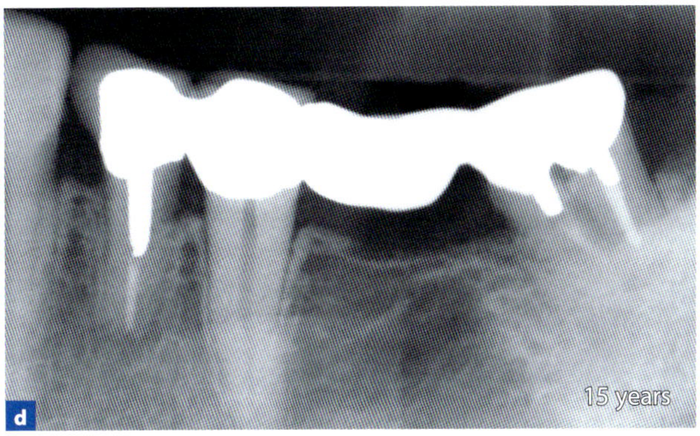

Fig 4-15d 15 years postoperative.

Definitive diagnosis of traumatized teeth

Teeth with crown-root fracture due to the traumatic injury can be extruded orthodontically or surgically to regain sufficient tooth structure above the crestal bone level. At this time, one may be able to detect more damages or issues with surgical extrusion which may not be detected with LOT[44].

3. Surgical reposition

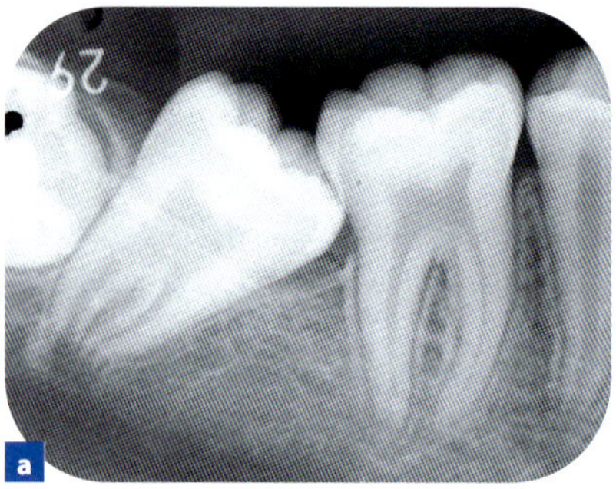

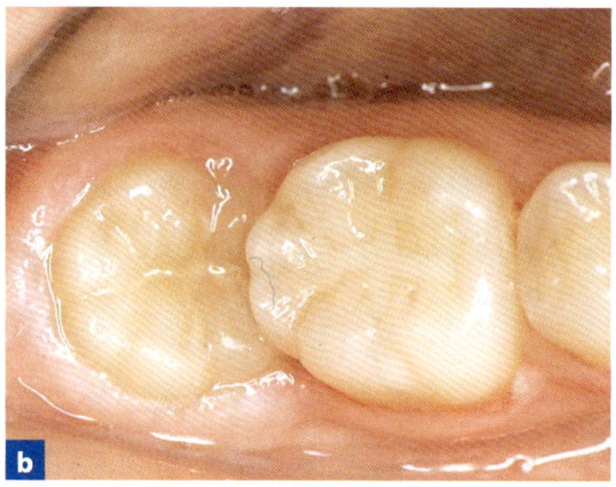

Fig 4-16a, b Preoperative radiograph and occlusal view of a 14-year and 5-month-old male. The chief complaint was issues around #47. Surgical reposition was chosen instead of orthodontic tooth movement because the tooth was immature and revascularization is possible and the patient could not afford orthodontic treatment and also we could save time on treatment.

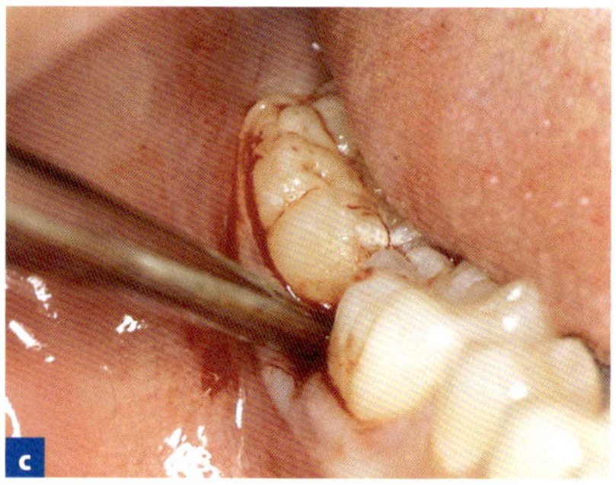

Fig 4-16c Intraoperative view. Under anesthesia, the tooth was repositioned surgically by an elevator.

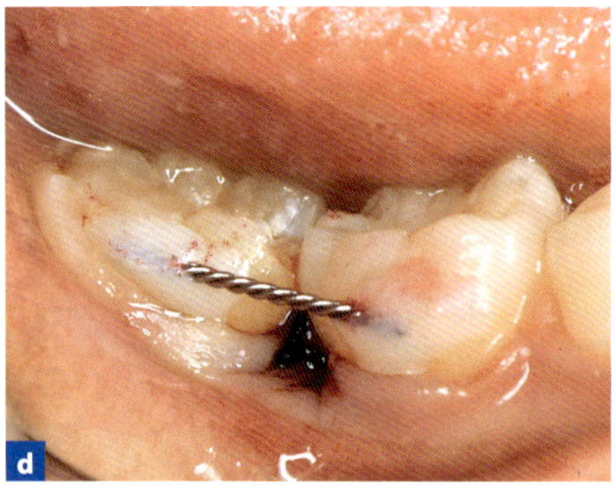

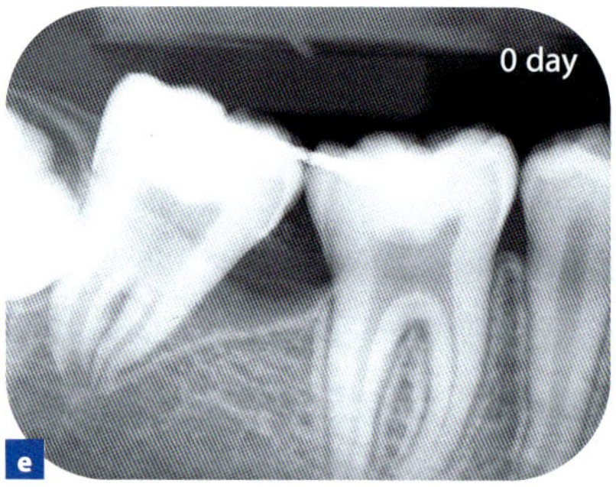

Fig 4-16d, e Immediately after surgery.

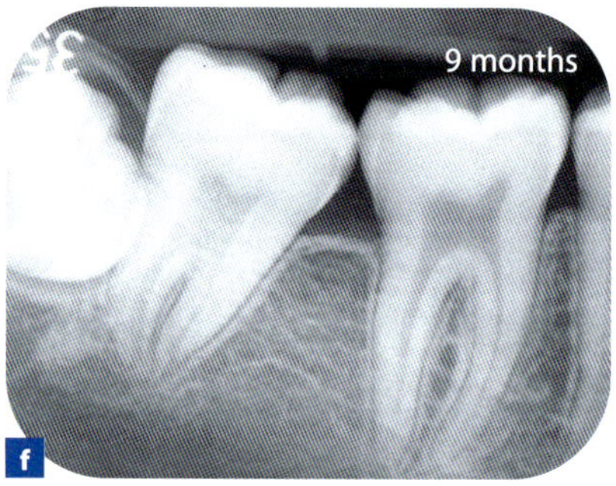

Fig 4-16f Nine months postoperative. The bony defect on the mesial aspect has already filled in with new bone, and the lamina dura has appeared. EPT response for #47 is positive.

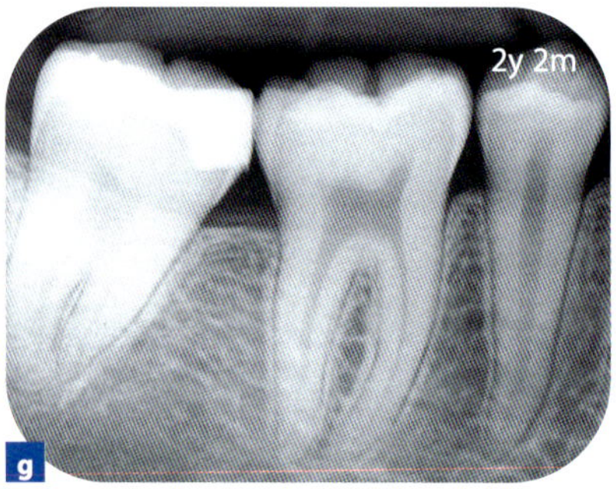

Fig 4-16g Two years and 2 months postoperative. The EPT response remains positive and pulp canal obliteration (PCO) has progressed. The mesial caries has been restored with CR.

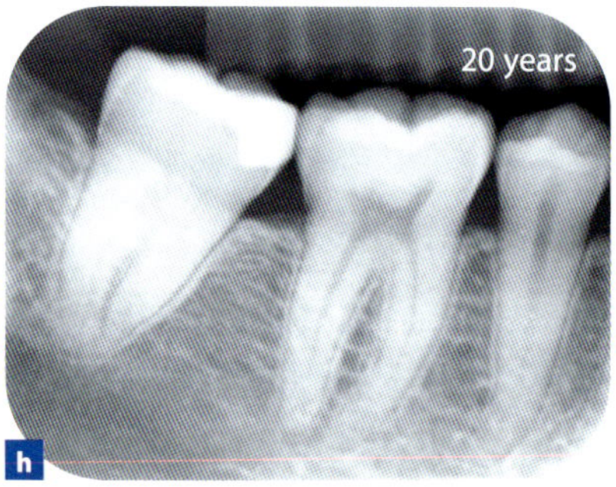

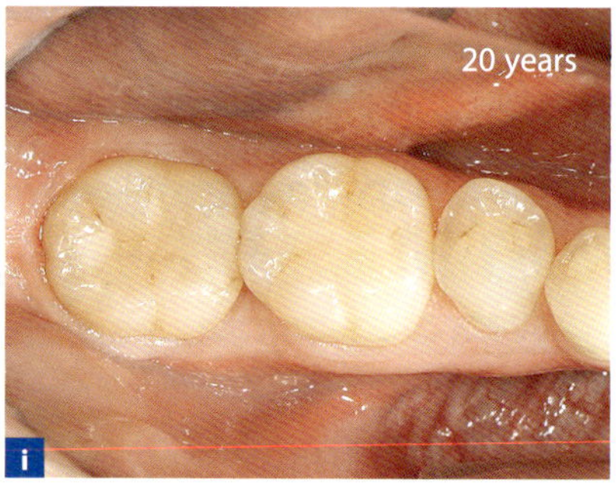

Fig 4-16h, i 20 years postoperative. Although PCO is observed, the EPT response is still positive.

Indications and criteria for intentional replantation

Intentional replantation is usually one of the last options to resolve root canal problems that cannot be treated by conventional orthograde endodontics or surgical endodontics such as apicoectomy (**Fig 4-17**). For example, if there is a problematic apical lesion in a tooth with a cast post that may be difficult or risky to remove, cases in which there are separated instruments, apical pulp space obliteration, lateral apical canals, zips, ledges, transportations, extraradicular biofilms, etc[7,8], intentional replantation would be indicated. Apicoectomy may be the first choice, but intentional replantation may be preferred in order to facilitate access to the affected tooth or to make a

A indication for intentional replantation

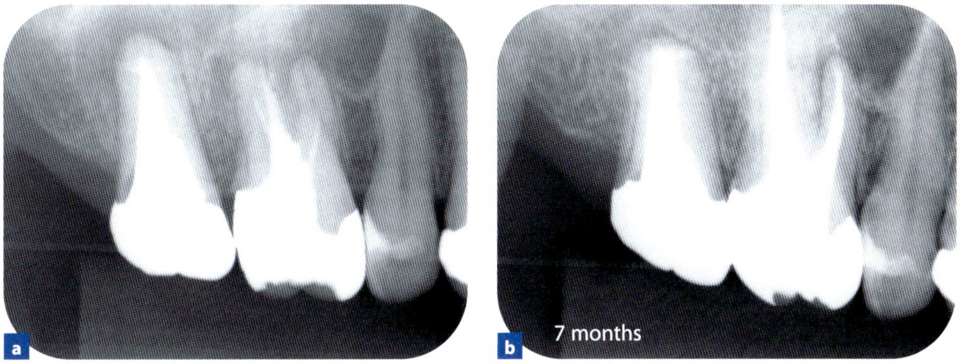

Fig 4-17a Preoperative radiograph around the right maxillary molars of a 24-year-old female. Apical radiolucencies were observed on #16 and #17. Because #17 was treated with a long and large post (removing it increases the risk of fracture and further weakening), and the root form was simple and single shaped, intentional replantation was indicated.
Fig 4-17b Seven months after intentional replantation of #17. Orthograde retreatment of #16 was performed.

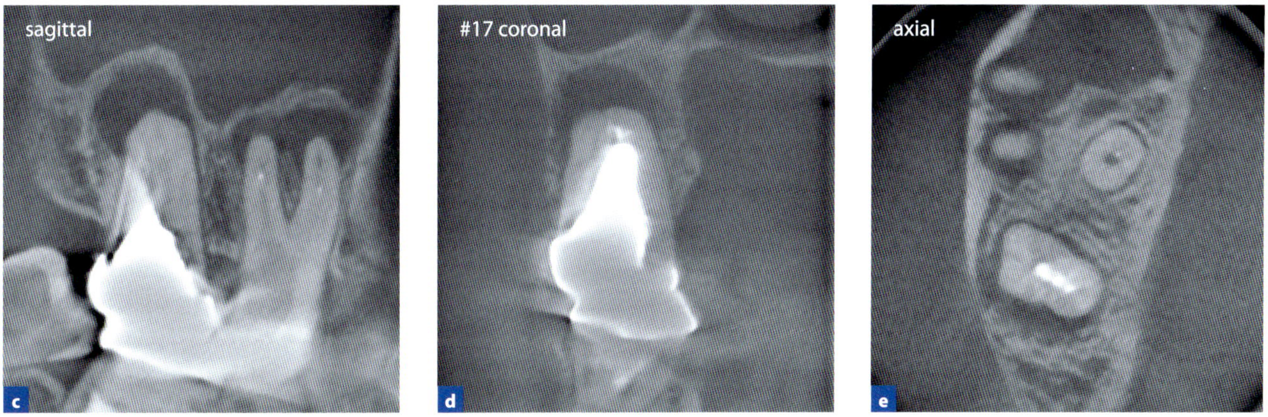

Fig 4-17c-e Preoperative CBCT images. All of the roots of #16 and #17 showed periapical radiolucent findings.

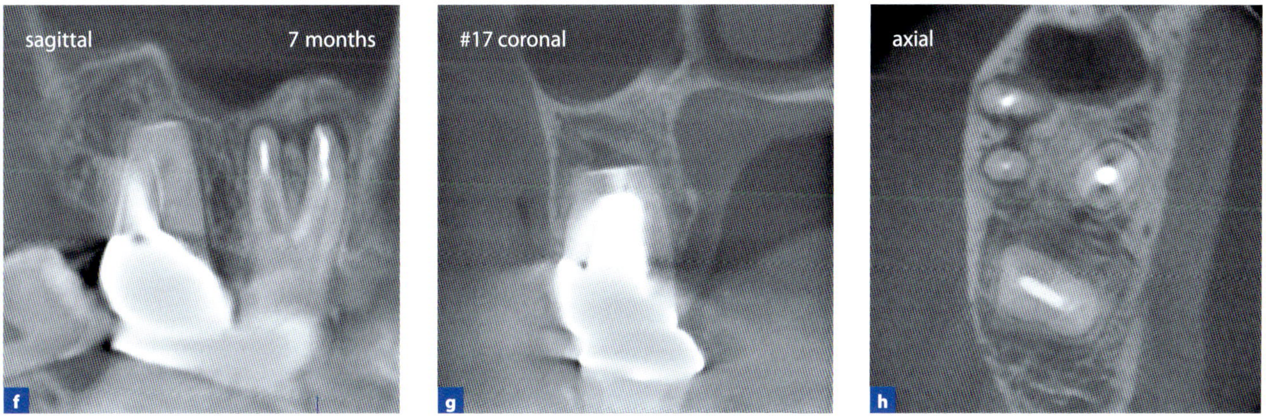

Fig 4-17f-h CBCT images 7 months after intentional replantation of #17. There is significant reduction in the size of the PARL findings.

definitive diagnosis of the affected tooth. If there are apical problems and or cervical problems such as deep caries, intentional replantation and surgical extrusion can be indicated. Indications for intentional replantation often depend on root morphology, as was discussed in cases of surgical extrusion. Teeth of single and tapered root are less susceptible to postoperative problems such as root resorption due to less PDL damage during extraction. Further details are discussed in **Chapter 10**.

Autotransplantation Across Multiple Disciplines

Prosthodontics and edentulism

Looking at the history of tooth transplantation, the main purpose for its use was to treat edentulous sites.[20-25,27,28,47,48]. If there are intact, non-functional teeth such as third molars, it is worth considering the possibility of transplantation before removable dentures, fixed bridges, and implants (**Fig 4-5** to **4-8**).

Orthodontics

If orthodontic alignment of displaced, mal-aligned, and or impacted teeth is difficult, or if treatment time is an issue, then surgical reposition or transplantation can be another option [34-39, 41, 42] (**Fig 4-7, 4-14** to **4-16**). If a patient who is going to start orthodontic treatment and has congenitally missing teeth or has lost teeth due to trauma, tooth transplantation can be indicated if there are teeth (e.g. premolar) that were to be removed for orthodontic treatment[28-33] (**Fig 4-23** and see **Chapter 9**).

Pediatrics and trauma

In cases that an anterior tooth has been avulsed due to a trauma and replantation has not been successful, the treatment to replace the missing or hopeless tooth with an appropriate donor tooth can be of great benefit in a young patient[20, 26, 27, 44]. When tooth decay or fracture due to trauma extends to or below the crestal bone, the tooth can be saved by surgical extrusion[3-6,26,27,44,46](**Fig 4-19**). Implant treatment is contraindicated in growing children (**Fig 4-21**).

Endodontics

If endodontic problems cannot be resolved with conventional root canal therapy or apicoectomy, intentional replantation with treatment done extra-orally can help save the tooth[8] (**Fig 4-17** and see **Chapter 10**).

Restorative dentistry

If caries has progressed deep under the gingival margin, the involved tooth may be surgically extruded to re-establish biological width and gain adequate ferrule (see **Chapter 10**). When caries has progressed deep enough that it cannot be predictably restored, transplantation can be performed if there is an available donor tooth[21, 24, 25, 45, 46, 48] (**Fig 4-5** and **4-6**).

Periodontics

It may be possible to treat areas of bone loss and tooth loss due to advanced periodontitis with tooth transplantation. The PDL of the transplanted tooth may be able to successfully generate bone and establish a healthy periodontal environment[49] (see **Chapter 6 Fig 6-6** and **6-7**).

A case of orthodontic extrusion to preserve a deeply fractured maxillary central incisor

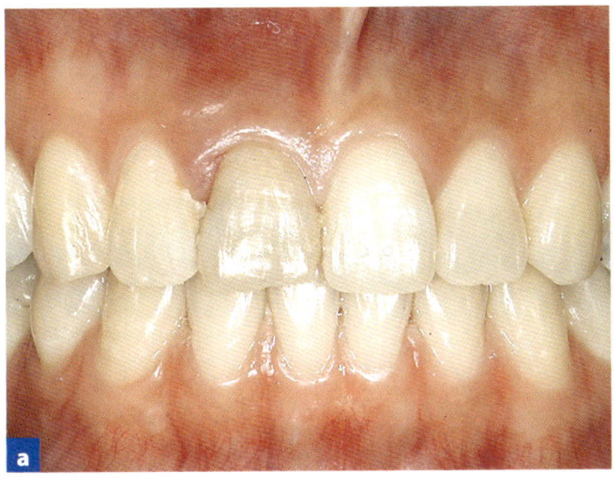
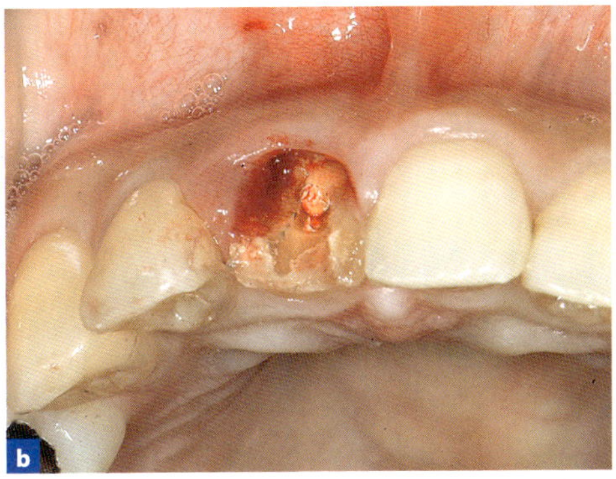
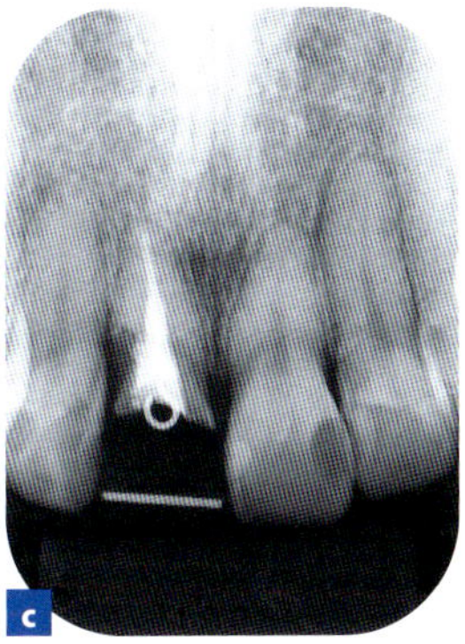

Fig 4-18a Frontal view at the first visit of a 32-year-old female, who has suffered a crown-root fracture of #11.
Fig 4-18b View after removal of the fragment under anesthesia. The fracture occurred at a deeper position than expected, and it was considered to have a poor prognosis but the patient wanted to try and save her tooth. Orthodontic extrusion was chosen.
Fig 4-18c Radiograph at the start of the orthodontic extrusion.

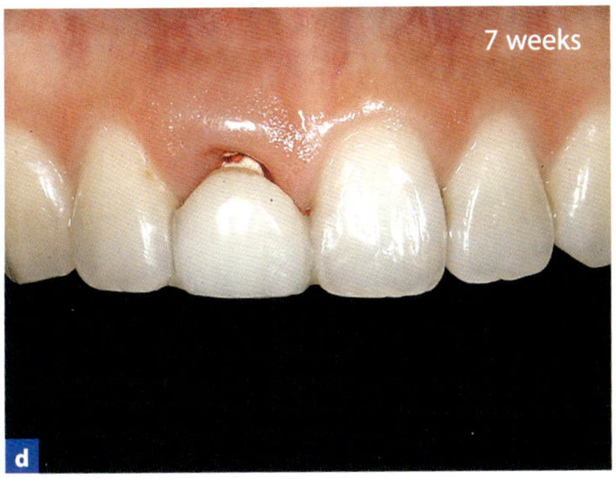

Fig 4-18d View after 7 weeks. As the root is extruded, the gingiva also has come up coronally. Therefore, it is necessary to perform gingival surgery to align the level of the gingiva with that of the adjacent teeth.

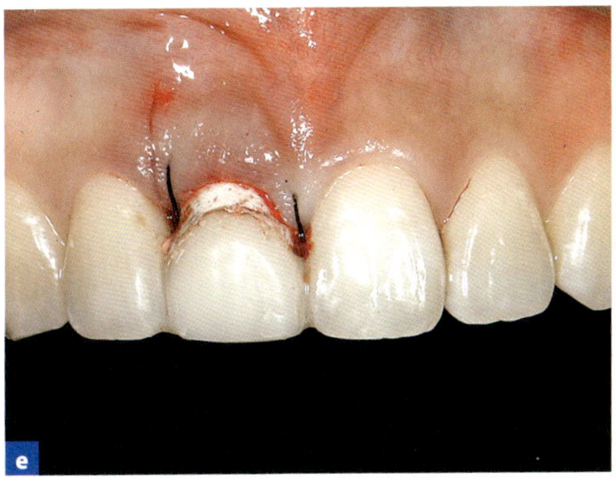

Fig 4-18e Immediately after the gingival surgery.

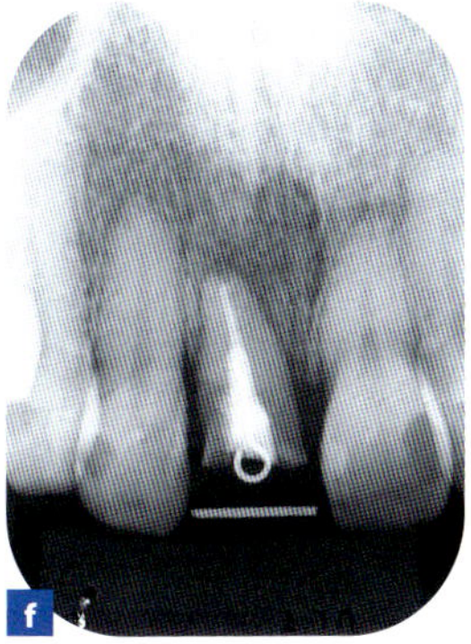

Fig 4-18f Radiograph on the same day as **Fig 4-18e**.

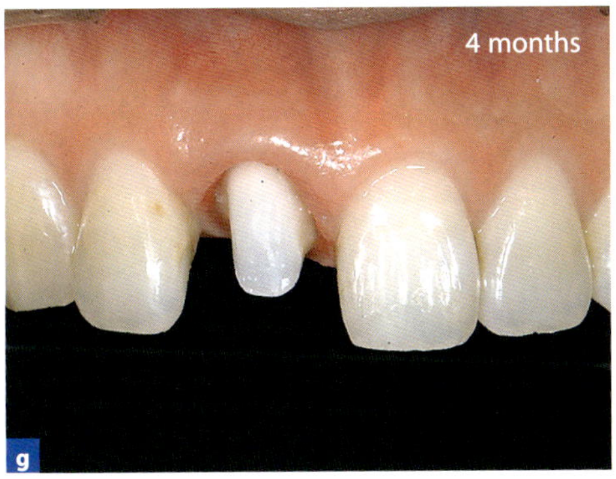

Fig 4-18g About 4 months after surgery. The tooth is restored with a fiber post and resin core.

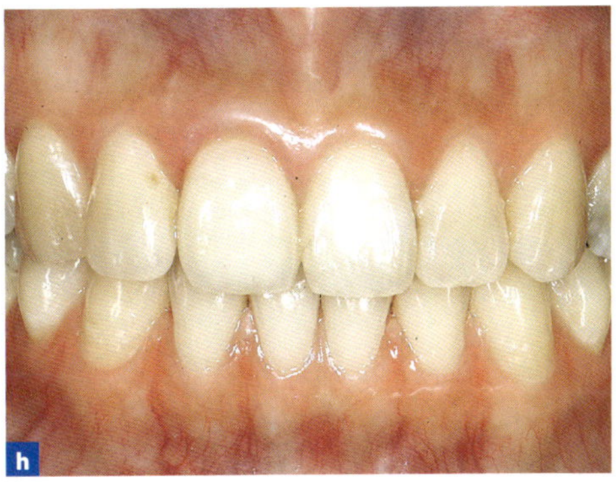
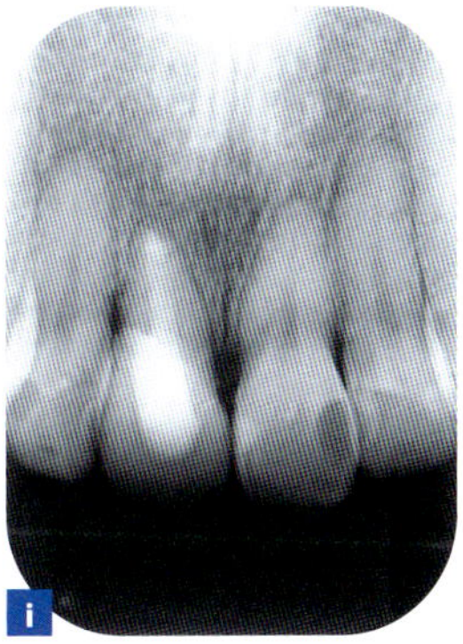

Fig 4-18h, i After fabrication of the final prosthesis (ceramic jacket crown). Tooth mobility and the probing depth were normal.

A case of surgical extrusion of a traumatized maxillary central incisor

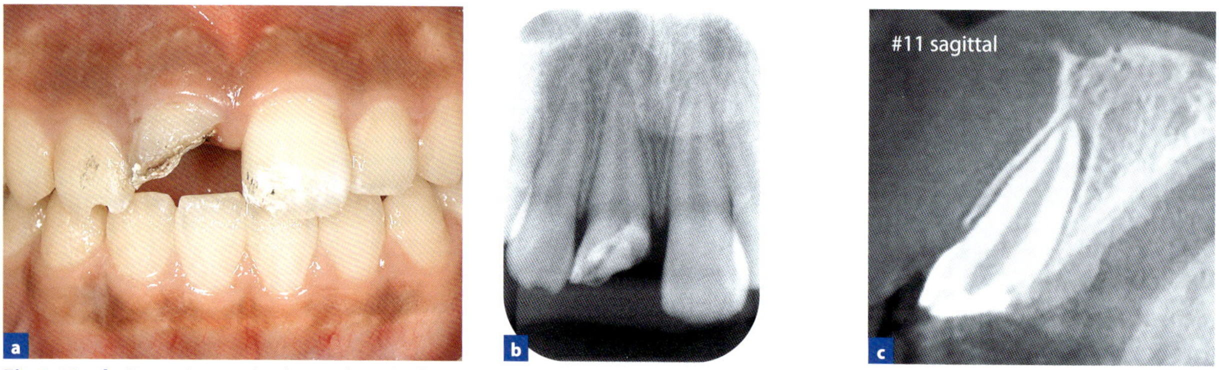

Fig 4-19a, b Front view and radiograph at the first visit of an 11-year-old male who was referred to our clinic. #11 suffered a crown-root fracture due to trauma.

Fig 4-19c CBCT image of #11 at the first visit. The fracture appears to reach below the alveolar crest on the palatal aspect. When trying to preserve the tooth, re-establishment of the biological width and gaining ferrule by surgical extrusion for the subsequent crown restoration were thought to be appropriate.

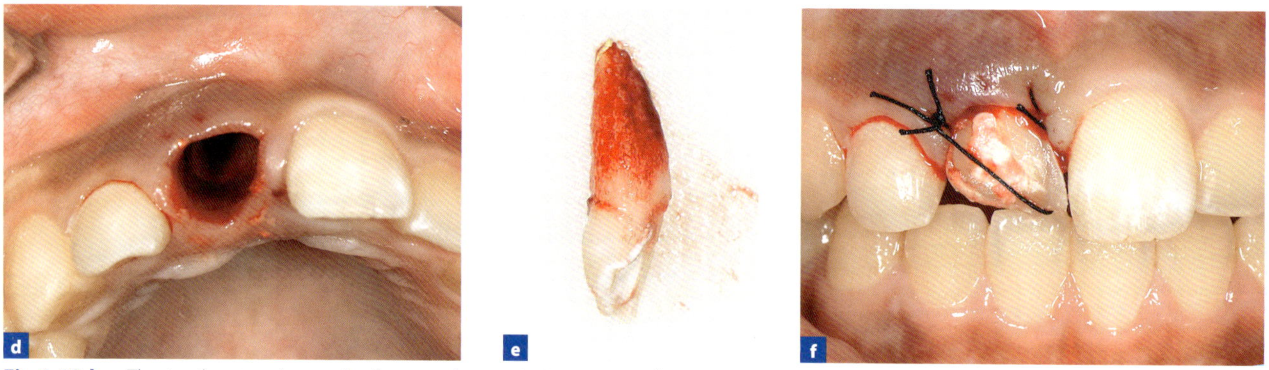

Fig 4-19d, e The tooth extraction as the first step for surgical extrusion of #11.

Fig 4-19f Immediately after the surgery. The tooth was rotated 180 degrees and positioned to an extruded position so that a certain amount of healthy tooth structure could be secured above the crest. Sutures were used to close the gingival flap and stabilize the replanted tooth at the same time.

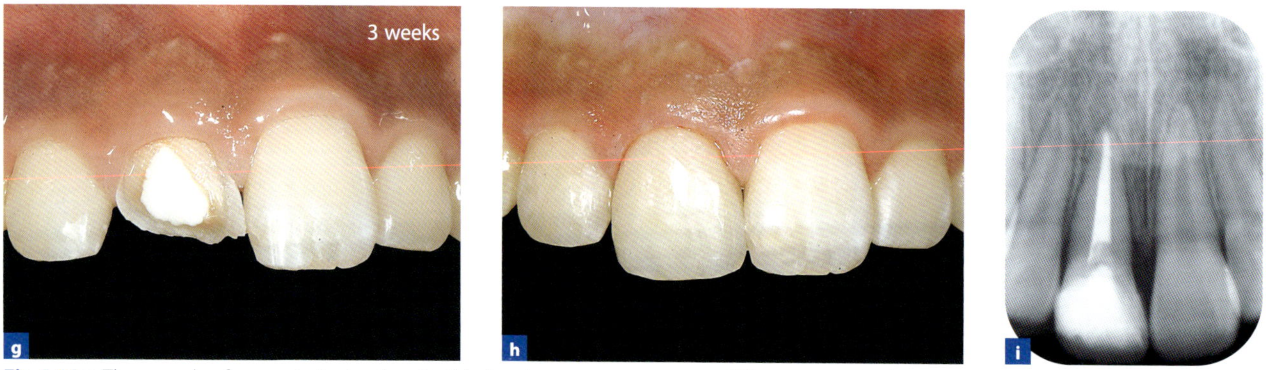

Fig 4-19g Three weeks after surgical extrusion. On this day, the temporary root canal filling material (calcium hydroxide preparation) was replaced with sealer and gutta-percha, and crown was restored with CR (direct method) on the same day.

Fig 4-19h, i Immediately after the restoration.

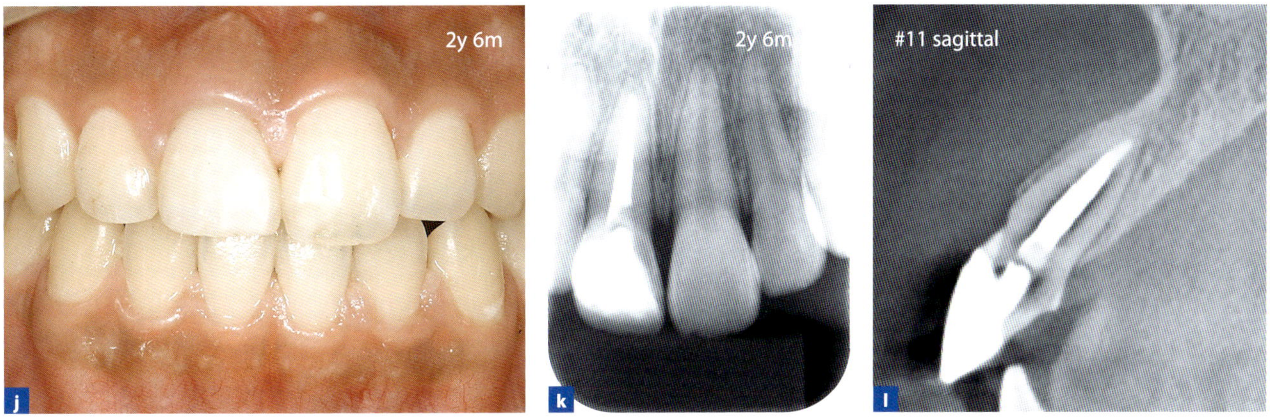

Fig 4-19j, k Two and a half years after surgery. Tooth mobility and probing depth were normal.
Fig 4-19l CBCT image after 2 and a half years. No evidence of root resorption and an intact lamina dura is observed around the root.

Efficacy of transplantation in treating maxillary central incisors

The efficacy and benefit of transplantation should be considered when comparing various available treatment options.

Fig 4-18 shows a case in which a crown-root fracture occurred so deeply that the prognosis may be considered hopeless by many practitioners. Since there was little remaining tooth structure (**Fig 4-18b** and **4-18c**), it was considered for tooth extraction, but the patient wanted to try and save the tooth. Prosthetic treatment was performed after LOT (orthodontic extrusion) and the gingival surgery to reestablish the biological width and ferrule. Although the treatment took about 6 months, the esthetics and function were recovered nicely (**Fig 4-18g** and **4-18h**).

Fig 4-19 is a case of crown-root fracture of #11 due to trauma. Crown-root fracture by trauma usually result in deeper fracture on the palatal aspect, and surgical extrusion associated with 180° rotation has several advantages over LOT (see **Chapter 10 Fig 10-1**). Since the healing occurs fairly quickly after surgical extrusion, it is possible to restore the crown about 1 month after the surgery. Considering treatment time, cost, and the ability to make a better diagnosis during surgery, surgical extrusion is considered to have more advantages than orthodontic extrusion in a case such as this.

Fig 4-20 shows a case in which a central incisor that was difficult to preserve due to root fracture was treated with an implant supported crown. If tooth preservation is not possible, there is no suitable donor tooth, and the patient can afford it, implants have many advantages over bridges and removable dentures. However, esthetic results can be difficult to achieve. Implant treatment is not indicated for younger patients because of problems such as infra-occlusion (**Fig 4-21**).

Fig 4-22 is an example of root resorption which occurred in a central incisor due to delayed replantation done in another clinic when the patient was 7 years old. At the start of the second stage of orthodontic treatment, four premolars were planned to be extracted. So, the option of transplanting one of the premolars to the central incisor was considered. However, space closure by orthodontic tooth movement was chosen (**Fig 4-22g** to **4-22i**). The right lateral incisor was orthodontically moved to the extracted central incisor site and composite resin was used to improve esthetics (**Fig 4-22j**).

Fig 4-23 is a 13 and 10 month-year-old patient who visited our clinic for orthodontic treatment (chief complaint was crowding and narrow dental arch). The tooth #11 had trauma and treated with delayed replantation 3 years and 7 months prior and ankylosis occurred. With the consent of the patient's mother, ATT was performed using #35 to replace #11 (**Fig 4-23d** to **4-23f**). The transplanted tooth responded to orthodontic tooth movement and provided sufficient esthetics and functional results (**Fig 4-23g** to **4-23l**). One of the advantages of ATT is alveolar bone regeneration. Immediately after surgery, the bone on the labial aspect of the transplanted tooth was not observed (**Fig 4-23f**), but after healing, it was regenerated by the PDL of the transplant (**Fig 4-23l**). Since the transplant can move naturally as the other natural teeth, transplantation is suitable for young patients.

A case of implant therapy of a hopeless maxillary central incisor

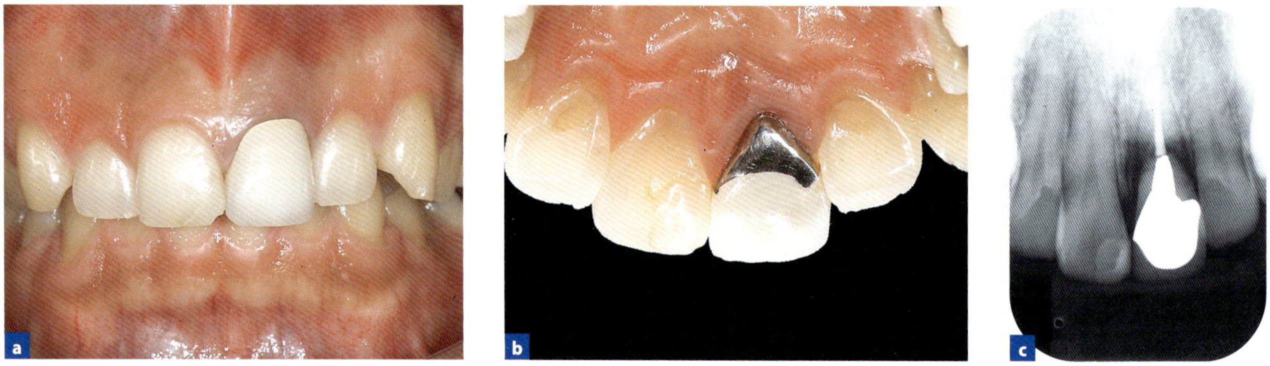

Fig 4-20a-c Oral views and radiograph at the first visit of a 30-year-old male. #21 had RCT due to dental trauma when he was young and horizontal fracture had occurred at the middle of the root. The tooth was considered hopeless and the patient chose implant therapy.

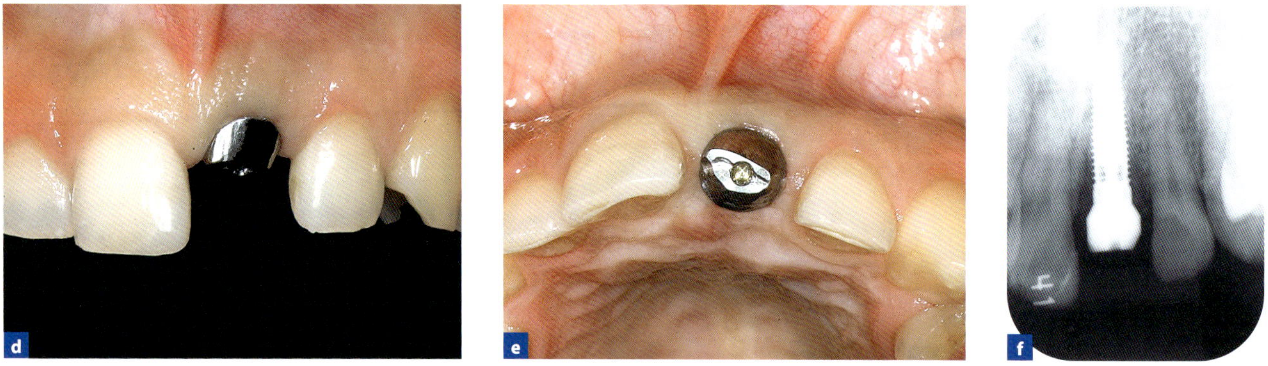

Fig 4-20d-f Six weeks after tooth extraction and immediately after placement of the fixture and healing abutment.

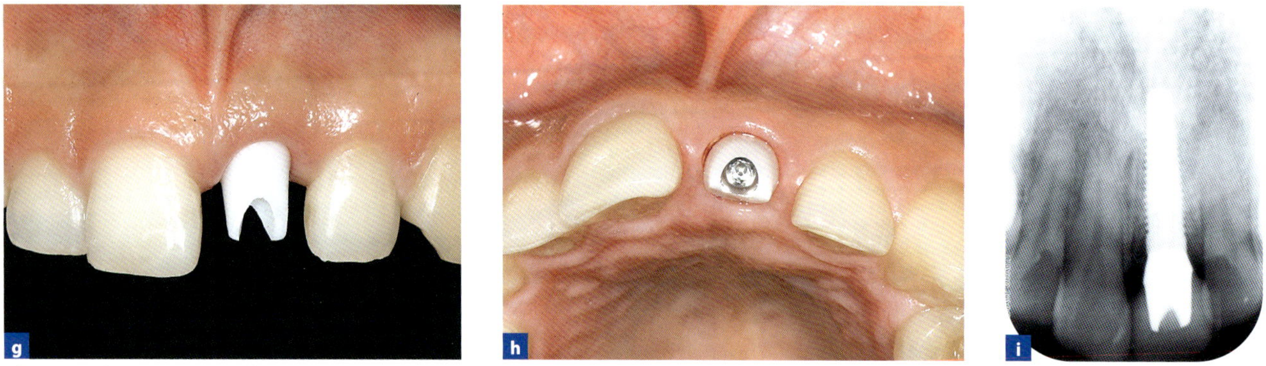

Fig 4-20g-i Four months after surgery. A zirconia abutment is placed.

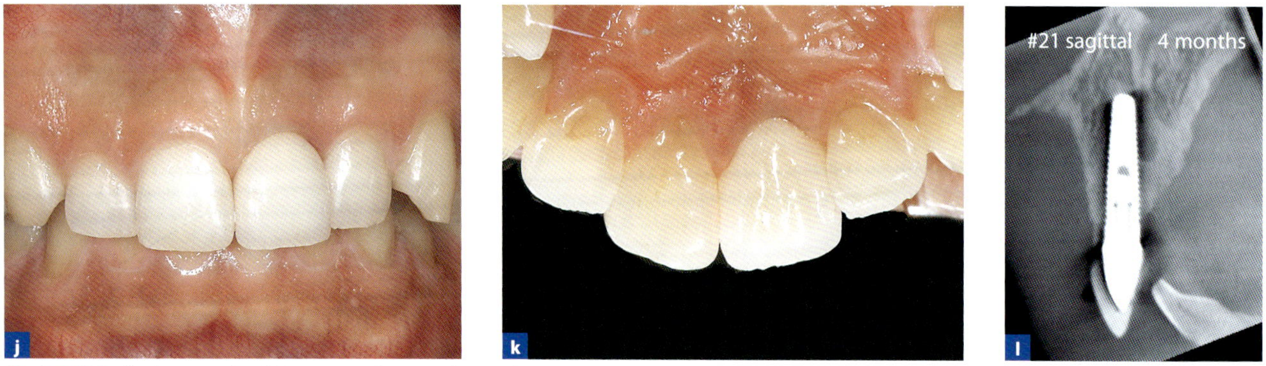

Fig 4-20j, k Oral views after fabrication of a porcelain jacket crown.

Fig 4-20l CBCT image in 4 months after surgery. Fortunately, the width of the alveolar ridge was wide enough that it was not difficult to complete the case esthetically at this stage of healing. However, long-term issues may develop as seen in **Fig 4-21**.

Implant and infra-occlusion

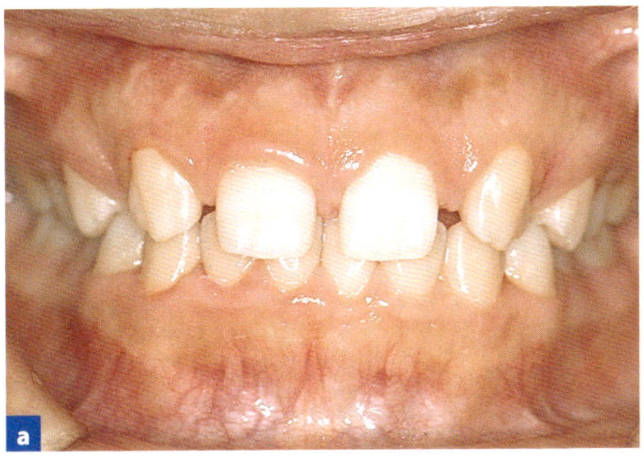
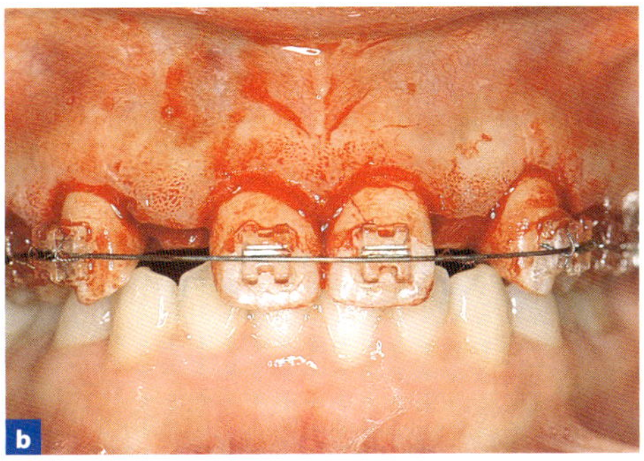

Fig 4-21a Frontal view before treatment of a 16-year-old female whose chief complaint was to improve the esthetics of the maxillary anterior area.
Fig 4-21b Gingivectomy was performed after orthodontic alignment.

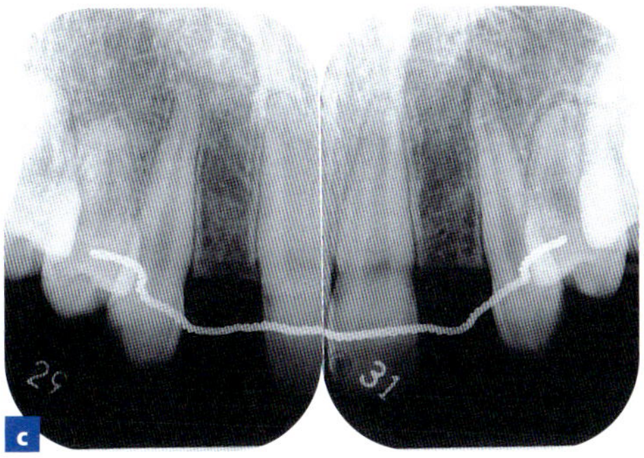

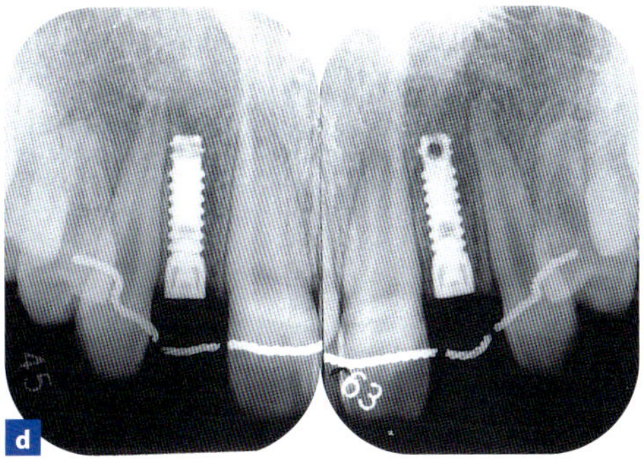

Fig 4-21c Radiograph immediately before implant fixtures were placed.
Fig 4-21d Radiograph 4 months after the implant surgery. The patient was 17 years and 9 months old.

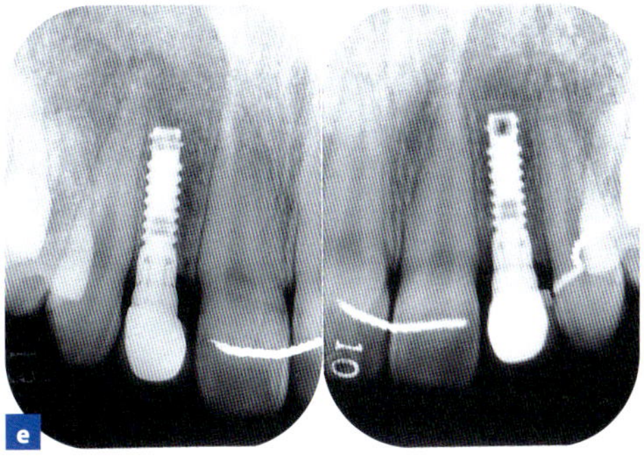

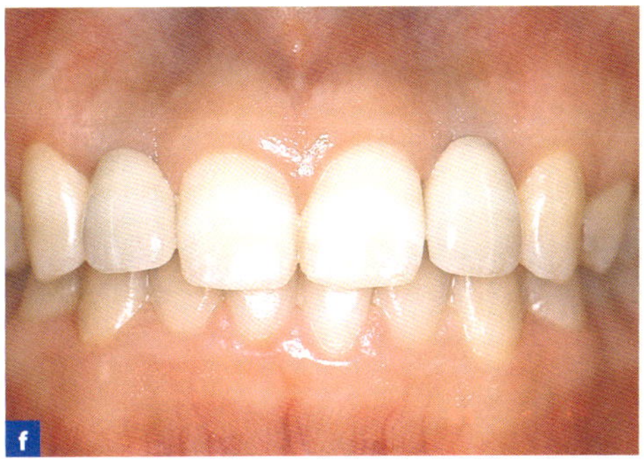

Fig 4-21e, f Seven months postoperative.

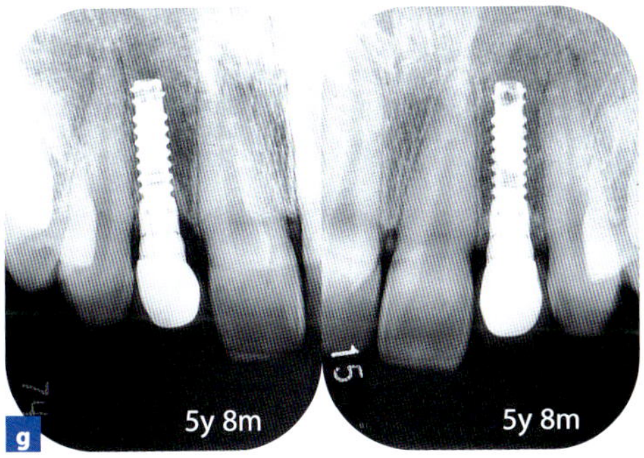

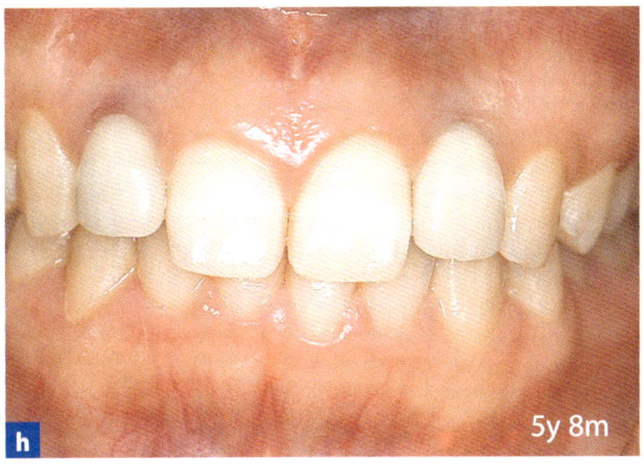

Fig 4-21g, h Five years and 8 months postoperative. The patient was 23 years and 1 month old. Infra-occlusion of the implant occurred. Such a problem can take place however old the patients are due to continued remodeling and skeletal changes that occur over one's lifetime.

A case of space closure of a maxillary central incisor by orthodontics

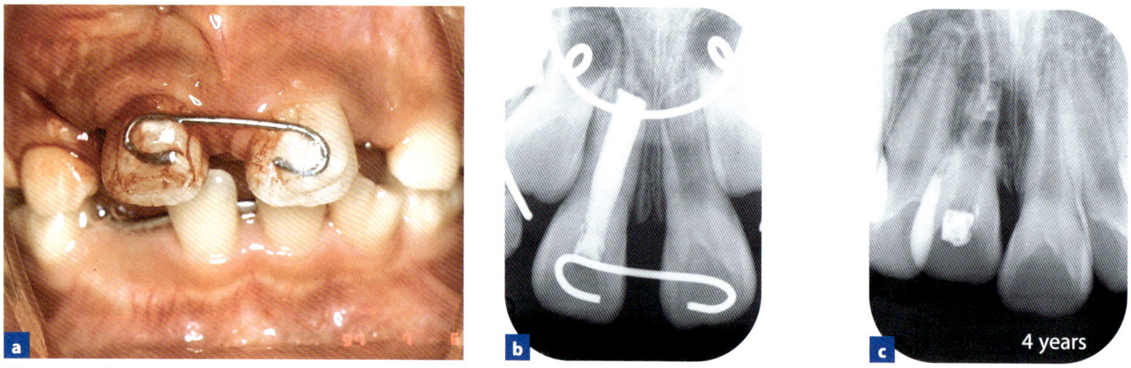

Fig 4-22a, b Frontal view and radiograph at the first visit of an 8-year and 10-months-old male. The patient visited our clinic after undergoing delayed replantation at another clinic on the same day.

Fig 4-22c Radiograph 4 years after replantation. Inflammatory root resorption and replacement root resorption has progressed severely, and the intracanal medicament (calcium hydroxide) has been resorbed.

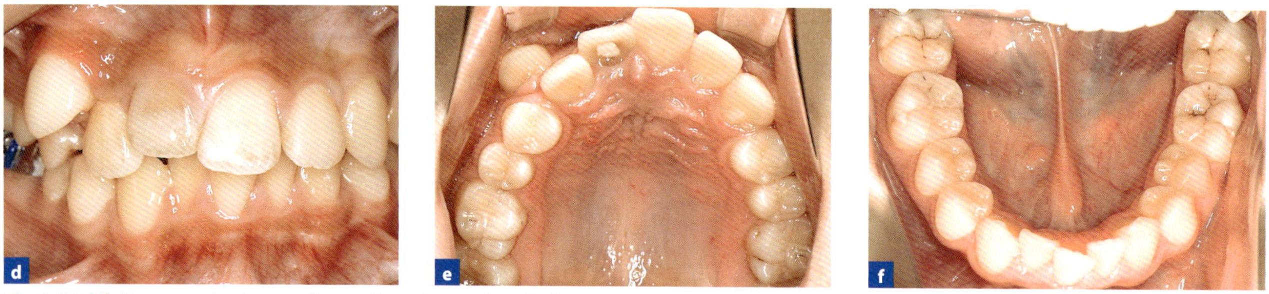

Fig 4-22d-f Photographs 4 years after replantation and just before initiating the second-stage orthodontic treatment. Discoloration and infra-occlusion of the crown are evident. In this case, orthodontic space closing after the extraction of #11 was chosen.

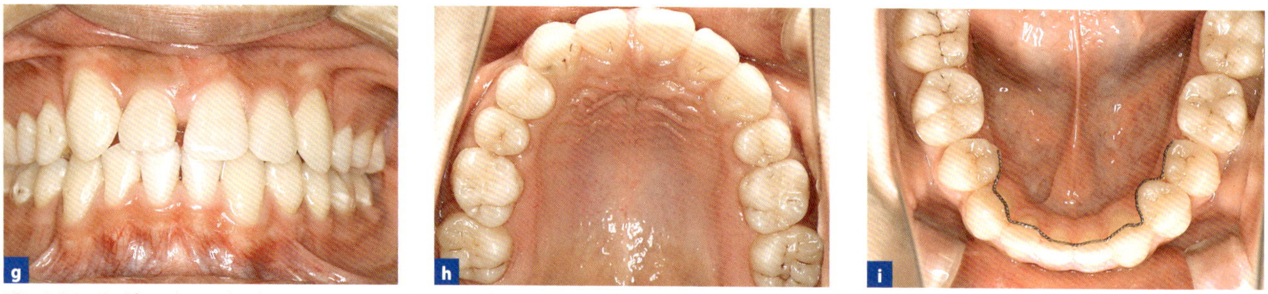

Fig 4-22g-i After the orthodontic treatment (3 years after the start of the second-stage orthodontic treatment).

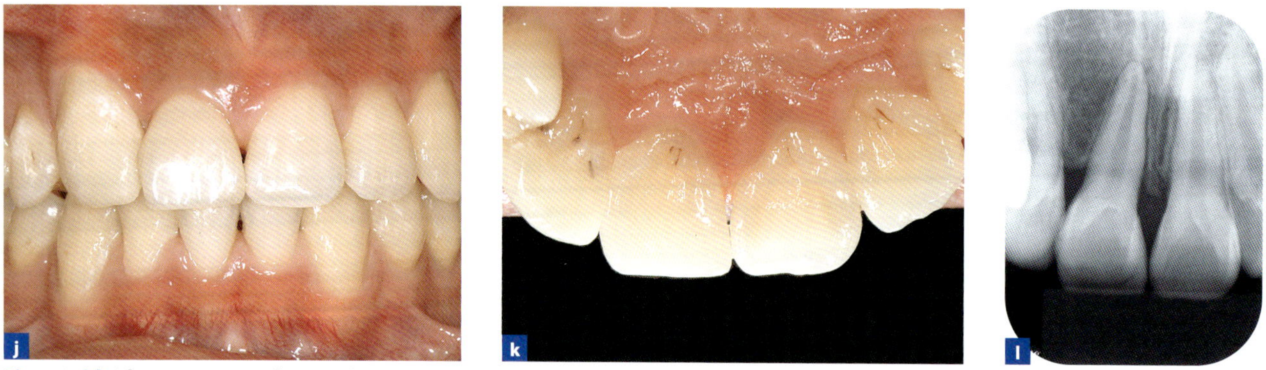

Fig 4-22j-l After restoration of #12 and #13 with CR.

A case of ATT to replace a maxillary central incisor involved in ankylosis

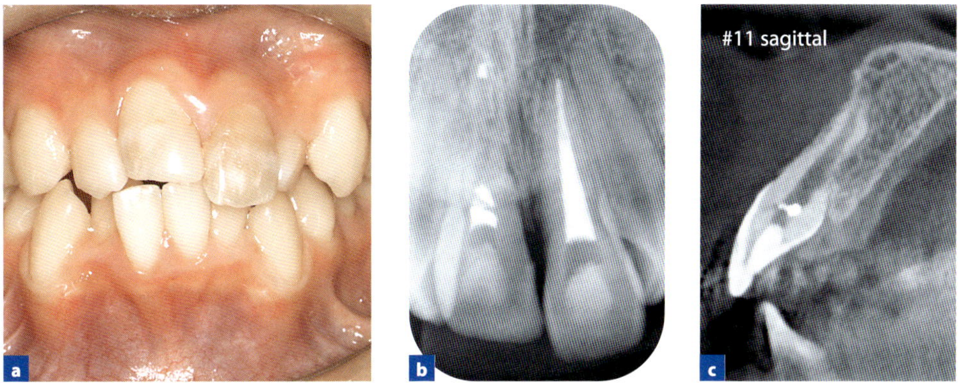

Fig 4-23a, b Frontal view and radiograph before treatment of a 13-year and 10-month-old male. The patient was referred for orthodontic treatment. At the age of 10 years and 3 months, #11 developed ankylosis due to delayed replantation. Infra-occlusion and root resorption were evident.
Fig 4-23c CBCT image of #11 showing findings consistent with root resorption progression.

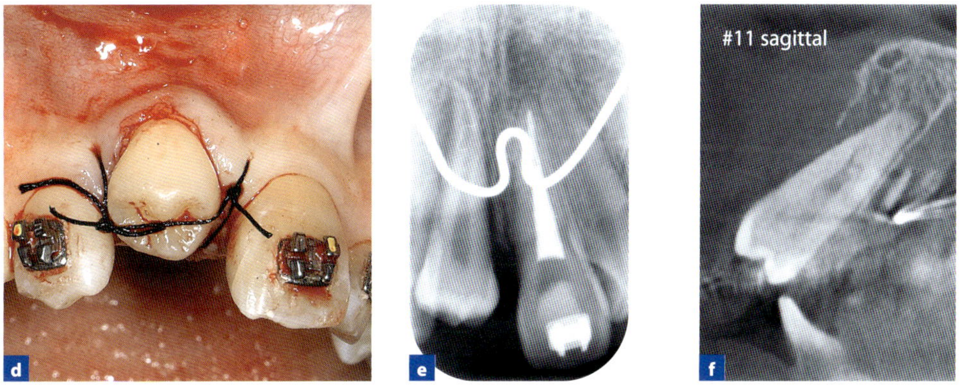

Fig 4-23d Immediately after transplantation. Extraction of #11 and the transplantation of #35 were performed on the same day. #35 had been planned for extraction as part of the orthodontic treatment plan.
Fig 4-23e Radiograph immediately after transplantation.
Fig 4-23f CBCT image of the transplant immediately after the surgery. Note the absence of alveolar bone on buccal aspect.

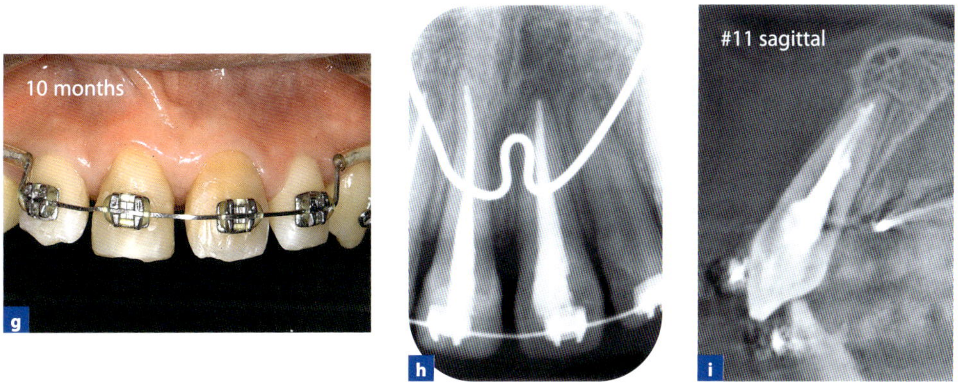

Fig 4-23g, h 10 months after transplantation. Orthodontic treatment was started 3 months after the surgery. The transplanted tooth was temporarily restored with CR.
Fig 4-23i CBCT image of the transplant 10 months after transplantation. The labial bone shows evidence of regeneration.

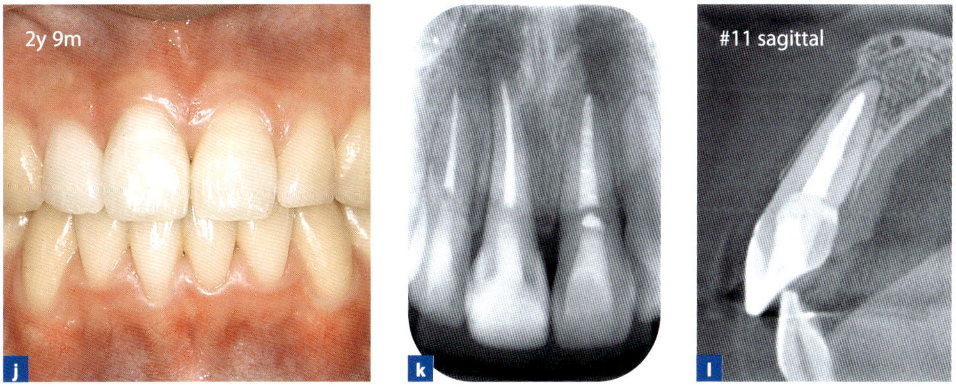

Fig 4-23j, k Two years and 9 months postop. Orthodontic treatment was completed 2 months prior. The transplanted tooth was restored with CR for esthetics.
Fig 4-23l CBCT image of the transplant after 2 years and 9 months. The PDL space along the root and a newly formed labial bone have been maintained.

A case of compromised surgical extrusion

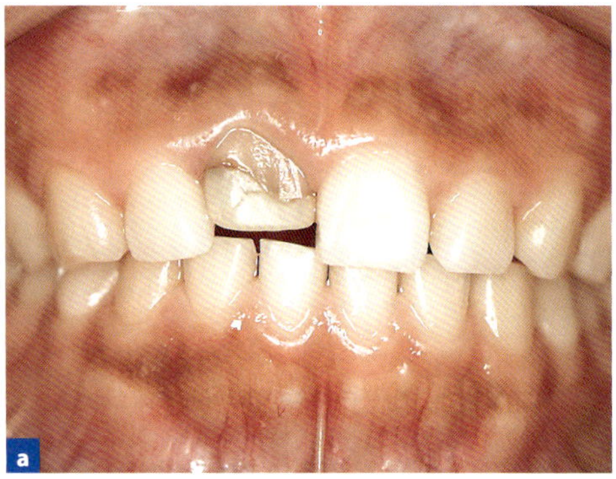
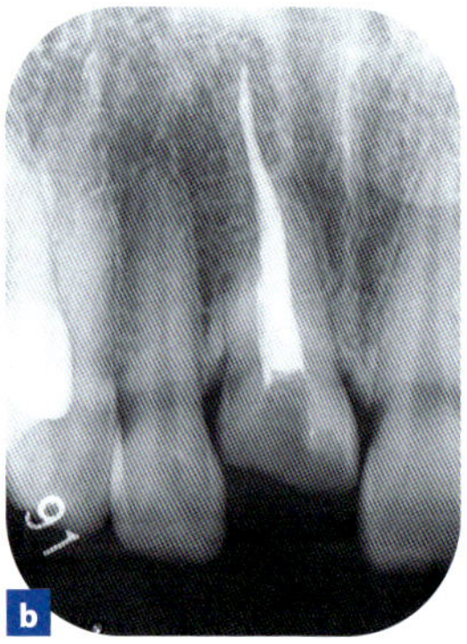

Fig 4-24a, b Frontal view and radiograph at the first visit of a 19-year-old female, with the chief complaint of the esthetic issues with #11. Though there were no symptoms, the tooth had a history of trauma when she was about 8 years old (treated at another clinic). Since the patient did not want to have a fixed bridge or an implant, it was decided to attempt surgical extrusion and restoration.

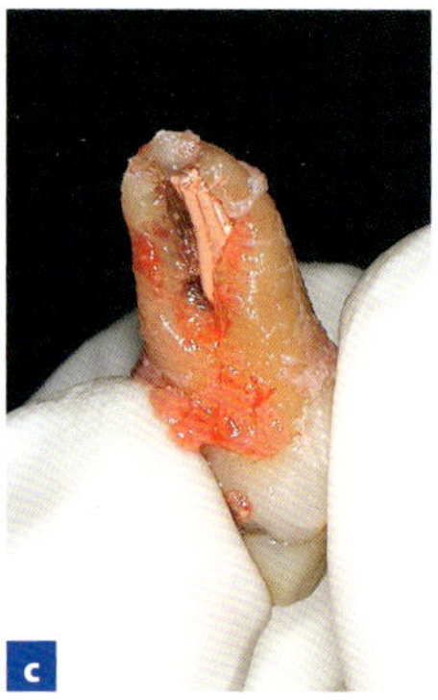

Fig 4-24c Extraction of #11. The tooth was extracted fairly smoothly. Although the PDL remained in some places, there were clear areas of root resorption.

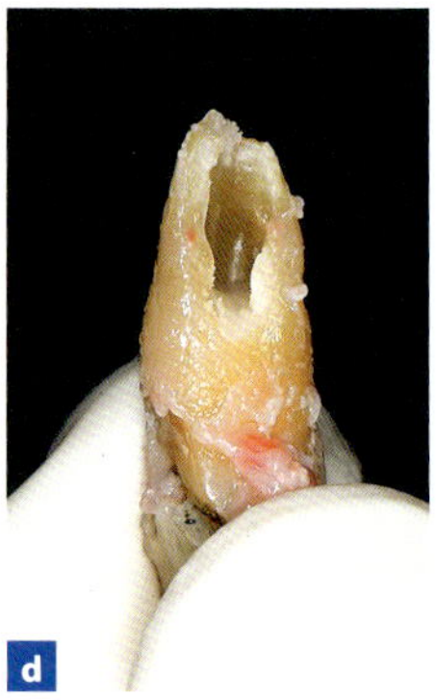

Fig 4-24d View after the extra-oral treatment of #11. The root canal filling material was removed from the apical side, and the root canal was filled with light-curing glass ionomer cement.

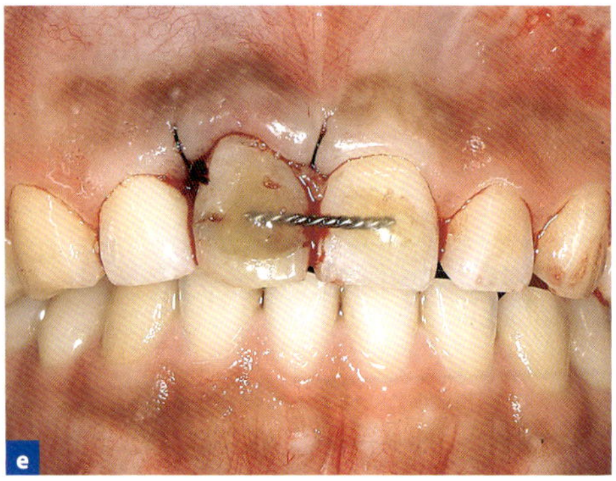
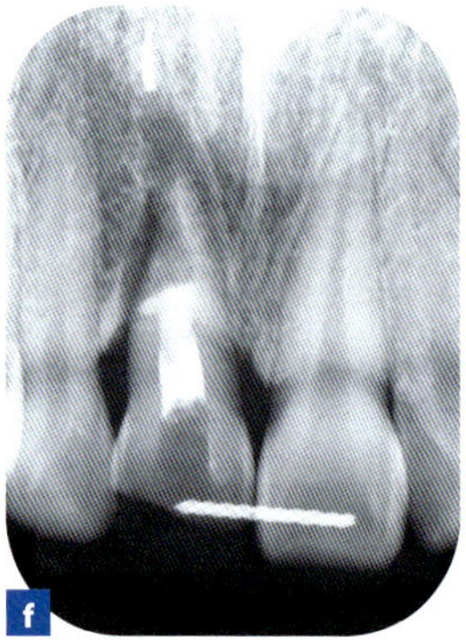

Fig 4-24e, f Immediately after surgical extrusion and fixation.

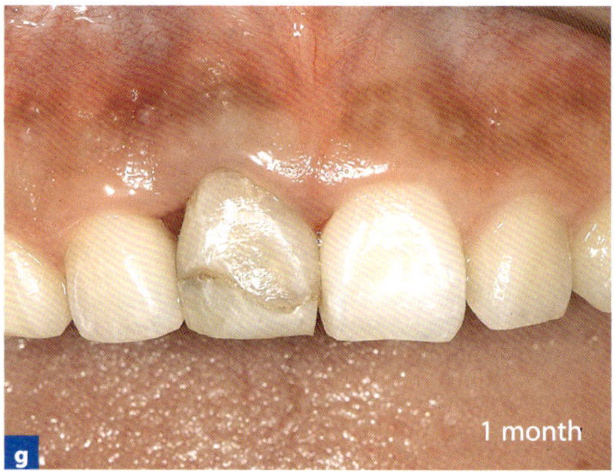

Fig 4-24g One month postoperative. The tooth mobility is close to normal. Bleaching of the crown (walking bleaching) was started.

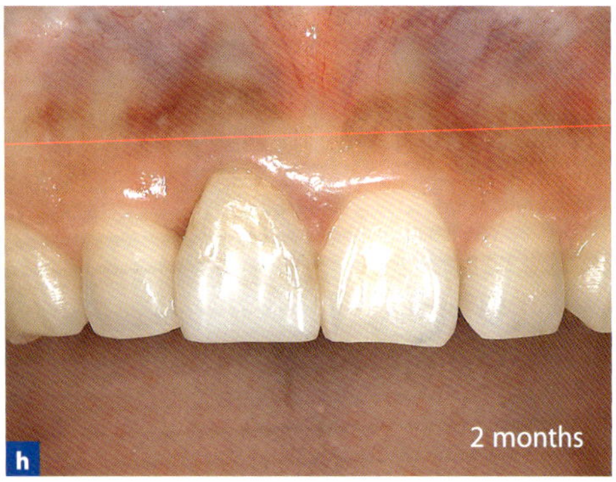

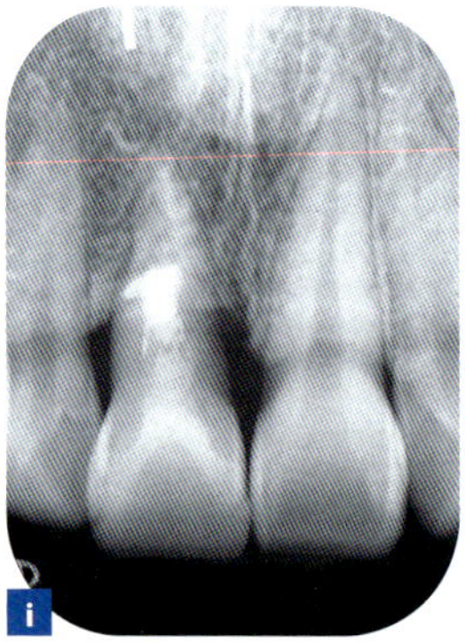
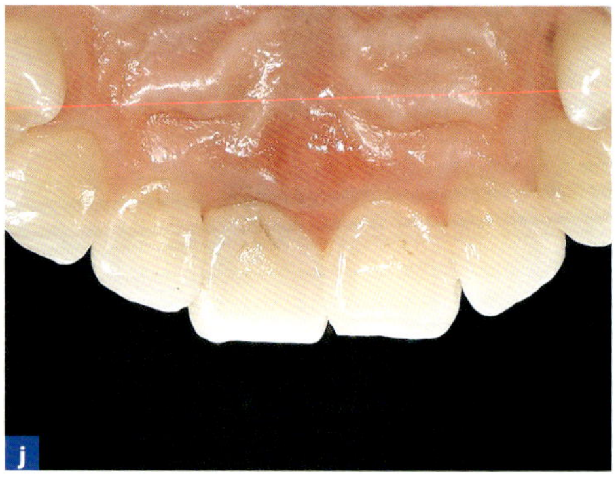

Fig 4-24h-j Two months postoperative. After 2 rounds of bleaching, the tooth was restored with CR.

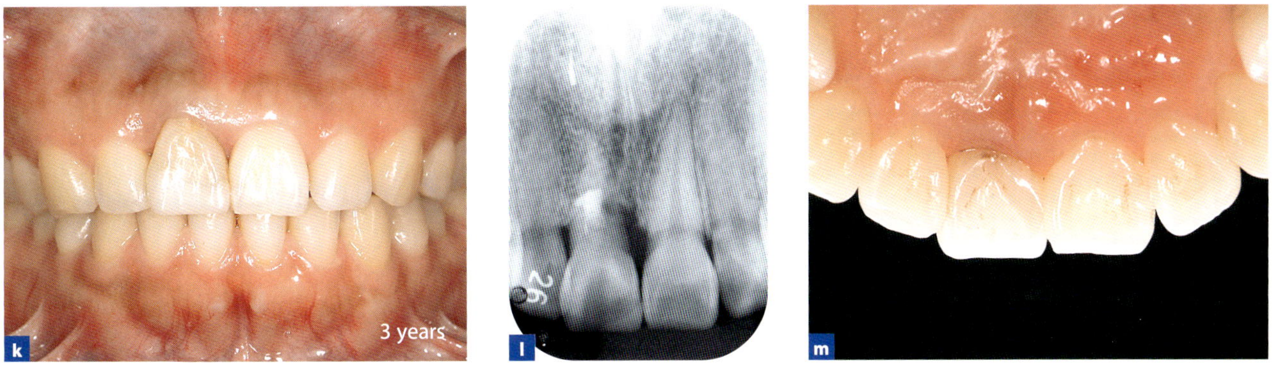

Fig 4-24k-m Three years postoperative. There is no clinical symptom, and the probing depth is normal. Root resorption may have progressed to some extent, but the speed of root resorption is slower in adults, and it is expected that esthetics and function will be maintained for more than 10 years until the root gets replaced.

Fig 4-24a, b shows a case of a 19-year-old female who came to our clinic for treatment of an ankylosed central incisor which occurred due to trauma when she was around eight years old. A removable denture was not accepted for functional and esthetic reasons, an implant was not accepted for the cost, and a fixed bridge was not accepted because she did not want to compromise her adjacent teeth. She decided on attempting surgical extrusion, understanding the risk-benefit and possibly guarded prognosis given the tooth was already ankylosed. In the surgical extrusion of such a tooth, ankylosis will likely occur again after the healing. However, considering that the patient is about 20 years old, the speed of root resorption due to ankylosis may be slow enough to maintain the tooth with proper function and esthetics for some years (possibly 10 years or more). Thus surgical extrusion was performed (**Fig 4-24c-g**). After healing the tooth was restored with walking bleach and composite resin (**Fig 4-24h-j**). The patient was satisfied with the result. Although this case may have a guarded prognosis (**Fig 4-24k-m**), it was also a conservative option that satisfied the patient.

References

1. Natiella J, Armitage J, Greene G. The replantation and transplantation of teeth. Oral Surg. 1970; 29: 397.
2. Iijima K. Surgical extrusion. In: Mori K (ed). Current Orthodontic Extrusion in General Practice [in Japanese]. Tokyo: Edition Gnosis, 1987; 96-101.
3. Kahnberg KE. Intraalveolar transplantation of teeth with crown-root fractures. J Oral Surg. 1985; 43: 38-42.
4. Kahnberg KE. Surgical extrusion of root fractured teeth: a follow-up study of two surgical methods. Endod Dent Traumatol. 1988; 4 : 85-9.
5. Tegsjo U, Valerius-Olsson H, Olgart K. Intra-alveolar transplantation of teeth with cervical root fractures, Swed Dent J. 1978; 2 : 73-82.
6. Tegsjo U. Clinical evaluation of intra-alveolar transplantation of teeth with cervical root fractures. Swed Dent J. 1987; 11: 235-50.
7. Grossman LI. Intentional replantation of teeth. J Am Dent Assoc. 1966; 72: 1111-8.
8. Grossman LI. Intentional replantation of teeth. In:Robinson Pj, Guernsey LH, eds. Clinical transplantation in dental specialities. St Louis:CV Mosby, 1980; 65-76.
9. Tsukiboshi M. The criteria of implant or transplant [in Japanese]. The Quintessence Yearbook. 1995; 132-44.
10. Shimada T. Effect of periodontal ligament curetted in alveolar socket for autotransplantation of tooth in adult monkeys [in Japanese]. J Jpn Soc Oral Implantol. 1998; 11: 492-500.
11. Ichinokawa H, et al. The pathological analysis in the experiments on autotransplantation of teeth [in Japanese]. Jpn J Conserv Dent. 1998; 41 (spring) : 38.
12. Ichinokawa H, et al. The pathological analysis in the experiments on autotransplantation of teeth: Part 4. The microstructural changes in the healing process [in Japanese]. J Jpn Soc Oral Implantol. 1999; 12: 131.
13. Heithersay GS. Combined endodontic-orthodontic treatment of transverse root fractures in the region of the alveolar crest. Oral Surg. 1973; 36: 404-15.
14. Ingber JS. Forced eruption, Part 2. A method of treatment nonrestorable teeth-periodontal and restorative considerations. J Periodontol. 1976; 47: 203-16.
15. Delivanis P, Delivanis H, Kuftnec MM. Endodontic-orthodontic management of fractured anterior teeth. J Am Dent Assoc. 1978; 97: 483-5.
16. Iijima K. Extrusion for deep carious teeth. In: Mori K(ed). Contemporary Dental Practice in Endodontics [in Japanese]. Tokyo: Ishiyaku, 1980; 225-34.
17. Malmgren O, Malmgren B, Frykholm A. Rapid orthodontic extrusion of crown root and cervical root fractured teeth. Endod Dent Traumatol. 1991; 7 : 49-54.
18. Mori K, Takahashi K. Intentional Extrusion [in Japanese]. Tokyo: Edition Gnosis, 1997.
19. Shimoji I. Criteria between orthodontic extrusion and surgical extrusion [in Japanese]. Dental Diamond. 1993; 18: 104-9.
20. Andreasen JO. Atlas of Replantation and Transplantation of Teeth. Philadelphia: Saunders, 1992.
21. Tsukiboshi M. The possible clinical applications of autotransplantation of teeth [in Japanese]. The Quintessence Yearbook. 1993; 15-9.
22. Miyazaki M, Sanada H. Science and the state of the art of autogenous tooth transplantation. Possible applications of autogenous tooth transplantation in partial edentulism [in Japanese]. The Quintessence. 1992; 11: 1147-65.
23. Miyazaki M. Treatment planning and techniques for autotransplantation of teeth [in Japanese]. Pract Prosthet. 1994; 27(1)-(5).
24. Tsukiboshi M, Inoue T, et al. Clinical application of autotransplantation of teeth [in Japanese]. The Quintessence. 1996; 15 (supplemental issue): 28-38, 193-9.
25. Shimoji I. Color Atlas. Basis and Practice of Autogenous Tooth Transplantation [in Japanese]. Kyoto: Nagasue, 1995.
26. Andreasen JO, Andreasen FM. Essentials of Traumatic Injuries to the Teeth. Copenhagen: Munksgaard, 1990.
27. Slagsvold O, Bjercke B. Autotransplantation of premolars in cases of missing anterior teeth. Trans Eur Orthod Soc. 1970; 66: 473 85.
28. Slagsvold O, Bjercke B. Indications for autotransplantations in cases of missing premolars. Am J Orthod. 1978; 74: 241-57.
29. Paulsen HU, Andreasen JO. Autotransplantation in orthodontic treatment. Nederlandse Vereniging Woor Orthodontische Studie, Studieweek. 1985; 248-64.

30. Andreasen JO, Paulsen HU, Yu Z, Ahlquist R, Bayer T, Schwartz O. A long term study of 370 autotransplanted premolars. Part 1. Surgical procedure and standardized techniques for monitoring healing. Eur J Orthod. 1990; 12: 3 -13.

31. Andreasen JO, Paulsen HU, Yu Z, Bayer T, Schwartz O. A long term study of 370 autotransplanted premolars. Part 2. Tooth survival and pulp healing subsequent to transplantation. Eur J Orthod. 1990; 12: 14-24.

32. Andreasen JO, Paulsen HU, Yu Z, Schwartz O. A long term study of 370 autotransplanted premolars. Part 3. Periodontal healing subsequent to transplantation. Eur J Orthod. 1990; 12: 25-37.

33. Andreasen JO, Paulsen HU, Yu Z, Bayer T. A long term study of 370 autotransplanted premolars. Part 4. Root development subsequent to transplantation. Eur J Orthod. 1990; 12: 38-50.

34. Holland DJ. A technique of surgical orthodontics. Am J Orthod. 1955; 41: 27.

35. Holland DJ. The surgical positioning of unerupted, impacted teeth (surgical orthodontics). Oral Surg Oral Med Oral Pathol. 1956; 9 (2):130-40.

36. BADEN E. Surgical management of unerupted canines and premolars. Oral Surg Oral Med Oral Pathol. 1956; 9 (2): 141-92.

37. Serling L. Surgical repositioning of an impacted mandibular bicuspid. J Am Dent Assoc. 1959; 59: 553.

38. Moss JP. The indications for the transplantation of maxillary canines in the light of 100 cases. Br J Oral Surg. 1975; 12: 268-74.

39. Oksala E, Kallionemo H. A longitudinal clinical and radiographic study of autotransplantation of the maxillary canine. Proc Finn Dent Soc. 1977; 73: 117-25.

40. Andreasen JO. Traumatic injuries of the teeth. 2 nd ed. Copenhagen: Munksgaard, 1981.

41. Andreasen GF. A review of the approaches to treatment of impacted maxillary cuspids. Oral Sug Oral Med Oral Pathol. 1987; 31: 479-84.

42. Tsukiboshi M, Tsukiboshi C. Treatment planning considering autotransplantation of teeth [in Japanese]. Dent Rev. 1994; 55 (special issue): 68-74.

43. Andreasen JO, Andreasen FM. Essentials of traumatic injuries to the teeth. Copenhagen: Munksgaard, 1990.

44. Tsukiboshi M. Treatment Planning for Traumatized Teeth. Chicago: Quintessence, 2000.

45. Tsukiboshi M. The expansion of indications for autotransplantation of teeth [in Japanese]. The Quintessence. 1995; 14: 90-4.

46. Tsukiboshi M. Autotransplantation of teeth as a conservative option in therapy [in Japanese]. The Quintessence Yearbook. 1997; 70-3.

47. Tsukiboshi M. Autotransplantation of third molars with complete root formation (p. 294- 5). In:Andreasen JO, Petersen JK, Laskin DM. Textbook and color atlas of tooth impactions. Copenhagen: Munksgaard, 1997.

48. Tsukiboshi M. Autogenous tooth transplantation:Reevaluation. Int J Periodont Rest Dent. 1993; 2 :120-49.

49. Baer PN, Gamble JW. Autogenous dental transplantation as a method of treating the osseous defects in periodontosis. Oral Surg. 1966; 22: 405.

50. Nagata M, Nagaoka S, Semba I. Combined treatment of autogenous tooth transplantation and sinus floor elevation technique for a high level bone resorption of maxilla: Experimental study in dogs [in Japanese]. J Jpn Soc Periodontol. 1998; 40: 180.

51. Nagata M, Nagaoka S, Semba I. Combined treatment of autogenous tooth transplantation and sinus floor elevation technique: Clinical study [in Japanese]. J Jpn Soc Periodontol. 1998; 40: 87.

52. Nagata M, Nagaoka S. Combined treatment of autogenous tooth transplantation and sinus floor elevation technique: Radiological study [in Japanese]. J Jpn Soc Periodontol. 1999; 41: 59.

CHAPTER 5

Sequence and Treatment Procedures

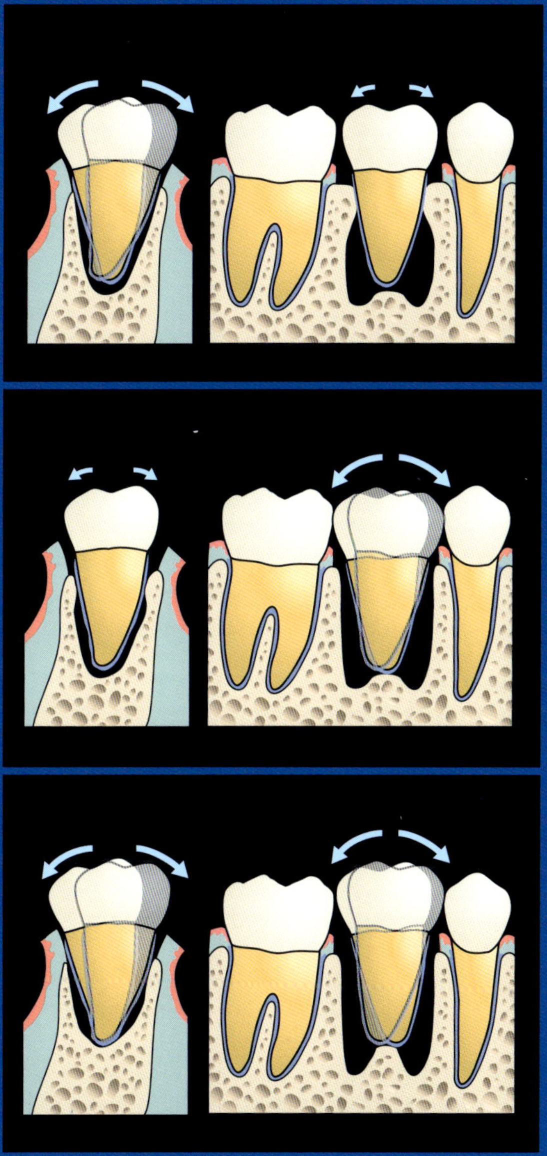

The sequence of autotransplantation of teeth (transplantation) includes clinical and radiographic examination, diagnosis, treatment planning, surgical procedure, endodontic treatment, orthodontic treatment, restorative treatment, and maintenance. The criteria and the indications have been discussed in detail in **Chapter 4**.

Cone-beam Computed Tomography (CBCT), which has been developed in more recent years, is very useful for transplantation procedures. It can help improve preoperative diagnosis and planning, risk reduction, and postoperative management. This chapter presents several cases of transplantation, and describes the sequence and the multi-disciplinary treatment procedures involved for conventional transplantation. The indications and surgical procedures for intra-alveolar transplantation and intentional replantation are explained in **Chapter 4** and **10**.

Sequence and Procedures of Conventional Transplantation

The sequence and procedures of several clinical cases are documented in **Fig 5-1** to **5-6**. The reader will note that a variety of treatment approaches have been used. In this chapter, basic and common procedures are discussed by sequence, and particular procedures of each case are explained with graphic illustrations.

Examination and Diagnosis

The examination of potential transplantation patients includes obtaining necessary radiographs and clinical photographs and performing periodontal and soft tissue evaluations, as well as reviewing medical history and obtaining informed consent. Detailed analysis of the donor tooth and the recipient side are important (**Fig 5-1a** to **5-1h**).

Analysis of donor teeth

Analyze whether the teeth planned for the donor are morphologically appropriate and whether they can be extracted with low risk. Ideally, the donor should be small enough to fit into the recipient site. If the donor tooth is immature, the developmental stage of the roots should ideally be stage 4 or 5 (**Fig 5-1a** and **5-1d**, see **Chapter 3 Fig 3-27**).

Analysis of recipient sites

Mesiodistal and buccolingual widths of the alveolar ridge of the recipient sites and position of the mandibular canal or maxillary sinus should be evaluated (**Fig 5-1a** to **5-1h**). Ideally, the recipient site is large enough to accommodate the donor tooth.

Treatment Planning

Oral hygiene instruction

Unless the caries or periodontal disease which has caused the tooth extraction of the recipient site is controlled, the transplanted tooth will have a higher risk of failure. Therefore, oral hygiene instruction, and scaling and root-planing must be performed prior to or concurrent with the surgical procedures, and the patient should demonstrate an ability to perform adequate oral hygiene[1,2].

Preparation of a replica

The success of transplantation depends much on the extraoral time and the mechanical damage of the PDL of a donor tooth during the surgery. A replica of a donor tooth can be fabricated and used to help reduce extraoral dry time and damage to the PDL when trial fitting the donor tooth into the recipient site (**Fig 5-1o** to **5-1v**, see **Chapter 3**)

Tooth extraction from the recipient site (immediate or delayed transplantation)

Timing of the tooth extraction from the recipient site should be carefully determined. If the tooth is extracted prior to the date of transplantation, transplantation should be performed 3 to 4 weeks after the extraction (see **Fig 5-2**). Indication for immediate transplantation (same day tooth extraction with transplantation) is determined by the availability of the gingival tissue for primary closure around the transplanted tooth. If the diameter of the extraction socket and cervical area of the transplanted tooth are similar, immediate transplantation is indicated (see **Fig 5-1**, **5-3**, and **5-4**), thus sparing the patient the inconvenience of undergoing surgery twice. Another advantage of immediate transplantation is that periodontal ligament tissue in the extraction socket can help with reattachment and the healing process (see **Chapter 3**).

The indication for delayed transplantation is when there is a discrepancy between the size of the extraction socket and that of the transplanted tooth, which would result in the lack of gingival tissue for primary closure. By about three weeks after extraction, the socket will be covered with enough keratinized tissue to achieve primary closure. Transplantation should be performed within 2 months after the extraction because bone resorption will begin to occur. Therefore, in delayed transplantation the ideal timing for transplantation is 3 to 4 weeks after the extraction, considering the amount of the keratinized soft tissue formation as well as easier preparation of recipient sites.

Thus, if transplantation is a possibility, the timing of tooth extraction from the recipient site and choosing between immediate or delayed transplantation should be considered during the treatment planning phase.

Timing of root canal treatment

For fully developed teeth (mature teeth), it is necessary to

Treatment sequence of an immediate transplantation of an immature third molar

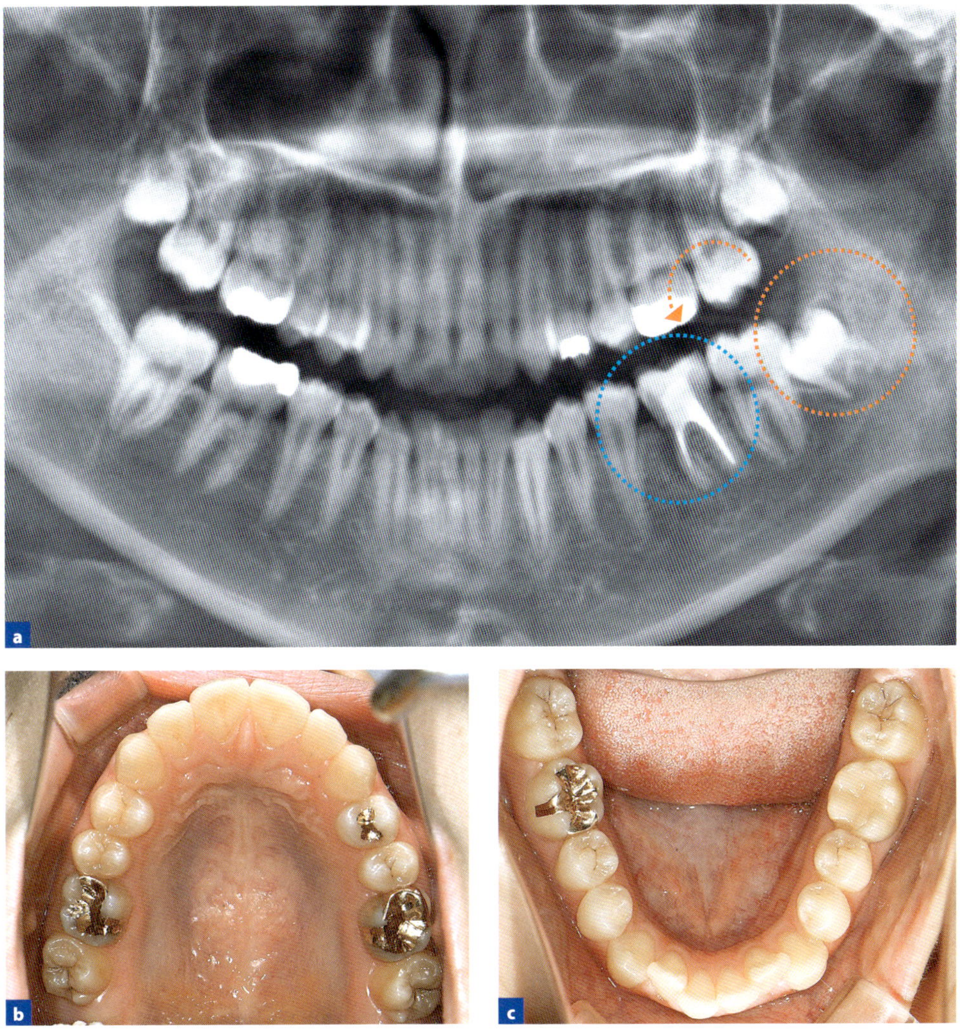

Fig 5-1a to 5-1c Preoperative views of an 18-year-old female. The patient had root canal treatment of #36 when she was 8 years and 11 months old at another clinic. The tooth developed progressive external root resorption on the mesial aspect. It was suggested that the transplantation of a third molar at an appropriate time in the future would be beneficial to the patient. An appropriate for time for transplantation time when the donor tooth (#38) has approximately 60 - 80% of root development completed.

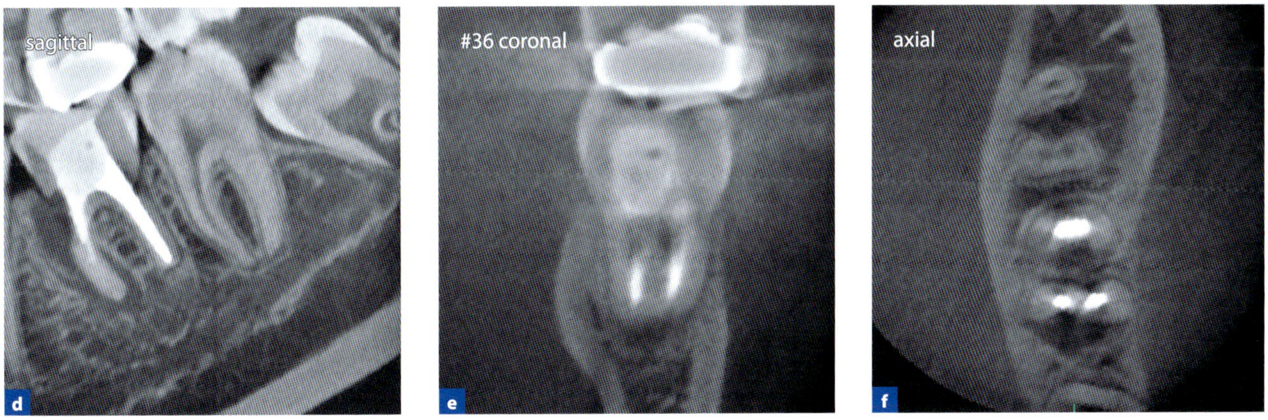

Fig 5-1d to 5-1f Preoperative CBCT images. Findings are consistent with root resorption of #36, and it appears that the degree of root development of the donor tooth is appropriate. It also appears that the mesiodistal and buccolingual width on the recipient site is sufficient to accommodate the donor.

complete root canal treatment before transplantation, or to start root canal treatment about 2 weeks after the surgery (**Fig 5-3** and **5-4**) to prevent inflammatory resorption (see **Chapter 3**).

Orthodontic treatment

If transplantation is included as part of the orthodontic treatment, the position or direction of transplanted teeth can be flexible (see **Chapter 9**). If there is insufficient spacing of the recipient site, orthodontic treatment can be performed prior to transplantation (**Fig 5-4**). Orthodontic treatment can help to correct malpositioned transplanted teeth or problems of alveolar bone (i.e. vertical bony defects) around transplanted teeth (See **Chapter 3 Fig 3-58**, **Chapter 6 Fig 6-7**).

Restorative treatment

Restoration of the crown of the transplanted tooth may be necessary. However, unnecessary preparation of the transplanted tooth (i.e. fabricating indirect prosthetics) can be avoided by careful restorative treatment planning before transplantation (**Fig 5-3** and **5-4**).

Surgical procedures

The sequence of the surgical procedures is as follows:

1. Preoperative administration of antibiotics
2. Setting up operatory and instruments
3. Disinfection and anesthesia of the surgical sites
4. Preparation of the recipient socket
5. Extraction of the donor tooth
6. Try-in of the donor tooth and radiographic evaluation
7. Suturing the flap and fixation of the transplant
8. Surgical dressing, home care instructions, antibiotics administration
9. Return for removal of dressing and suture, and wire splinting

1. Preoperative administration of antibiotics

The author advises having the patient take antibiotics a few hours prior to the surgery in order to have a desirable antibiotic level in the blood during and after surgery. Penicillin is recommended to achieve rapid increase of antibiotic levels of the blood[3]; tetracycline is recommended to maintain high levels of antibiotics in exudate of sulcus[4–7].

2. Setting up operatory and instruments

Surgical instruments required for transplantation include blades, blade holders, periosteal elevators, forceps, scissors, needle holders, sutures with needles, etc. used in conventional surgeries. Specific instruments for transplantation cases may be diamond forceps, surgical bone burs, fixation wire, adhesive resin, surgical dressings (packs), etc. Instrument setup is illustrated in **Fig 5-8**. It is also important for the operatory to be properly set up so that the doctor and assistant(s) can perform treatment safely, efficiently, and ergonomically.

3. Disinfection and anesthesia of the surgical sites

Thorough tooth cleaning should be performed before the surgery and the surgery sites should be disinfected. The donor tooth and recipient site are anesthetized at the same time. Generally, local anesthesia (including regional block) is adequate for both the donor site and the recipient site.

4. Preparation of the recipient socket

As discussed in the treatment planning section, a replica of a donor tooth can be very helpful in order to reduce the extra-oral time and possible damage to the periodontal ligament of the donor tooth (**Fig 5-1o** to **5-1q**). But if it is not available, the approximate morphology (length, width, etc.) of the donor tooth can be obtained through a CBCT study prior to the surgery. Preparation of the socket should be performed before extraction of a donor tooth.

① **Immediate transplantation**

In cases of immediate transplantation, the tooth in the recipient site is extracted first (**Fig 5-1i**). The granulation tissue in the socket should be removed thoroughly but the periodontal ligament on the socket walls should try to be preserved as much as possible.

② **Delayed transplantation**

If tooth extraction at the recipient site has been performed within a few weeks before the surgery, an incision is made on the alveolar ridge of the recipient site and in the sulcus of the adjacent teeth with a full-thickness flap to expose 3 to 5 mm of alveolar bone. The incision in the sulcus of the adjacent teeth should be minimal to prevent unnecessary attachment loss for those teeth. A vertical incision can be made on the distobuccal area of the adjacent tooth to expose more alveolar bone if needed.

After removing granulation tissue from the extraction socket, the alveolar septum is removed with a rongeur or round bur (**Fig 5-1j** to **5-1l**). If the depth or width of the extraction socket is not sufficient, the lateral wall can be removed with proper saline cooling so that a slightly larger socket is formed for a passive fit of the donor in the recipient site.

③ **Forming a new socket**

When the recipient site does not have an extraction socket (excluding tooth extraction sockets from deciduous teeth) and

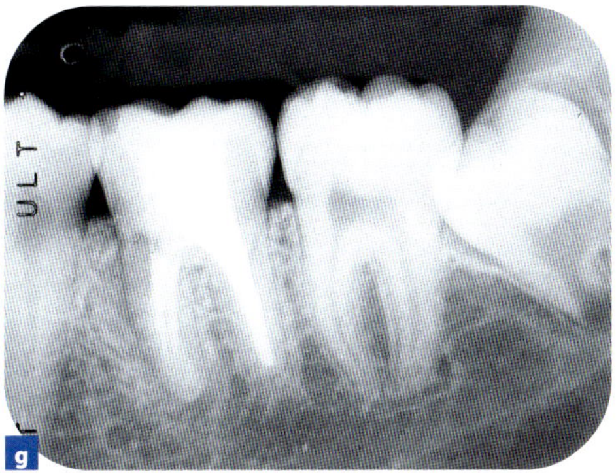
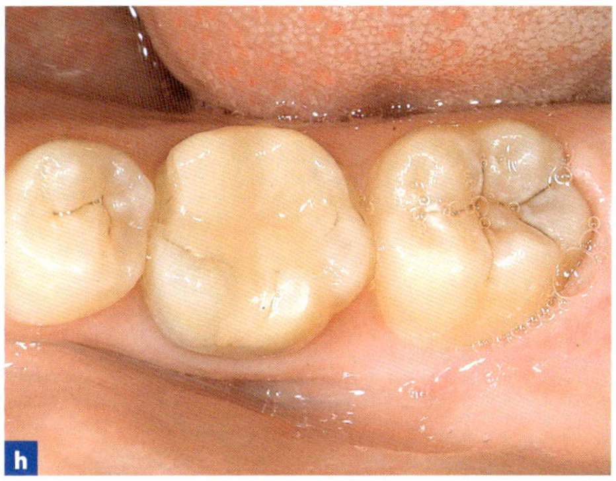

Fig 5-1g, h Preoperative views of the recipient site.

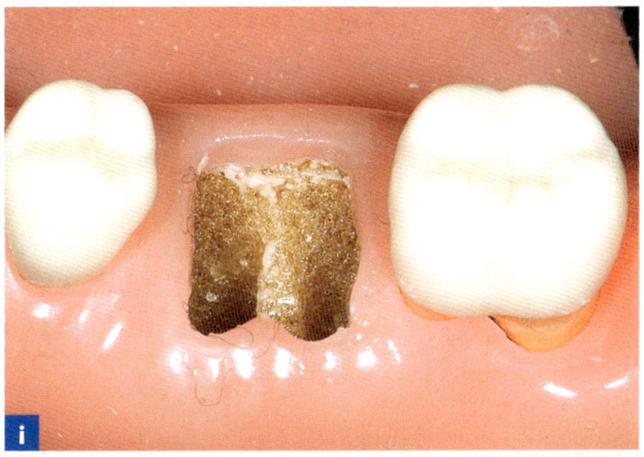
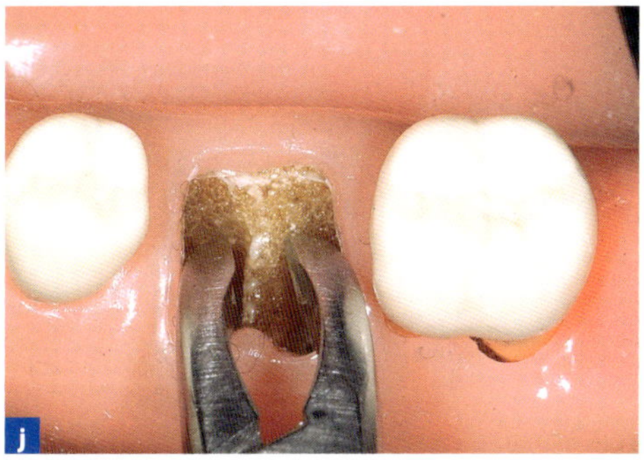

Fig 5-1i A model showing the condition immediately after the tooth extraction of a recipient site. In an immediate transplantation the tooth of the recipient site is extracted first.

Fig 5-1j Remove the alveolar septum in the furcal area with a forceps.

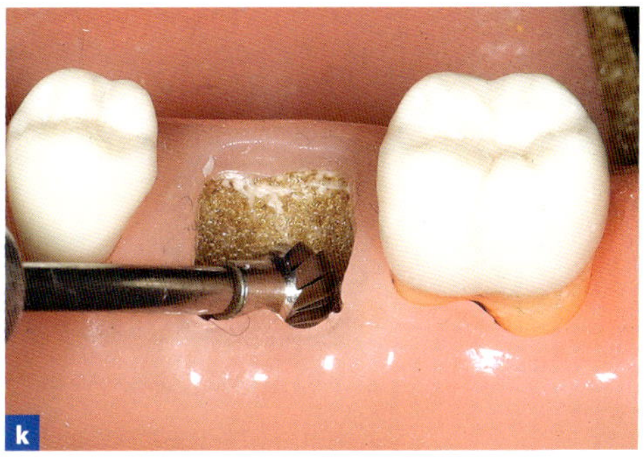
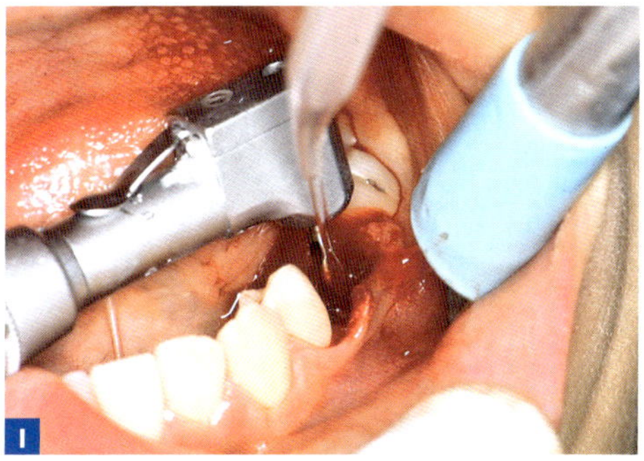

Fig 5-1k Form a recipient socket with a surgical round bur.

Fig 5-1l Drilling is performed with saline cooling, and the engine speed is about 2,000-6,000 rpm.

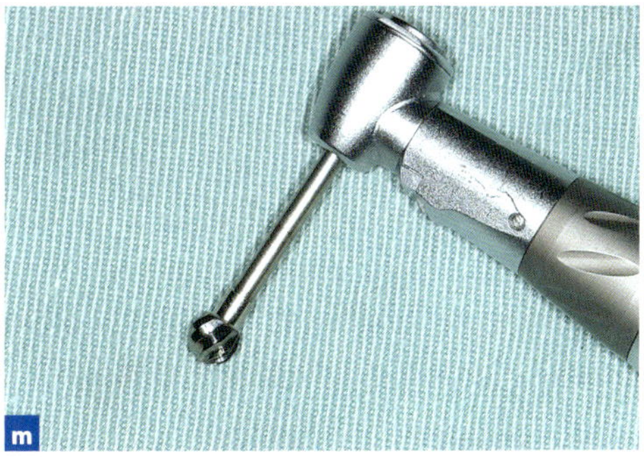
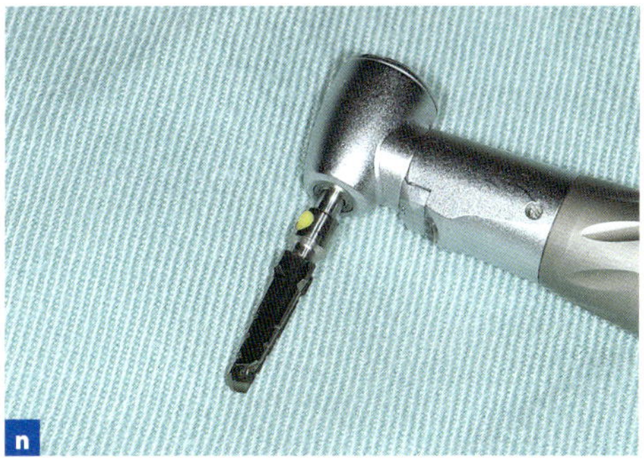

Fig 5-1m Round bur for drilling.

Fig 5-1n Implant bur can be useful for forming the socket.

must be prepared (see Fig 5-8 and 5-9), the position and size of the recipient site and direction of transplant should be well-planned by marking the measurements of the donor tooth on the alveolar bone surface. This can be done by creating a reference cut corresponding to the size of mesiodistal and buccolingual width of the donor tooth in the cortical bone (Fig 5-7a and 5-7b). Direction and depth are transferred using a bur (Fig 5-7d and 5-7e). An implant bur (Fig 5-1n) can be used when the donor tooth is a premolar, but a surgical round bur (Fig 5-1m) should be used when preparing for a molar or making minor adjustments to the recipient site. Preparation of the recipient site should be made with a lower-speed handpiece (about 2,000-6,000 rpm) while irrigating with saline (Fig 5-1l).

④ **Try-in of the replica and adjustment of the socket**

Regardless of the type of recipient socket, the final adjustment between the donor and recipient is performed with the replica in the contemporary technique (Fig 5-1o and 5-1p). The replica is placed into the formed socket and is moved buccolingually or mesiodistally (**Fig 5-1q**). If the replica is moves buccolingually but not mesiodistally, it is an indication that there may be an interference in the mesiodistal space. If this is the case, the socket should be enlarged more mesiodistally. If the replica moves mesiodistally but not buccolingually, the socket should be enlarged buccolingually. If the replica moves laterally but does not seat deep enough, the interference is likely located in the bottom area of the socket. If this is the case the socket should be deepened carefully being mindful of the proximity of the inferior alveolar nerve or other vital structures.

If the donor tooth cannot be positioned as initially planned, the tooth can be rotated 90 degrees to allow a more favorable fit.

⑤ **Discrepancy between the mesiodistal width of the recipient and the that of the crown of the donor**

When transplantation is performed into a site with two adjacent teeth, it is important to measure the difference between the mesiodistal distance of the recipient site and the crown width of the donor tooth (**Fig 5-3a** to **5-3d**). If the distance is insufficient, the discrepancy up to 2 mm can be adjusted by removing 0.5 mm from the proximal surfaces of both adjacent teeth and the donor tooth with a carbide bur[8] (**Fig 5-3e** and **5-3f**).

If there is inadequate mesiodistal distance of bone between the adjacent teeth, orthodontic treatment may be necessary to create enough space for the transplanted tooth to fit prior to transplantation (**Fig 5-4**).

⑥ **Insufficient buccolingual width of bone**

When the bone width is not sufficient buccolingually, it may be necessary to remove some of the buccal cortical plate of the recipient socket and to try and place the donor tooth as lingually as possible. Osteoinduction through the PDL of the transplant may be able to make new bone over the exposed root surface without graft materials (see **Chapter 3 Fig 3-54**).

If the bone width is significantly insufficient, the transplant is placed into the bone as deep as possible and may need to be angled with some inclination. Regeneration of alveolar bone can be expected by natural eruption of teeth or orthodontic extrusion 1 to 3 months after transplantation (see **Chapter 3 Fig 3-57** and **3-58**).

⑦ **Sinus elevation**

When the sinus floor is low and the height of the bone is shorter than the length of the donor tooth, a sinus lift procedure can be performed[9-13] (**Fig 5-5**) as follows:

1. The recipient site is prepared up to the cortical bone subjacent to the sinus floor.
2. Incision line is made with a round bur on the cortical bone in the area of the sinus floor, with care not to damage the Schneiderian membrane (sinus mucosa) (**Fig 5-5f**).
3. Cortical bone plate is slightly lifted into the sinus using an osteotome (**Fig 5-5g**).
4. Schneiderian membrane is gradually loosened from the sinus floor and gently lifted from the space created along the incision line of the cortical bone (**Fig 5-5h**).

⑧ **Trimming of gingival tissue**

After try-in of the replica in the recipient site, the fit of the gingival tissues around the replica (donor tooth) is checked. The success of transplantation depends much on the primary closure of the gingiva around the donor tooth (see **Chapter 3**). If excess soft tissue is present, the excess is trimmed and the remaining soft tissue is fitted around the donor tooth, making sure that adequate keratinized gingival tissue is available (**Fig 5-2f** and **5-2g**). If there is minimal keratinized tissue at the site, the fitting of the tissue must be done by creating an oblique incision to preserve all keratinized gingival tissue.

When a third molar is transplanted to the area of an adjacent second molar, it may be difficult to obtain a tight fit of the gingival tissue on the distal aspect of the donor tooth. By making a releasing incision, the flap can be brought in to create a more desirable fit around the tooth (**Fig 5-6**).

After completing the preparation of the recipient socket using the replica, the next step is the extraction of the donor tooth.

5. Extraction of the donor tooth

If an impacted donor tooth is to be extracted (**Fig 5-1a** to **5-1d**), the alveolar bone over the donor tooth must be removed with a surgical round bur with saline irrigation to avoid damage to the crown or the root. Before elevation of the donor tooth, an incision is made with a blade around the cervical area into the periodontal ligament to preserve as much periodontal ligament on the root as possible. The extracted tooth should be quickly placed into the prepared recipient socket.

6. Try-in of the donor tooth and radiographic evaluation

If transplantation is performed using a replica, the extracted donor tooth should ideally fit into the recipient socket with minimal additional adjustments. It is recommended to take a radiograph to check the fit. Then the donor tooth is removed from the socket and is placed into saline or the original socket until the second step of suturing. The try-in must be done carefully, as the periodontal ligament may be mechanically damaged if it is forced into place.

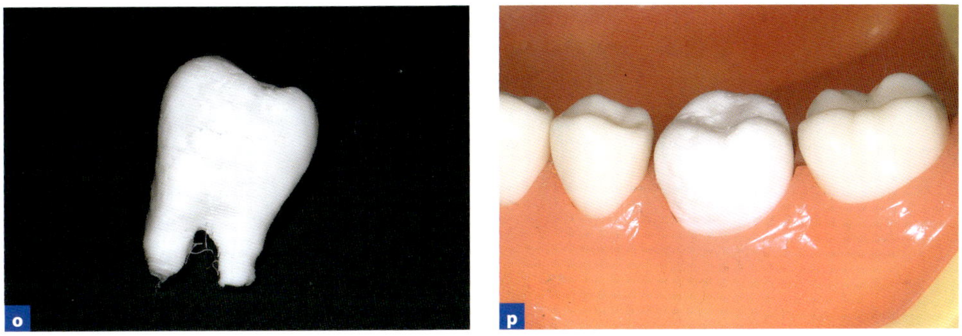

Fig 5-1o The plastic 3D replica of the donor tooth, which is made from the DICOM data of the CBCT.
Fig 5-1p Try-in of the replica into the approximately prepared socked.

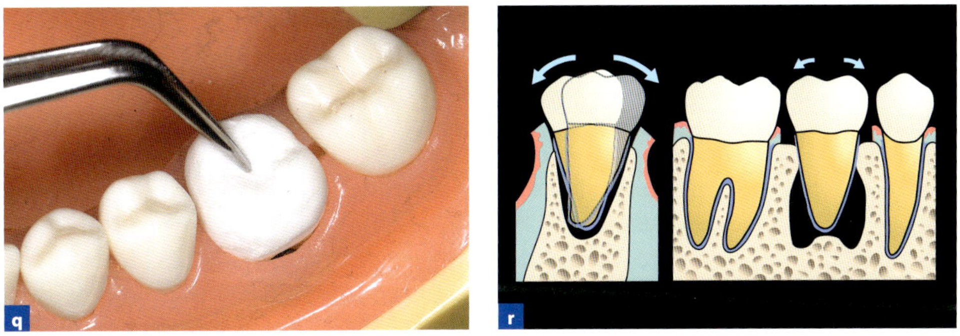

Fig 5-1q Move the replica in the mesiodistal and buccolingual directions with tweezers to find any interferences between with socket wall and replica.
Fig 5-1r If the replica moves buccolingually but not mesiodistally, it means there are interfering areas on the mesiodistal walls so the socket should be enlarged more mesiodistally.

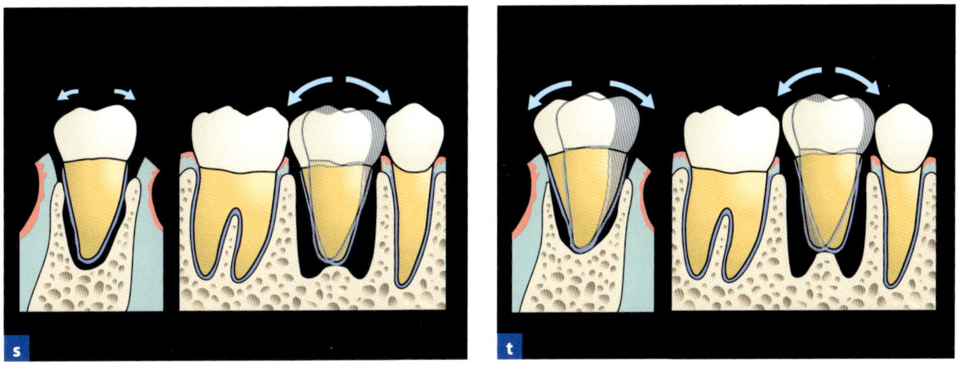

Fig 5-1s If the replica moves mesiodistally but not buccolingually, it means there are interfering areas on the buccolingual walls so the socket should be enlarged more buccolingually.
Fig 5-1t If the replica moves laterally but not to the planned depth, it means the bottom of the socket has interfering areas and should be deepened more with care not to damage vital structures (i.e. the inferior alveolar nerve).

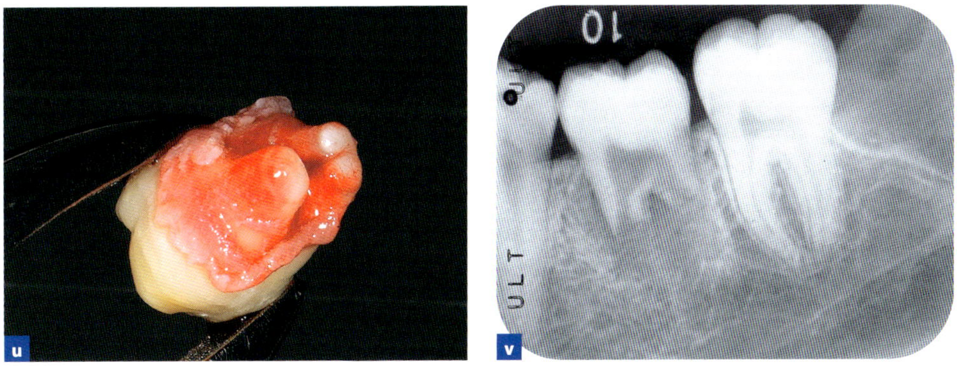

Fig 5-1u The extracted donor tooth (#38). The donor tooth is extracted after completing the preparation of the recipient socket using the replica. The donor tooth is placed into the prepared socket to check the final fit.
Fig 5-1v Check the fit with a radiograph if necessary.

7. Suturing the flaps and fixation of the transplant

It tends to be easier to suture the vertical incision and the interproximal area without the donor tooth in place (**Fig 5-1w** to **5-1z**) (the donor tooth should be preserved in physiologic saline or the original socket during this phase of suturing). The placement of the donor tooth after suturing the flap closed is not difficult because of the elasticity of the gingival tissue of the flap and a better fit can be obtained this way (**Fig 5-1aa**, **5-1bb**, and **5-1ll**). If the suture will be used to fixate the transplanted tooth for the first week, a longer length of the suture string should be left for the crossing and or crisscrossing the sutures (**Fig 5-1aa** to **5-1kk**).

① Flow of suture fixation

After the try-in of the donor tooth is complete, the tooth is preserved in physiological saline or the original socket, and suturing the flap and fixation with sutures are performed. The details of this are shown in **Fig 5-1w** to **5-1kk**.

1. Suture the flap on the distal aspect and place the knot on the buccal or lingual side. Leave about 4 cm of one of the ends of the string (**Fig 5-1w** and **5-1x**).
2. The mesia aspect is sutured, but only one knot is tied, and the knot is placed diagonally across from the knot of the distal side. Proceed to the next step without cutting the thread (**Fig 5-1y** and **5-1z**).
3. The donor tooth is now placed into the recipient socket (**Fig 5-1aa**). Then, a second knot is tied on the mesial aspect (**Fig 5-1bb**).
4. The string with the needle still on it is then tied to the diagonal string on the distal at the center of the transplant (**Fig 5-1cc** and **5-1dd**).
5. A horizontal mattress suture is added to the lingual aspect, and the knots are tied on the occlusal surface using the lingual gingiva as an anchor (**Fig 5-1ee** to **5-1gg**).
6. A horizontal mattress suture is added to the buccal aspect, and the knots are tied on the occlusal surface using the buccal gingiva as an anchor (**Fig 5-1hh** to **5-1kk**). This should result in the transplanted tooth being fixed evenly in the mesiodistal and buccolingual directions.

Since occlusal adjustment cannot be performed after suture fixation, any occlusal adjustments should be completed before transplantation extra-orally or before the extraction of the donor tooth. Suture fixation is usually removed at 1 week and replaced with wire and adhesive resin fixation which is described in the next section.

If the transplant is not stable because the root is too short or the fit between the transplant and the recipient socket is too loose, wire and adhesive resin fixation may be placed on the day of transplantation (**Fig 5-3** and **5-4**).

② Occlusal adjustment

The occlusion must be checked to ensure that no occlusal contact is present. If a suture is used for stabilization, the occlusal contacts should be reduced prior to tying the suture; if a wire splint is used, the adjustment is done after placing the splint. The occlusal surface of the donor tooth may need to be reshaped when there is excessive occlusal discrepancy or if suture fixation is used. The periodontal ligament must be protected with gauze soaked in physiologic saline during the adjustment. If the opposing tooth is supra-erupted, it must be recontoured prior to the surgical procedure.

③ Radiographic evaluation

After transplantation and fixation, postoperative radiograph should be taken to evaluate the transplanted tooth.

8. Surgical dressing, home care instruction, antibiotic administration

The reattachment between the gingival flap and periodontal ligament at the cervical region is one of the key steps to successful transplantation. In order to ensure reattachment at this area, it is important to prevent infection from saliva as well as possible impaction of debris. By protecting the area around the transplant with a surgical dressing for several days after surgery, healing around the cervical region can occur with less risks (**Fig 5-1oo**). The patient should be instructed to brush the teeth gently even over the dressing.

Although it has not been shown that there is a significant benefit to administering antibiotics after the transplantation, the author routinely prescribes tetracycline for 3 days postoperative.

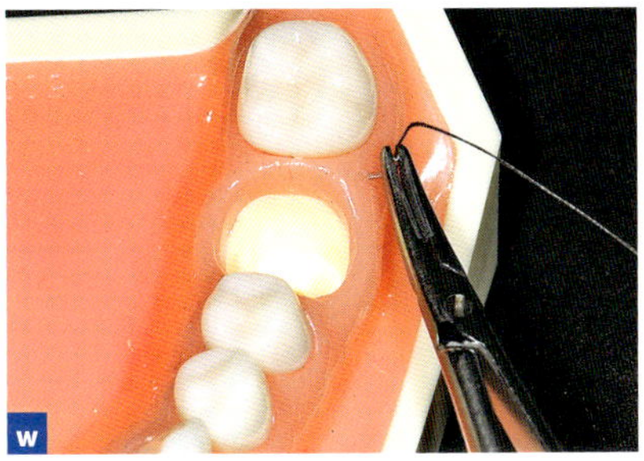

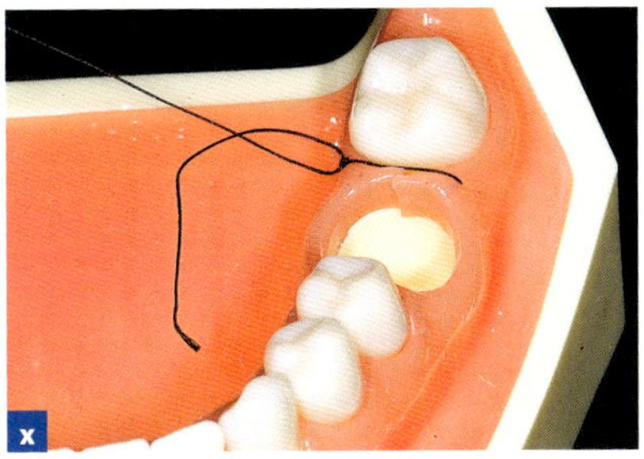

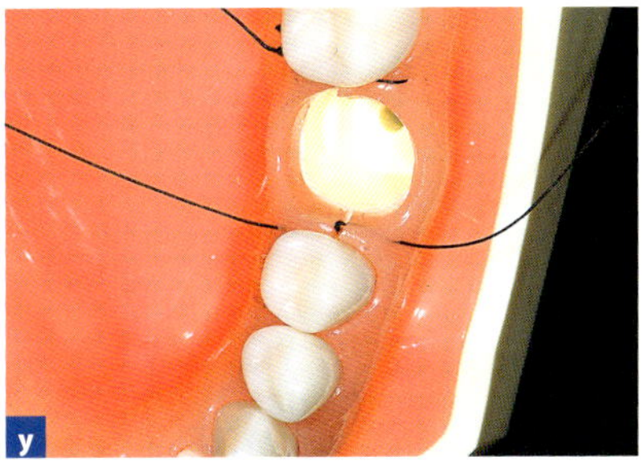

Fig 5-1w After the try-in of the donor tooth, the tooth is preserved in saline and the gingival flap is sutured.
Fig 5-1x, y Suture the distal interproximal area and place the knot on the buccal or lingual side. Leave about 4 cm of one of the suture ends.

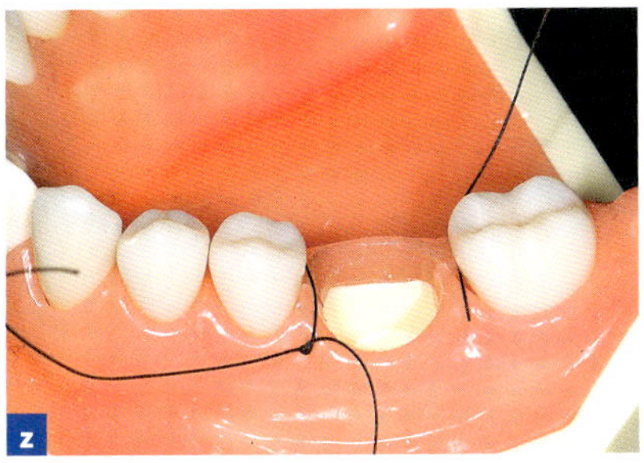

Fig 5-1z The mesial interproximal area is sutured, but only one surgical knot is made, and the knot is placed diagonally across from the distal one. Proceed to the next step without cutting the suture.

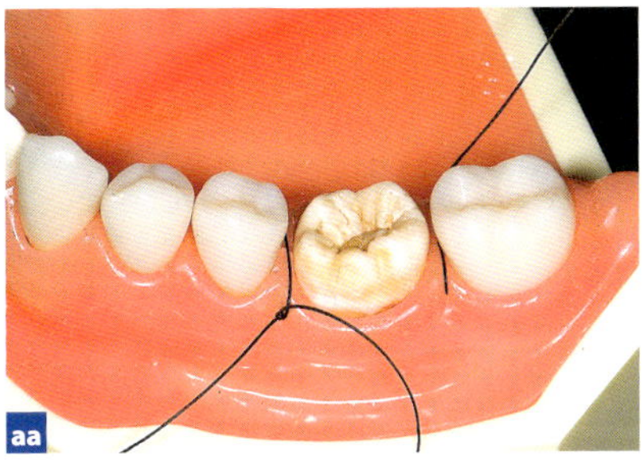

Fig 5-1aa The donor tooth is now placed into the socket.

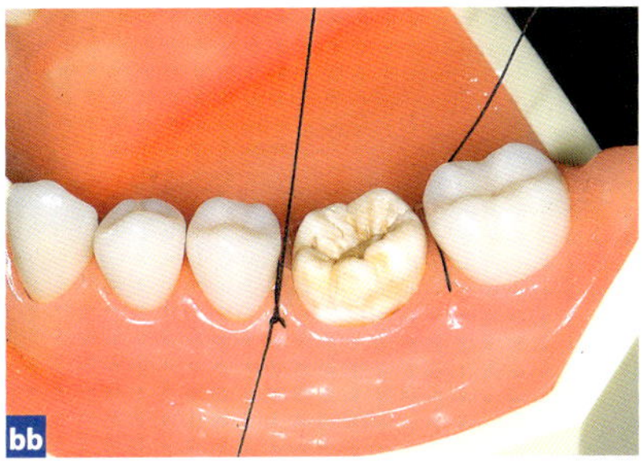

Fig 5-1bb Tie the second knot of the mesial suture. Do not cut the suture and move to the next step.

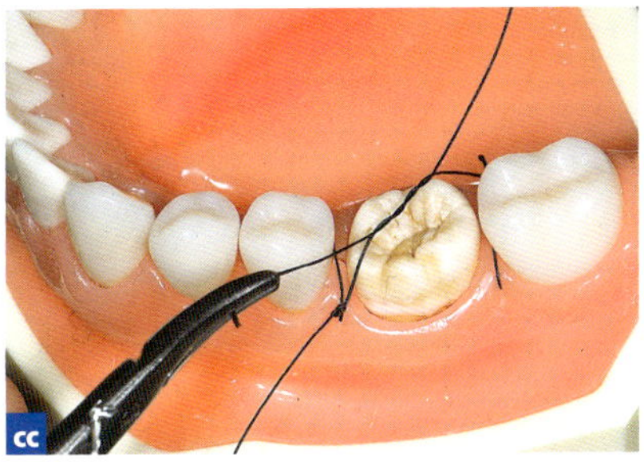

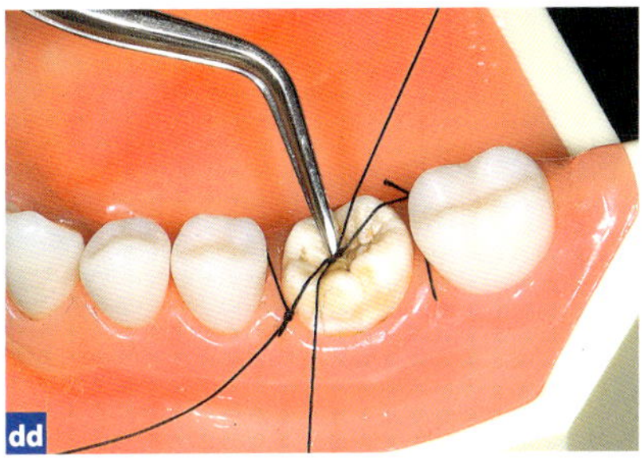

Fig 5-1cc, 5-1dd A cross suture is made between the mesial suture and the remaining distal suture. The knot should be placed in the center of the occlusal surface of the transplanted tooth. Holding the occlusal surface with tweezers prevents the thread from loosening when tying.

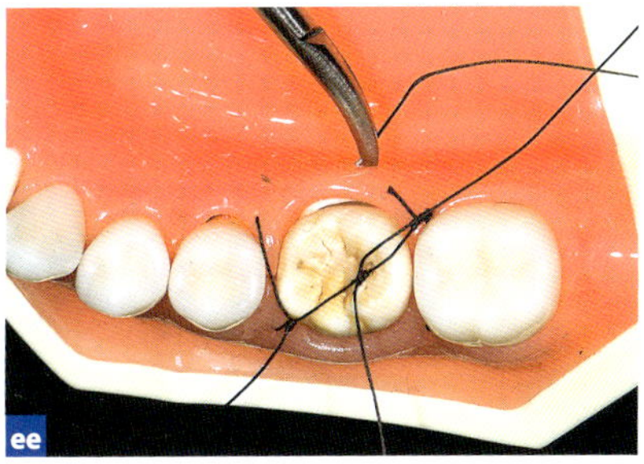

Fig 5-1ee Add a horizontal mattress suture on the lingual side.

9. Removal of dressing and suture, and splinting with bonded wire

The patient is usually asked to come for a check the day after the surgery. The dressing and sutures should be removed and the tooth and surrounding soft tissues cleaned with a cotton swab 5 to 7 days after surgery. The patient should be instructed to brush the area gently. As the mobility of the transplant is typically high after 7 days, wire and adhesive resin splinting can be placed as follows:

After removal of the sutures, the buccal side (or lingual side) of the transplant and the adjacent tooth (splinting to one tooth is typically enough) are etched. Then the two teeth are fixed with the adhesive resin such as "Super Bond®" (Sun Medical, Shiga, Japan) and a flexible wire such as "Twisted wire7" (3M Unitek, USA). The details of the procedure are explained in **Fig 5-1pp** to **5-1ss**.

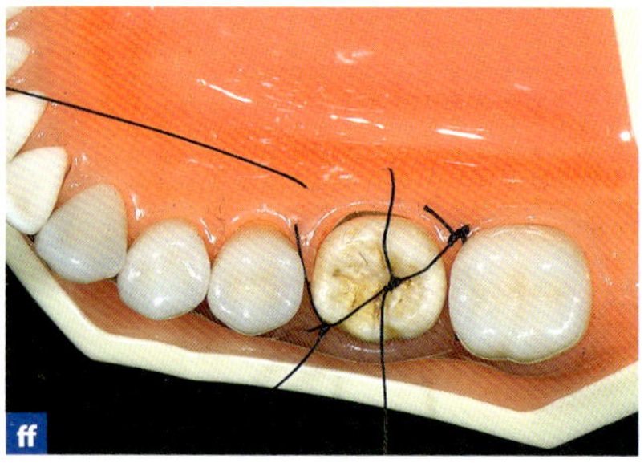
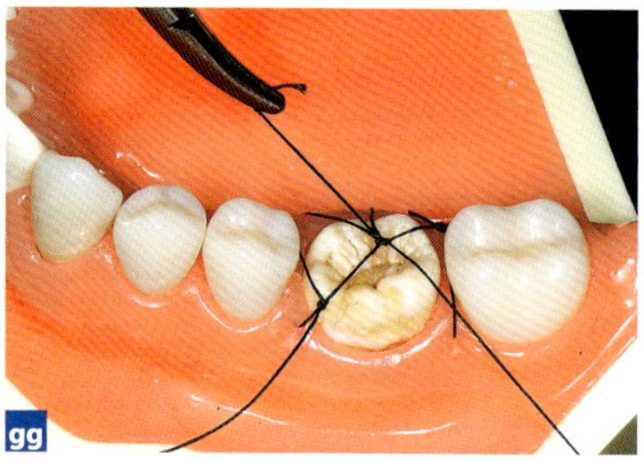

Fig 5-1ff, 5-1gg Using the gingiva on the lingual side as an anchor, knots are made on the occlusal surface.

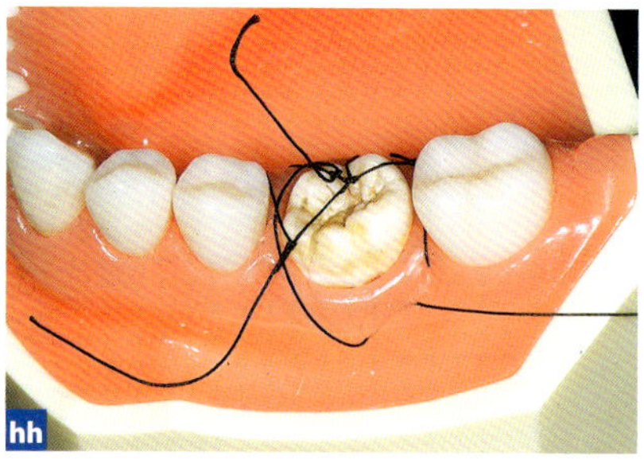

Fig 5-1hh Add a horizontal mattress suture on the buccal side.

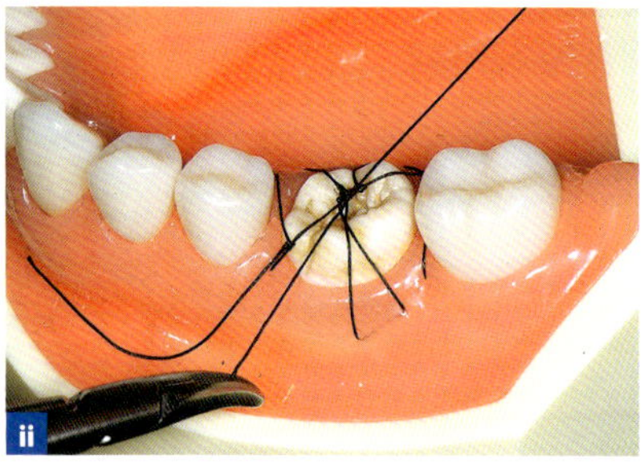
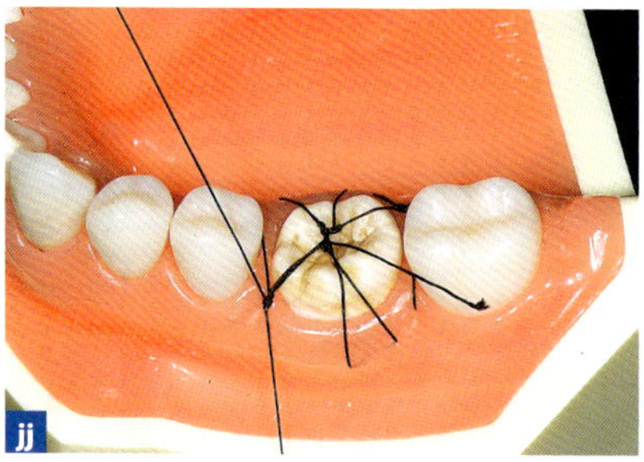
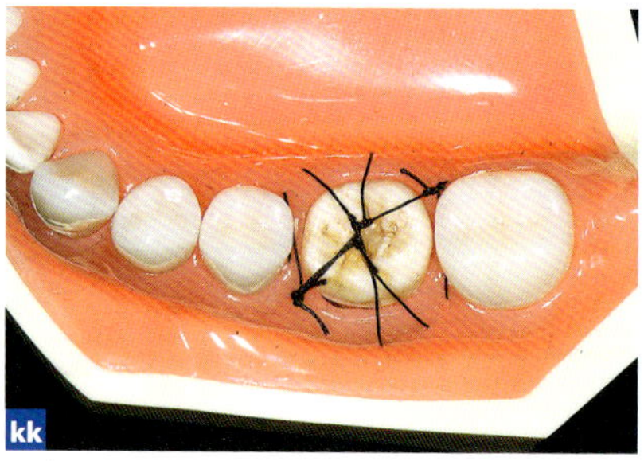

Fig 5-1ii to 5-1kk Using the buccal gingiva as an anchor, knots are made on the occlusal surface. The transplanted tooth is now tightly fixed in position.

1. Cut the wire so that it reaches from the transplant to the adjacent tooth (about 1 cm) (**Fig 5-1pp**).
2. Etch the buccal side of the adjacent tooth and the transplant for about 15 seconds with 37% phosphoric acid solution (**Fig 5-1qq**).
3. Rinse with water. Rinse the water from the gingival side and suction from the occlusal side so that the etchant does not enter the gingival sulcus. Air drying is performed in the same way (**Fig 5-1rr**).
4. Place adhesive resin on the etched surface with the wire and wait for setting (if it is a self-curing or dual-cure resin) or light cure (if it is a light-cured resin) (**Fig 5-1ss**).

There is no definitive answer as to what is the best type and duration of fixation of the transplant on the prognosis. From clinical experience, excessive movement of the transplant would likely be disadvantageous for obtaining reattachment (PDL healing). The literature suggests that long-term rigid fixation after replantation may induce ankylosis[14], but it is questionable whether this is the case for transplantation[15]. The author prefers suture fixation on the day of transplantation (**Fig 5-1aa** to **5-1kk**), and after 7 days, the fixation is changed to the bonded wire (**Fig 5-1pp** to **5-1ss**), which will help stabilize the tooth during chewing and root canal treatment which is usually started 2 weeks after transplantation. This bonded wire fixation is usually removed 1 to 2 months after transplantation.

The timing of removal is determined by the degree of mobility of the transplanted tooth. The tooth should be stable with low mobility by the time the wire splint is removed.

When performing root canal treatment of a transplanted mature tooth, it is easier to do so while keeping the wire splint on to help maintain stability and protection.

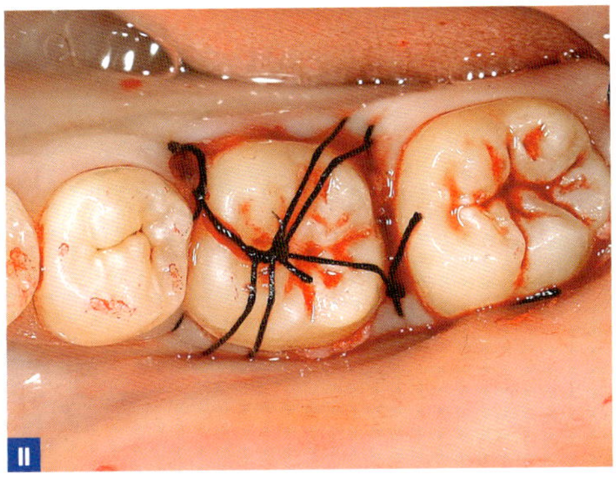

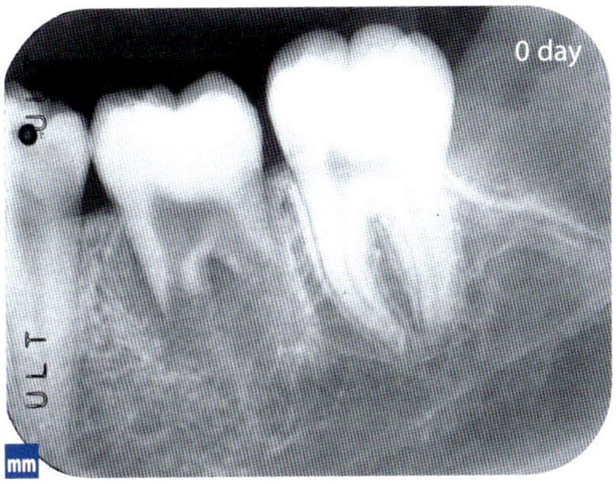

Fig 5-1ll Clinical photograph immediately after transplantation.
Fig 5-1mm Radiograph immediately after transplantation.

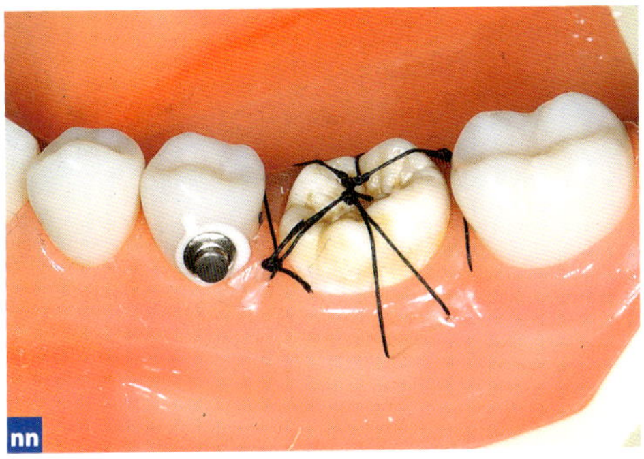

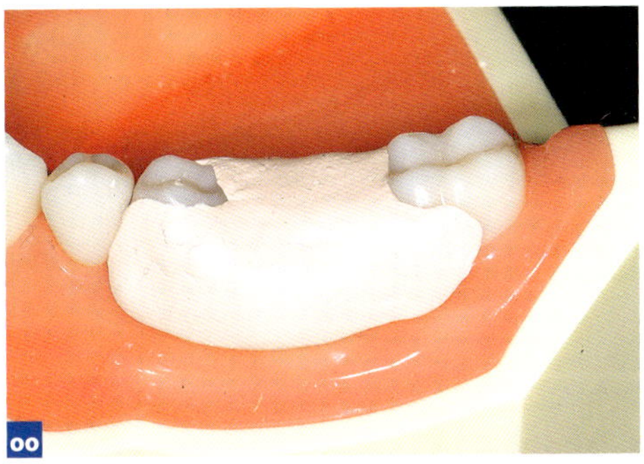

Fig 5-1nn Adhesion of a lingual button for dressing retention. It can be easily adhered with conventional glass ionomer cement without any bonding system.
Fig 5-1oo Surgical dressing. Surgical dressing and suture strings are usually removed in 7 days and wire and adhesive resin fixation is performed if the mobility of the transplant is high.

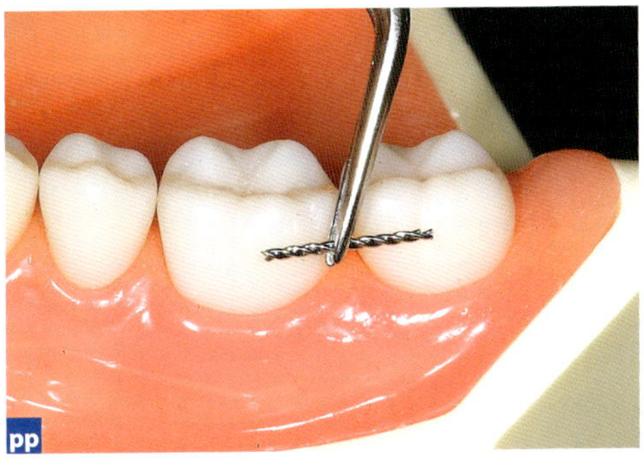

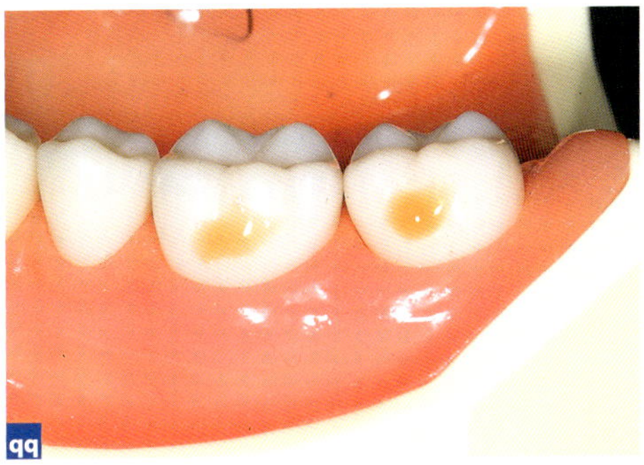

Fig 5-1pp Wire try-in. Cut the wire "Twisted wire 7" (3M Unitek) approximately 1 cm.
Fig 5-1qq Etch the surface of the teeth for about 15 seconds with 37% phosphoric acid.

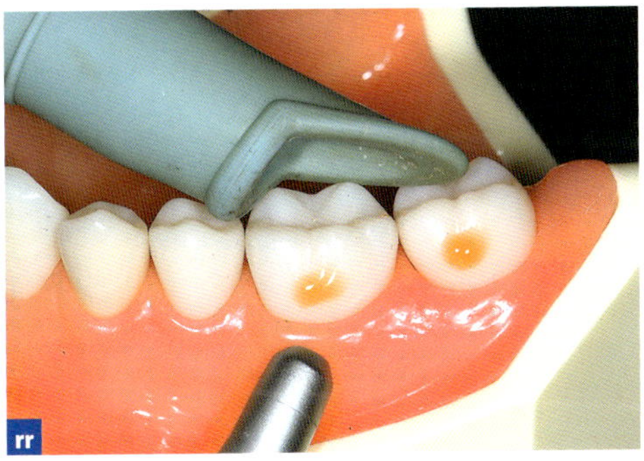

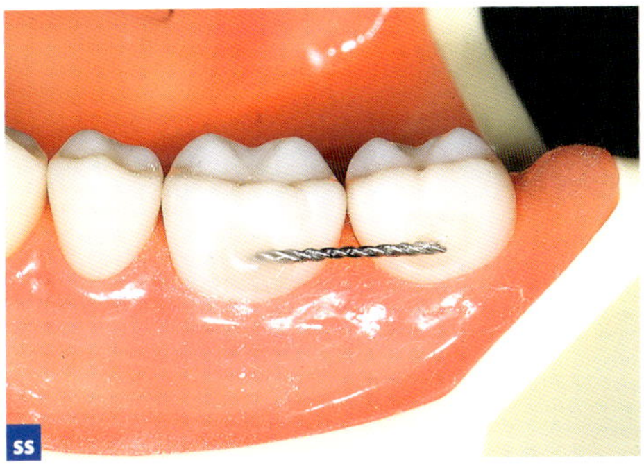

Fig 5-1rr Wash with water. Flow water from the gingival side to the occlusal side.
Fig 5-1ss After air drying, the wire is adhered to surface of the teeth with adhesive resin "Super Bond®" (Sun Medical) to splint the transplant to the adjacent tooth.

Root canal treatment for transplanted teeth

Root canal treatment is necessary for the fully developed donor tooth before or after transplantation because pulp healing cannot be expected after apical closure (**Fig 5-3** to **5-6**). In the case of an impacted donor tooth, RCT is performed 2 weeks after the transplantation. After cleaning and instrumentation of the root canal spaces, an interim dressing of calcium hydroxide is placed in the canals. About 1 to 2 months later, the calcium hydroxide is replaced with gutta-percha and sealer[16,17]. The reason RCT is started 2 weeks after the transplantation is that earlier RCT may negatively affect the attachment around the transplanted tooth and obturation material may damage the periodontal ligament. The advantage of using calcium hydroxide before final obturation is twofold: (1) if the tooth is not fully formed, the calcium hydroxide will promote apical closure (**Fig 5-5**) and (2) the calcium hydroxide is an excellent antiseptic that will keep the root canal system free from bacterial contamination during the important attachment phase of healing.

Root canal treatment performed extraorally at the time of transplantation can be both time- and cost-effective. However, there is the risk of damage to the periodontal ligament during the procedure, so extraoral RCT is not recommended unless the periodontal ligament can be kept intact during the procedure[18,19].

Pulpal healing is expected with transplantation of an immature tooth (**Fig 5-1tt** to **5-1yy**, see **Chapter 3**). Closure of the apex and positive response to electric pulp tests are expected and the roots should continue to develop (**Fig 5-1tt** to **5-1yy**, see **Chapter 3**). The pulp should be monitored closely for healing with transplanted teeth at developmental stage 6 (**Fig 5-2**). Root canal treatment should be started immediately if inflammatory root resorption is suspected (see **Chapter 3**), or if pulp infection is diagnosed. If there is suspected pulp necrosis and the apex is open, apexification can be performed to establish a hard tissue barrier apically before obturation (**Fig 5-5**, see **Chapter 3**).

Natural movement of transplanted teeth

After removal of the wire splint, the transplanted tooth should be allowed to naturally settle into its new position; however, it is advisable to continually check for and adjust any developing occlusal interference. This will help with the reattachment of the periodontal ligament and osseous healing around the transplant. During the natural movement and settling of the transplanted tooth, the whole arch will align in a functional manner, creating proximal contacts in most cases (**Fig 5-1tt** to **5-1aaa**).

Orthodontic movement of transplanted teeth

When the position or the angulation of the transplanted tooth in the arch is not ideal, or when orthodontic treatment had been planned prior to the surgery (see **Chapter 9**), orthodontic treatment can be initiated at the appropriate time. Not only the position of the transplanted tooth but also the height of the alveolar bone can be changed by orthodontic movement[20,21] (see **Chapter 3 Fig 3-58**). It is better to start orthodontic movement after complete healing of the periodontal ligament around the transplanted tooth (usually about 12 weeks) but before complete healing of the alveolar bone. Extrusive orthodontic movement can be started 1 month after the transplantation. The movement of the roots out of the alveolar bone may prevent early ankylosis.

Fig 5-1tt, uu One month after transplantation. In the transplantation of immature teeth, radiographs should be taken every month for 3 months after transplantation to confirm that inflammatory resorption has not occurred.

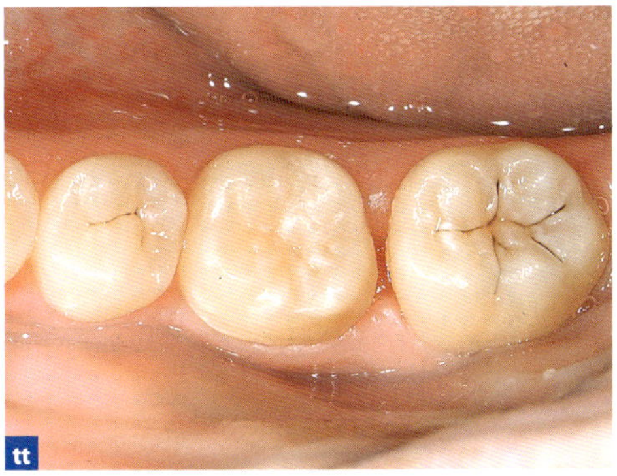

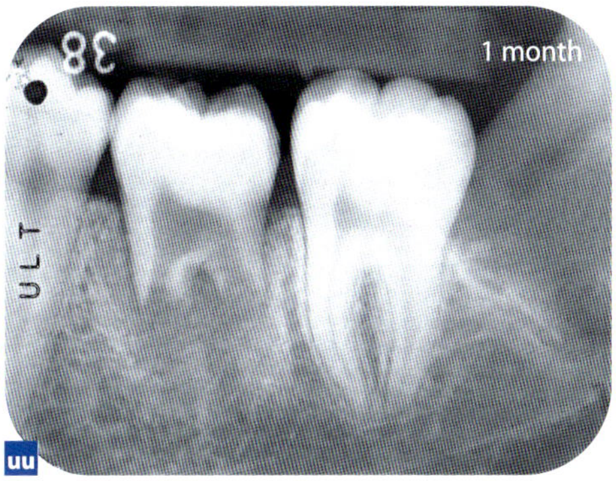

Fig 5-1vv, ww Two years after transplantation. Pulpal healing (pulp canal obliteration) and root development can be observed. The transplant responds EPT(+).

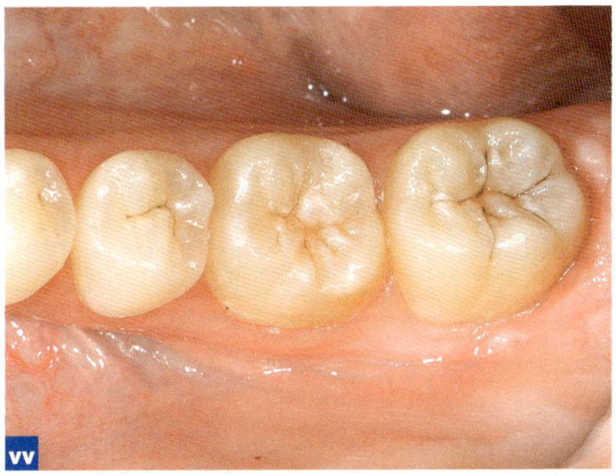

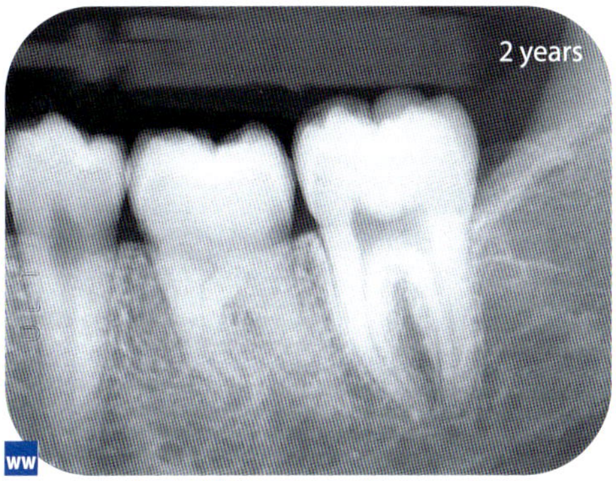

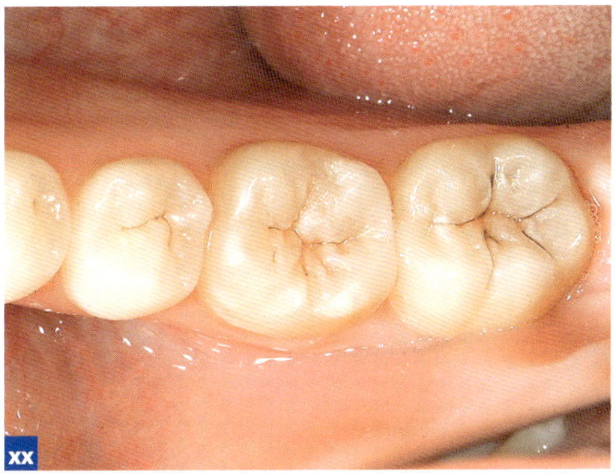

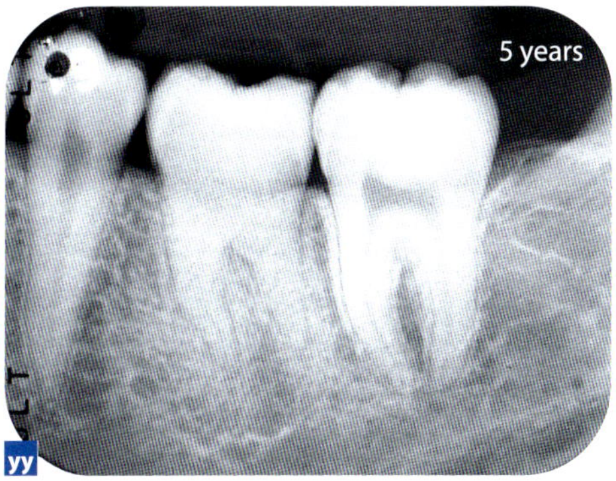

Fig 5-1xx to aaa Five years after transplantation. The transplant responds EPT(+). Pulpal healing and root development are evident. A functional occlusal relationship with the opposing tooth is maintained.

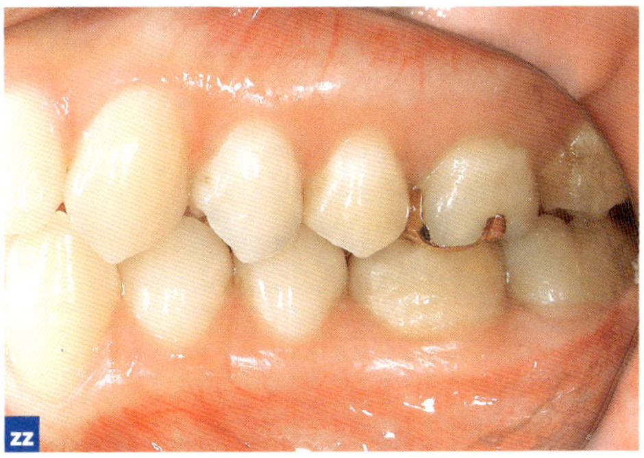

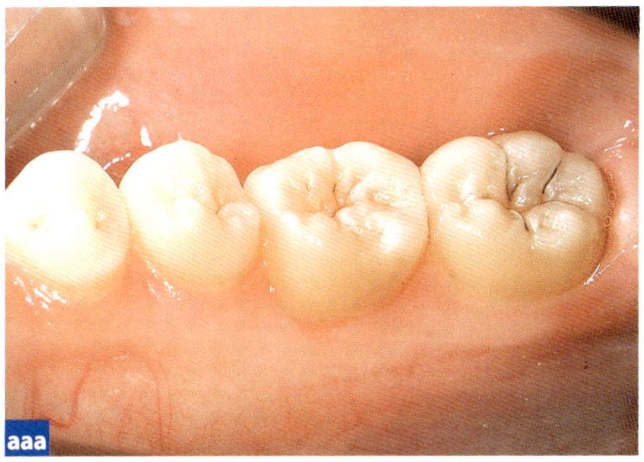

A case of delayed transplantation of an immature third molar

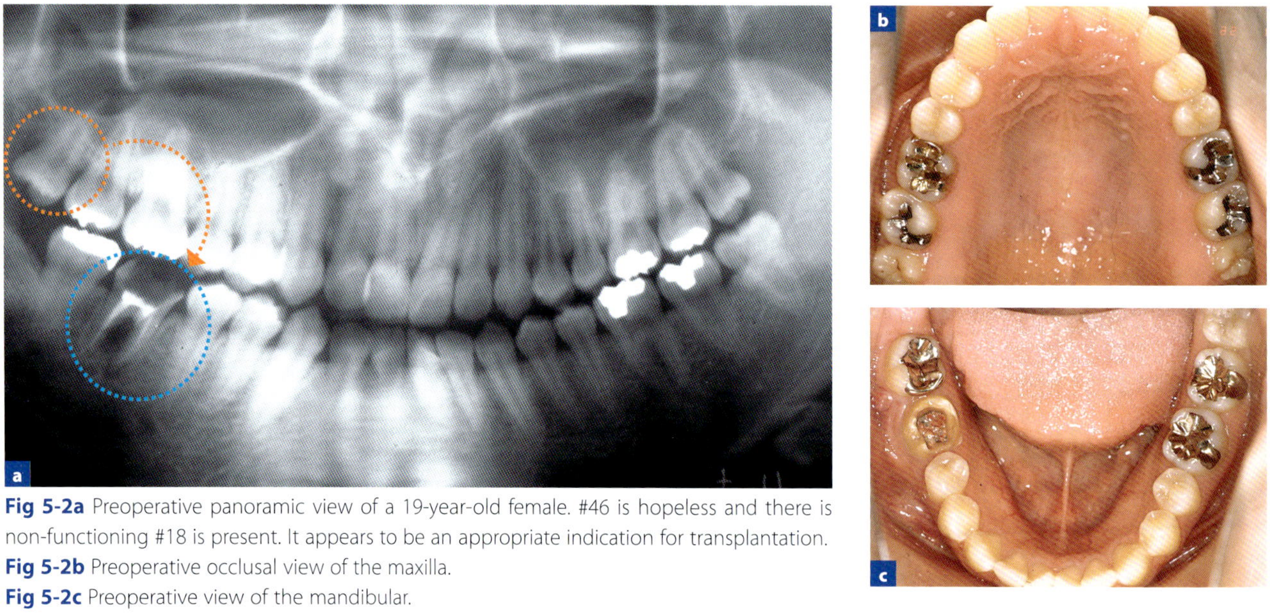

Fig 5-2a Preoperative panoramic view of a 19-year-old female. #46 is hopeless and there is non-functioning #18 is present. It appears to be an appropriate indication for transplantation.
Fig 5-2b Preoperative occlusal view of the maxilla.
Fig 5-2c Preoperative view of the mandibular.

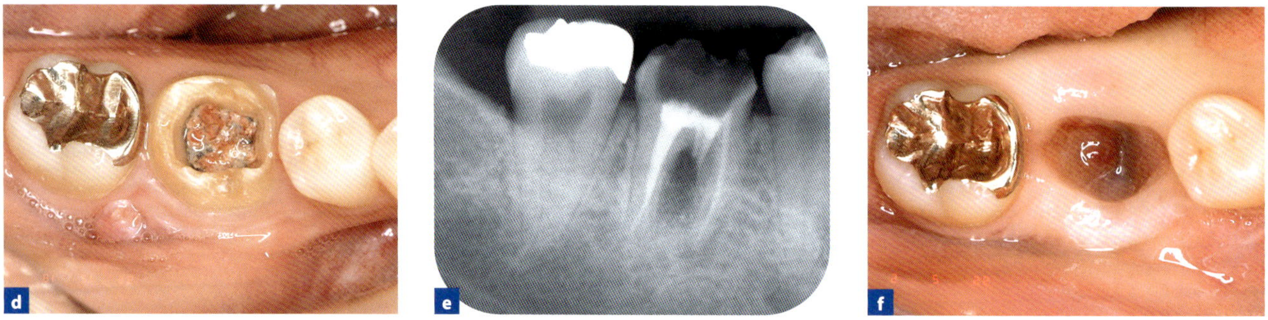

Fig 5-2d, e Recipient site before treatment. Her chief complaint was an abscess on the buccal aspect of the hopeless #46.
Fig 5-2f Three weeks after the extraction of #46. The recipient socket is closing with keratinized gingiva which will be of benefit when trying to close the flap more tightly around the transplant. Delayed transplantation is an option when the donor tooth is smaller compared with the recipient socket.

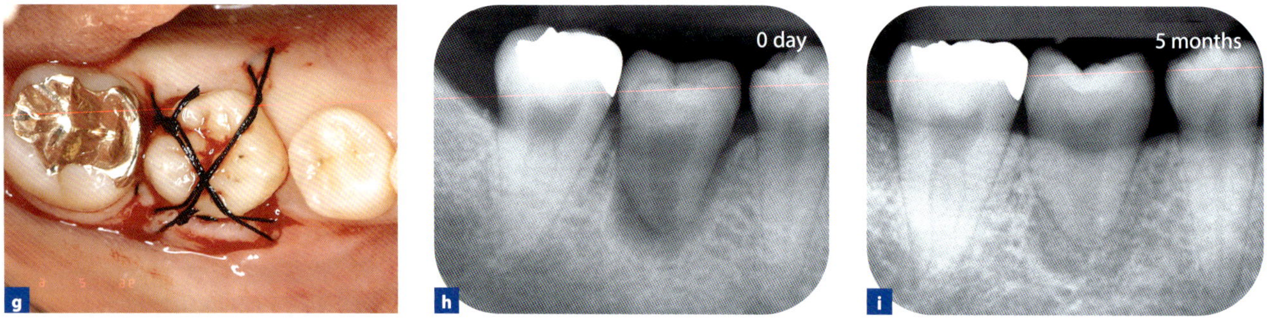

Fig 5-2g Immediately after the delayed transplantation which was performed 3 weeks after the extraction of #46. Delayed transplantation is optimal when performed 3 to 6 weeks after extraction. If waiting longer than 2 months, the alveolar ridge of the recipient site may be reduced, making it difficult to form a recipient socket. Note there is no gap between the transplant and the gingiva.

Fig 5-2h Radiograph immediately after transplantation. It appears that the apical foramen is wider than 1 mm, which indicates that pulpal healing can be expected.

Fig 5-2i Radiograph after 5 months. The PDL space around the transplant is becoming more even. The transplant responds EPT(+).

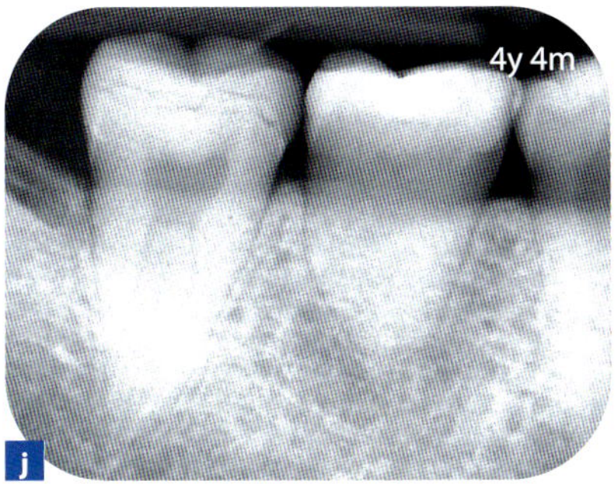

Fig 5-2j Four years and 4 months after transplantation. Pulp canal obliteration is evident.

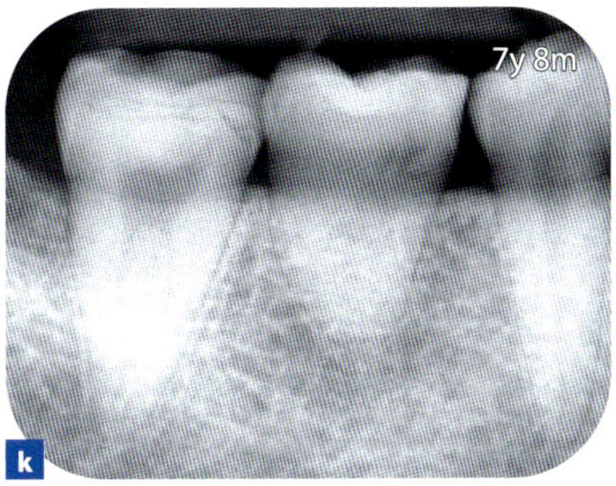

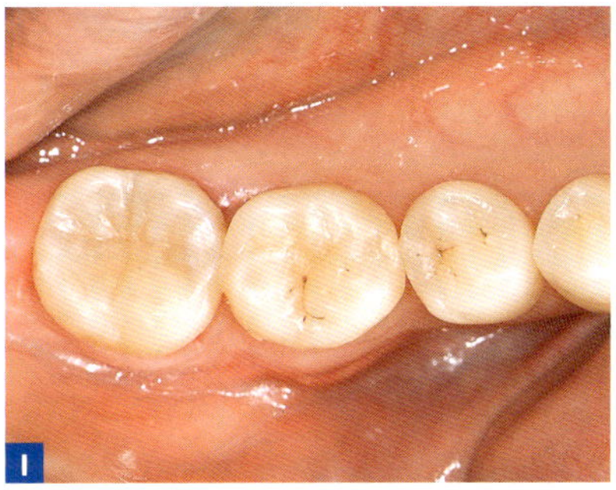

Fig 5-2k, l Seven years and 8 months after transplantation. The transplant responds EPT(+) and is restored (morphologically modified) with composite resin (CR).

Restorative treatment of transplanted teeth

In an ideal situation, when an immature third molar is transplanted to another site in the arch, restorative treatment does not become necessary, provided the pulp heals and no root canal therapy is needed (**Fig 5-1tt** to **5-1aaa**). But there are cases in which some aspect of restorative dentistry will be needed, such as restoring an access cavity after root canal treatment, establishing better interproximal contact, or recontouring the crown (e.g. when a premolar is used as an anterior tooth).

Transplanted teeth are one's own natural teeth and, thus all types of restorative treatments can be performed. For the author, CR restorations are the first choice of material considering the cost of treatment and preservation of esthetics and structure of enamel (**Fig 5-1** to **5-5**).

Internal bleaching can be performed before the restorative treatment of an endodontically treated anterior transplanted tooth (see **Chapter 8 Fig 8-1** and **8-3**). If it requires extensive recontouring, an all-ceramic restoration can be fabricated.

In the case of developing teeth, any preparation should be kept within enamel, or if the preparation is into dentin, then it should be restored as soon as possible because microbial infiltration can progress more easily through the dentin. If endodontic infection develops later on a tooth that has developed canal calcification, then endodontic treatment becomes more difficult (see **Chapter 3 Fig 3-31**).

Maintenance

Transplanted teeth should be monitored on a schedule: at 1, 2, 3, 6 and 12 months, then yearly. Evidence of pulpal healing in immature transplants is continued root formation and pulp canal obliteration (**Fig 5-1** and **5-2**). Lack of pulpal healing and infection will lead to periradicular lesions (see **Chapter 3 Fig 3-31** and **3-35**) with or without inflammatory root resorption (see **Chapter 3 Fig 3-20**). Gingival healing can be improved and maintained by daily good oral hygiene by patients.

Successful transplantation will show uniform PDL space along the root surfaces on radiographs and normal tooth mobility. Percussion test is reliable for assessing ankylosis of transplants. Two major problems leading to transplants failure are progressive root resorption and loss of attachment (see **Chapter 11**).

Conventional sequence and treatment procedures in transplantation were explained in this Chapter. However, the same surgical technique may not be applicable to all clinical cases. It is necessary to modify procedures little by little depending on each case. More details are diecussed in **Chapter 6** to **Chapter10**.

Transplantation of a mature tooth into a recipient site with two adjacent teeth

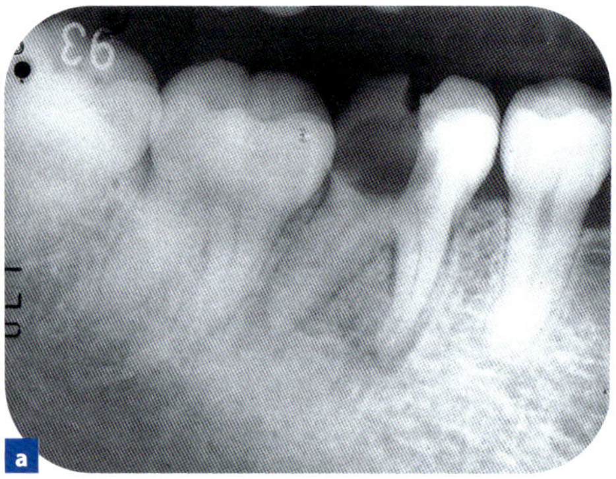

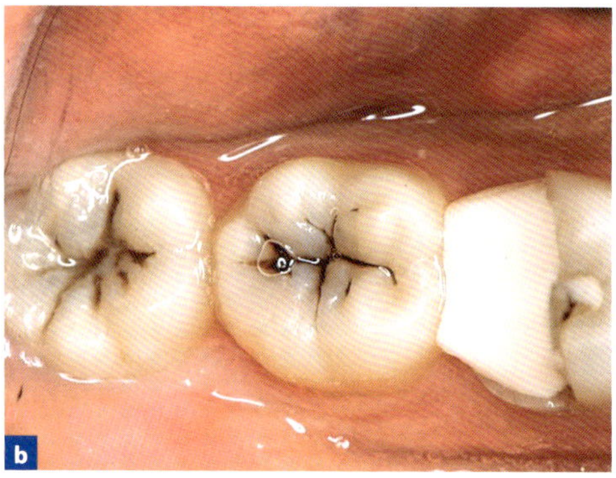

Fig 5-3a, b Views of a 24-year-old female, Treatment plan was accepted to transplant #48 to the hopeless #46 site.

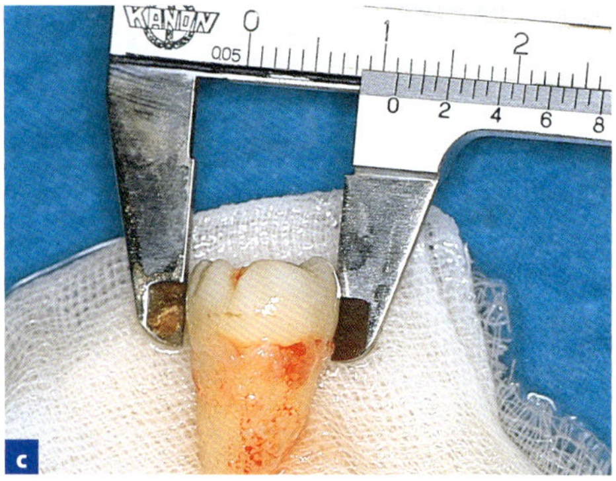

Fig 5-3c Measurement of the mesiodistal width of the crown of the donor tooth.

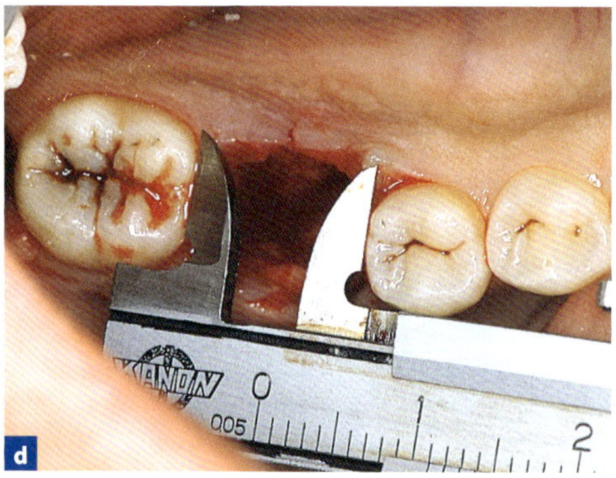

Fig 5-3d Measurement of mesiodistal width on the recipient site.

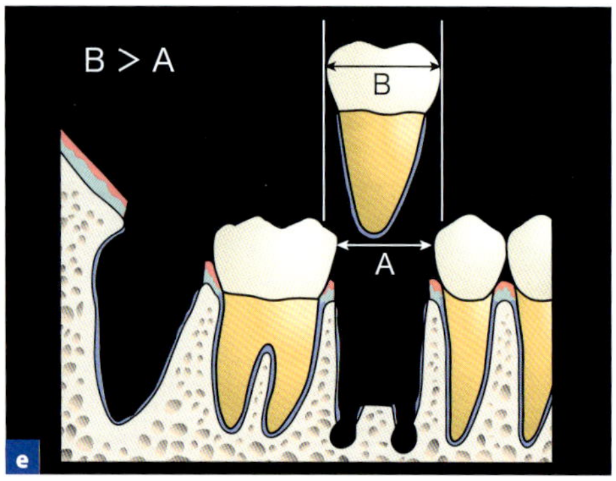

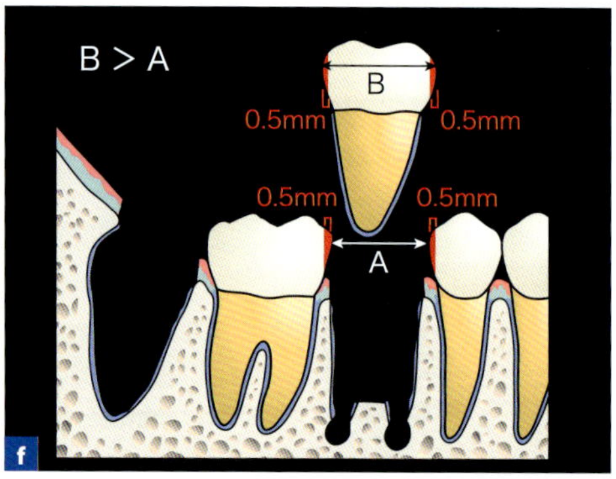

Fig 5-3e, f If the mesiodistal width of the door tooth is slightly larger than that of the recipient site, the proximal surfaces of the donor tooth and both adjacent teeth can be conservatively reduced (not to exceed 0.5 mm of preparation) to adjust and fit into the space.

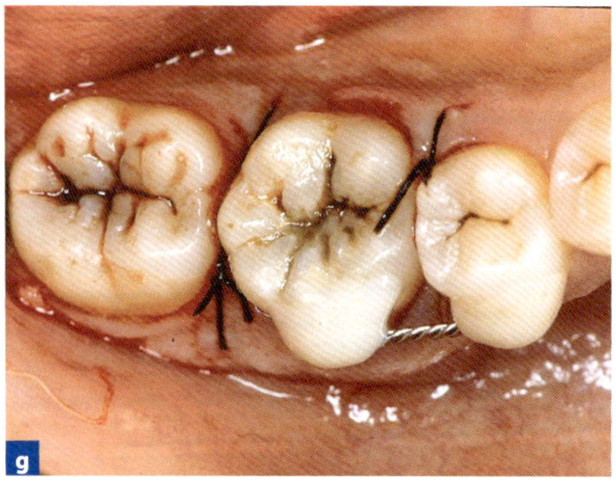

Fig 5-3g After surgery and fixation.

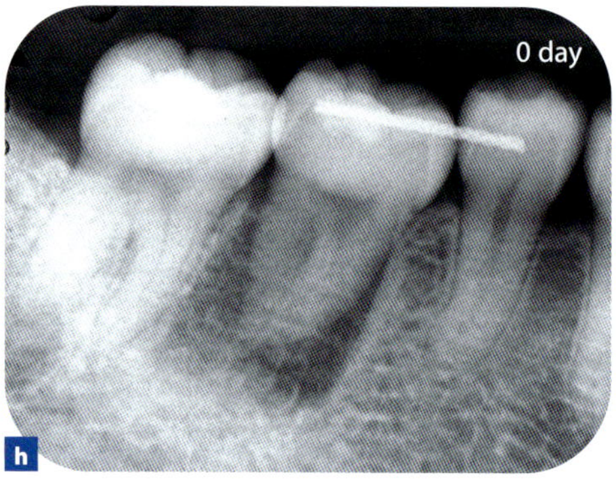

Fig 5-3h Radiograph immediately after transplantation.

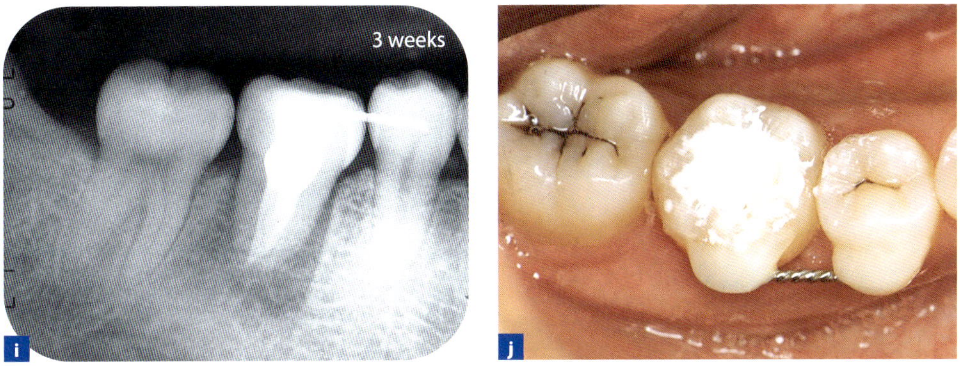

Fig 5-3i, j Three weeks after transplantation. Root canal treatment is started 2 weeks after transplantation, and the root canal is cleaned and filled with a calcium hydroxide preparation "Vitapex®" (NEO Dental chemical products). Root canal filling with sealer and gutta-percha is performed 4 to 5 weeks after transplantation. The fixation is removed immediately after the RCT.

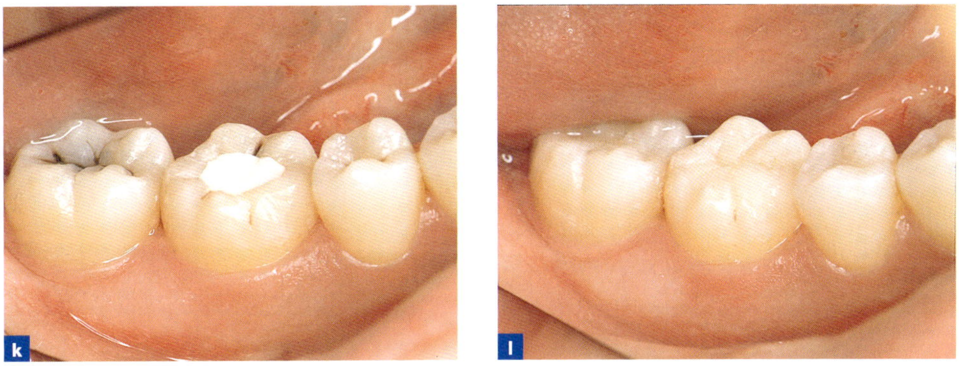

Fig 5-3k 75 days after transplantation. There is evidence of natural movement (drifting) of the transplant.
Fig 5-3l After crown restoration with CR.

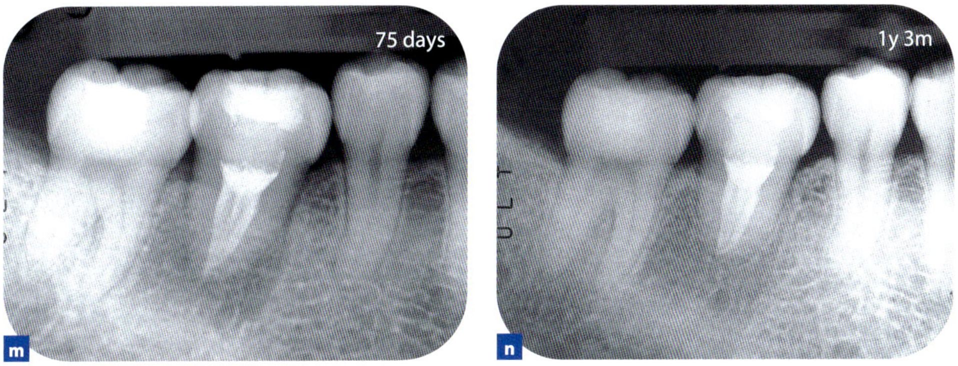

Fig 5-3m Radiograph 75 days after transplantation.
Fig 5-3n Radiograph 1 year and 3 months after transplantation. Normal periodontal ligament space and alveolar bone proper are observed.

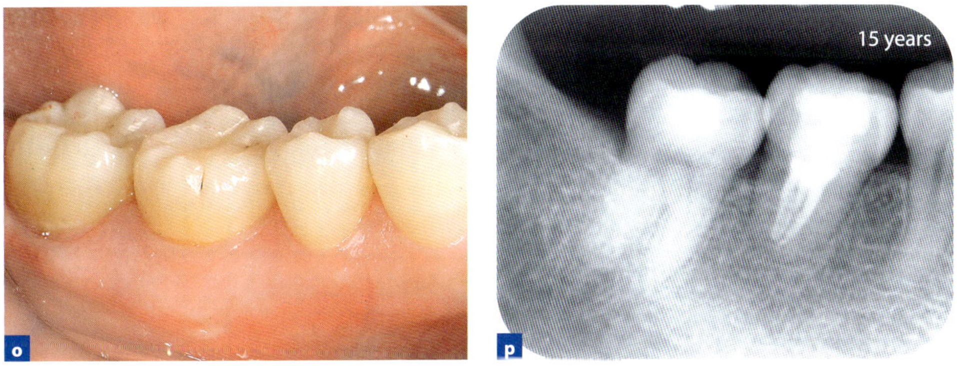

Fig 5-3o, p 15 years after transplantation. Slight progression of periodontitis is observed throughout the dentition, but no apparent abnormalities are detected for the transplant.

Transplantation when the mesiodistal width on the recipient site is 2 mm less than that of the width of the donor tooth

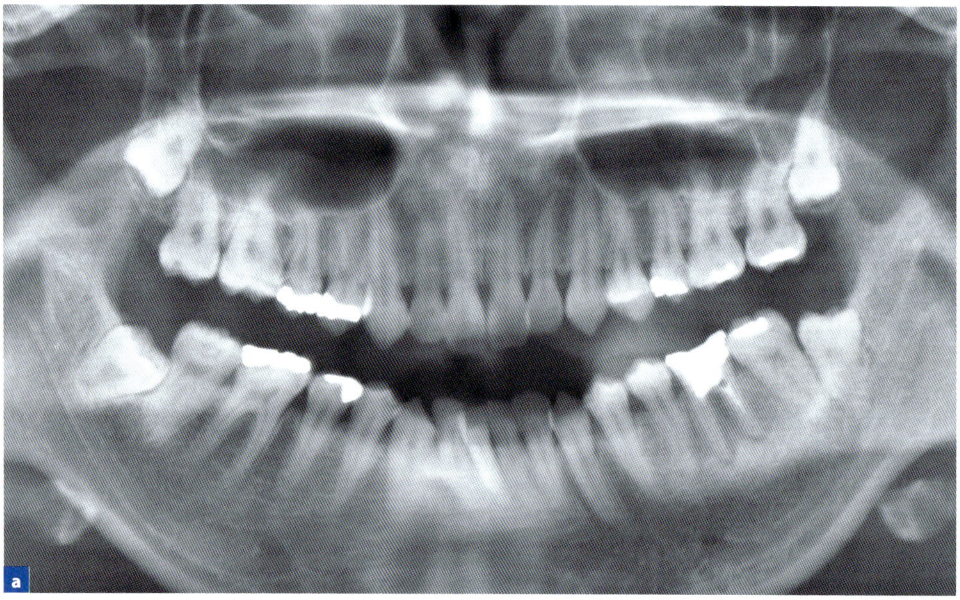

Fig 5-4a Preoperative panoramic radiograph of a 27-year-old female. Treatment plan was accepted to perform transplantation of #38 to the site of the #36 which has an unfavorable prognosis.

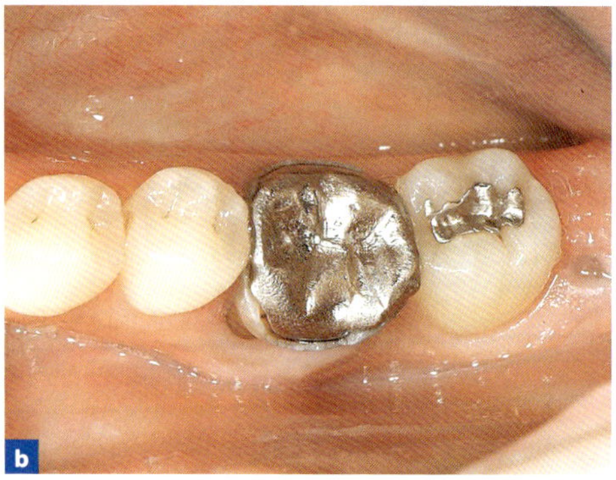

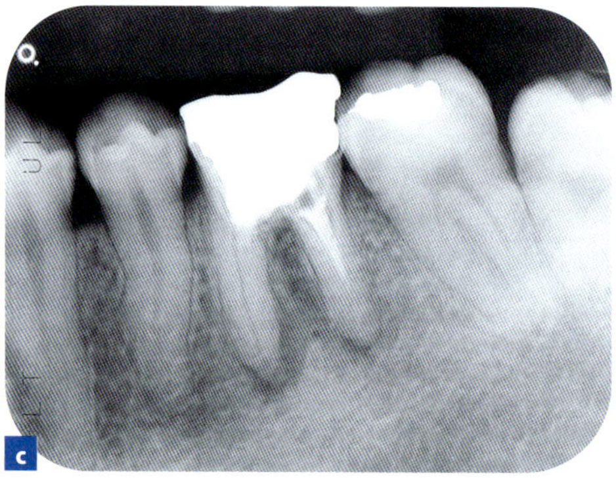

Fig 5-4b Occlusal view of the recipient site before treatment.
Fig 5-4c Preoperative radiograph.

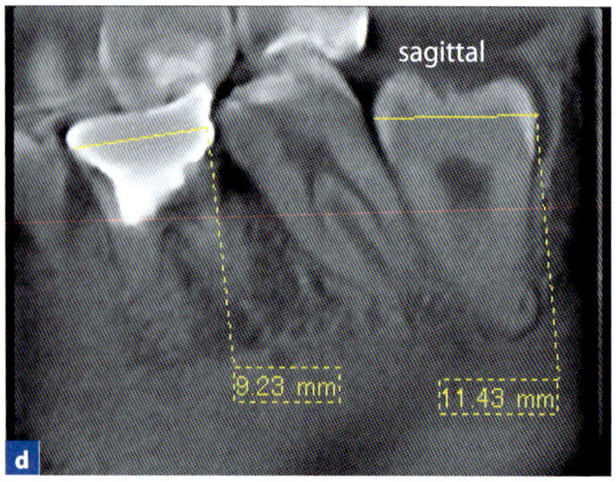

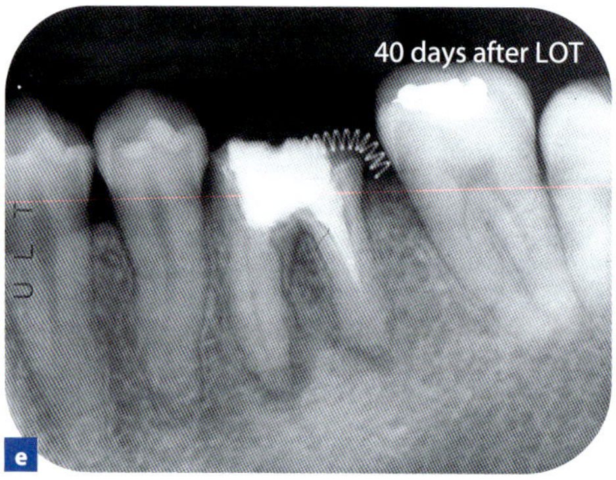

Fig 5-4d Sagittal CBCT image before treatment. The mesiodistal width of the recipient site is more than 2 mm shorter than that of the donor tooth.
Fig 5-4e 40 days after starting LOT. Sufficient space is regained by up-righting #37.

Fig 5-4f Occlusal view of the LOT device at the end of up-righting. A temporary crown is made of self-curing MMA resin on the recipient tooth in which a coil is placed to push the adjacent tooth.
Fig 5-4g Extracted donor tooth. **g1**: the lingual aspect. **g2**: the mesial aspect.

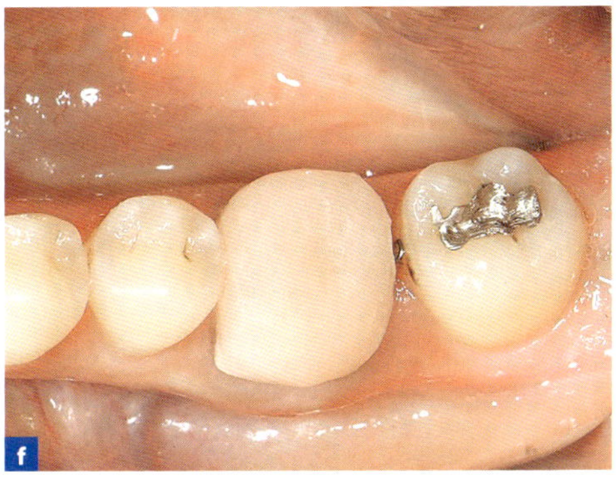

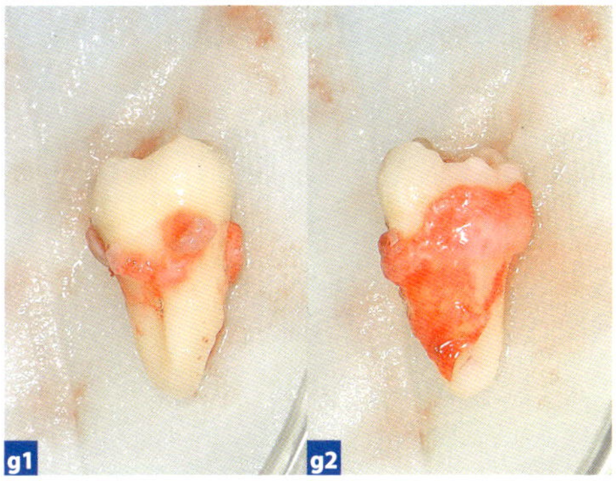

Fig 5-4h Radiograph immediately after transplantation.
Fig 5-4i Five months after transplantation.

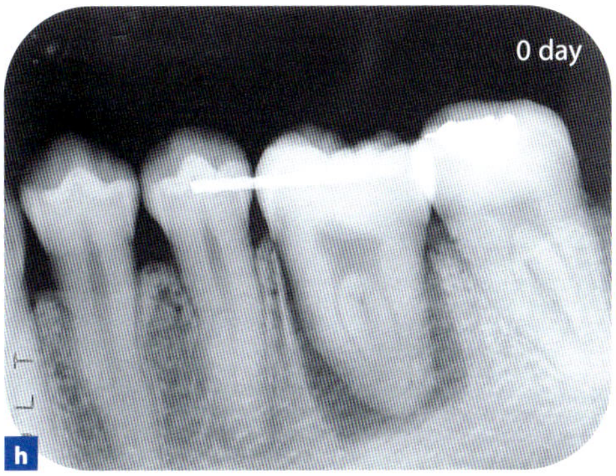

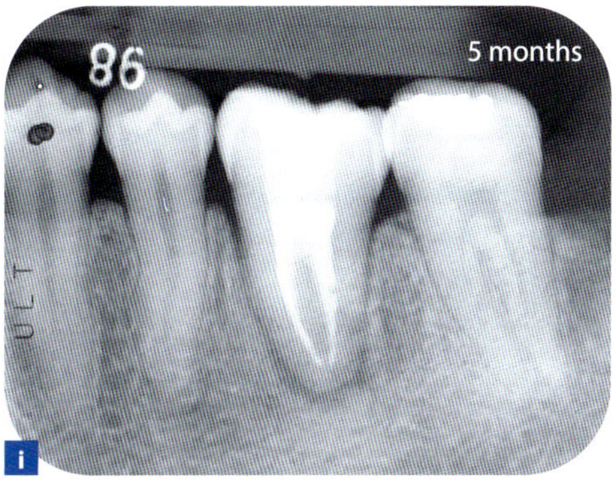

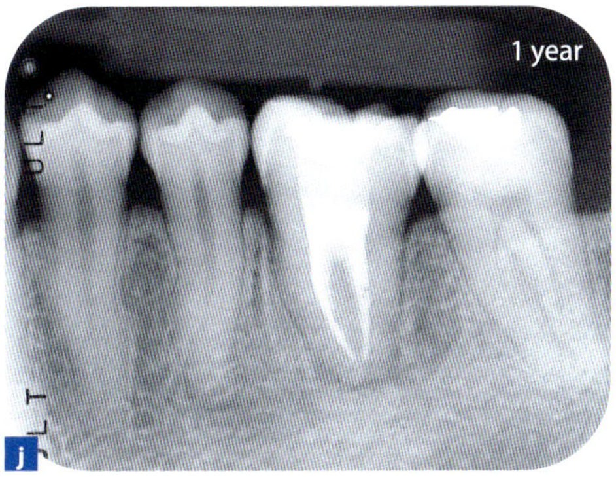

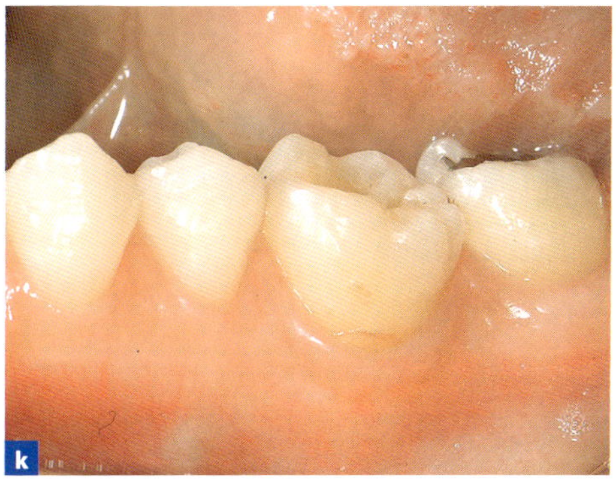

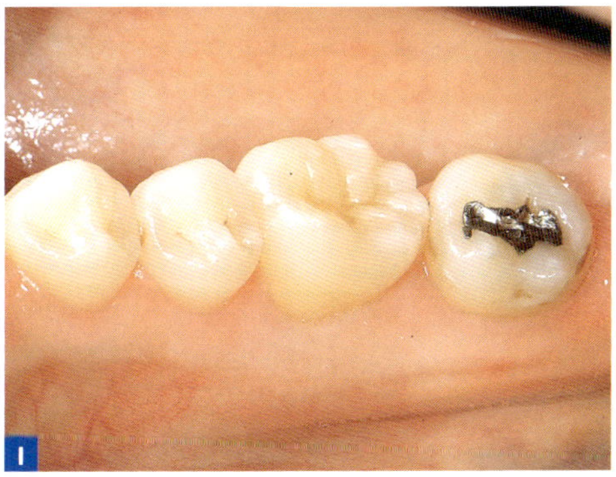

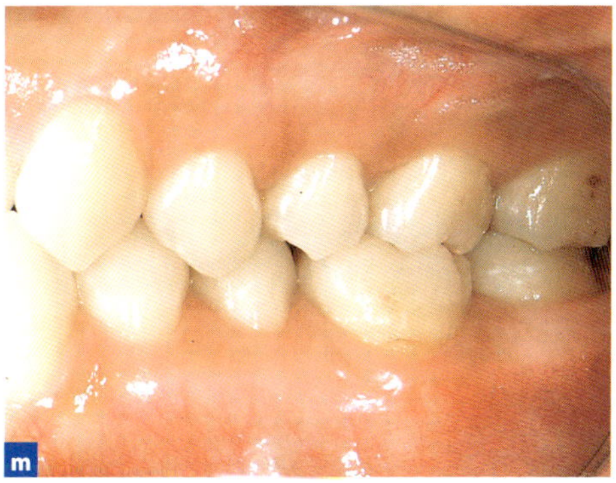

Fig 5-4j to m One year after transplantation. No evident abnormalities are observed.
The transplanted tooth has been restored with CR.

Transplantation with maxillary sinus floor elevation

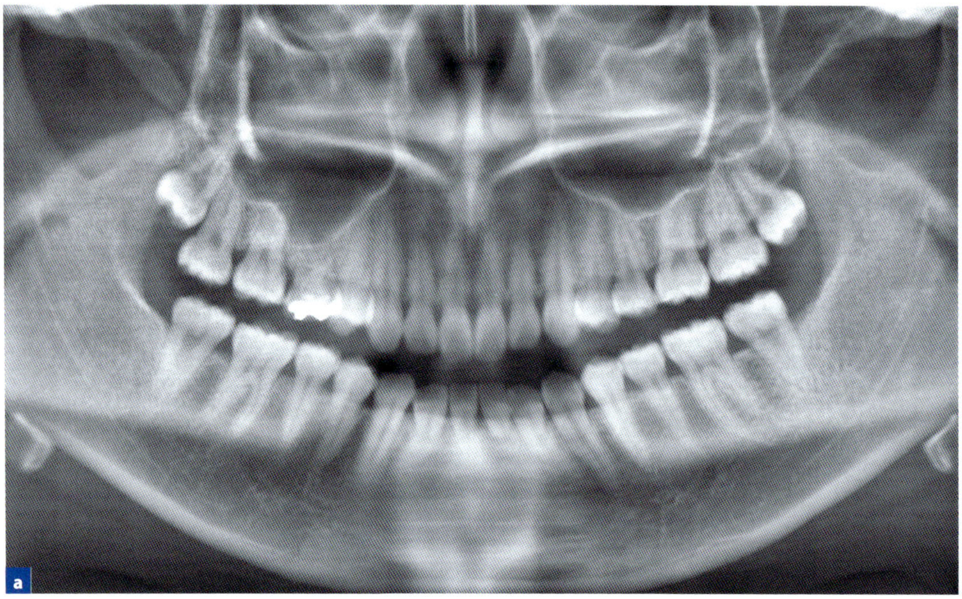

Fig 5-5a Preoperative panoramic radiograph of a 24-year-old female. She herself presented with a desire to have #28 transplanted into #15 site, which was congenitally missing.

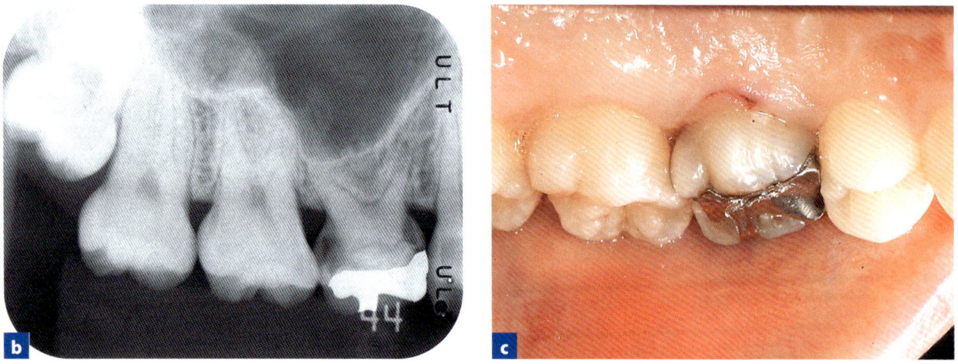

Fig 5-5b Radiograph before treatment. The distance from the alveolar crest to the maxillary sinus floor of the recipient site (#55) is short.
Fig 5-5c Oral view before treatment.

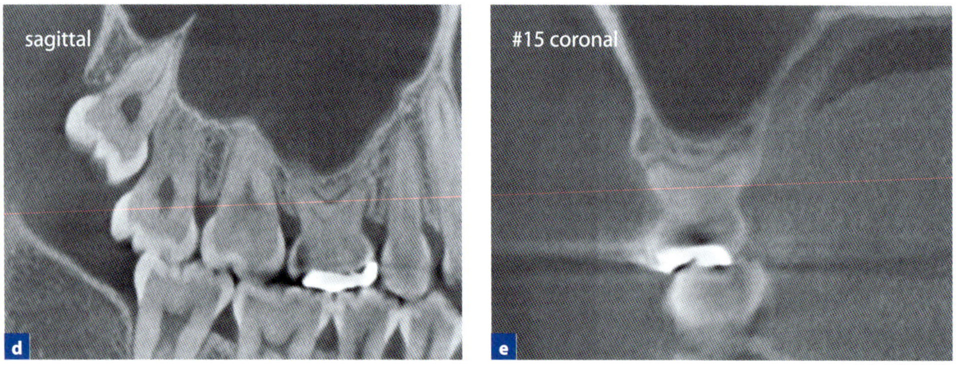

Fig 5-5d, e Preoperative CBCT images of the recipient site. The height of the recipient bone is clearly less compared to #18.

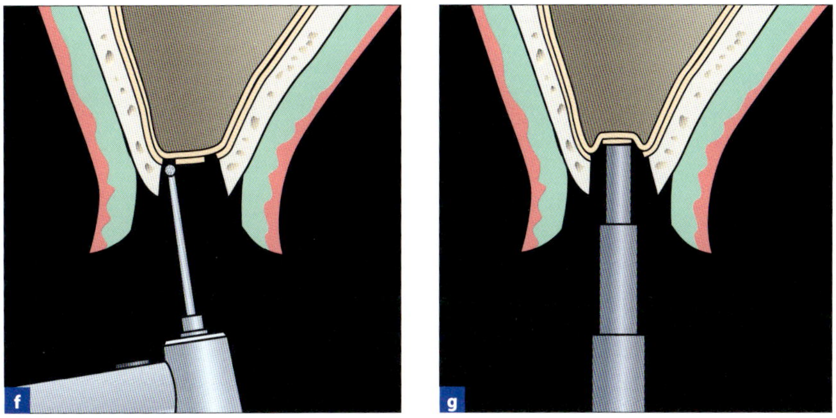

Fig 5-5f Maxillary sinus floor elevation. First, a groove is made in the shape of the cross-section of the donor tooth using a round bur on the alveolar bone surface of the extraction socket.
Fig 5-5g Gently push up the maxillary sinus floor with an osteotome.

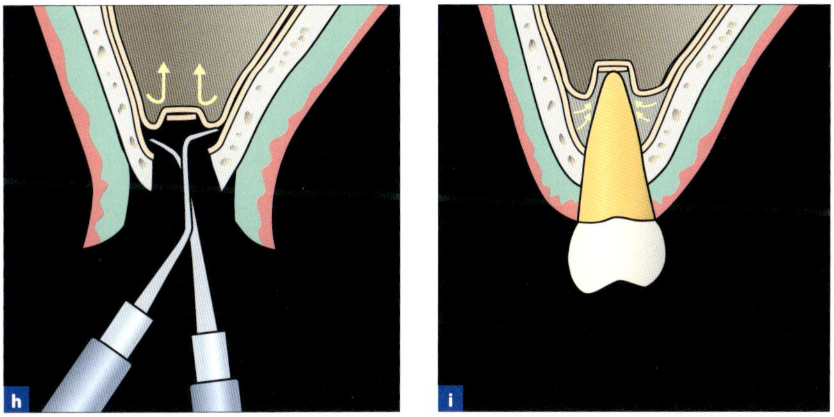

Fig 5-5h Insert an elevator into the gap between the bone and maxillary sinus mucosa (Schneiderian membrane) and lift it up being careful not to tear the membrane.
Fig 5-5i When the membrane is elevated to a sufficient distance, the lateral socket walls are prepared, and the donor tooth (replica) is tried in. The space around the root will be filled with new bone within several months.

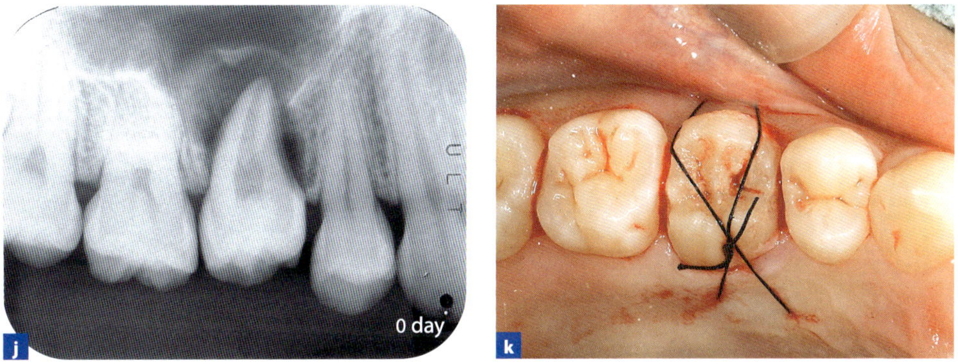

Fig 5-5j Radiograph immediately after transplantation. No bone grafting material was used.
Fig 5-5k View immediately after transplantation.

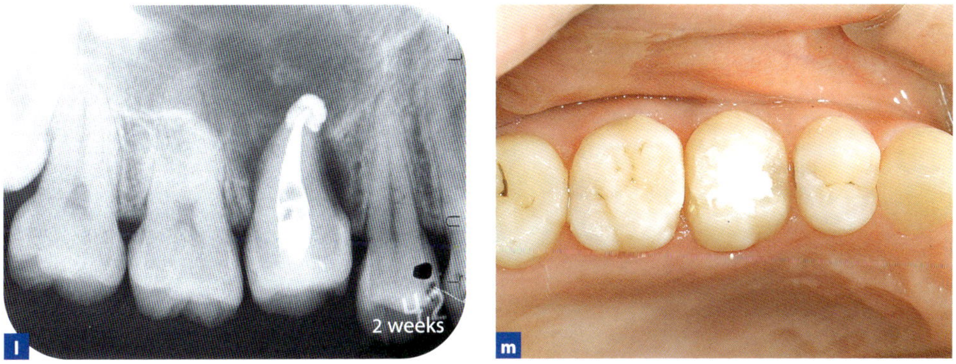

Fig 5-5l, m Two weeks postoperative. As the root apex was slightly open but not wide enough for expected pulpal healing, root canal treatment was initiated and filled with a calcium hydroxide preparation "Vitapex" for apexification.

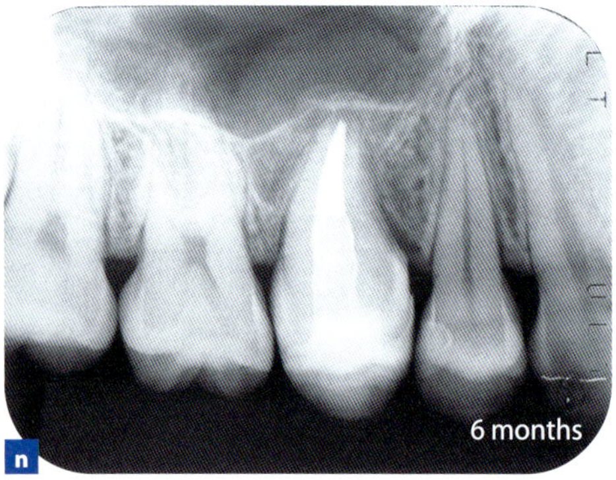

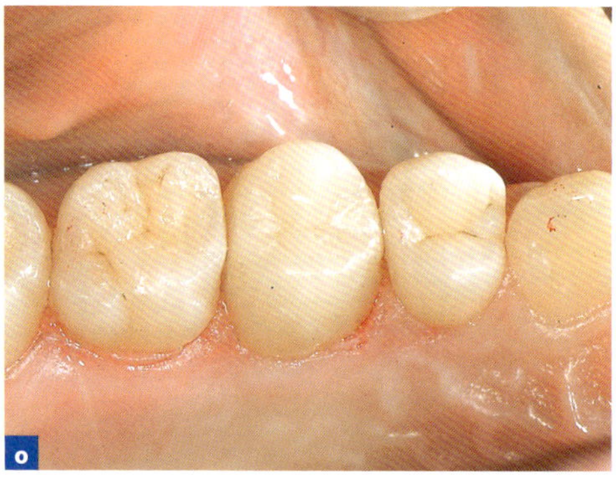

Fig 5-5n, o Six months after transplantation. The pictures were taken just after the root canal filling with sealer and gutta-percha and the crown restoration with CR on the same day.

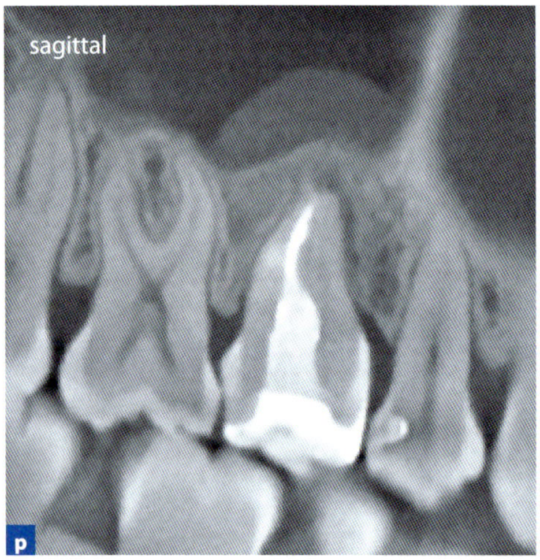

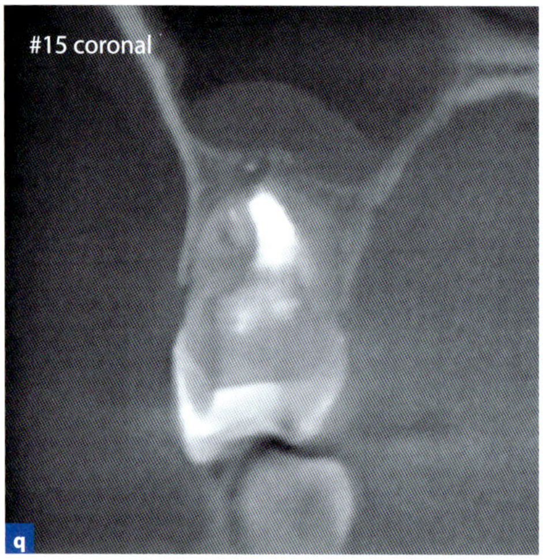

Fig 5-5p, q CBCT images 6 months after transplantation. It will take a little more time for the maxillary sinus membrane and periodontal ligament to completely heal, but there is evidence that the root of the transplant has been surrounded by new bone, indicating that the sinus elevation with transplantation was successful.

Transplantation of a horizontally impacted third molar to the adjacent second molar site

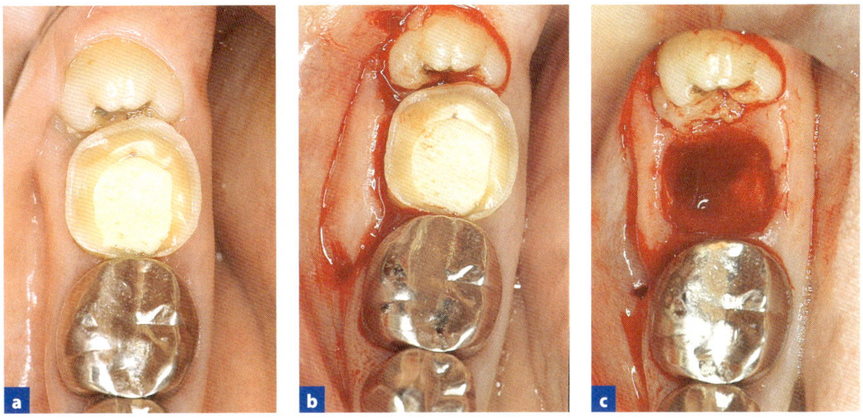

Fig 5-6a Preoperative view of a 22-year-old female. #48 is to be transplanted into the adjacent #47 site on the same day. A key point for success depends on closing the flap on the distal aspect without leaving any space.
Fig 5-6b Incision and reflection of the gingival flap. Incision is made in the gingival sulcus around the tooth at the recipient site and the donor tooth. A vertical incision is made in the distobuccal corner of the first molar. Horizontal incisions in the sulcus are made in the buccal corners of the donor tooth and the gingival flap is reflected.
Fig 5-6c After extraction of the second molar from the recipient site.

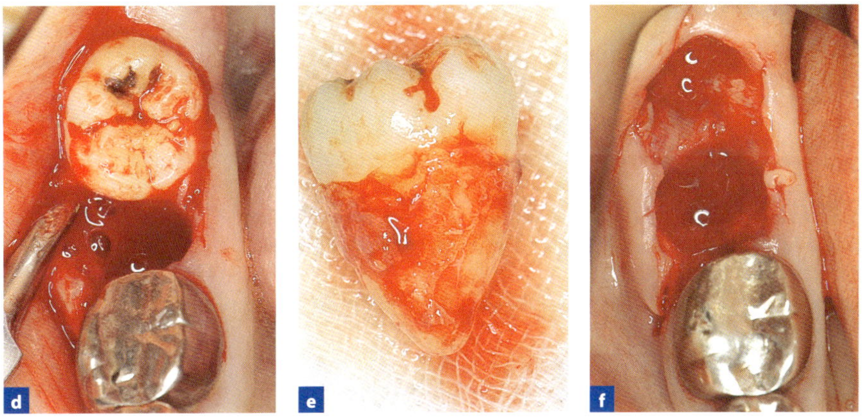

Fig 5-6d Extraction of the donor tooth.
Fig 5-6e Donor tooth.
Fig 5-6f After modification of the recipient socket.

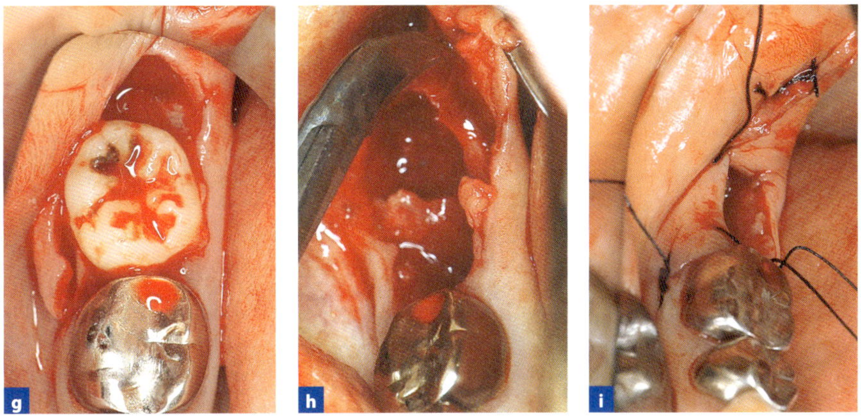

Fig 5-6g Try-in of the donor tooth.
Fig 5-6h Releasing incision of the flap. The releasing incision is made in the lingual gingival tissue of the extraction socket of the third molar to achieve better fit of the gingival flap.
Fig 5-6i Suture of gingival flap. Without placing the donor tooth, the flap of the horizontal incision and the area of the mesial proximal wall are sutured. One end of each suture cut and is left at about 4cm while the other end of the suture is left uncut.

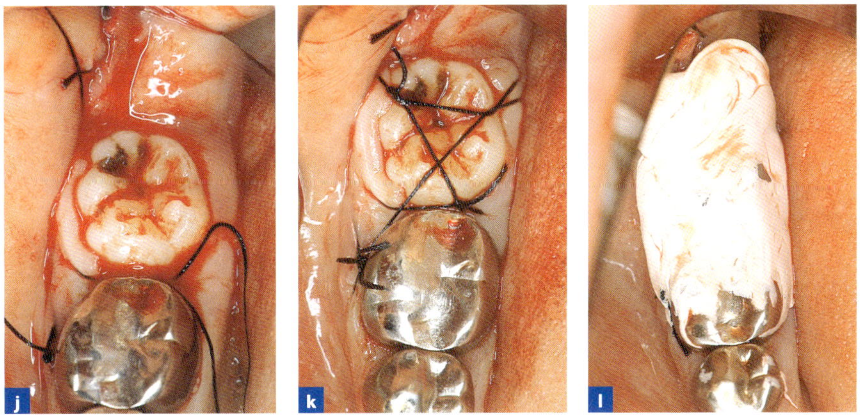

Fig 5-6j Placement of the donor tooth. The donor tooth is sealed tightly by the gingival flap due to the flap's elasticity.
Fig 5-6k Fixation of the donor tooth by suture strings. The extra suture of the distolingual site is used for fixation of the donor tooth.
Fig 5-6l After application of the surgical dressing to protect the surgical area.

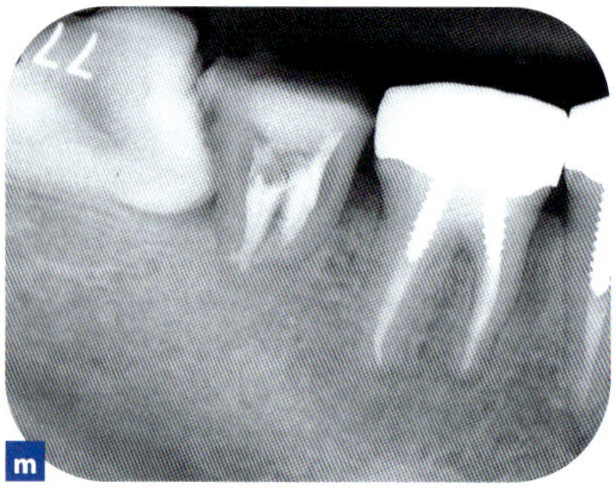

Fig 5-6m Preoperative radiograph.

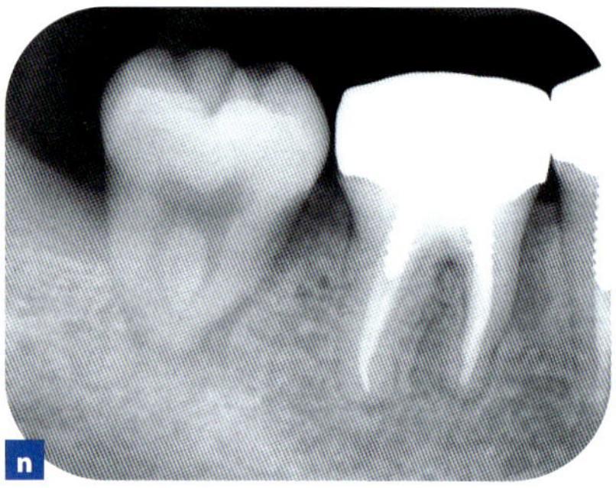

Fig 5-6n Immediately after transplantation.

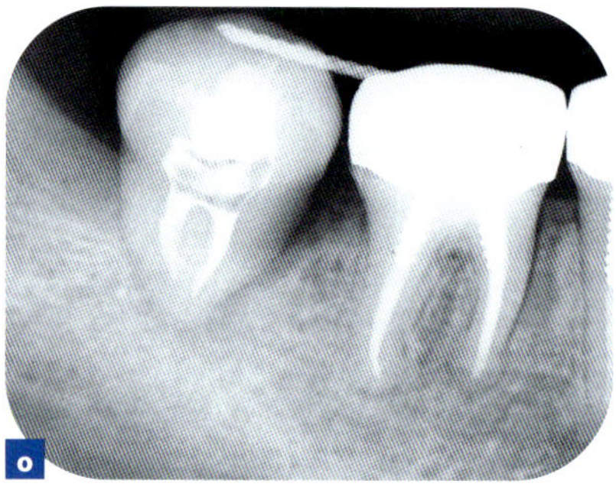

Fig 5-6o One month after surgery and immediately after temporary root canal filling with "Vitapex".

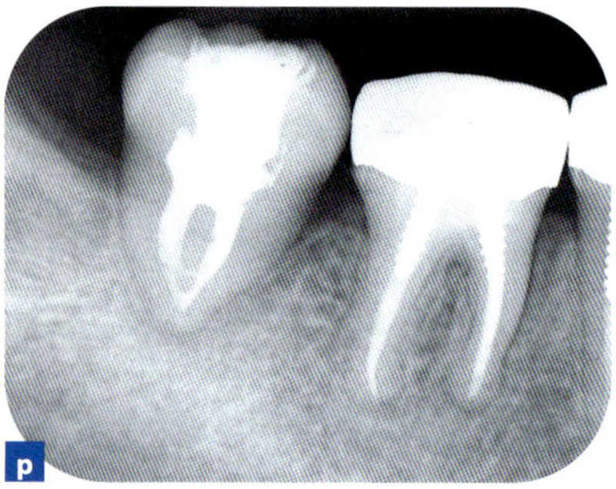

Fig 5-6p Four months postop and immediately after root canal filling with sealer and gutta-percha.

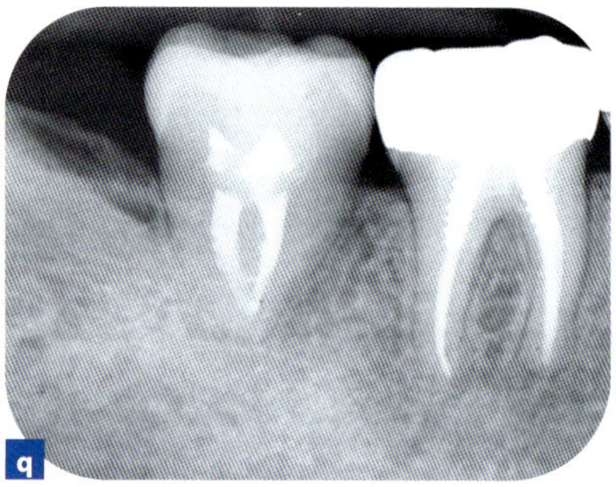

Fig 5-6q Two years postop. Note the increased bone level on the distal aspect.

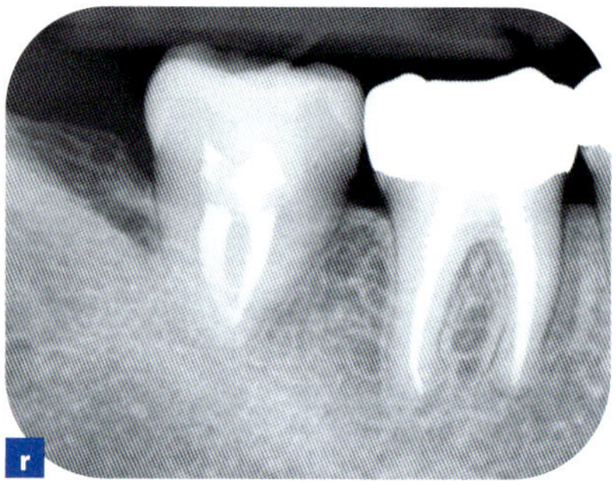

Fig 5-6r Five years after transplantation.

The sequence of preparation of the recipient site in an area without a prior extraction socket

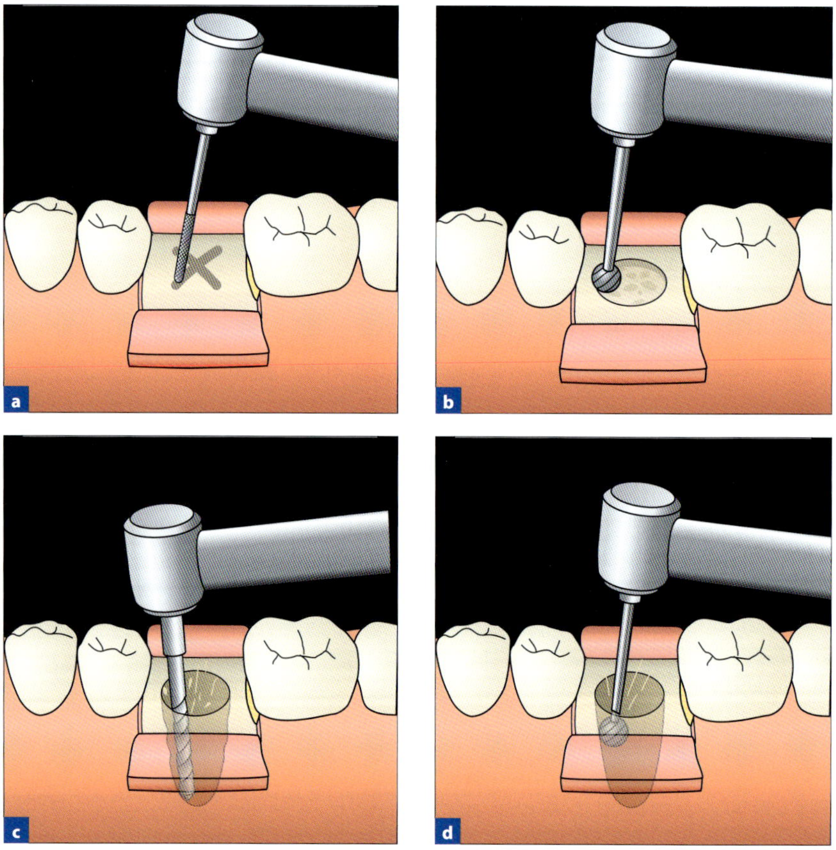

Fig 5-7a Use of a bur to mark the size of the socket to be prepared.
Fig 5-7b After removal of the cortical plate from the crest of the bone.
Fig 5-7c Preparation of the recipient site. The recipient site is prepared slightly larger than the dimension of the root of the donor tooth; surgical round burs or implant burs can be used for this purpose, running at about 2,000-6,000 rpm.
Fig 5-7d If the donor tooth is too large to be accommodated into the prepared socket, the socket should be further enlarged.

Surgical instruments used for transplantation

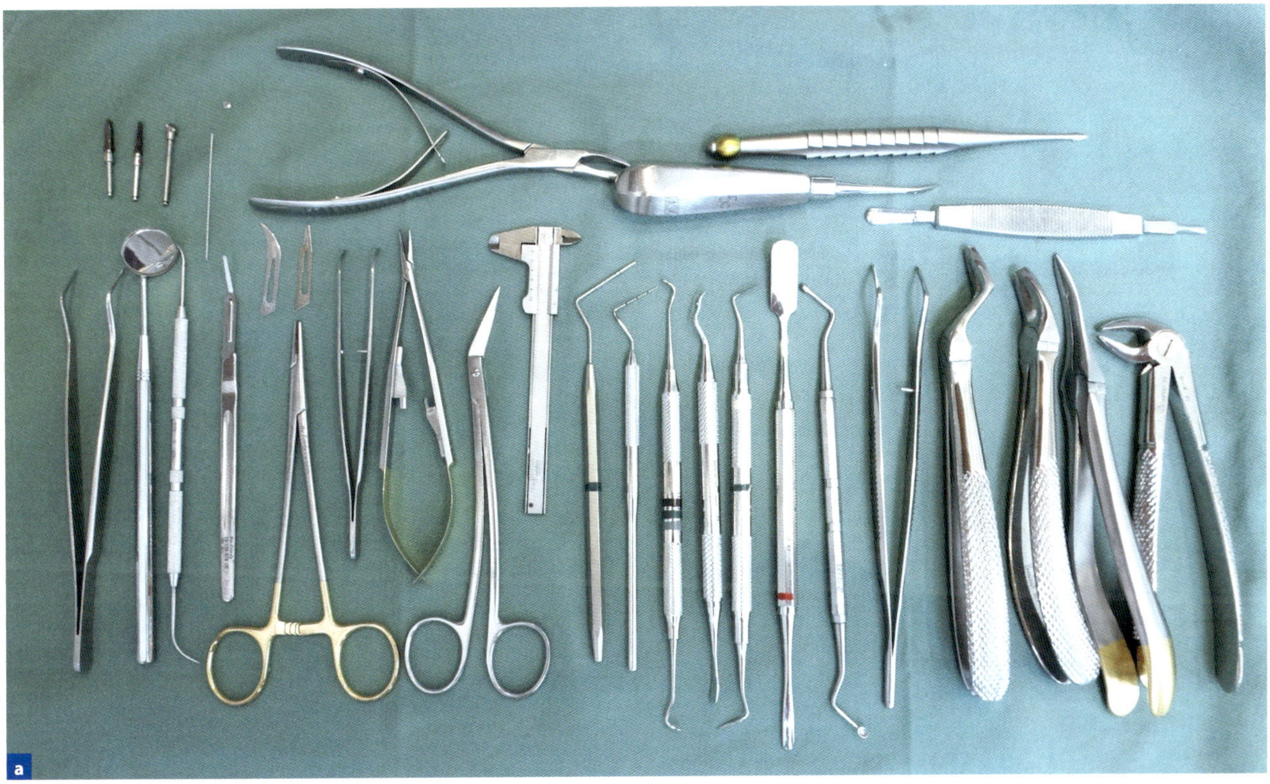

Fig 5-8a List of surgical instruments.

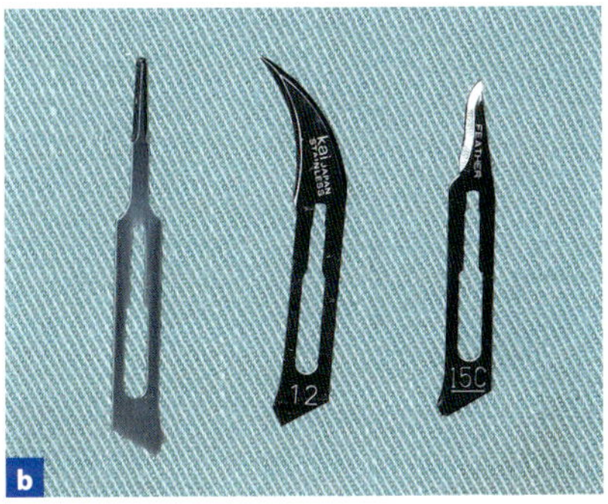

Fig 5-8b Blades. From the left No.390, 12D, 15C.

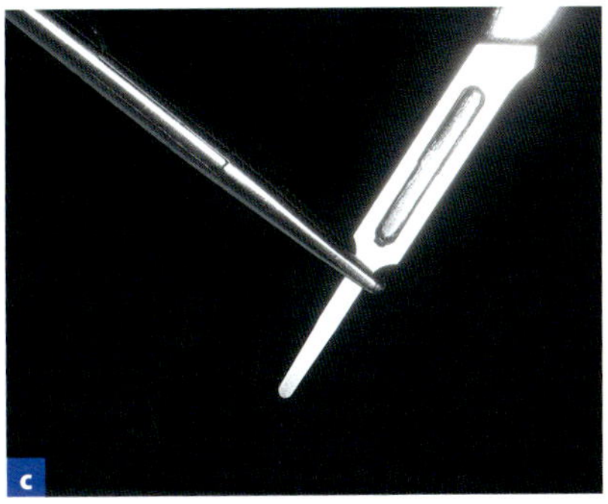

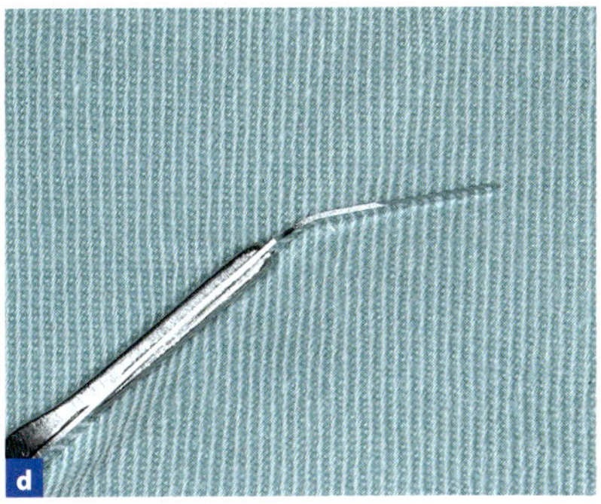

Fig 5-8c, d No.390 is easy to use if it is bent about 30 to 45 degrees.

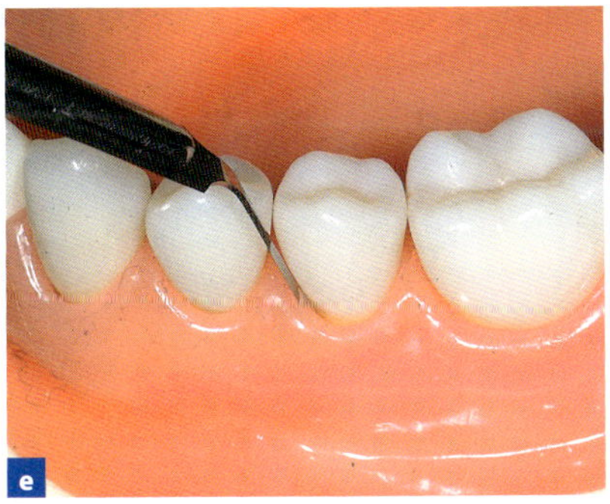

Fig 5-8e Making an incision into sulcus using No.390.

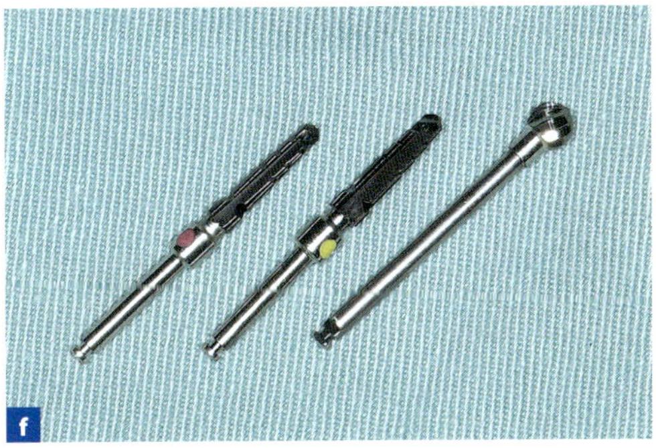

Fig 5-8f Implant drills and a surgical round bur used for preparation of a recipient socket.

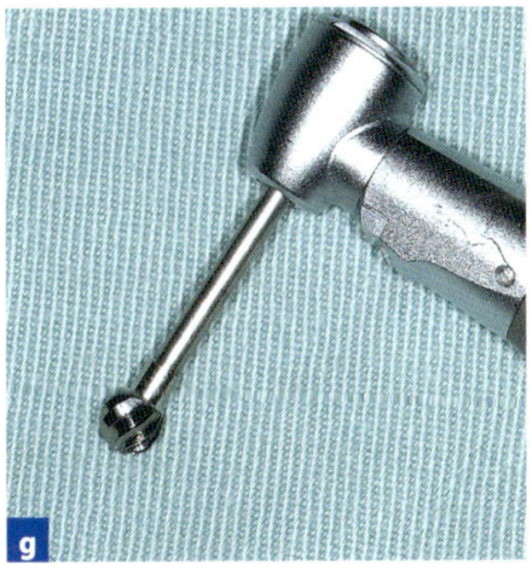

Fig 5-8g A round bur is attached to an electric engine and used at about 2,000-6,000 rpm.

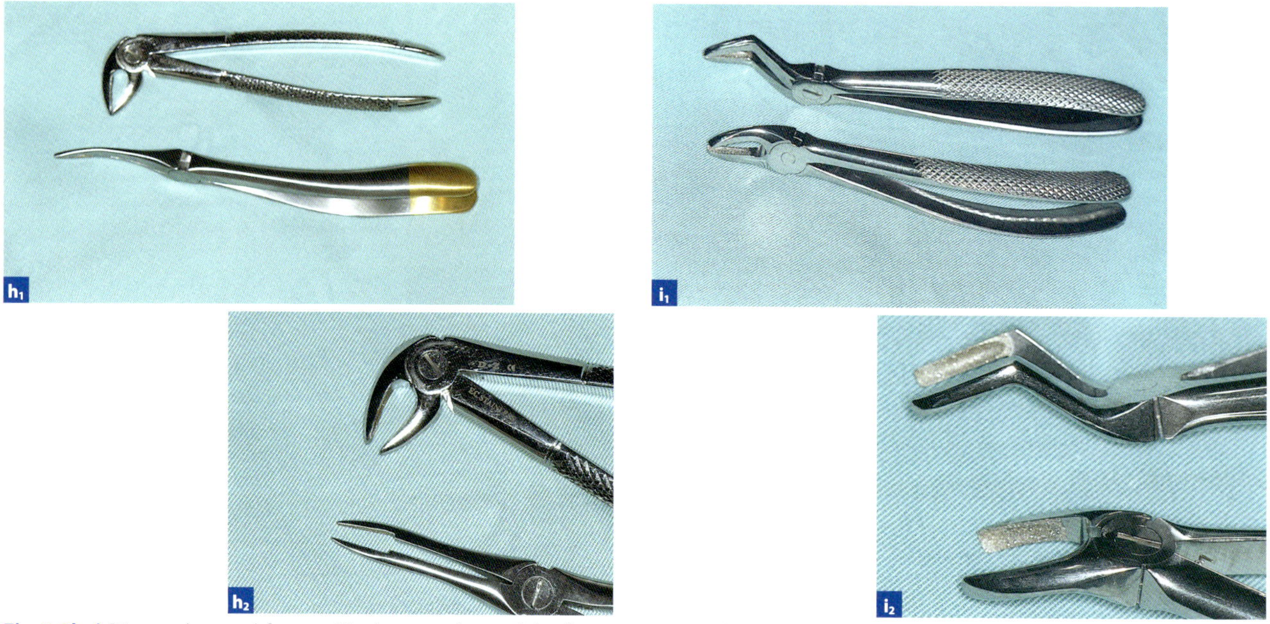

Fig 5-8h, i Diamond-coated forceps. The inner surfaces of the forceps are coated with diamond to allow for better hold on the tooth during extraction.

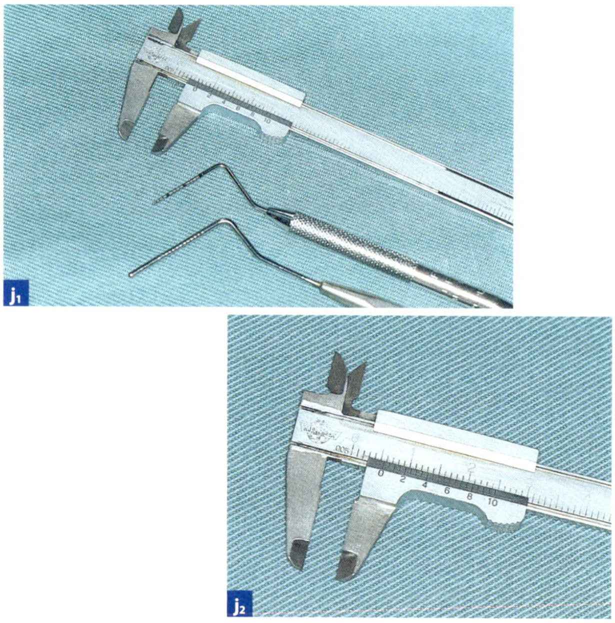

Fig 5-8j A caliper and probes. It is used to measure the size of a donor tooth and a recipient site.

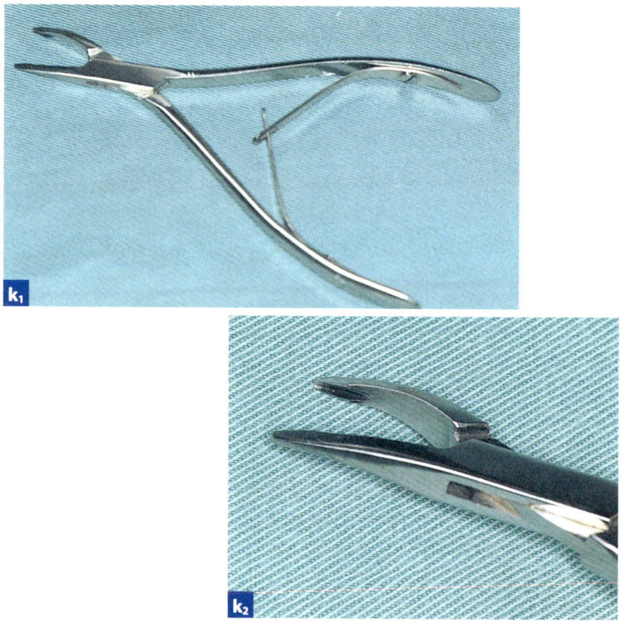

Fig 5-8k A bone removal forceps. Rongeur mini is useful.

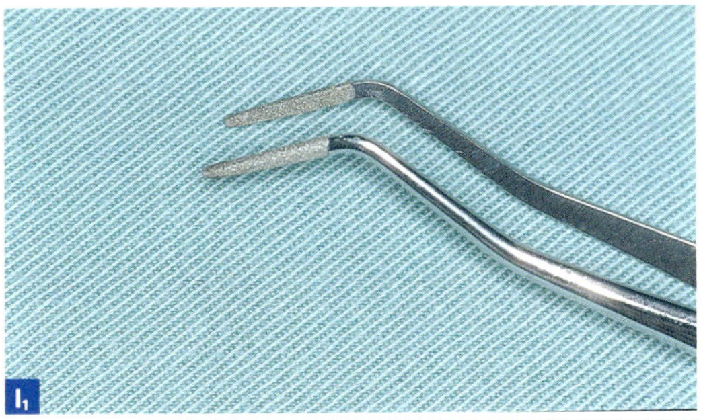

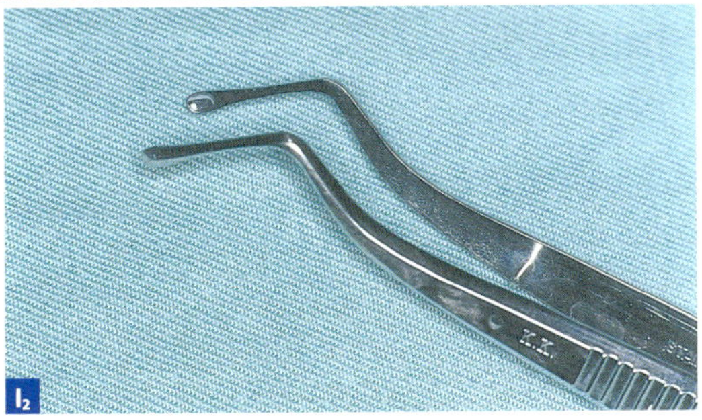

Fig 5-8l_1 A diamond-coated tweezers for holding flaps (upper).
Fig 5-8l_2 An excavator-type tweezers for removing granulation tissues or holding a tooth (lower).

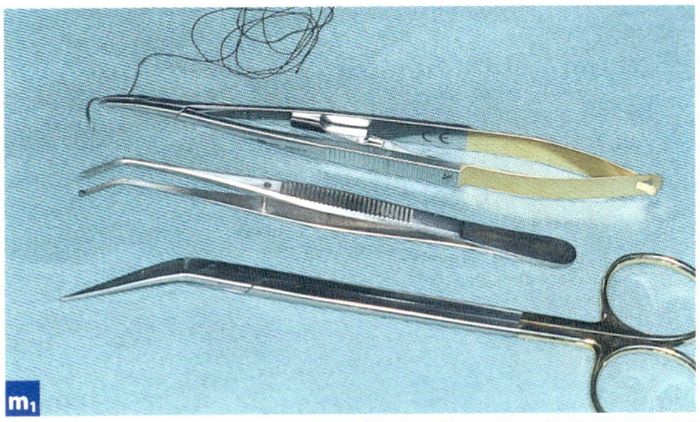

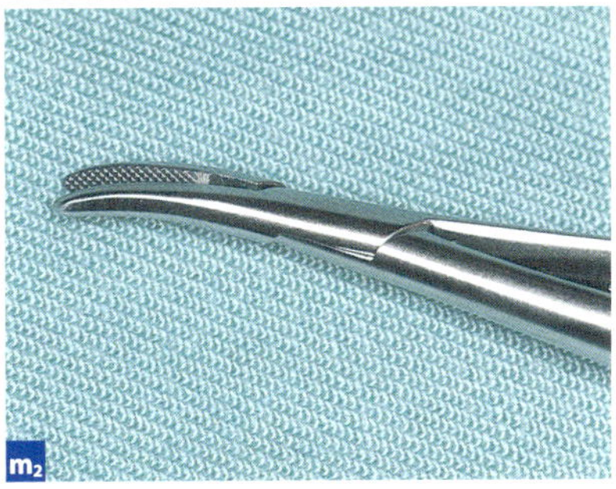

Fig 5-8m (top to bottom) Needle holders (Castroviejo type), soft tissue tweezers (tissue forceps), scissors.

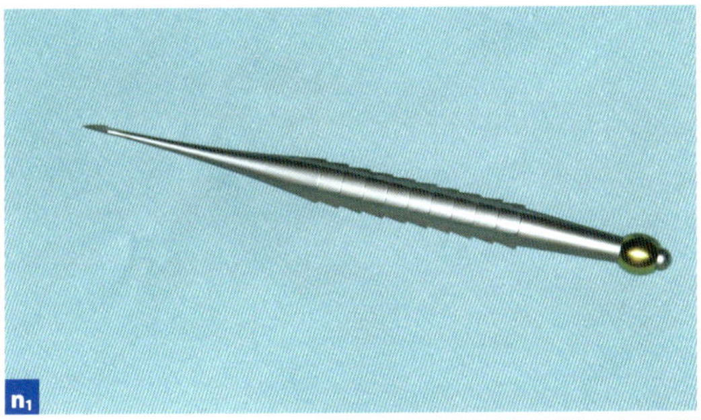

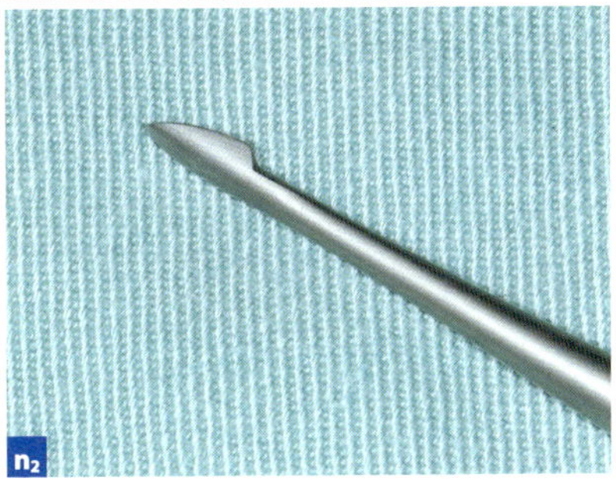

Fig 5-8n "X Desmo Tool 1" (Micro tech). It is useful for tooth extraction, surgical extrusion, and intentional replantation.

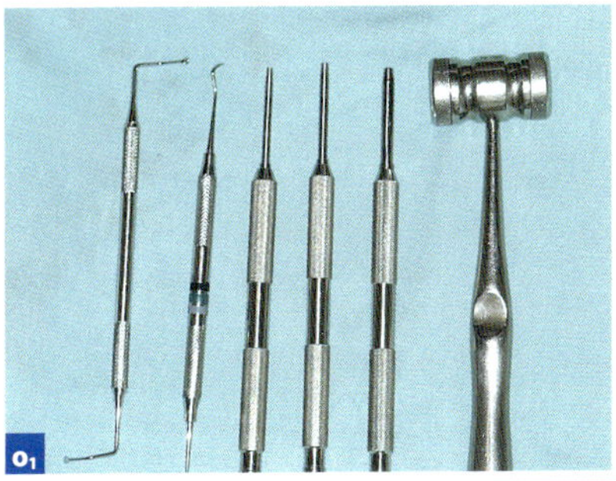

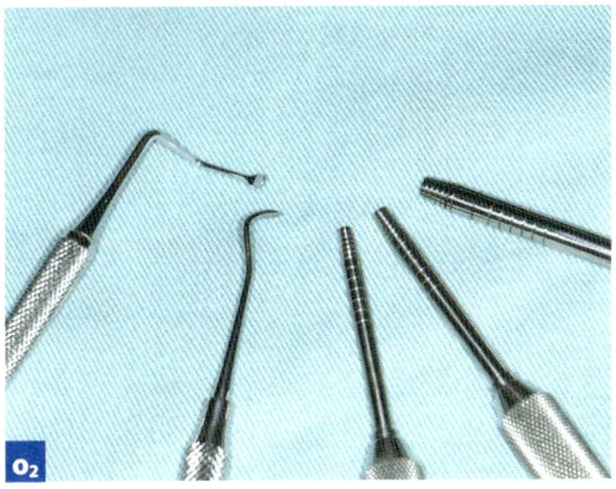

Fig 5-8o Kits for sinus elevation. Hammer used for socket lifting (right), osteotome (middle), mucosal elevator (left).

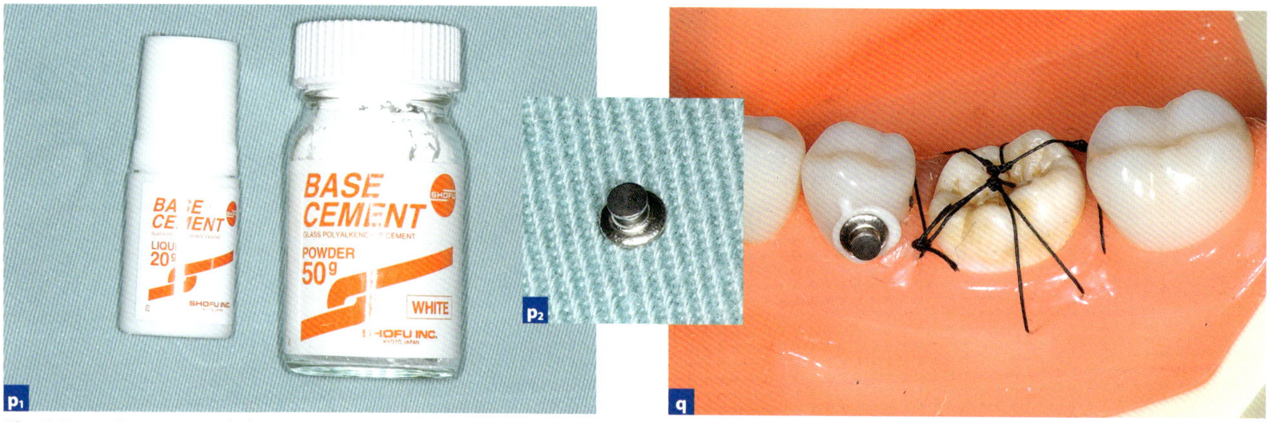

Fig 5-8p, q Conventional glass ionomer cement "BASE CEMENT" (Shofu, Kyoto, Japan) and "lingual buttons" (TOMY Inc. Tokyo, Japan). Buttons are attached on adjacent teeth with glass ionomer cement to retain surgical dressing after transplantation.

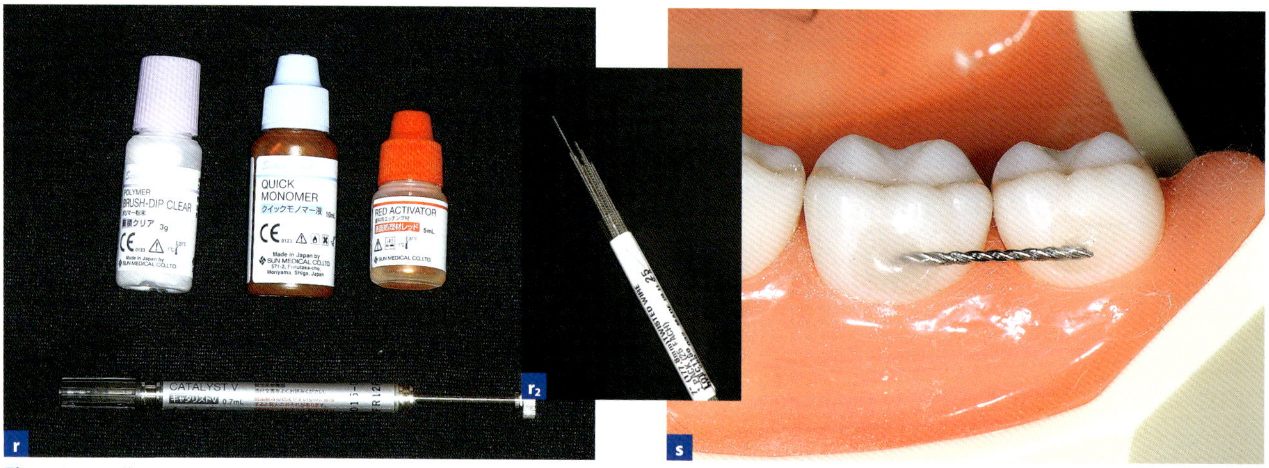

Fig 5-8r, s Adhesive resin "Super Bond" (Sun Medical), fixing wire "Twisted wire7" (3M Unitek).

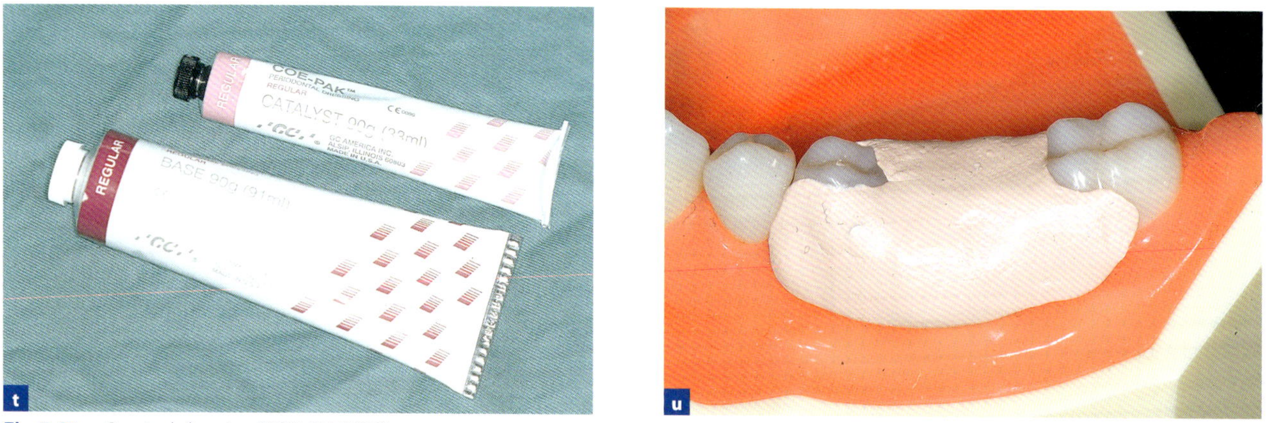

Fig 5-8t, u Surgical dressing "COE-PAK" (GC).

*Note that the above instruments and materials may not be available outside Japan.

References

1. Lindhe J, Nyman S. The effect of plaque control and surgical pocket elimination on the establishment and maintenance of periodontal health. A longitudinal study of periodontal therapy in cases of advanced disease. J Clin Periodontol. 1975; 2 : 67.
2. Nyman S, Rosling B, Lindhe J. Effect of professional tooth cleaning on healing after periodontal surgery. J Clin Periodontol. 1975; 2 : 80.
3. Holroyd SV, Wynn RL. Clinical pharmacology in dental practice. (4 th ed). St Louis: CV Mosby, 1998.
4. Preus HR, Lassen J, Aass AM, Christersson LA. Prevention of transmission of resistant bacteria between periodontal sites during subgingival application of antibiotics. J Clin Periodontol. 1993; 20: 299-303.
5. Gordon JM, Walker CB, Murphy JC, Goodson JM, Socransky SS. Concentration of tetracycline in human gingival fluid after single doses. J Clin Periodontol. 1981; 8 : 117-21.
6. Gordon JM, Walker CB, Murphy JC, Goodson JM, Socransky SS. Tetracycline: Levels achievable in gingival crevice fluid and in vitro effect on subgingival organisms. Part 1. Concentrations in crevicular fluid after repeated doses. J Periodontol. 1981; 52: 609-12.
7. Walker CB, Gordon JM, McQuilkin SJ, Niebloom TA, Socransky SS. Tetracycline: Levels achievable in gingival crevice fluid and in vitro effect on subgingival organisms. Part 2. Susceptibilities of periodontal bacteria. J Periodontol. 1981; 52: 613-6.
8. Andreasen JO. Atlas of replantation and transplantation of teeth. Philadelphia: WB Saunders, 1992.
9. Summers RB. A new concept in maxillary implant surgery: The osteotome technique. Compendium. 1994; 15: 152-60.
10. Nagata M. Teeth loss and autotransplantation of teeth. the Quintessence. 1994; 13(3): 561-74.
11. Nagata M, Nagaoka S, Semba I. Combined treatment of autogenous tooth transplantation and sinus floor elevation technique for a high level bone resorption of maxilla: Experimental study in dogs [in Japanese]. J Jpn Soc Periodontol. 1998; 40: 180.
12. Nagata M, Nagaoka S, Semba I. Combined treatment of autogenous tooth transplantation and sinus floor elevation technique: Clinical study [in Japanese]. J Jpn Soc Periodontol. 1998; 40: 87.
13. Nagata M, Nagaoka S. Combined treatment of autogenous tooth transplantation and sinus floor elevation technique: Radiological study [in Japanese]. J Jpn Soc Periodontol. 1999; 41: 59.
14. Andreasen JO. The effect of splinting upon periodontal healing after replantation of permanent incisors in monkeys. Acta Odont Scand. 1975; 33: 313-23.
15. Kristerson L, Andreasen JO. The effect of splinting upon periodontal and pulpal healing after autotransplantation of mature and immature permanent incisors in monkeys. Int J Oral Surg 1983; 12: 239-49.
16. Tsukiboshi M. Science and art of autotransplantation of teeth. the Quintessence. 1992; 11(1): 47-75.
17. Tsukiboshi M, Tsukiboshi C. Treatment planning considering autotransplantation of teeth [in Japanese]. Dent Rev. 1994; 55 (special issue): 68-74.
18. Andreasen JO, Hjørting-Hansen E, Jølst O. A clinical and radiographic study of 76 autotransplanted third molars. Scand J Dent Res. 1970; 78: 512-23.
19. Schwartz O, Bergmann P, Klausen B. Resorption of autotransplanted human teeth: a retrospective study of 291 transplantations over a period of 25 years. Int Endod J. 1985; 18: 119-31.
20. Miyazaki M. Treatment planning and techniques for autotransplantation of teeth [in Japanese]. Pract Prosthet. 1994; 27(1)-(5).
21. Tsukiboshi M, Miyazaki M. Orthodontic teeth movement of replanted and transplanted teeth. [in Japanese]. Dent Rev. 1994; 55 (special issue): 201- 3

CHAPTER 6

Autotransplantation of teeth in molar regions

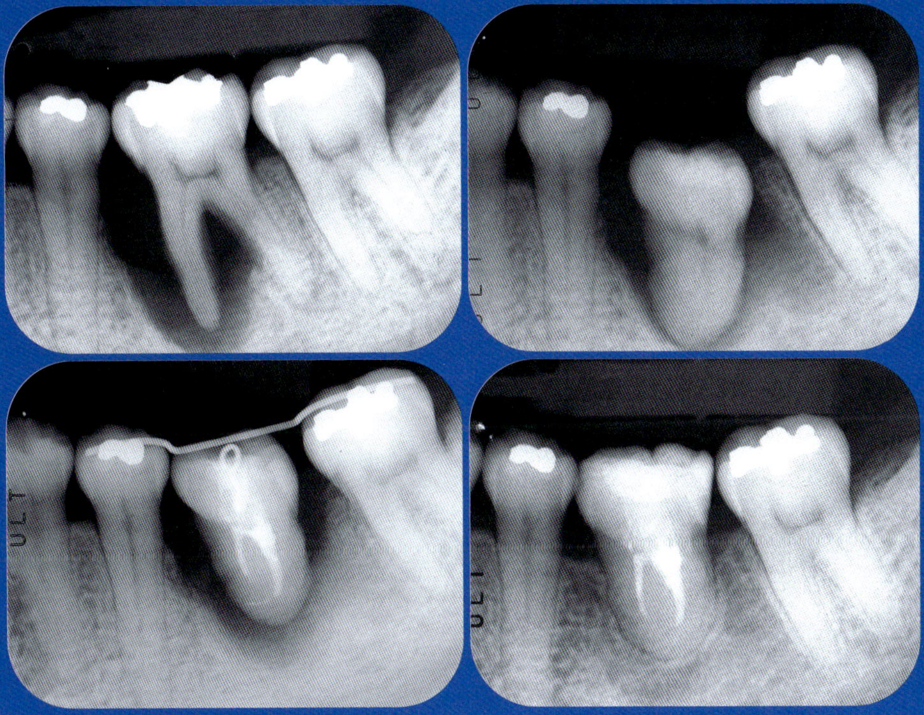

In order to demonstrate the efficacy of transplantation, it would be helpful to present different case types, their indications and the flow of treatment by presenting them based on the region or type of treatment. So **Chapter 6** will present molar cases, **Chapter 7** will present premolar cases, **Chapter 8** will present anterior cases, **Chapter 9** will present those cases involving orthodontic treatment, and **Chapter 10** will present cases of surgical extrusion and replantation. The wound healing in transplantation has already been discussed in **Chapter 3**, so in **Chapters 6** through **10**, the treatment benefits and important technical points will be explained based on authors' clinical experiences.

General indications for transplantation

The general indications for transplantation, including intentional replantation and surgical extrusion, are often present when treating various dental problems such as "advanced caries", "inadequate root canal treatment", "root resorption", "root fracture", "dental trauma", "congenitally missing teeth", and "advanced periodontitis". In other words, transplantation is indicated if there is a tooth with an unfavorable prognosis and there is a donor suitable for transplantation in the same mouth. And transplantation is chosen if transplantation can provide more favorable benefit over other treatment options such as fixed bridges, implants, removable dentures, and orthodontic tooth movement.

In the authors' practice, there are many indications for transplantation found in the molar regions since they often had prior treatments with problems that are difficult to retreat or repair with a favorable prognosis.

Furthermore, countries such as Japan have dental insurance plans that cover molar transplantation procedures.

Case 1. Transplantation of an immature third molar to the site of a second molar involved in external root resorption

Fig 6-1 is a case of a 17-year-old female whose second molar which had developed root resorption was replaced with the adjacent impacted third molar. The stage of root development of the donor tooth was early stage 4 (see **Fig 3-27** in **Chapter 3**), which was thought to be a little early for transplantation. However, in this case if the root developed more, the extraction would be more difficult (**Fig 6-1a** and **6-1d**). The transplantation was performed successfully, but the root did not develop fully (partial arrest, **Fig 6-1e** to **6-1o**). The reason was thought to be damage to Hertwig's epithelial sheath during the extraction. A positive response to the electrical pulp test (EPT) developed six months after transplantation (**Fig 6-1f**), and no clinical problems occurred throughout the 18 years of follow-up (**Fig 6-1h** to **6-1o**).

When transplanting a third molar to the adjacent second molar site, orthodontic tooth movement should be taken into consideration as an alternative option. However, taking into consideration the difficulty and risk to move molar teeth, the treatment period, treatment cost, and discomfort of orthodontic appliances, and the high predictability of transplantation of immature teeth (success rate of about 95%), an immediate transplantation may be more advantageous than orthodontic treatment in these case types.

Another frequent indication for transplantation in molar regions is caries that has progressed too deep to be treated with a good outcome (see **Chapter 5 Fig 5-2**). Although dental caries prevention is improving, there are still young people who present to the dentist with extensive caries of their molars. In such cases, transplantation of immature third molars may often times be a better option, especially for young patients. Often times molars that have undergone poor root canal procedures at an early age will have an increased likelihood of structural failure (i.e. root fracture) in the future. So, before extracting third molars, it is important to check in advance whether there are any treated molars that have guarded to unfavorable long-term prognosis (see **Chapter 1 Fig 1-1**).

Case 1. Transplantation of an immature third molar to the site of a second molar involved in external root resorption

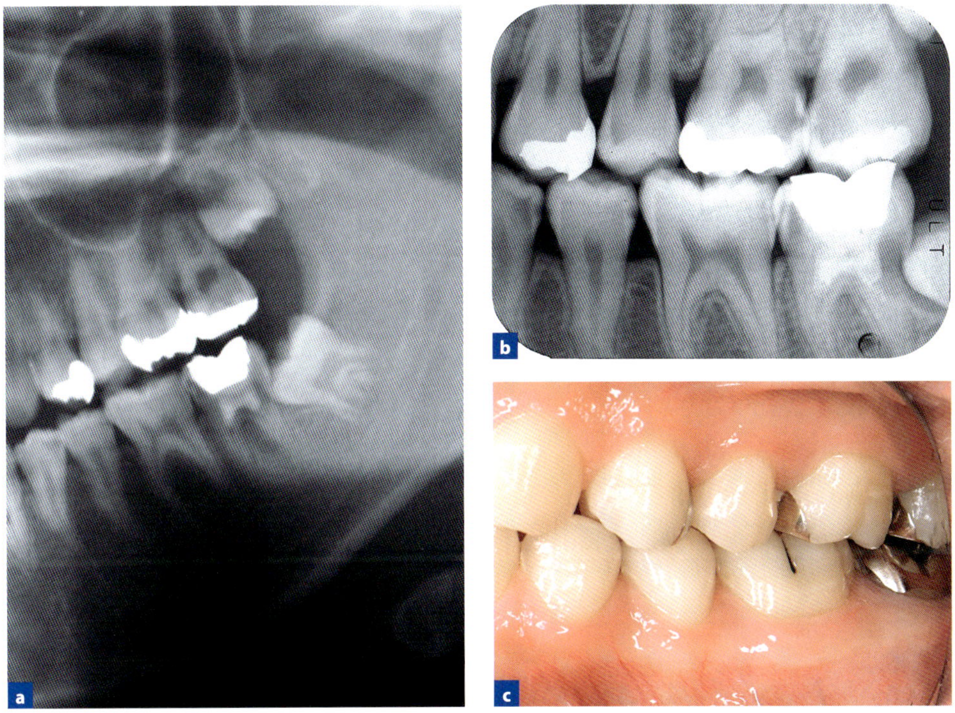

Fig 6-1a to 6-1c Preoperative views of a 17-year-old female who presented with a chief complaint of having dental caries. The panoramic radiograph and the bitewing radiograph revealed that #37 was involved in external root resorption. Because of the difficulty of preserving it, the transplantation using the impacted #38 was indicated.

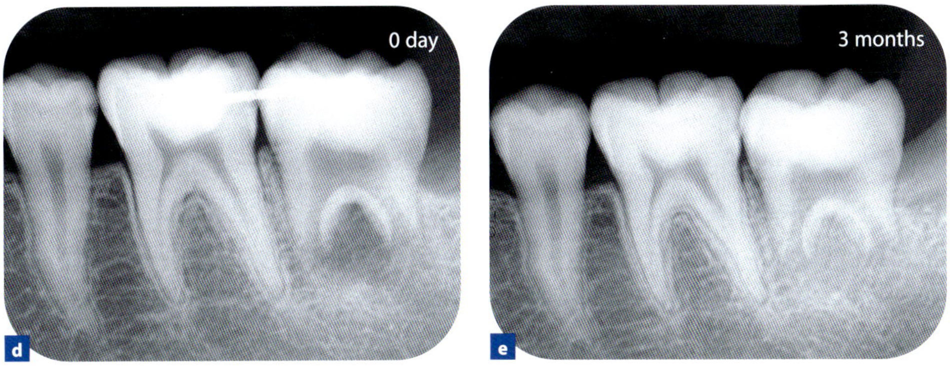

Fig 6-1d Radiograph immediately after transplantation. The stage of root development is about the first half of stage 4 and pulpal healing and root development can be expected.
Fig 6-1e Three months postop. There is no evidence of inflammatory resorption or other pathologies.

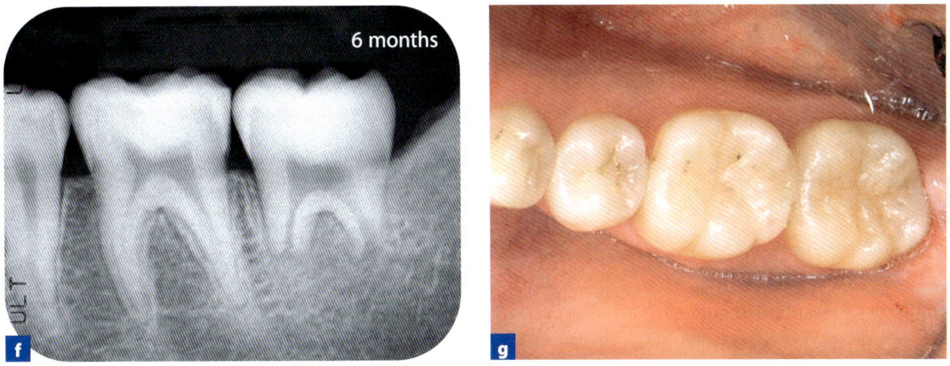

Fig 6-1f and 6-1g Six months postop. The transplant responds EPT(+), and there appears to be pulpal healing.

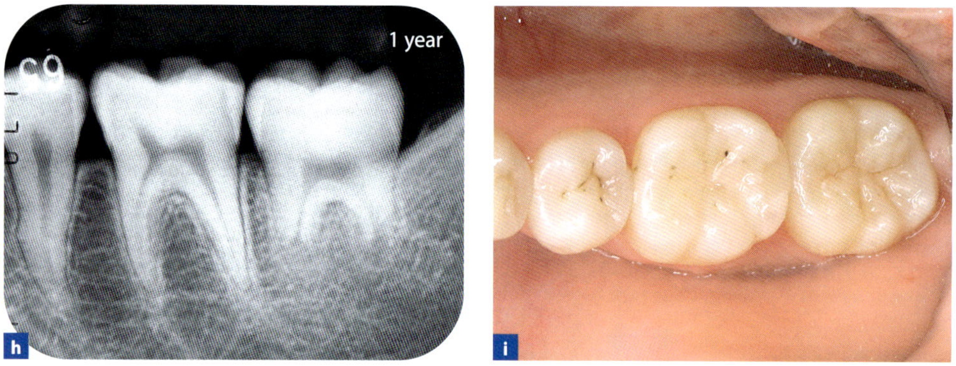

Fig 6-1h and 6-1i One year postop. Pulp canal obliteration is developing.

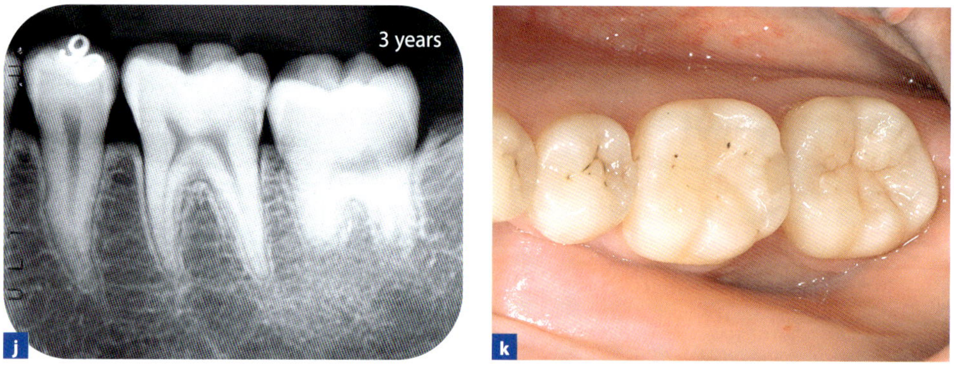

Fig 6-1j and 6-1k Three years postop. Root development seems to have arrested, but no other problems are observed.

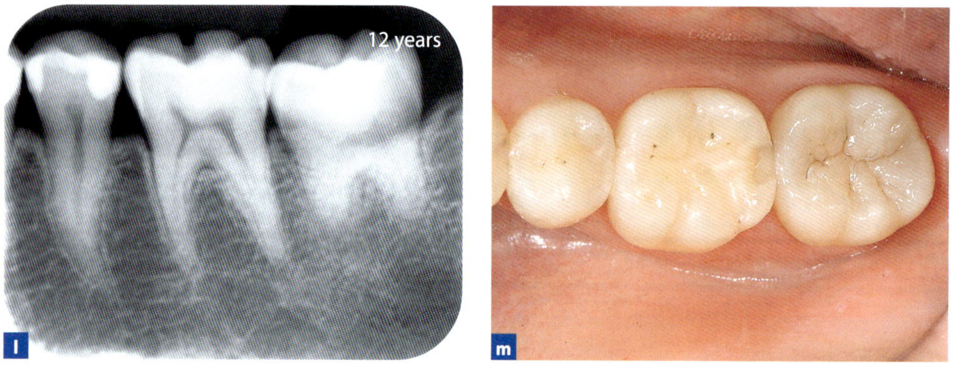

Fig 6-1l and 6-1m 12 years postop. The transplant responds EPT(+).

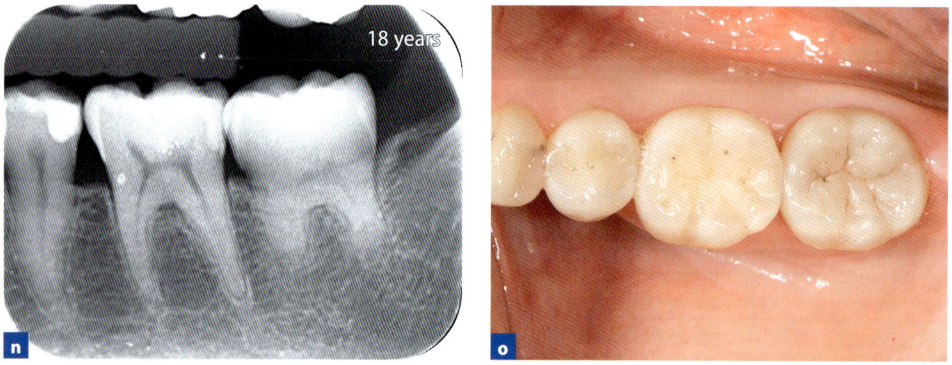

Fig 6-1n and 6-1o 18 years postop. The tooth is asymptomatic, functional and shows no apparent abnormalities.

Case 2. Transplantation of a mature third molar to the site of a second molar involved in crown-root fracture

Fig 6-2 shows a case of a 33-year-old female who presented with crown-root fracture of #27. If the fracture had stopped around the bone margin, crown lengthening might have been performed before restoration, or it might have been possible to proceed directly to restoration without it. In addition, it might have been possible to preserve the tooth by orthodontic extrusion (see **Chapter 4 Fig 4-18**) or surgical extrusion if the root morphology is appropriate (see **Chapter 4 Fig 4-19**). However, as a suitable donor tooth was available, transplantation had several advantages. In case 2, a single-rooted third molar was available on the opposite side of the jaw, making it an ideal morphology for transplantation .

In the transplantation of a mature tooth, pulpal healing cannot be expected, so root canal treatment is necessary after transplantation (**Fig 6-2j**). RCT is initiated 2 weeks after transplantation, and the root canal filing is finished after 1 month. The wire splinting is removed on the same day, and after waiting for natural movement of the transplant for about 3 months, the crown is restored with composite resin (CR) (**Fig 6-2i**).

Case 3. Transplantation of a maxillary molar to a mandibular molar

Fig 6-3 is a case of a 27-year-old female who presented with crown-root fracture of #47. Fortunately, an appropriately shaped third molar was available in the upper jaw. After discussion of the risk-benefit and cost-benefit of transplantation or trying to treat and save a compromised tooth, the patient chose to have transplantation. From the author's point of view, transplantation in this case would have a much greater benefit than risk ratio than any other treatment alternative.

Case 2. Transplantation of a mature third molar to the site of a second molar involved in crown-root fracture

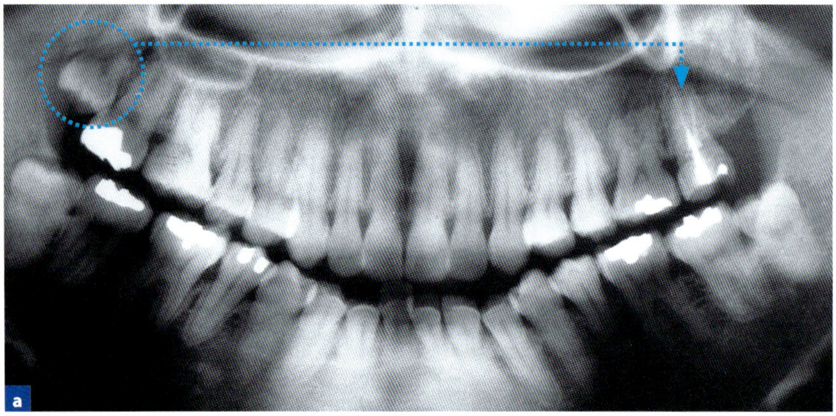

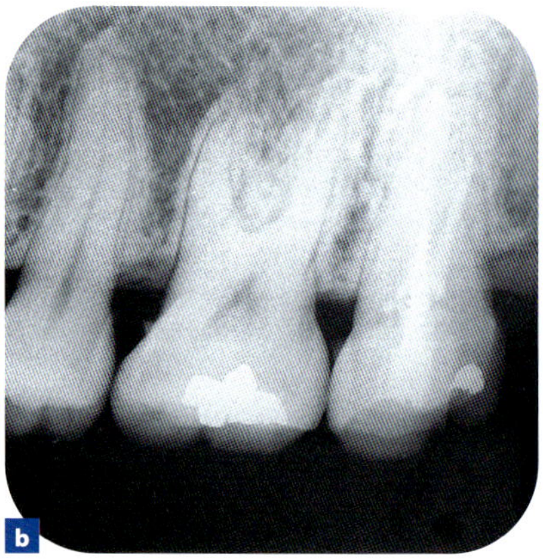

Fig 6-2a and 6-2b Preoperative radiographs of a 33-year-old female, who presented with crown-root fracture of #27. It was considered an indication for transplantation because an appropriate donor tooth (#18) was available.

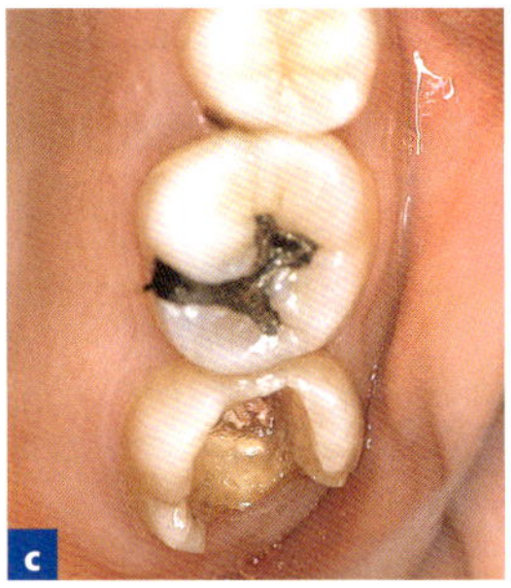

Fig 6-2c Preoperative occlusal view.

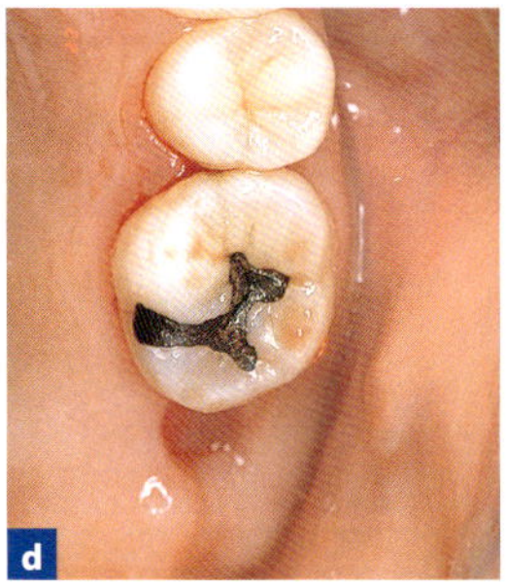

Fig 6-2d 45 days after the extraction of #27 and the day of transplantation. Sufficient keratinized gingiva is present.

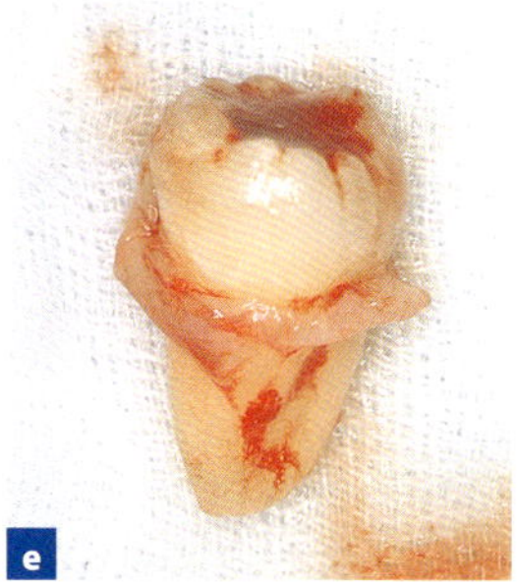

Fig 6-2e Donor tooth (#18). The root form is appropriate and the size seems to be similar to #27.

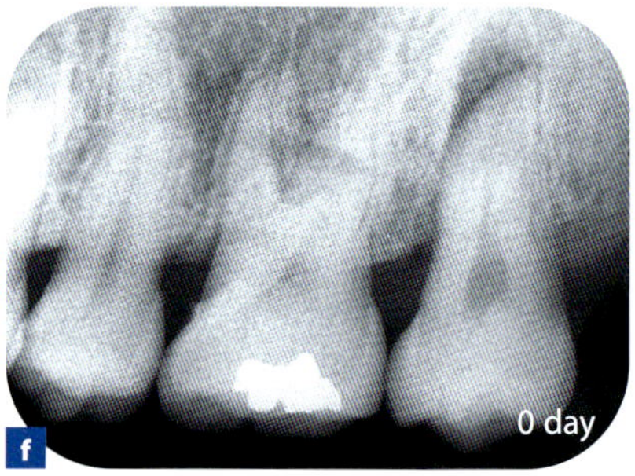

Fig 6-2f Radiograph immediately after transplantation.

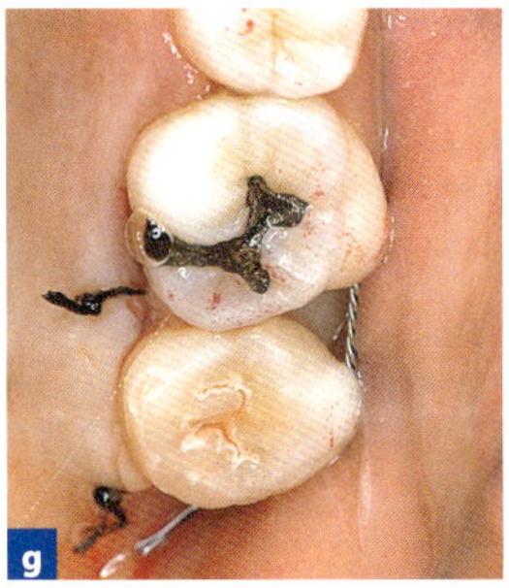

Fig 6-2g View immediately after transplantation. Wire fixation was placed on the day of transplantation.

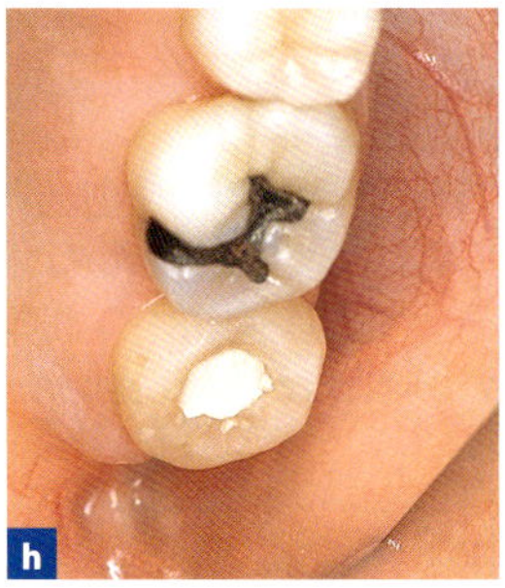

Fig 6-2h Five months postop. Immediately before crown restoration.

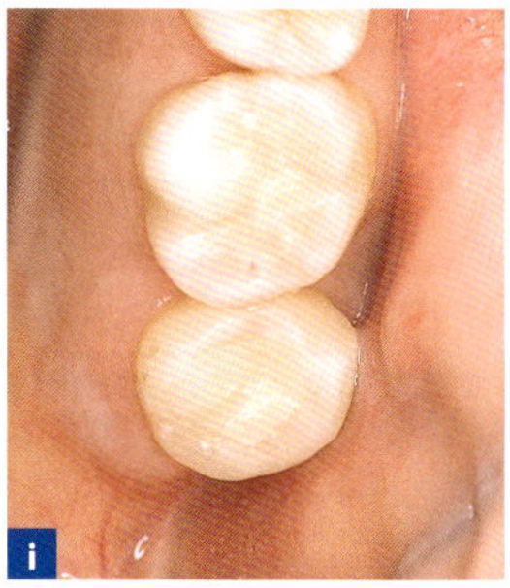

Fig 6-2i Immediately after crown restoration with composite resin (CR).

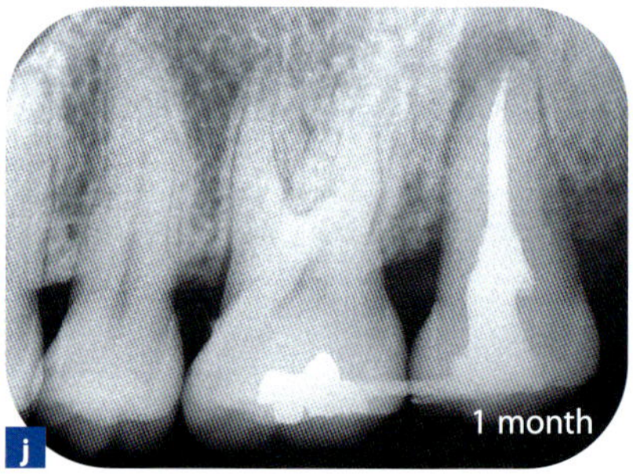

Fig 6-2j Radiograph 1 month after transplantation.

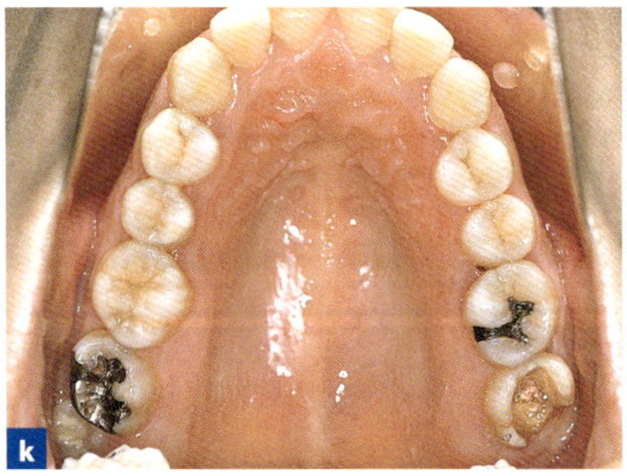

Fig 6-2k Occlusal view of the maxillary before surgery.

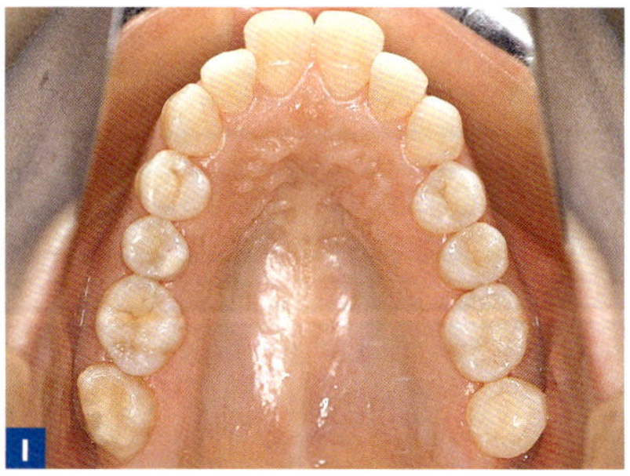

Fig 6-2l Occlusal view after surgery.

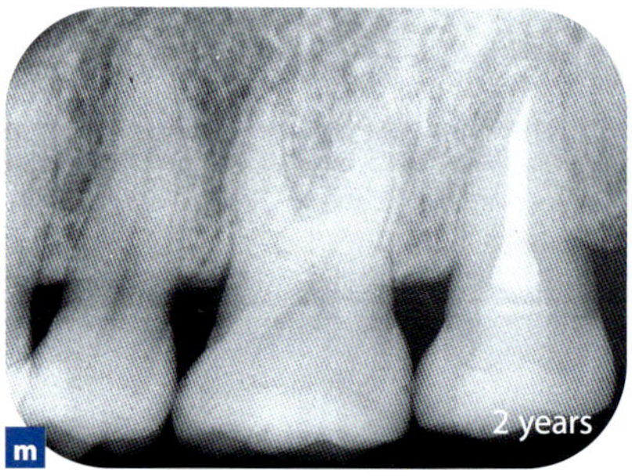

Fig 6-2m Radiograph 2 years after transplantation.

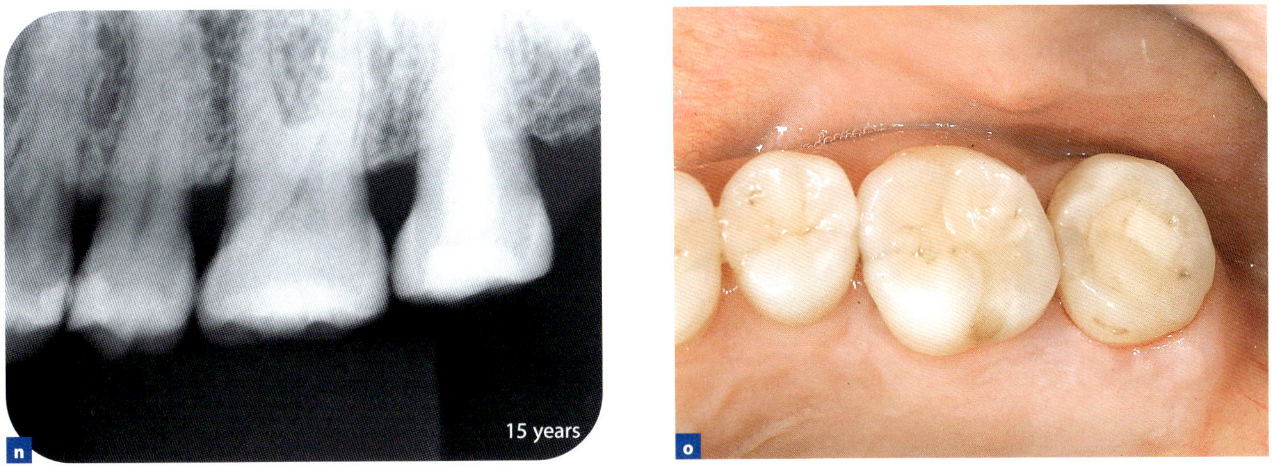

Fig 6-2n and 6-2o Views 15 years after transplantation.

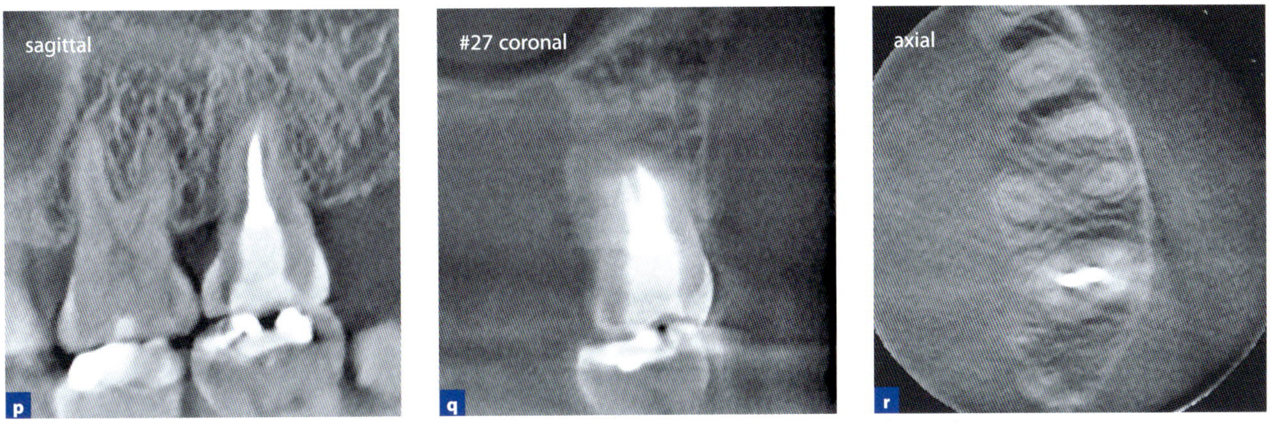

Fig 6-2p to 6-2r CBCT images 15 years after transplantation. There are no apparent abnormalities detected.

Case 3. Transplantation of a maxillary molar to a mandibular molar

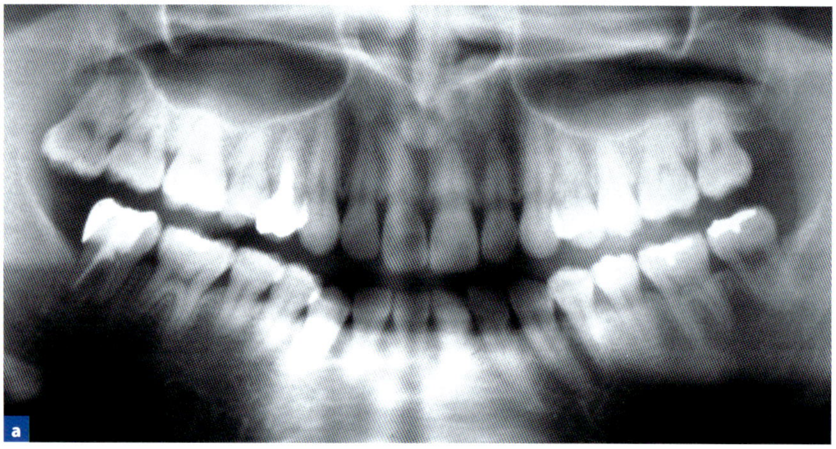

Fig 6-3a Preoperative panoramic radiograph of a 27-year-old female. The chief complaint was pain on #47.

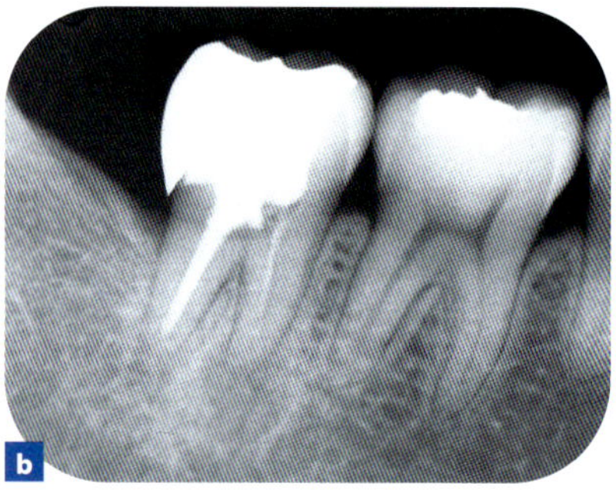

Fig 6-3b Preoperative radiograph. Inadequate root canal treatment of the mesial root of #47 was observed.

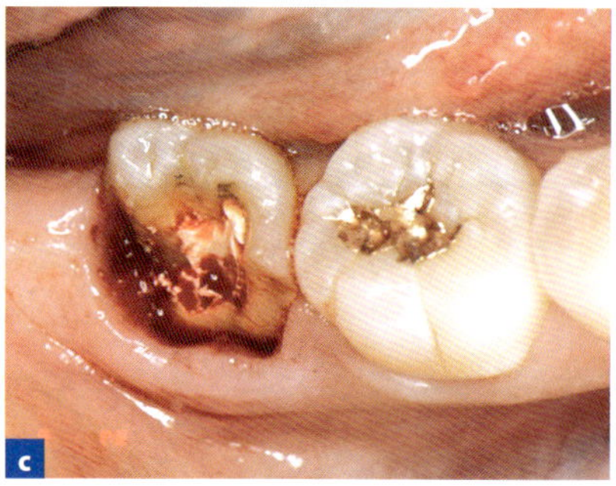

Fig 6-3c The likely cause of the pain was crown-root fracture. The preservation and prognosis of #47 was thought to be unfavorable.

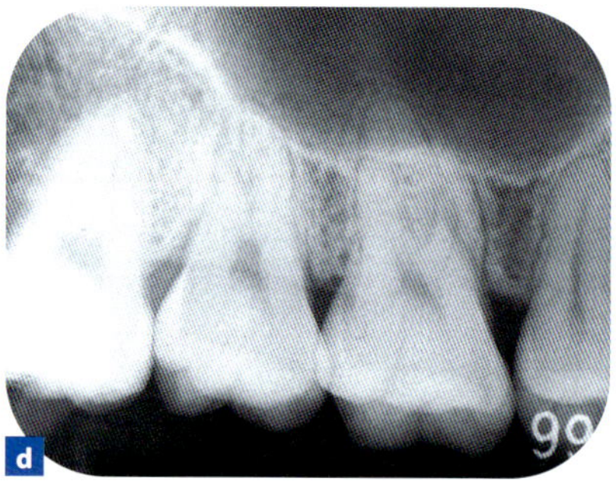

Fig 6-3d Radiograph of the maxillary third molar as a donor candidate. It was judged to be an appropriate donor tooth because the root form was favorable and there was not an opposing tooth.

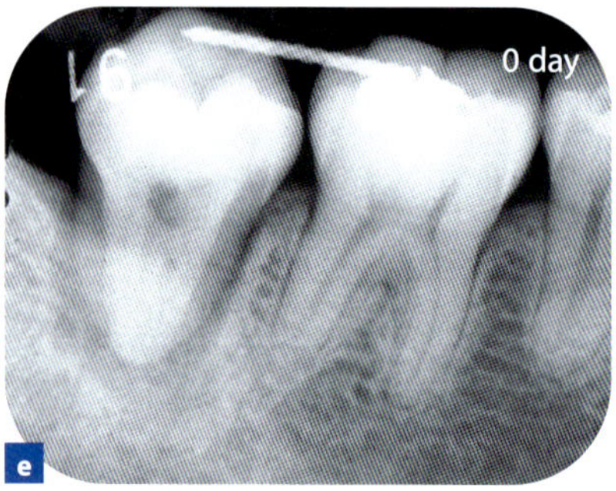

Fig 6-3e Immediately after transplantation.

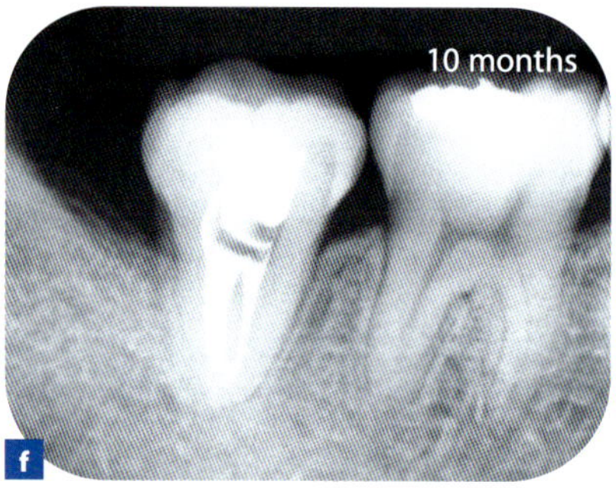

Fig 6-3f 10 months postoperative.

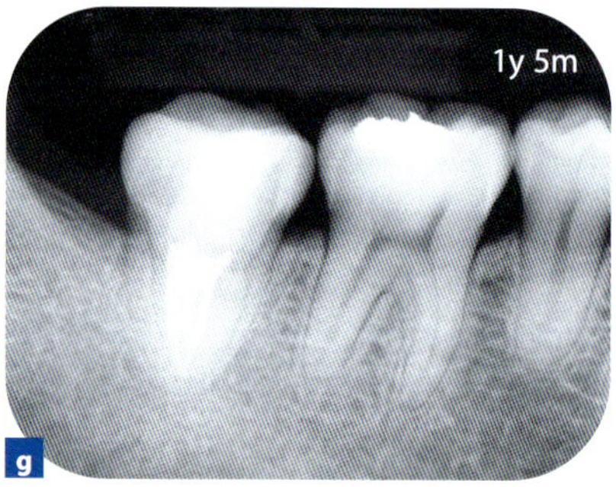

Fig 6-3g One year and 5 months postop.

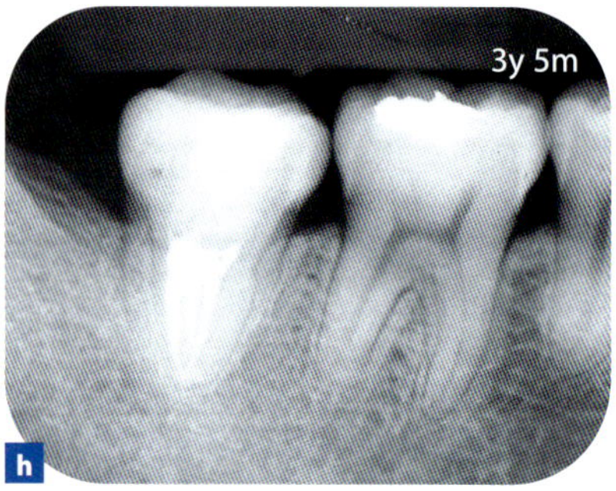

Fig 6-3h Three years and 5 months postop.

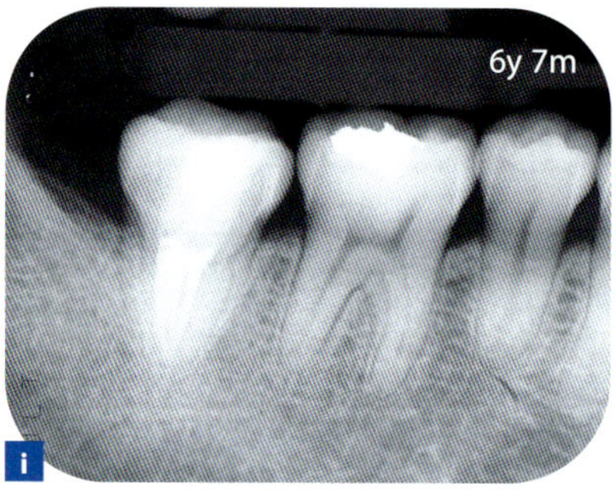

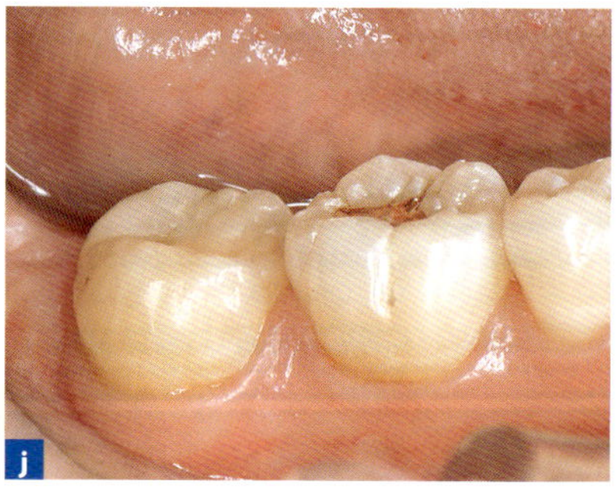

Fig 6-3i and 6-3j Six years and 7 months postop. The tooth is functional and appears esthetically normal.

Case 4. Transplantation to replace two compromised adjacent molars

Fig 6-4 shows a case of a 32-year-old female that presented with the chief complaint of deep dental caries and periodontitis in the left mandibular molar region. #36 and #37 were involved in inadequate root canal therapy and moderate periodontitis, but the treatment to restore health and function to these teeth was possible (**Fig 6-4a** to **6-4e**). If there had been no donor teeth available, the teeth might have been able to be saved with endodontic retreatment and periodontal therapy, possibly including periodontal surgery. However, since the patient had available third molars, transplantation was chosen. Four third molars were preserved in the mouth, but since the occlusion between the upper and lower third molars was maintained on the right side, the right third molars were not chosen to be donors (**Fig 6-4a** to **6-4c**). In addition, if the left-sided wisdom teeth had large, spread root forms then transplantation may not have been a favorable treatment option. In transplantation, there sometimes must be some favorable or lucky situations that are present in the patient for it to work, but it is important to be able to recognize and visualize the possibility of transplantation as an available treatment alternative. When transplanting two donor teeth into one molar region, it is better not to perform two transplantations at the same time. The reason is that it becomes difficult to close the gingival flap around the two consecutive transplanted teeth at once and that reattachment (PDL healing) may result in attachment loss (pocket formation). Therefore, each transplantation should be performed on a separate day, but priority should be given to the first molar site (**Fig 6-4n** to **6-4q**). The reason is that transplantation placed into the second molar site first can create difficult spacing mesiodistally for the second transplant going into the first molar site. If the second molar that cannot be preserved and has created a tight space for the recipient site of the first molar to be transplanted, one can simply reduce the mesial surface of the hopeless second molar to create more space. Usually, the second transplantation should be performed about two months after the first one (**Fig 6-4r** and **6-4s**).

In addition, when the donor tooth cannot be placed in the ideal buccolingual and mesiodistal direction, it is acceptable to rotate it 90 degrees or 180 degrees in relation to the width of the bone of the recipient site (**Fig 6-4s** and **6-4y**).

One of the problems with transplantation of third molars is root canal treatment after transplantation (**Fig 6-4t**, **6-4x** to **6-4aa**). The root canals of third molars have large degree of curvature and more complex morphology. The clinician must have the knowledge and skill to perform high level endodontic treatment. In order to avoid such complexity, some dentists adopt the procedure of extraoral apicoectomy when the transplant is out of the mouth. This may help with complex anatomy and saving time and cost for endodontic treatment later, but increase the risk of damage to the PDL, affecting the prognosis for reattachment.

The authors usually try to complete crown restoration with CR such as in this case (**Fig 6-4v** and **6-4w**). However, there are cases where indirect prosthetic treatment can be a better treatment.

Case 4. Transplantation to replace two compromised adjacent molars

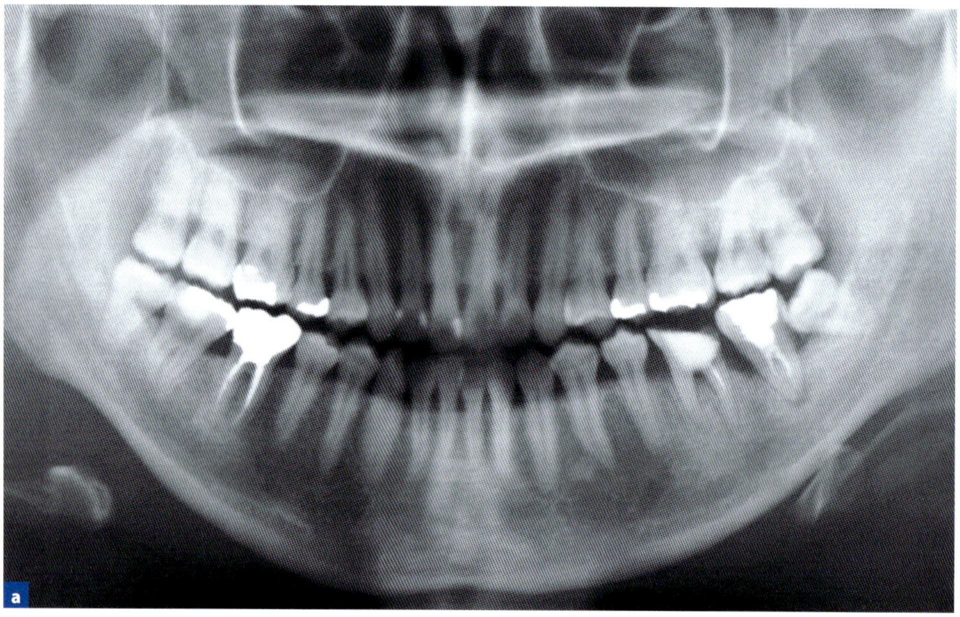

Fig 6-4a to 6-4e Preoperative views of a 32-year-old female. #36 and #37 had severe caries and moderate periodontitis. Although the affected teeth may have been able to be treated, the prognosis was guarded to unfavorable long-term and it was considered an indication for transplantation because the patient had donor teeth with appropriate morphology.

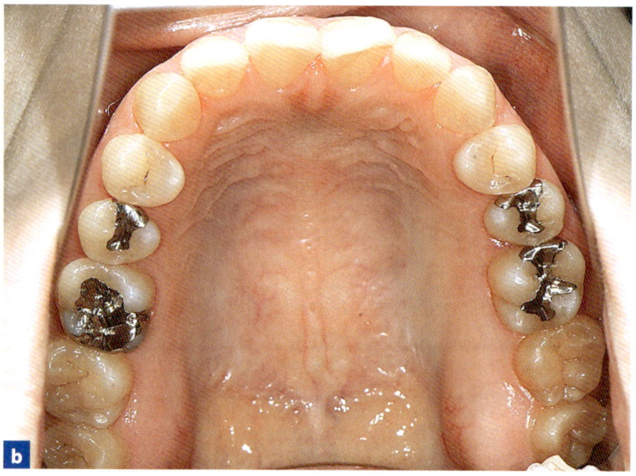

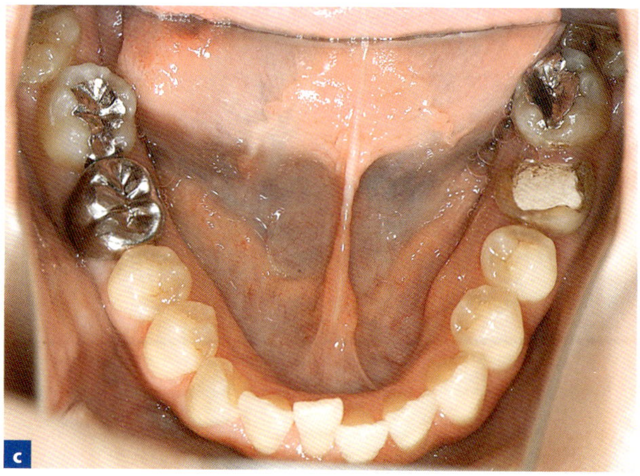

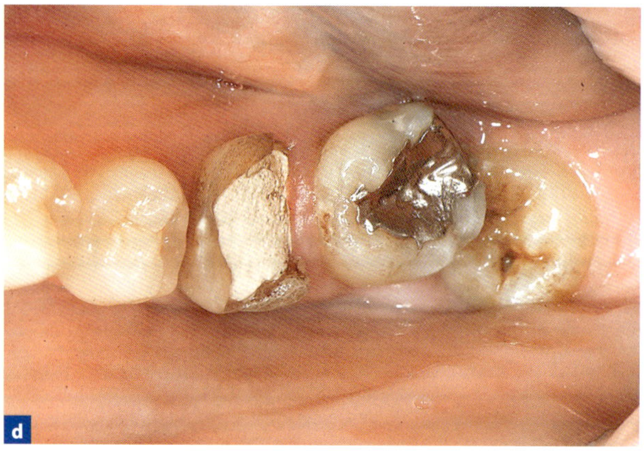

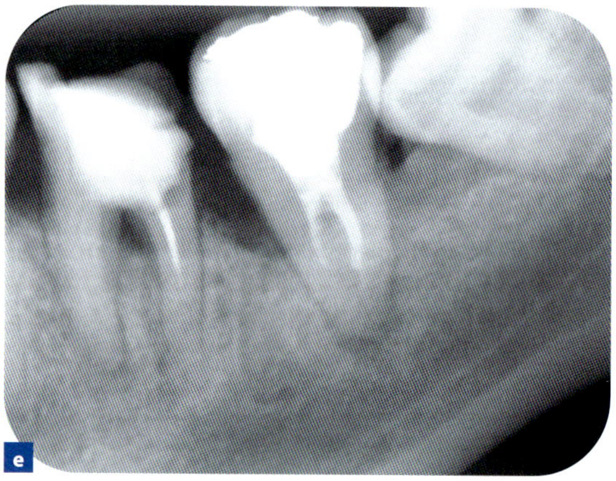

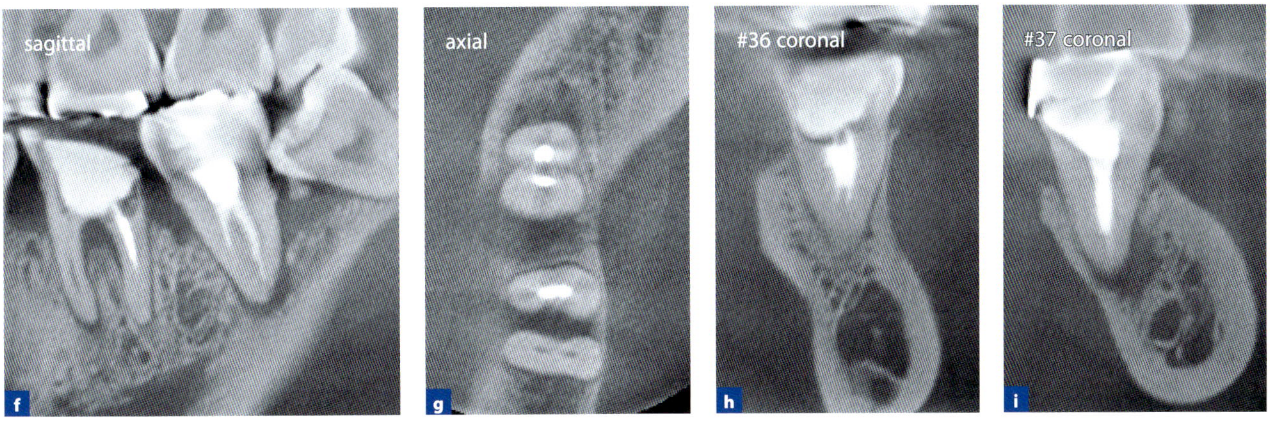

Fig 6-4f to 6-4i Preoperative CBCT images of the recipient site (#36 and #37). The bone width is wide enough to accommodate donor teeth.

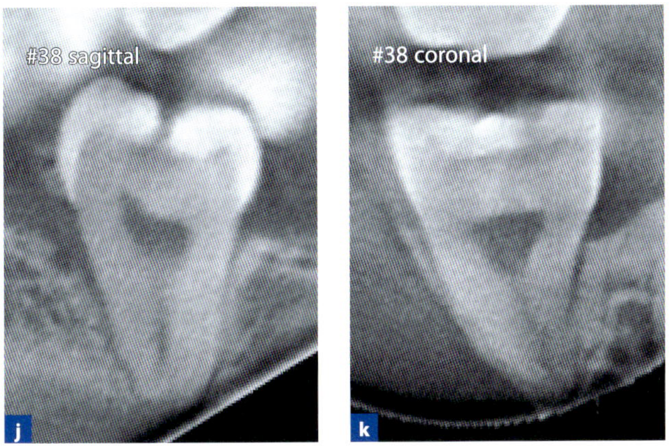

Fig 6-4j and 6-4k CBCT images of #38. It has an appropriate morphology as a donor tooth (to be transplanted to #36 site).

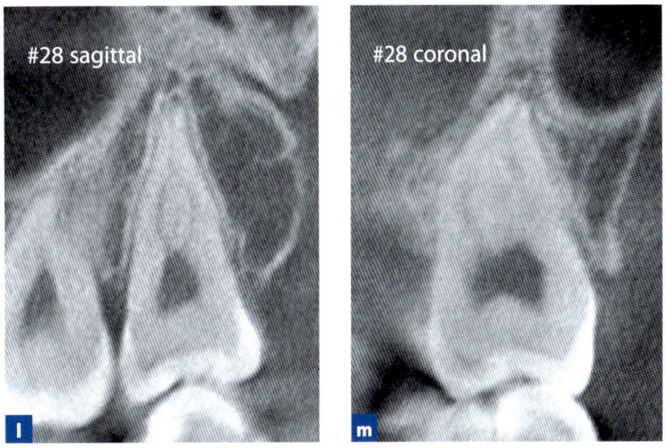

Fig 6-4l and 6-4m CBCT images of #28. It has an appropriate morphology as a donor tooth (to be transplanted to #37 site).

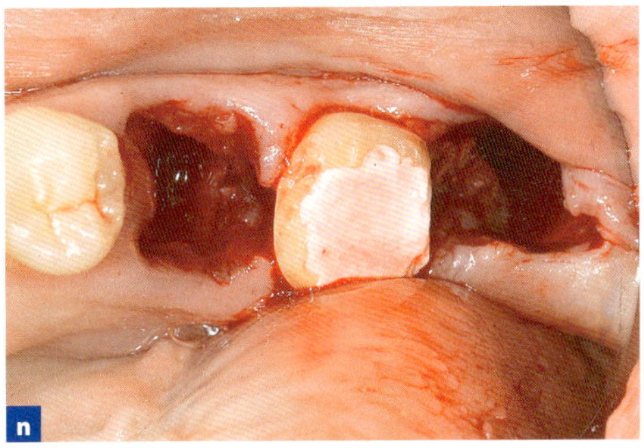

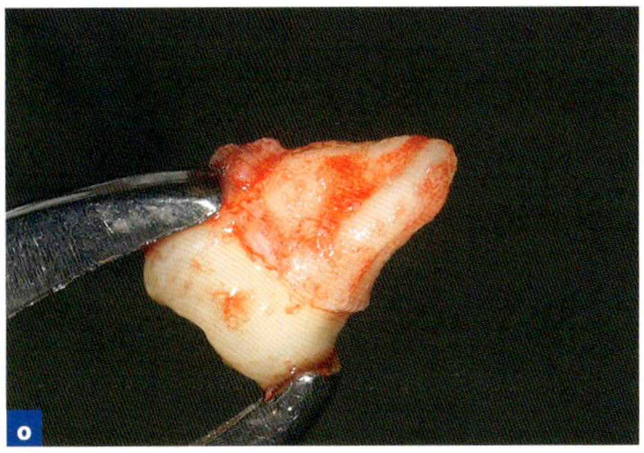

Fig 6-4n View during surgery. #36 and #38 were extracted, and the recipient socket was roughly formed.
Fig 6-4o Extracted #38 as a donor.

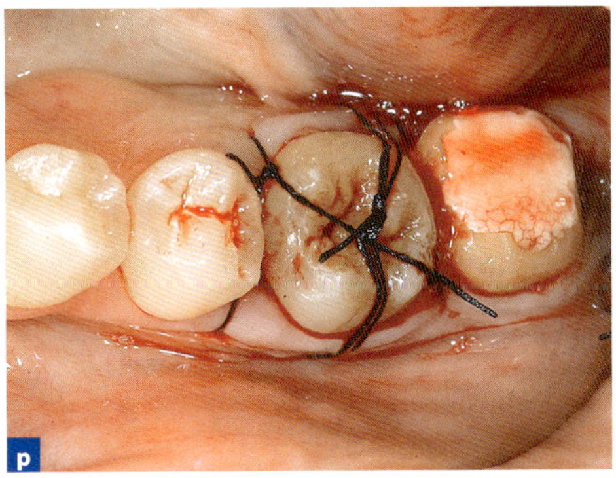

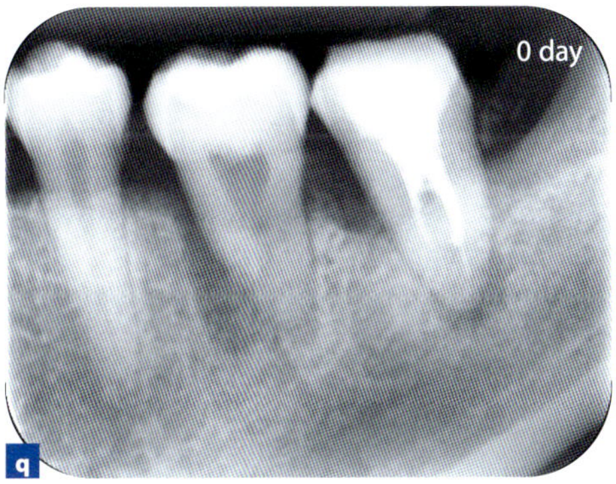

Fig 6-4p Immediately after transplantation.
Fig 6-4q Radiograph immediately after transplantation. Ideally, it should have been placed a little deeper.

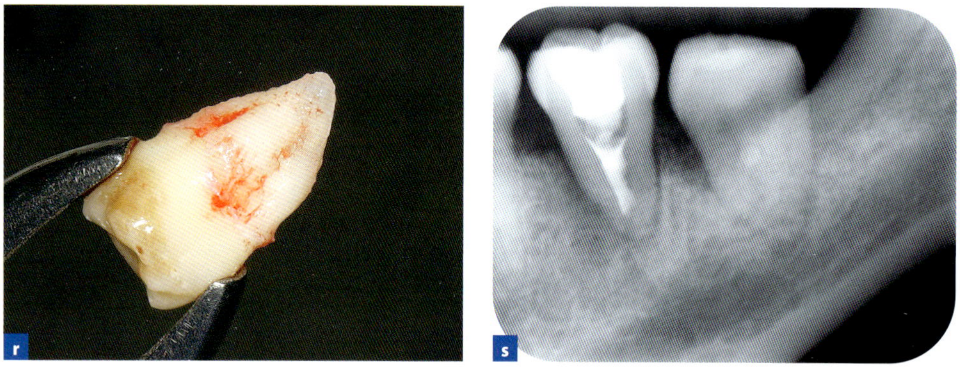

Fig 6-4r At the second surgery which was performed 2 months after the first one. This is the extracted #28 as a donor.
Fig 6-4s Radiograph immediately after the second transplantation. The transplant has been rotated by 90 degrees.

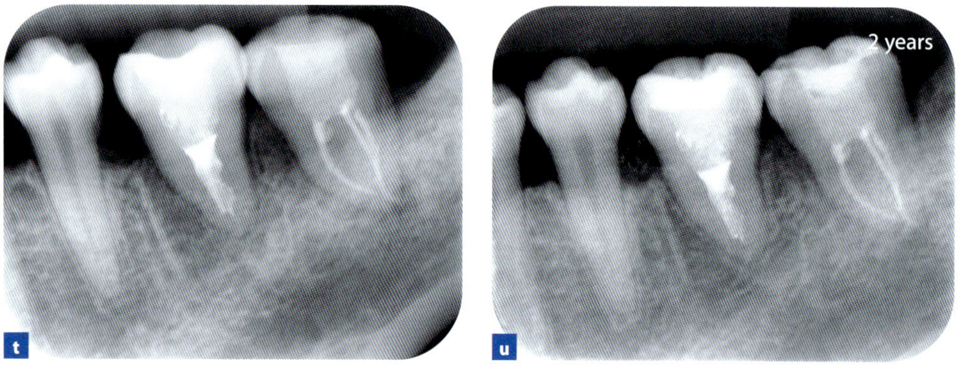

Fig 6-4t Seven months after the first transplantation.
Fig 6-4u Two years postoperative. There appears to be adequate PDL and osseous healing.

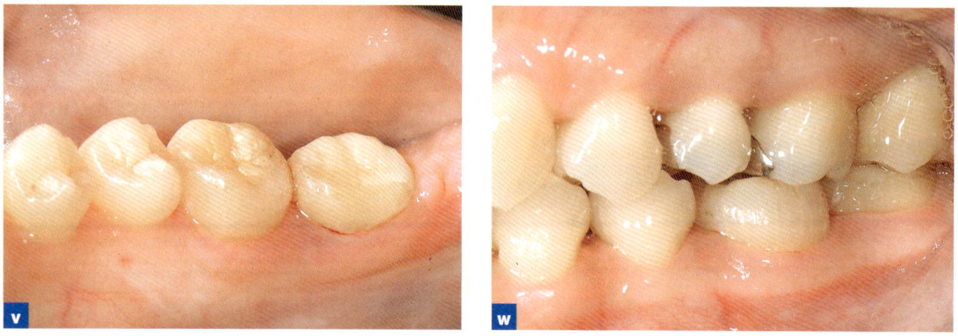

Fig 6-4v and 6-4w The 2 transplants were restored with CR for improved function and aesthetics.

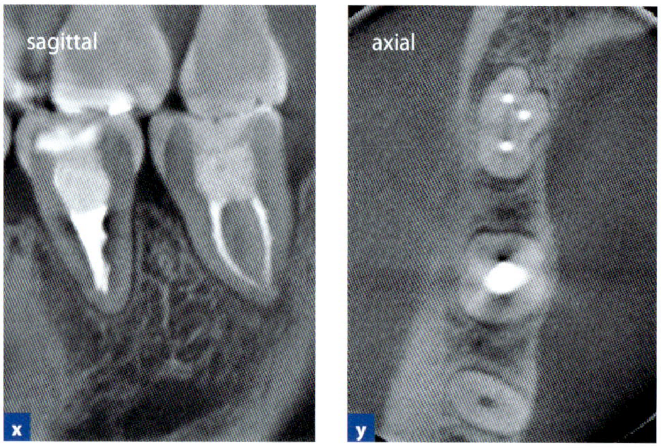

Fig 6-4x and 6-4y CBCT images (sagittal image, axial image) of the transplants (#36 and #37) 2 years after transplantation. Nice healing is maintained.

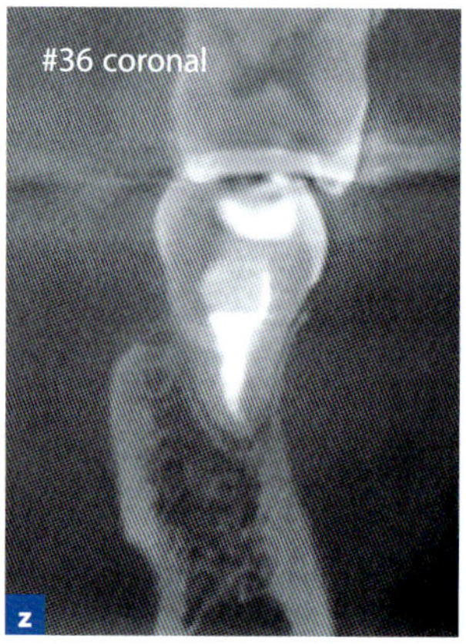

Fig 6-4z Coronal CBCT image of the transplant #36.

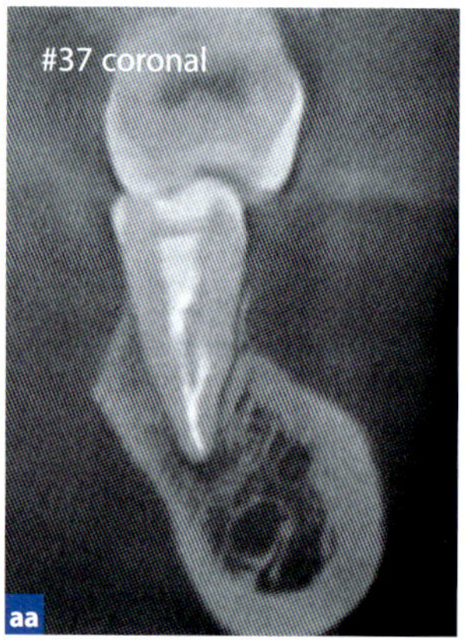

Fig 6-4aa Coronal CBCT image of the transplant #37.

Case 5. Transplantation combined with maxillary sinus floor elevation

Fig 6-5 is a case of a 45-year-old female who presented with crown-root fracture of #26. The fracture reached deep below the bone crest, and it was considered to have an unfavorable prognosis (**Fig 6-5a** to **6-5c**). Fortunately, a third molar with appropriate morphology was impacted and available, so it was considered as a favorable indication for transplantation. As can be seen in the radiograph after tooth extraction of #26, the floor of the maxillary sinus is located very close to the socket (**Fig 6-5d**). In such a case, implant therapy needs more treatment, time and cost. However, since bone induction by the periodontal ligament of the transplant can be expected, the combination of transplantation and sinus lifting (crestal approach) has more advantages than going the implant route. Bone can be formed and maintained around the transplant rapidly and predictably without any graft materials (**Fig 6-5n** to **6-5y** and see **Chapter 3**).

In addition, since the recipient socket is large (the access hole is wide), it is easier to perform sinus elevation surgery by the crestal approach. Detailed surgical procedures are explained in **Chapter 5 Fig 5-5**.

Case 6. Transplantation to replace a tooth involved in advanced periodontitis

Fig 6-6 is a case of a 39-year-old male who presented with a chief complaint of tooth mobility and pain of #37. It was considered to have an unfavorable prognosis due to advanced periodontitis (**Fig 6-6a** to **6-6c**). The preserved third molar may have caused some negative effect on the second molar. In general, tilted and impacted third molars may frequently cause caries, root resorption, and periodontitis on the adjacent second molars. Thus, early extraction of such teeth is recommended.

In transplantation to a recipient site with such larger bony defect, the success seems to be higher when the transplant is placed deeper and slightly distal (**Fig 6-6g** and **6-6h**). The reason for this is that the distal part of the transplant can be more easily closed with the gingival flap, and natural extrusion and mesial movement of the transplant can be expected during healing. In addition, bone healing (bone induction) can be expected to occur as the tooth moves (**Fig 6-6k** to **6-6r**). Wire splinting of a transplant is usually removed after 1 month, but if tooth mobility of the transplant is still high as in this case, the splinting may be removed much later (in this case after 3 months). It should be noted that no bone graft material was used in this case.

Case 5. Transplantation combined with maxillary sinus floor elevation

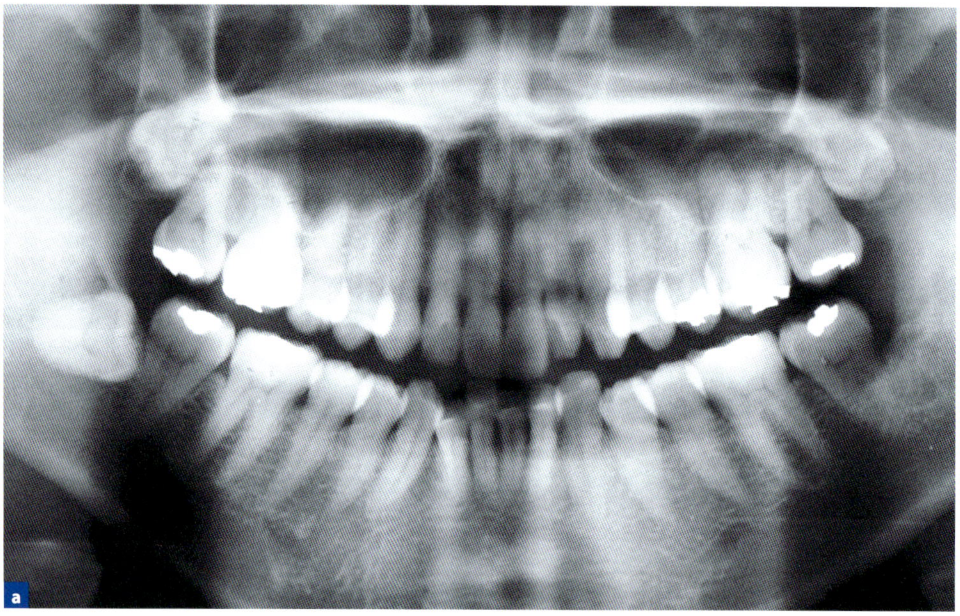

Fig 6-5a Preoperative panoramic radiograph of a 45-year-old female who presented with pain to #26 which was involved in a crown-root fracture and thought to have an unfavorable prognosis. Fortunately, #28 of simple root form was present and the case was thought to be a good indication for transplantation.

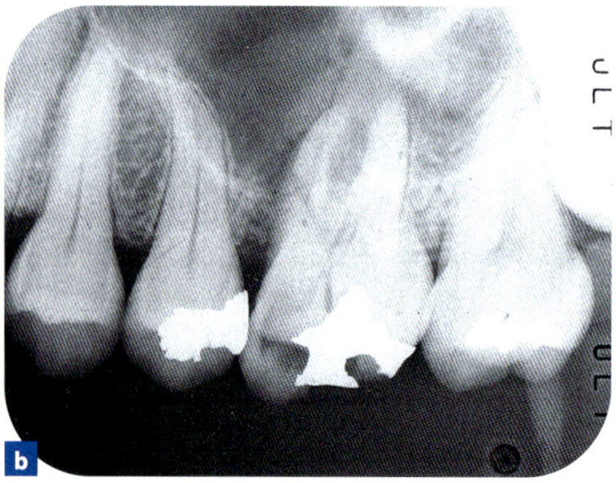

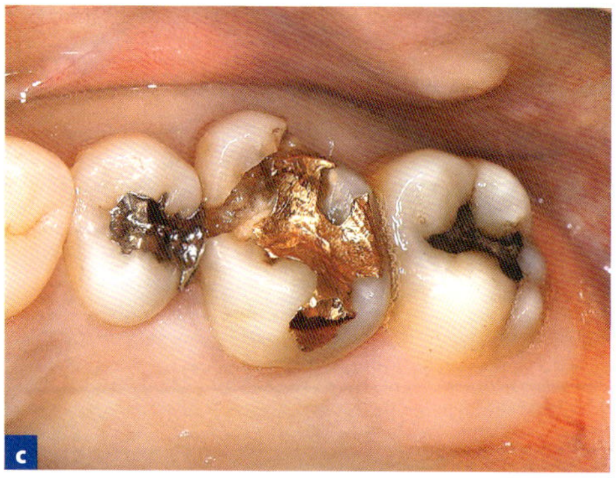

Fig 6-5b Preoperative radiograph of #26. The fracture extended deep below the crest.

Fig 6-5c Preoperative view around the surgery area. #26 was extracted on this day.

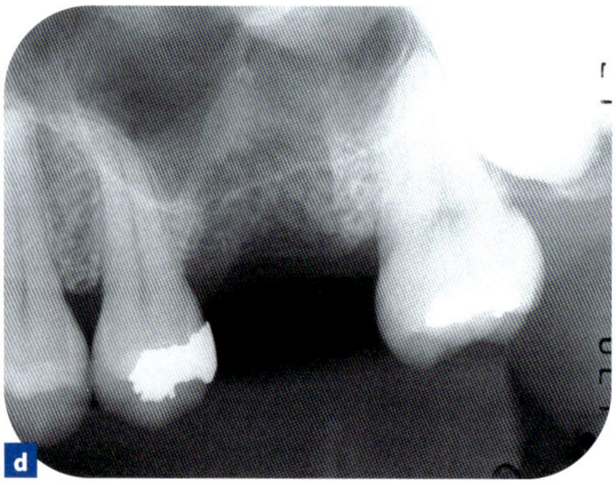

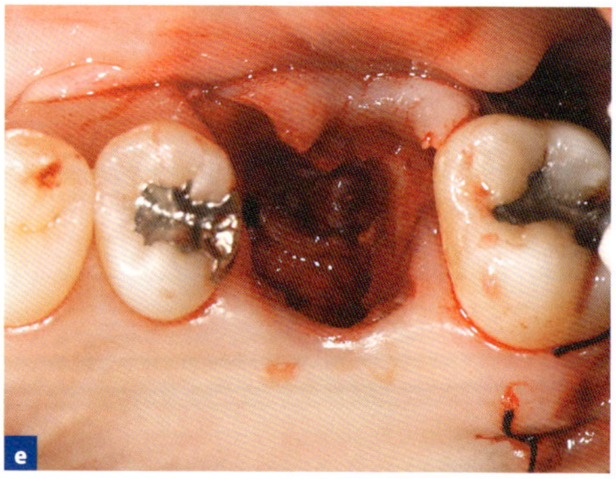

Fig 6-5d Radiograph just before transplantation. Note that the sinus floor deeply pneumatized and very close to the root apices.

Fig 6-5e Transplantation was performed 3 weeks after extraction of #26. At the same time sinus elevation was performed. Refer to **Chapter 5 Fig 5-5** for detailed surgical procedures.

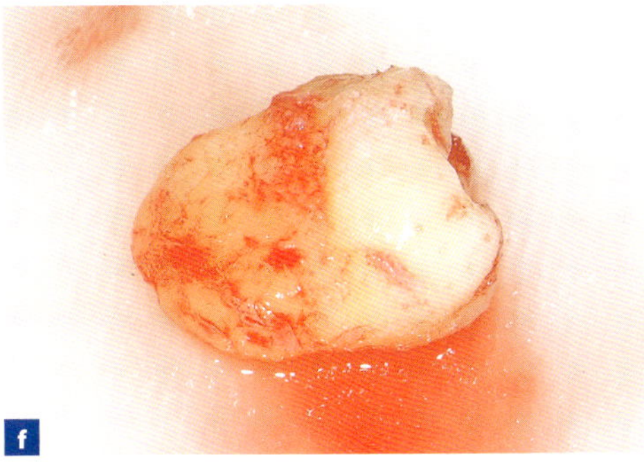

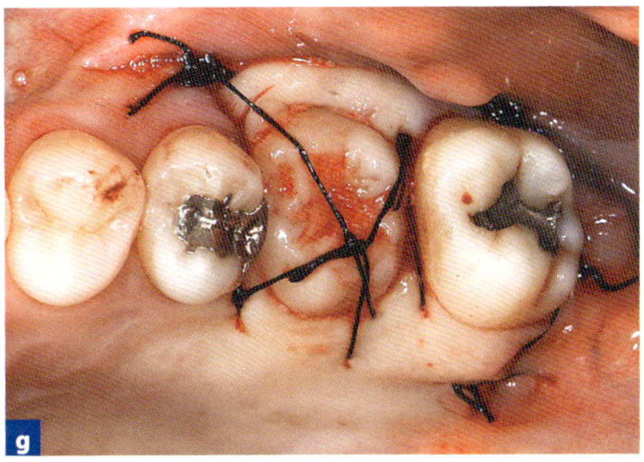

Fig 6-5f #28 extracted as a donor tooth.
Fig 6-5g Immediately after transplantation.

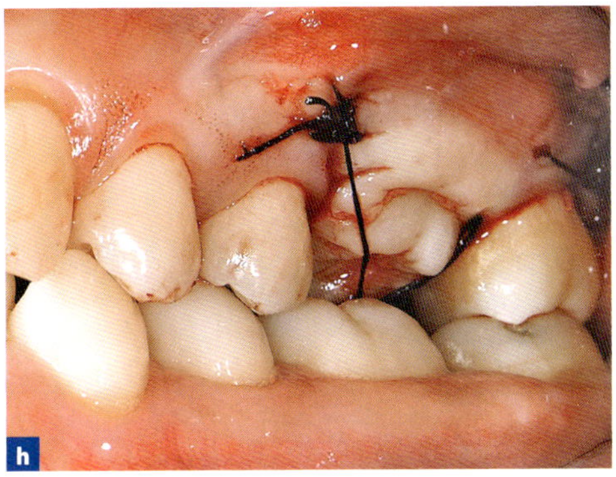

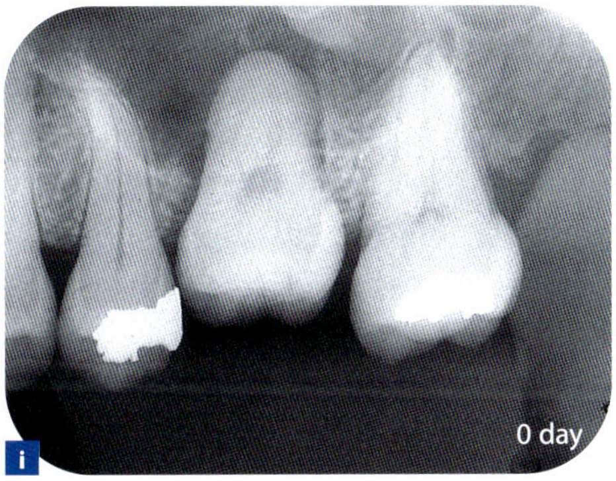

Fig 6-5h Occlusal relationship immediately after transplantation.
Fig 6-5i Radiograph immediately after transplantation. Note that there is no bone tissue around the apex of the transplant.

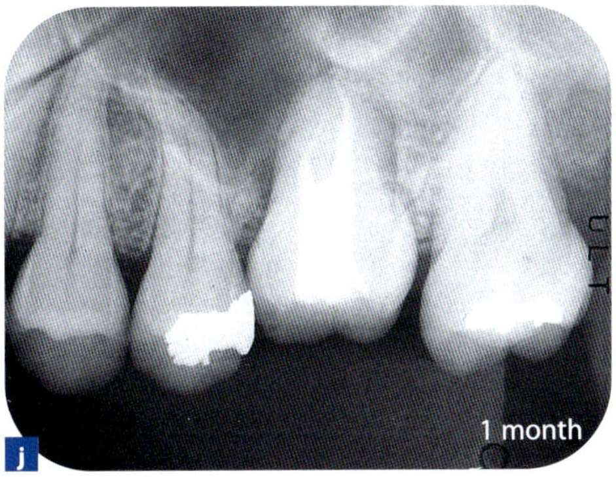

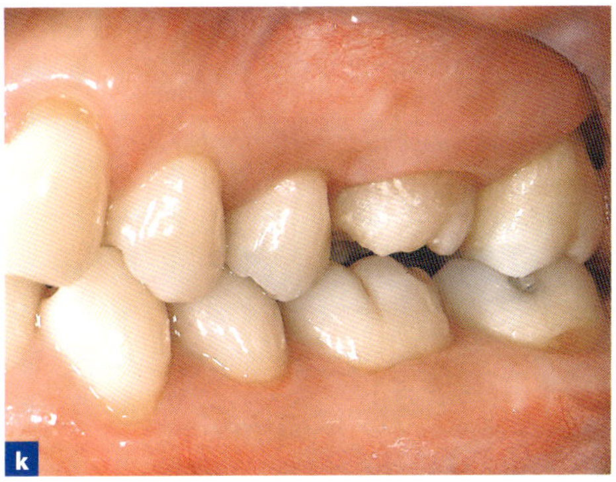

Fig 6-5j One month postop and immediately after final root canal filling.
Fig 6-5k Occlusal relationship after about 4 months. Spontaneous eruption has started to occur.

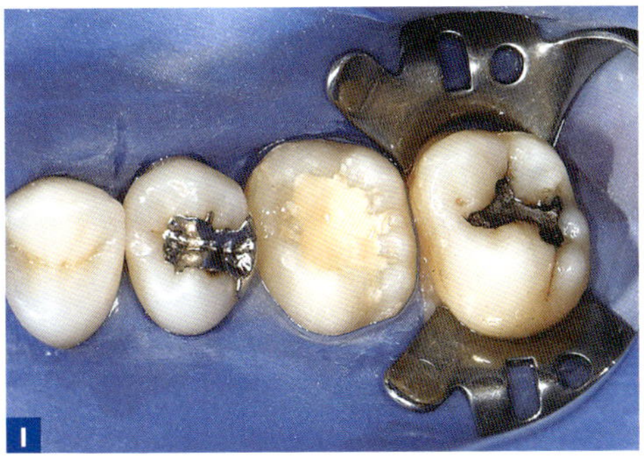

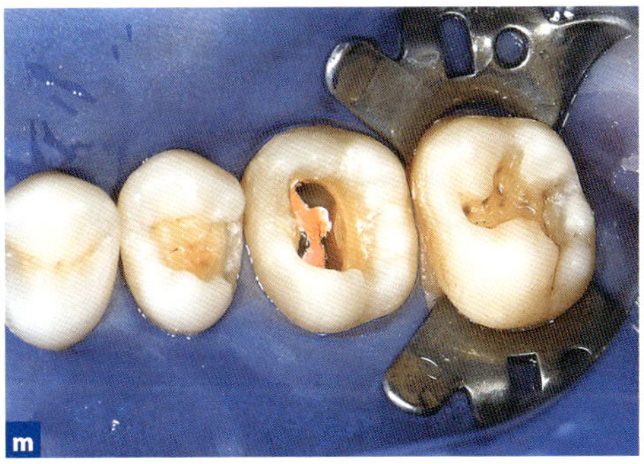

Fig 6-5l Before restoration of the transplant with CR. Same day as **Fig 6-5k**.
Fig 6-5m After preparation. The patient wanted to replace the metal restorations of the adjacent teeth with CR at the same time.

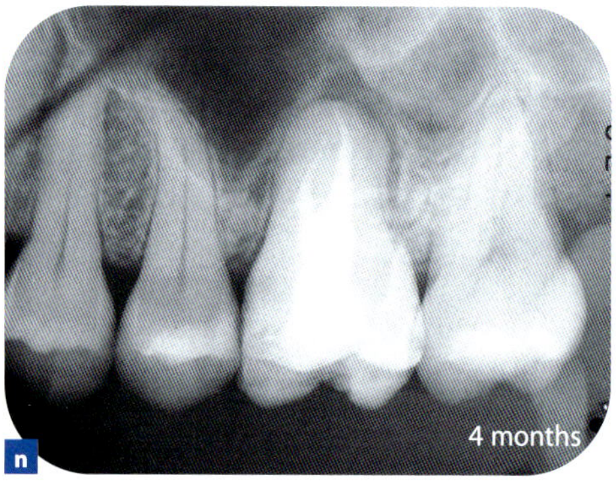

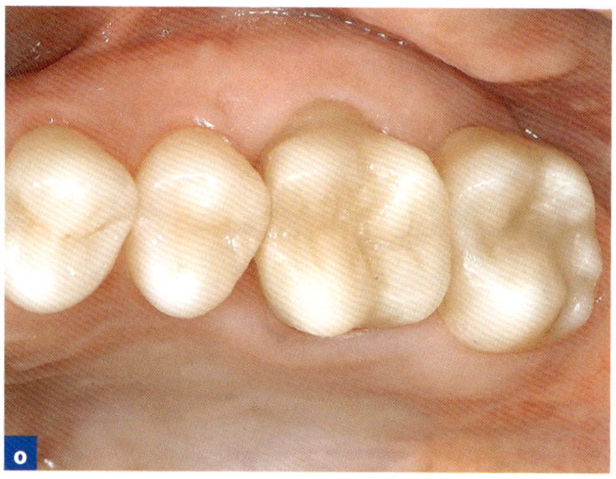

Fig 6-5n and 6-5o After CR restoration of #25, #26 and #27.

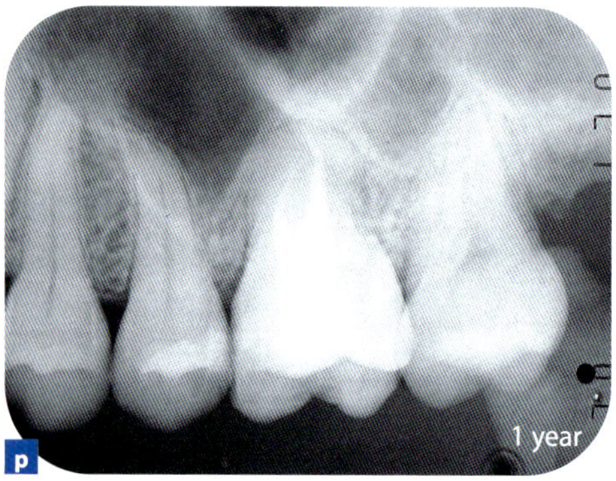

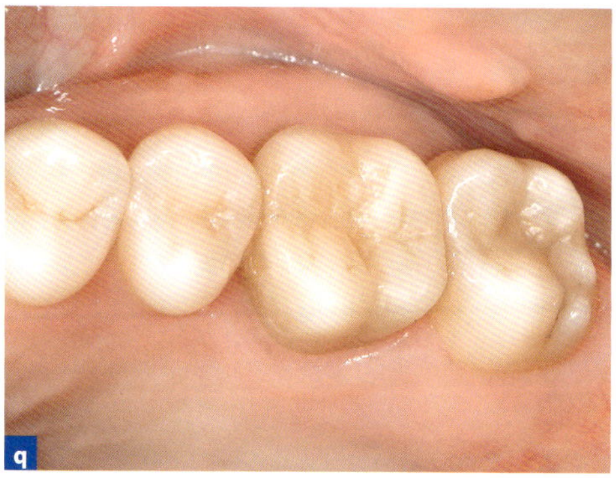

Fig 6-5p and 6-5q One year postoperative. No root resorption was observed. Bone formation is observed around the root of the transplant.

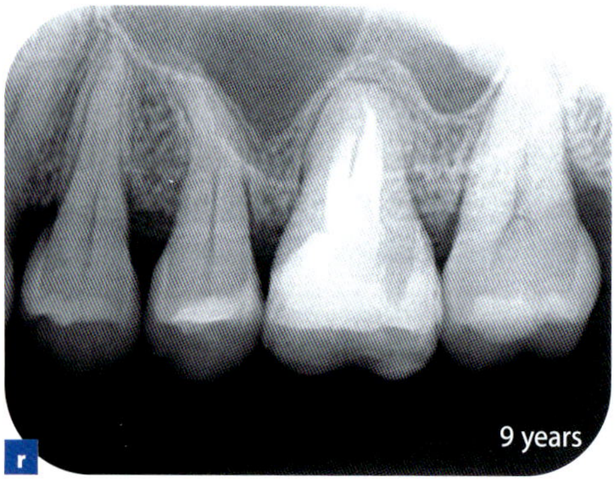

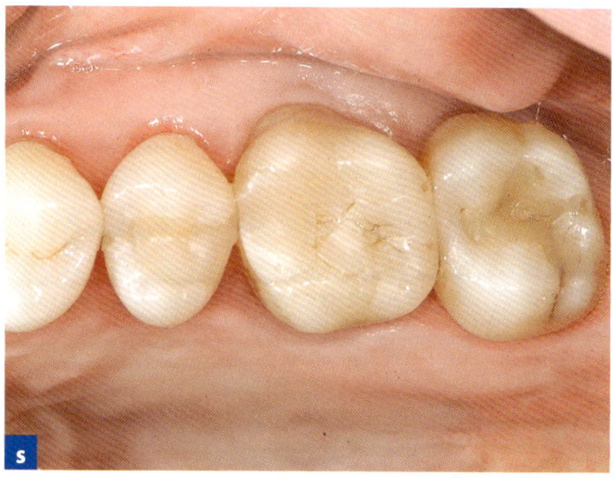

Fig 6-5r and 6-5s Nine years postop.

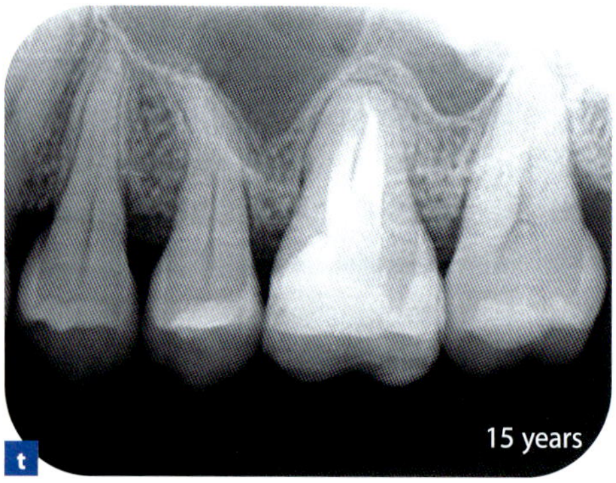

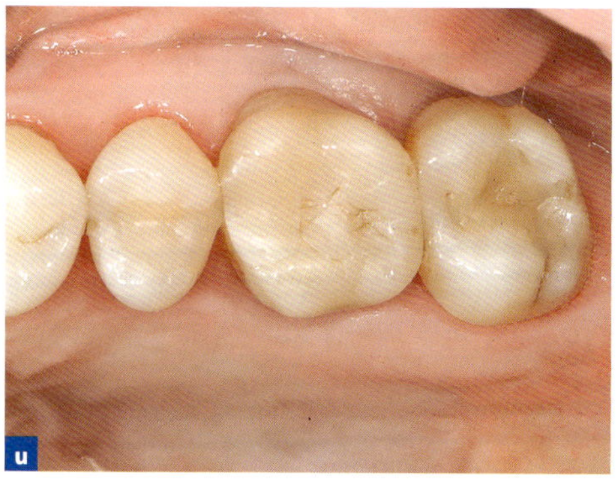

Fig 6-5t and 6-5u 15 years postop.

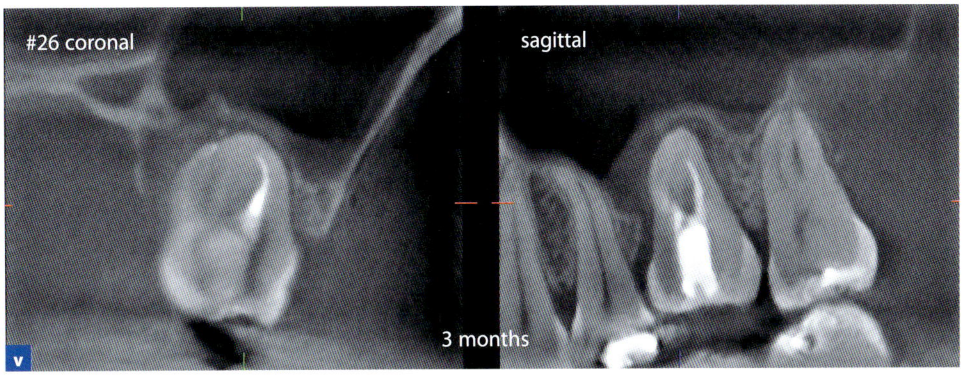

Fig 6-5v CBCT images 3 months after transplantation. The area around the transplant is not yet covered with new bone.

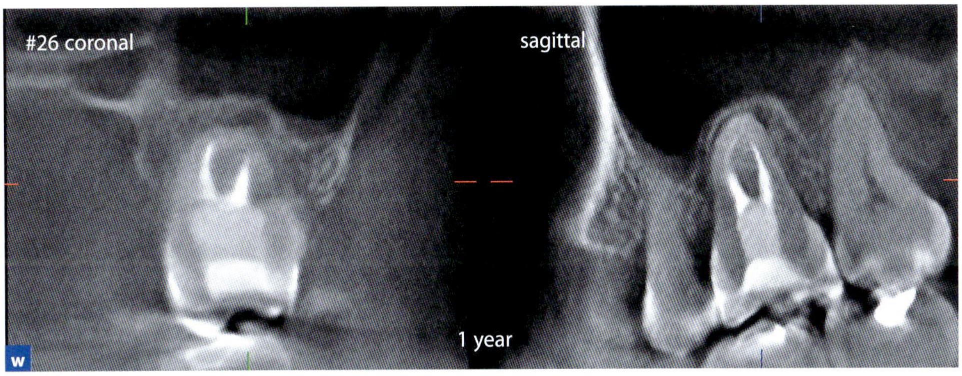

Fig 6-5w CBCT images after 1 year. New bone formation around the transplant is evident.

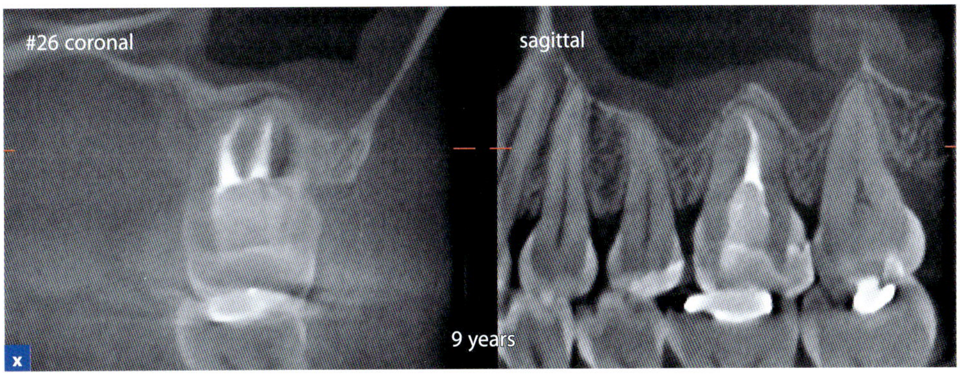

Fig 6-5x CBCT images after 9 years. The newly formed bone and periodontal ligament space is maintained around the root.

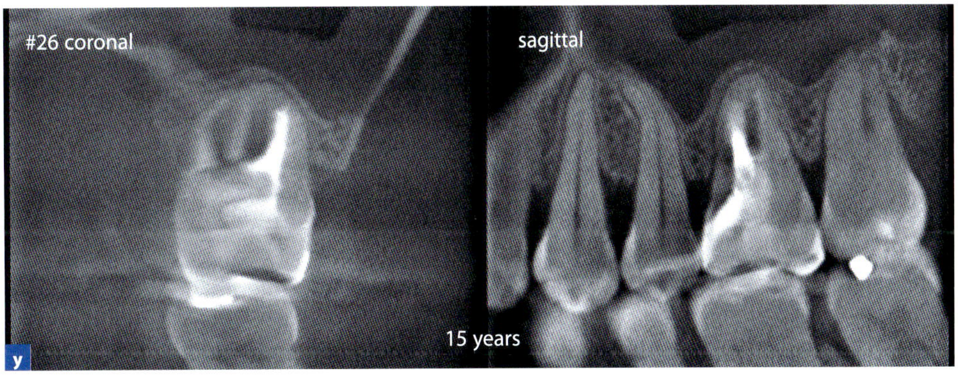

Fig 6-5y CBCT images 15 years after transplantation. No abnormalities are evident.

Case 6. Transplantation to replace a tooth involved in advanced periodontitis

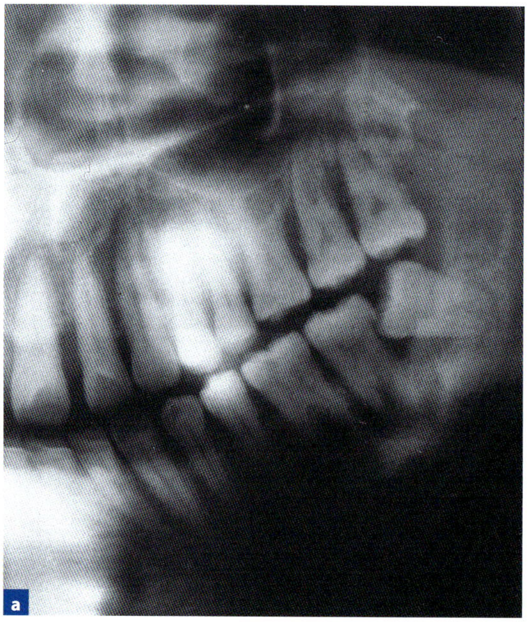

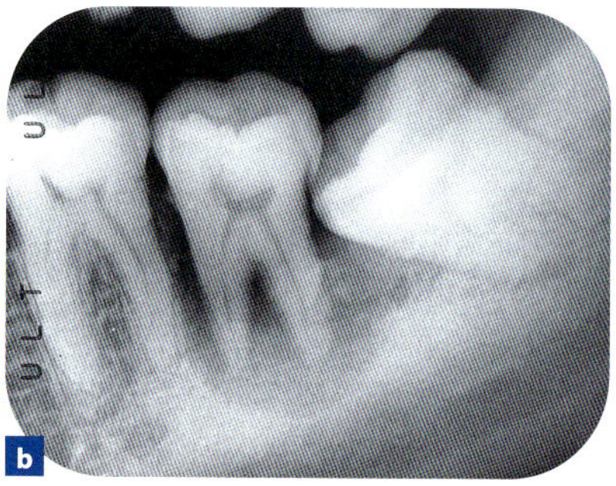

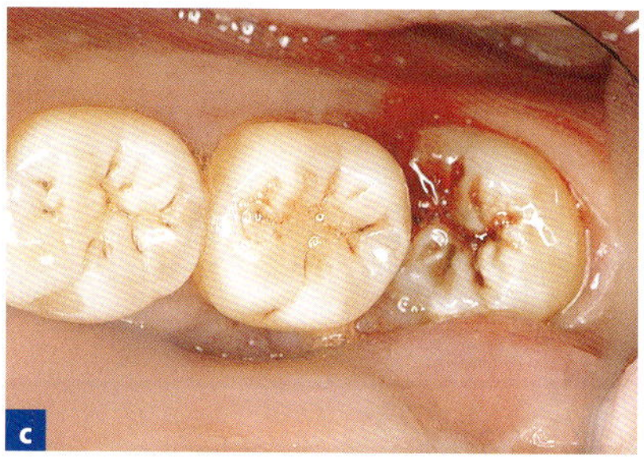

Fig 6-6a Preoperative panoramic radiograph of a 39-year-old male who suffered from advanced periodontitis.
Fig 6-6b Radiograph at the first visit. Severe bone loss around #37 has progressed. Transplantation using the adjacent partially impacted third molar was considered a good treatment option.
Fig 6-6c Surgical area before surgery.

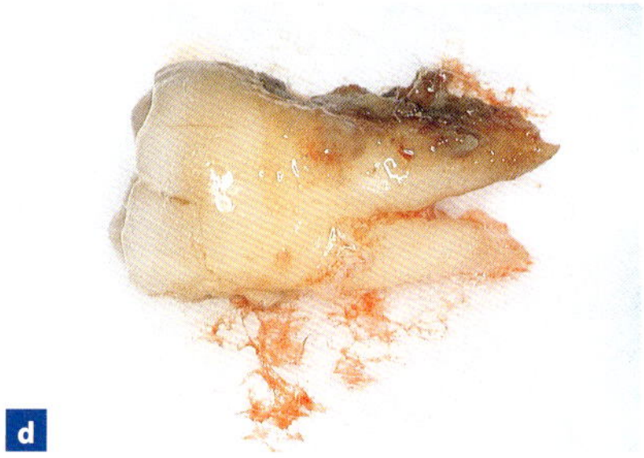

Fig 6-6d #37 was extracted 6 weeks before transplantation.

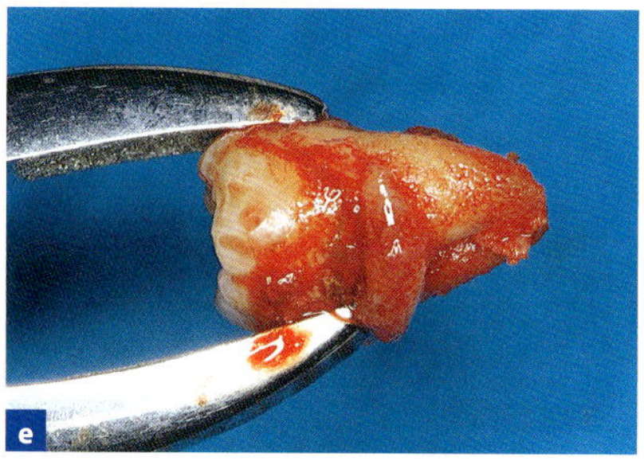

Fig 6-6e #38 extracted as a donor tooth. There appears to be adequate and healthy periodontal ligament attached.

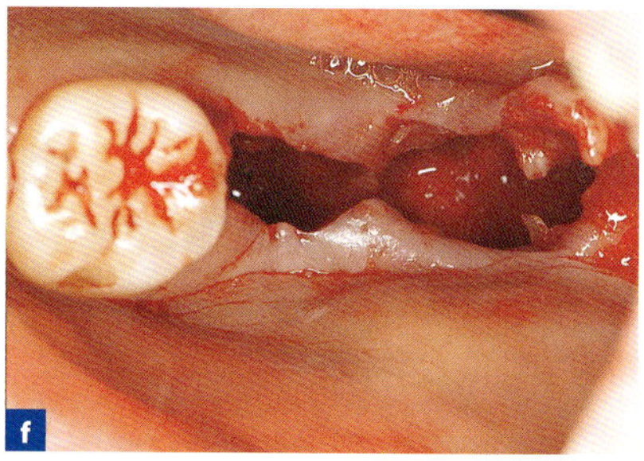

Fig 6-6f After extraction of the donor tooth and formation of the recipient socket.

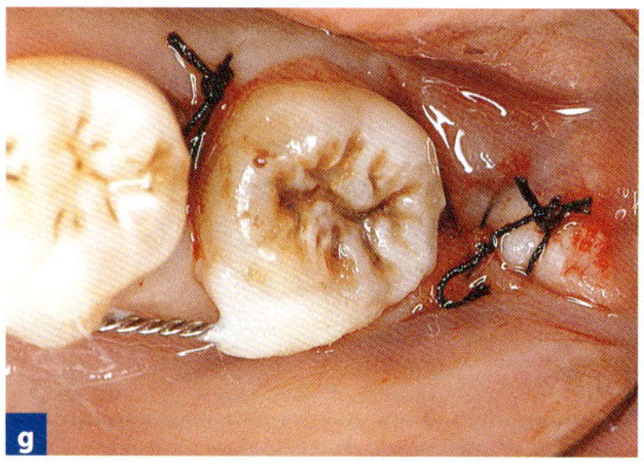

Fig 6-6g After suturing the gingival flap and splinting the transplant to the adjacent tooth. The distal aspect of the flap was able to be sutured tightly.

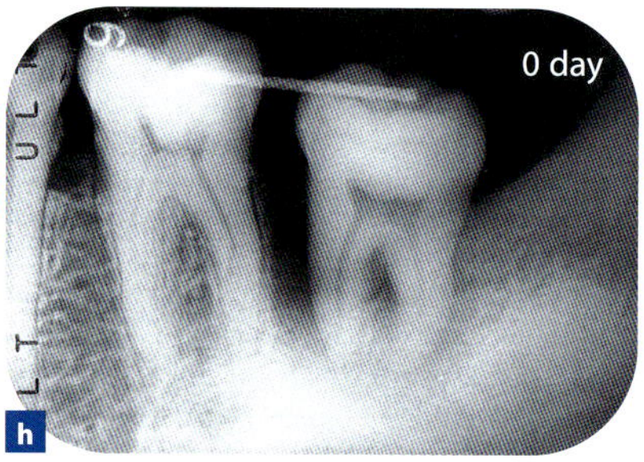

Fig 6-6h Radiograph immediately after transplantation.

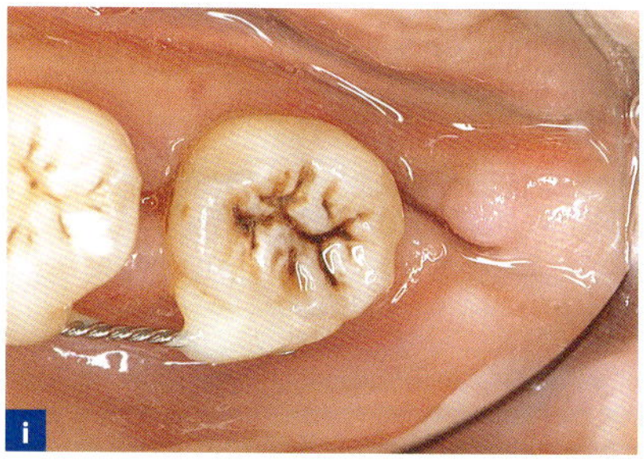

Fig 6-6i Two weeks postop.

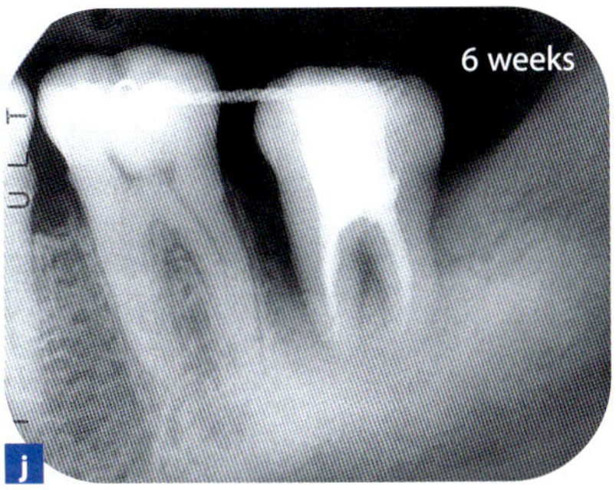

Fig 6-6j Six weeks postop. The root canal has been filled temporarily with calcium hydroxide preparation.

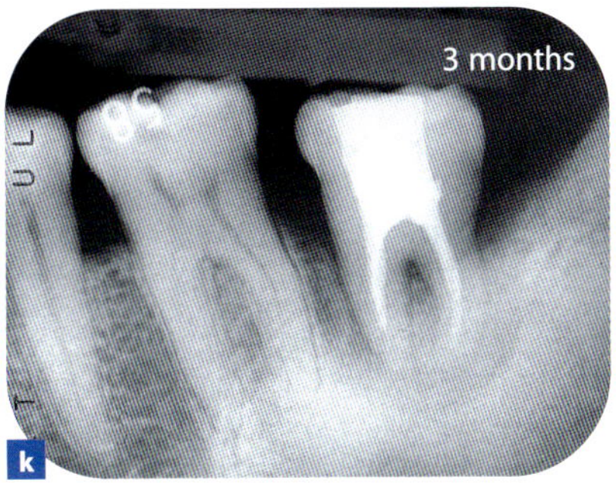

Fig 6-6k Three months postop. Immediately after removal of the splinting.

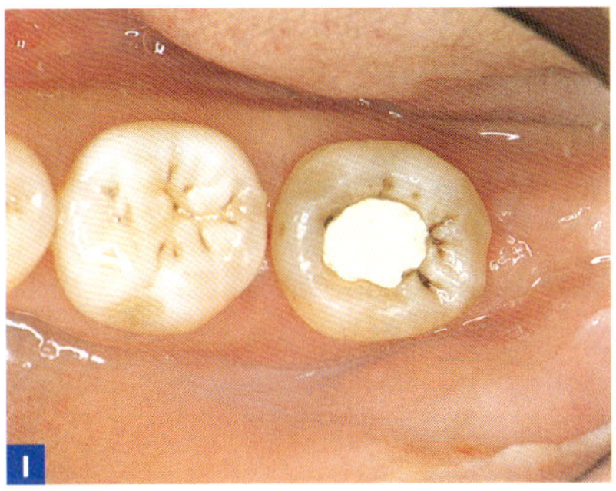

Fig 6-6l Seven months postop.

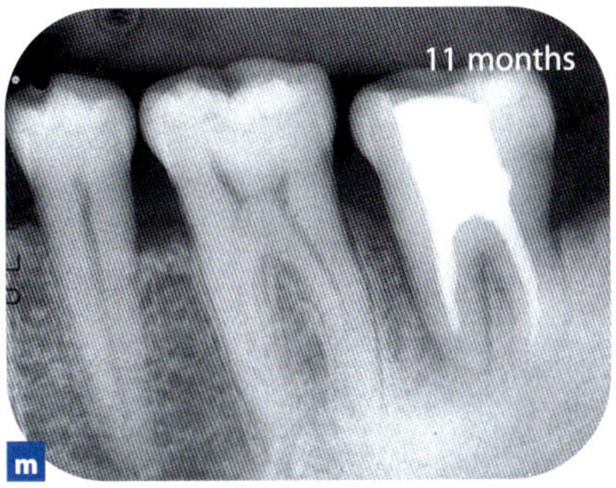

Fig 6-6m 11 months after transplantation and just before root canal filling with sealer and gutta-percha.

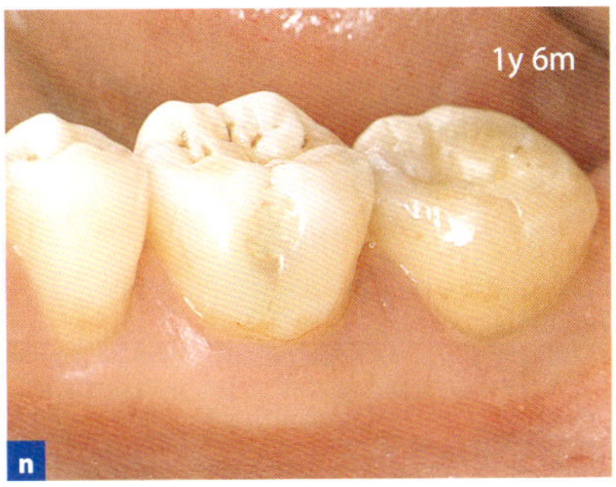

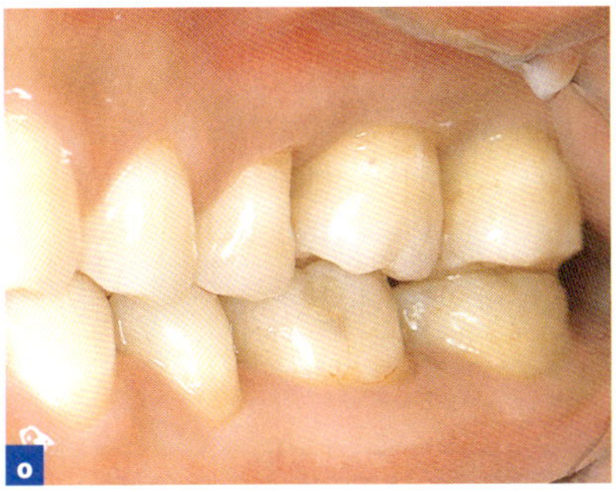

Fig 6-6n and 6-6o One year and 6 months postop. The transplant has been restored with CR.

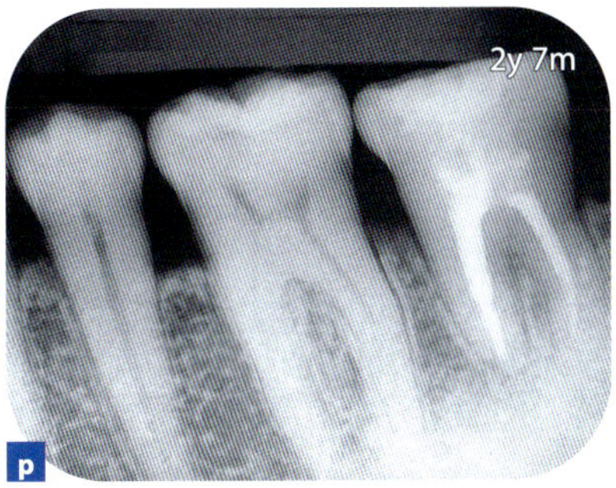

Fig 6-6p Two years and 7 months postop.

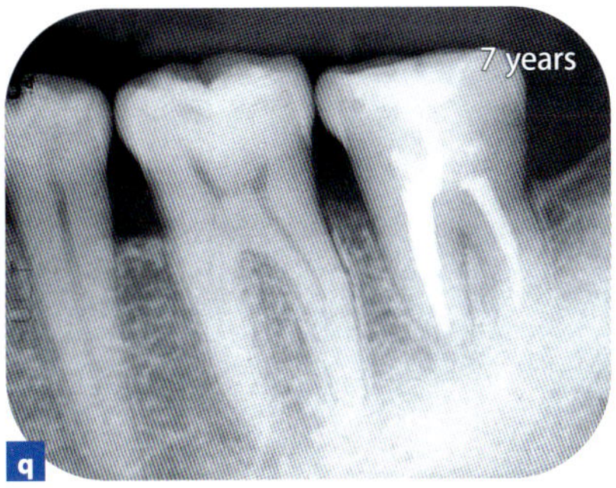

Fig 6-6q Seven years postop.

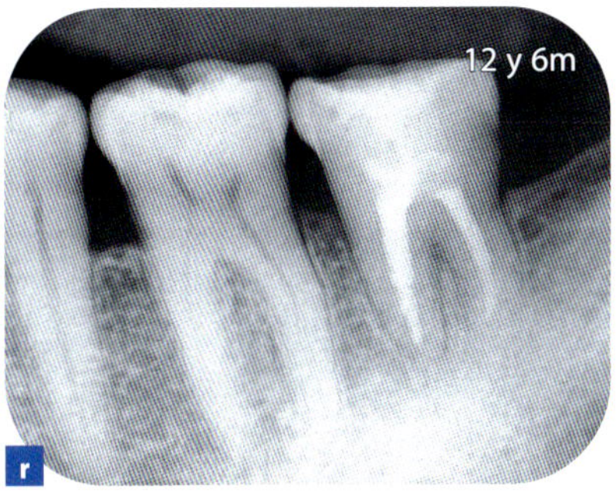

Fig 6-6r 12 years and 6 months after transplantation.

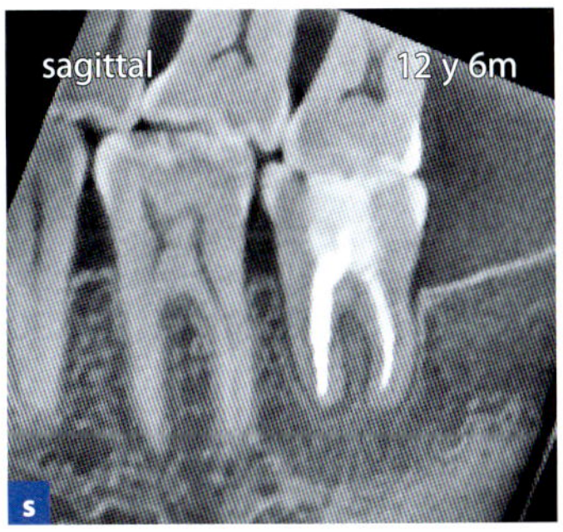

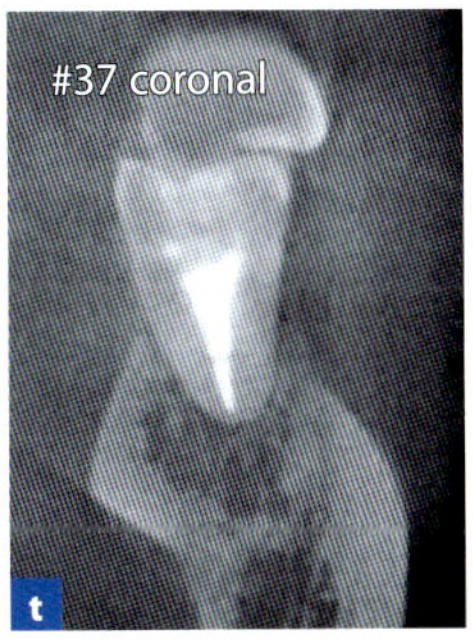

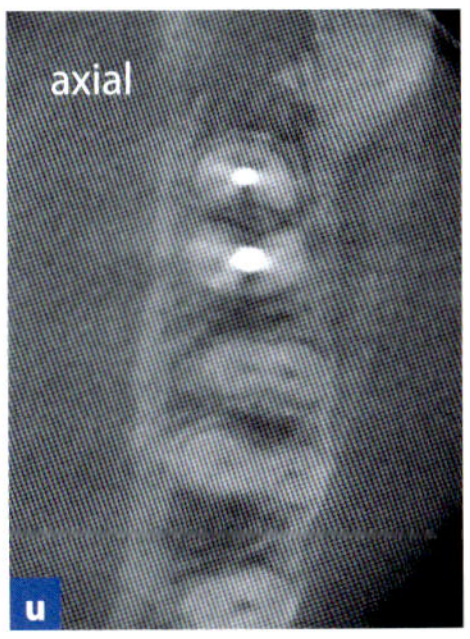

Fig 6-6s to 6-6u CBCT images 12 years and 6 months after transplantation. Regenerated bone around the transplant is maintained and no evidence of abnormalities such as root resorption is observed.

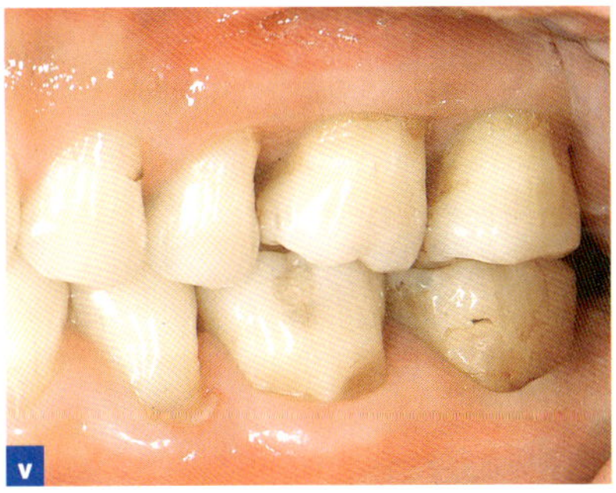

Fig 6-6v Occlusal relationship 12 years and 6 months after transplantation.

Case 7. Efficacy of transplantation in juvenile periodontitis

Fig 6-7 is a 46-year-old female who has been visiting our clinic intermittently for treatment and maintenance of juvenile periodontitis since she was 20 years old. **Fig 6-7a** to **6-7c** were the views taken 7 years after the last maintenance visit. The periodontal destruction had progressed too much to preserve the tooth. However, since the third molar (#18) was impacted and preserved in the maxilla, transplantation to replace the involved tooth (#36) with #18 was indicated.

Transplantation was performed about 3 weeks after the tooth extraction on the recipient site (**Fig 6-7d** and **6-7e**). The transplant was unintentionally placed deep into the socket (**Fig 6-7e** and **6-7f**), but in cases where bone destruction of the recipient site has progressed, it will be better to place the donor tooth deeper into the recipient socket and wait for the natural eruption of the transplant.

In this case, natural eruption did not occur sufficiently (**Fig 6-7g**), so orthodontic extrusion was performed two and a half months after transplantation (**Fig 6-7h** and **6-7i**). The transplant was extruded to its proper position in about 1 month (**Fig 6-7j** and **6-7k**), but it looked as if it had protruded from the socket. However, the periodontal ligament of the transplant induced bone around the transplant, and postoperative follow-up observation by CBCT confirmed that the bone around the transplant was regenerated three-dimensionally (**Fig 6-7l** to **6-7ee**). Transplantation can be so advantageous because it can not only replace the tooth but also rebuild periodontal tissues.

This patient visited our clinic for the first time when she was 20 years old and at that time had juvenile periodontitis already present. At her first visit, #46 was extracted because of severe bone destruction such as **Fig 6-7b**. However, an immature #48 wisdom had been preserved at that time. Retrospectively, if we had the knowledge and techniques related to transplantation back then, we would have been able to provide similar treatment for #46.

Through seeing the cases in this chapter, one may notice the efficacy and advantages of preserving third molars. When treating hopeless molars, transplantation using third molars can be of great benefit especially for young patients. Therefore, it is important for dental practitioners to have clear criteria and reasoning when deciding to extract or preserve third molars.

In general, for patients who are around the age of 20 and have low caries risk, have no teeth that have undergone extensive treatments , and have low risk of periodontitis, impacted third molars in the lower jaws should be extracted. This is because mandibular molars may adversely affect adjacent teeth (dental caries, root resorption, periodontitis), as well as affect the entire dentition (malalignment).

Contrarily, since maxillary molars are unlikely to cause future problems, we don't often have to extract them. We would like to save them as a natural tooth bank for possible future transplantation (see **Case 2** to **Case 5** and **Case 7**).

Case 7. Efficacy of transplantation in juvenile aggressive periodontitis

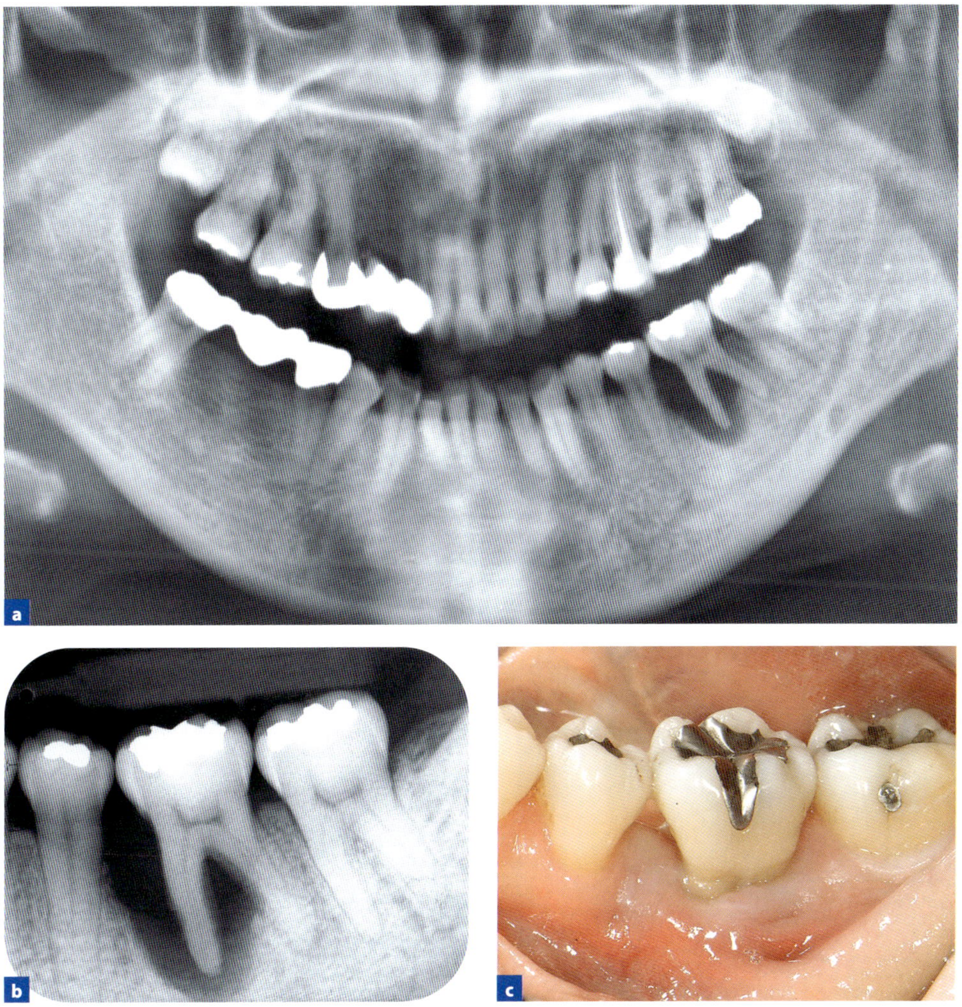

Fig 6-7a to 6-7c Preoperative views of a 46-year-old female. The patient had intermittent visits for treatment and maintenance of juvenile periodontitis since the age of 20. Unfortunately, #36 was continued to develop severe bone loss while the patient moved away and did not come for 7 years. Fortunately, the patient had an impacted third molar (#18), which was thought to be a candidate as a donor tooth for transplantation.

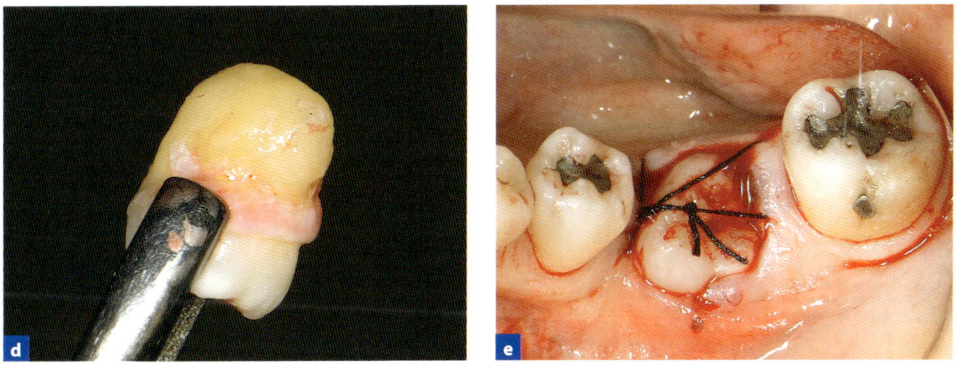

Fig 6-7d #18 extracted for transplantation. At a glance, clinically it appeared that there was not much periodontal ligament tissue attached around the root surface, but it was assumed that a thin cementoblast layer was attached.

Fig 6-7e Immediately after transplantation. Since the bony defect of the recipient site was large, the transplant was unintentionally placed in deep position (no bone graft material was used).

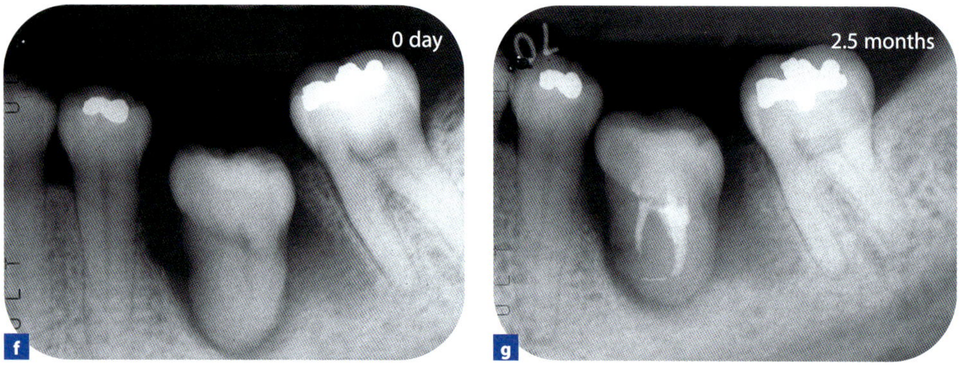

Fig 6-7f Radiograph immediately after transplantation.
Fig 6-7g Two and a half months postop. Spontaneous extrusion of the transplant does not seem to be occurring as desired.

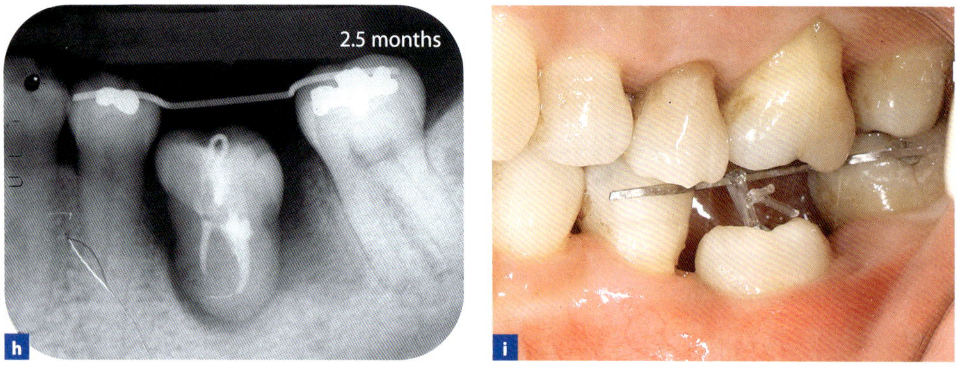

Fig 6-7h and 6-7i Two and a half months postop and just before orthodontic extrusion. Extrusion was performed in order to help align the gingival margin and correct the bony defect. The orthodontic device was simple using bonded wire and elastic thread.

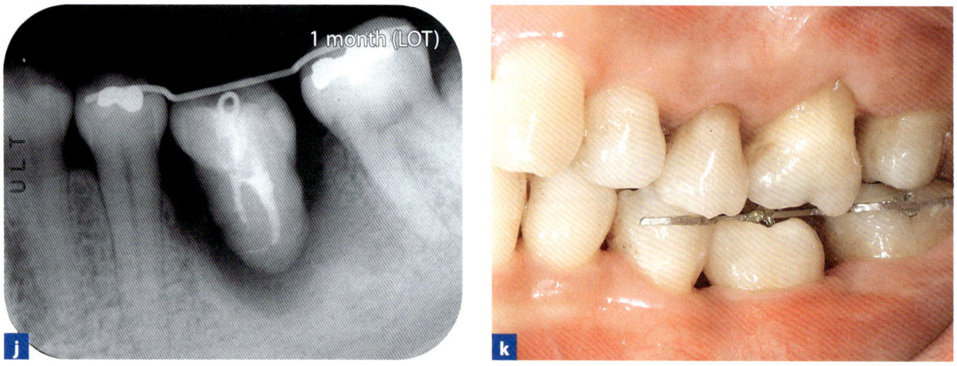

Fig 6-7j and 6-7k One month after initiation of the extrusion. The transplant has already moved to the desired position so it was bonded and stabilized in place. The gingival tissue moved up to the coronal side along with the tooth eruption, but the bony defect is still large.

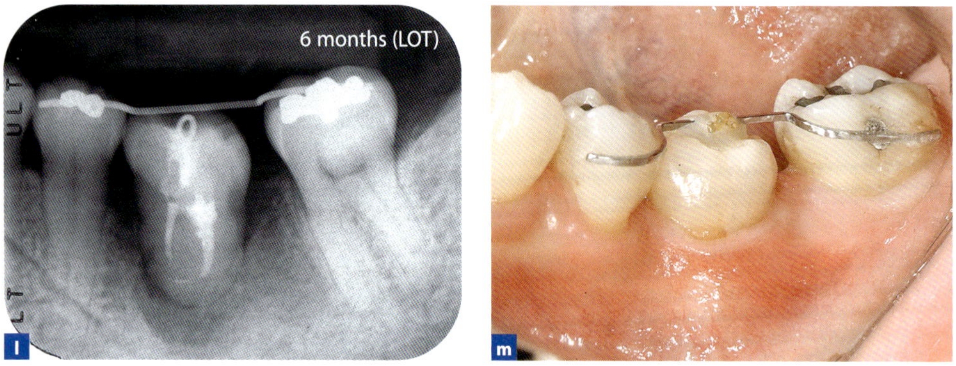

Fig 6-7l and 6-7m Six months after extrusion. Bone appears to be gradually regenerating around the transplant.

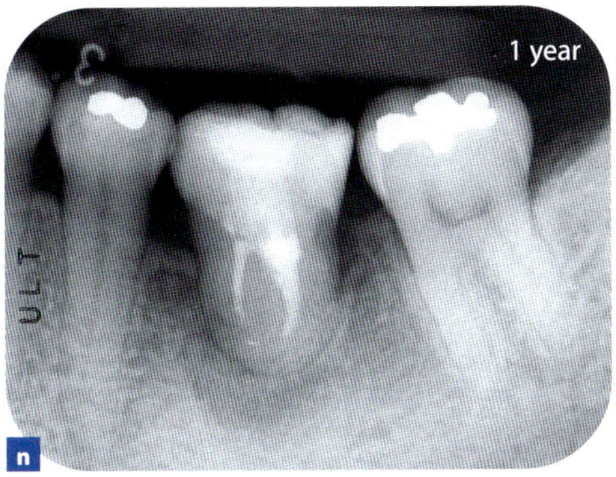

n

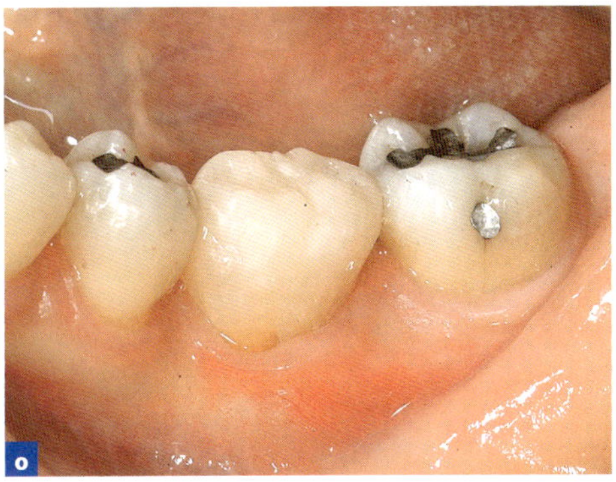

o

Fig 6-7n and 6-7o One year after transplantation. The transplant was restored with CR.

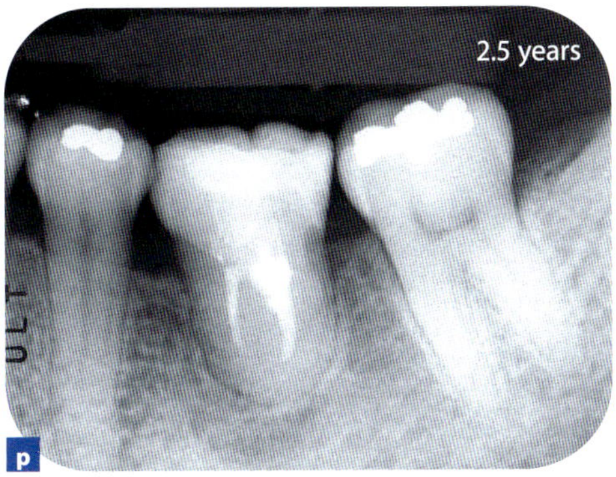

p

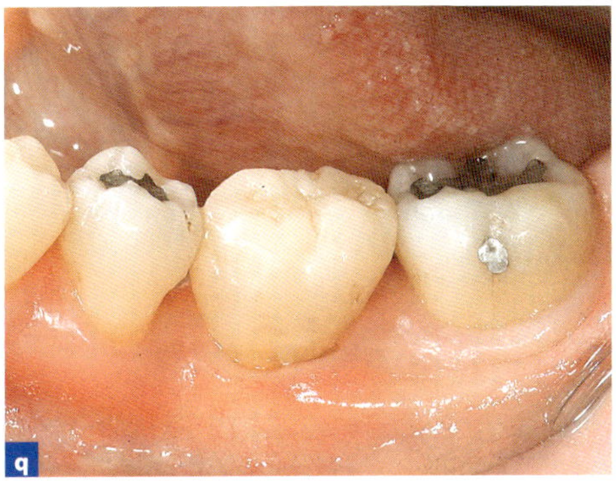

q

Fig 6-7p and 6-7q Two and a half years postop. The periodontal tissues seem to have been fully regenerated.

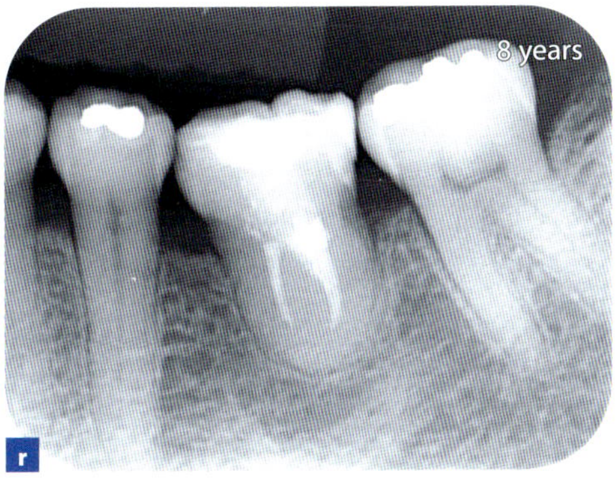

r

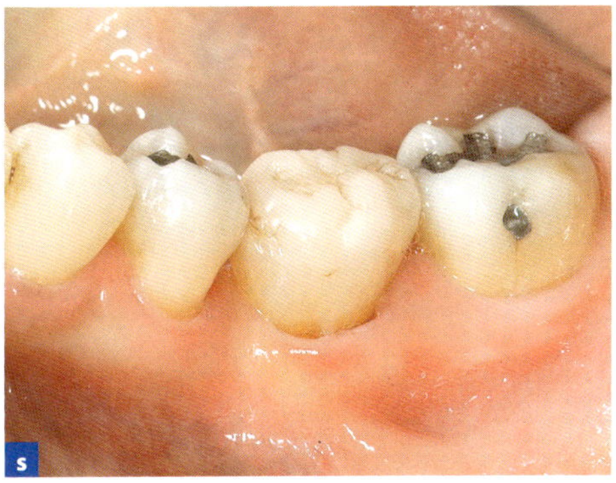

s

Fig 6-7r and 6-7s Eight years postop. There are no apparent abnormalities observed.

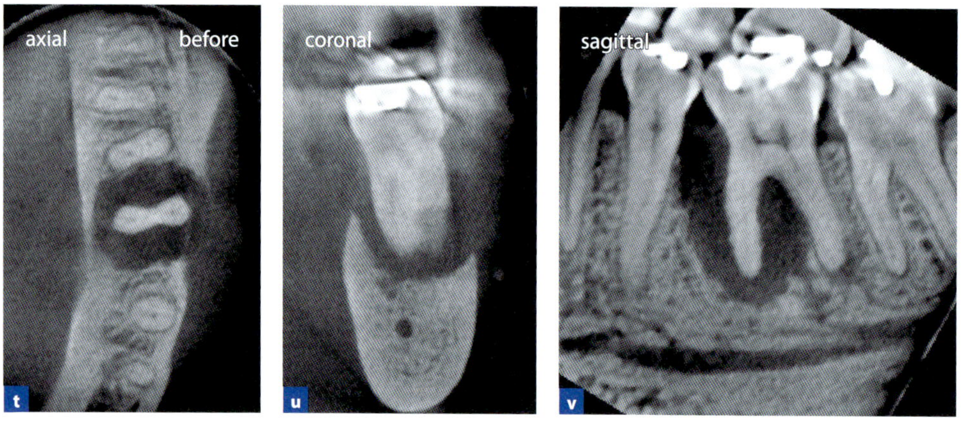

Fig 6-7t to 6-7v Preoperative CBCT images of the recipient site. Bone loss has progressed and there is loss of the buccal cortical plate around the mesial root of #36.

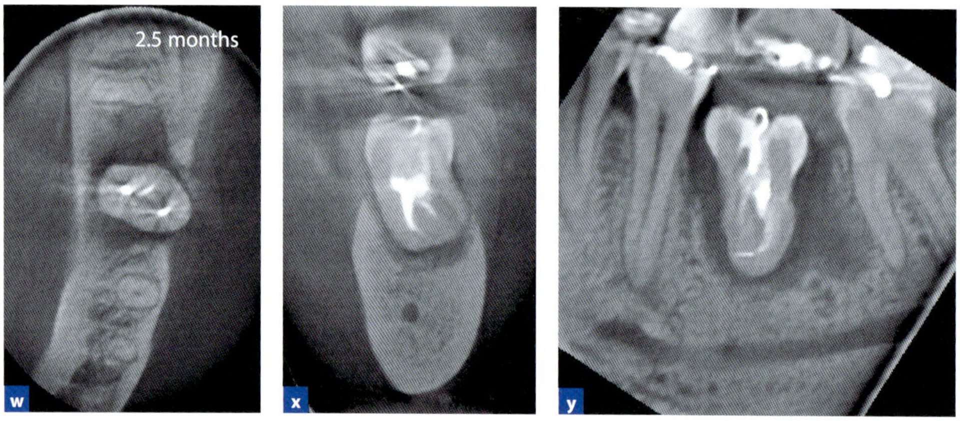

Fig 6-7w to 6-7y CBCT images 2 and a half months after transplantation. Note that the transplant is exposed out of the socket (bony housing) through the buccal dehiscence and is not yet covered with new bone.

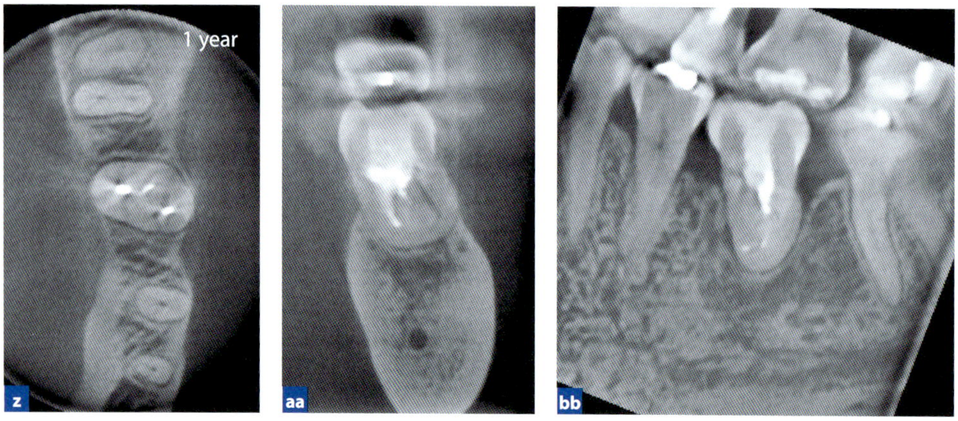

Fig 6-7z to 6-7bb One year postop. The exposed root is being covered with new bone, which is thought to be formed by osteoblasts derived from the periodontal ligament.

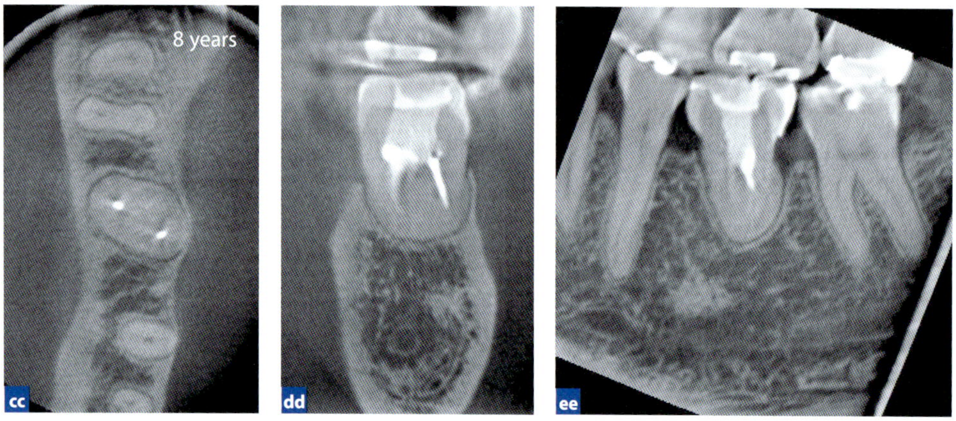

Fig 6-7cc to 6-7ee Eight years after transplantation. The newly formed bone is maintained.

CHAPTER 7

Autotransplantation of teeth in premolar regions

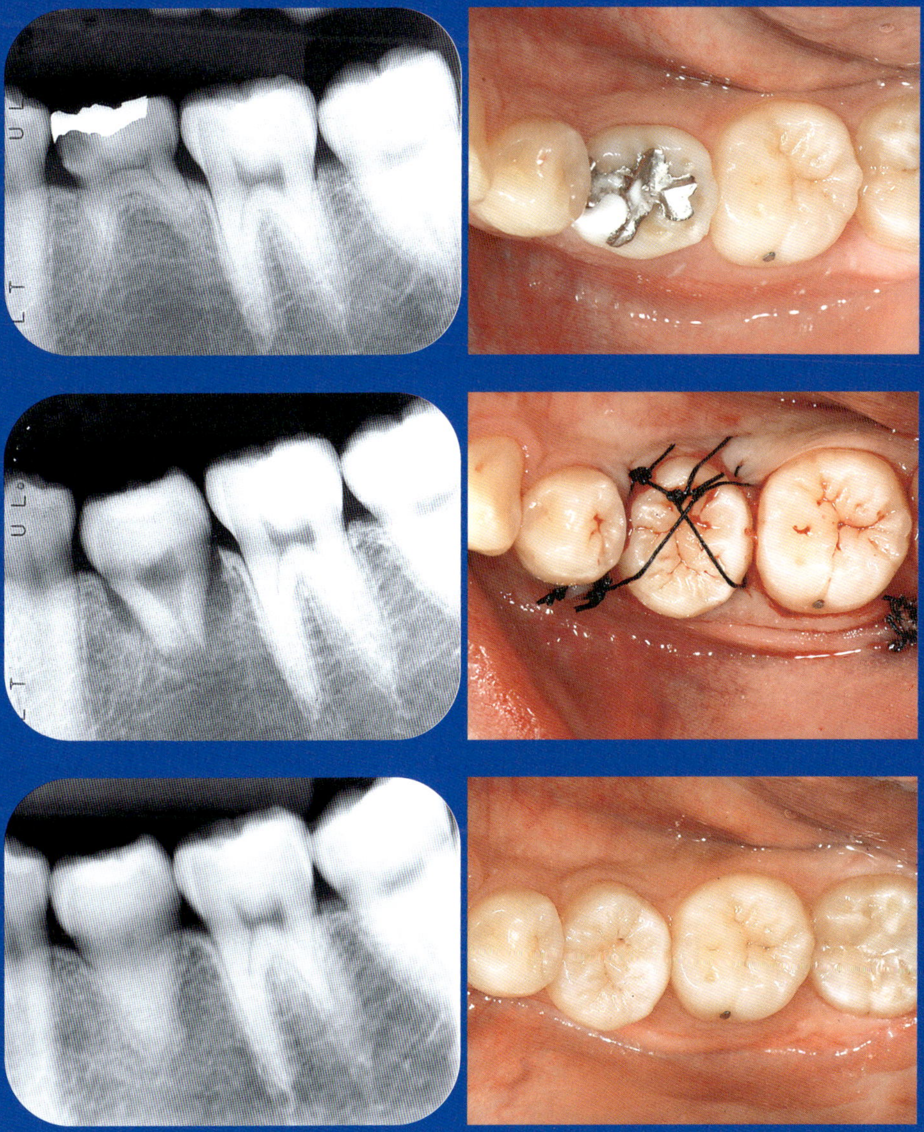

Most of the indications of transplantation in premolar regions are for cases in which there are congenitally missing second premolars. Although third molars are most frequently used as donor teeth, ectopic second premolars and premolars that are extracted for orthodontic treatment can be used as well. In this chapter, surgical techniques and indications for transplanting immature third molars into congenitally missing second premolars sites are discussed. Indications and cases involving transplantation with orthodontic treatment are discussed in **Chapter 9**.

Case 1. Transplantation of immature third molars to sites of congenitally missing mandibular second premolars

Fig 7-1 shows a case of a 19-year-old male whose mandibular second premolars were congenitally missing. The congenitally missing teeth were discovered when the patient was 9 years old and transplantation was discussed. He and his family accepted the treatment and waited for the appropriate timing for transplantation (**Fig 7-1a** and **7-1g** to **7-1j**).

For dentists who are not familiar or comfortable with transplantation, the surgery may seem aggressive or heroic, but this can be performed with predictability and low risks and long-term benefit for the patient. Many children regularly visit their family doctors and dentists from preschool age for prevention and routine checkups. Once a year, bitewing dental radiographs are taken to diagnose caries and other conditions. If no premolars are found under primary molars when the child is in the upper grades of elementary school, a panoramic radiograph will be taken to further evaluate (**Fig 7-1g**), and discussion of possible future transplantation can be discussed with the patient and family.

Appropriate timing for transplantation

For these case types the appropriate timing for transplantation is when an immature donor tooth's root development is about three-fourths to four-fifths complete. For teeth that are too immature, there is a higher risk in the predictability of root development and length after transplantation (see **Chapter 3**). For teeth with complete root formation, there is very little chance for pulpal healing. Therefore, it is necessary to check the presence or absence of third molars (as possible donor teeth), the stage of root development, the morphology, and the direction of eruption every 2 years starting around the age of 15, and to monitor the appropriate timing for transplantation (**Fig 7-1h** to **7-1j**). If the development and morphology of the root are judged to be suitable for transplantation, it should be performed according to the surgical procedure discussed in **Chapter 5 Fig 5-1**.

In clinical practice, there are various reasons (root size, morphology, eruption position and direction of the donor tooth, bone morphology of the recipient site, patient's time constraints, etc.), which may make it very difficult to perform transplantation at the ideal stage of root development. Therefore, in transplantation of immature third molars to premolar sites, transplantation can be performed when the root development is around one-half to just before completion (still having an open apex).

Selection of donor teeth – size and position

If there are a multiple numbers of donor teeth in the mouth available, it is necessary to have good selection criteria. In general, teeth with a single root and round cross section (little concavity) are considered to have a better prognosis. In addition, considering the transplantation to the premolar region, the smaller the width of the crown, the easier placement into the recipient site. If similar teeth exist in the mandible, a donor tooth in the same jaw and the same side should be the first choice. Therefore, in this case, #38 was the first choice for the site of #35 (**Fig 7-1o** to **7-1mm**). But on the right side, #18 was selected as a donor tooth to be transplanted into the #45 site (**Fig 7-1ee** to **7-1bbb**).

Surgical procedure

There are no special precautions taken for the surgical technique, but if the root morphology of the donor tooth and the recipient site can be evaluated with a CBCT study, the donor tooth can be extracted and transplanted after the recipient site is prepared with less risk and more predictable outcomes. Having the CBCT information will also help to minimize the handling and dry time of the transplant (**Fig 7-1o** to **7-1x**). The transplanted tooth should be positioned slightly deeper so that occlusal adjustment is not necessary (**Fig 7-1z**). It is also important that teeth should not be prepared or adjusted to expose dentin, especially in teeth with immature root development. Fixation is performed with sutures on the day of transplantation, and is changed to fixation with wire and adhesive resin after 7 days (**Fig 7-1bb**). Wire fixation should be removed 1 month after transplantation.

Dental pulp healing can be expected in transplanted teeth with immature roots, but radiographs should be taken every month for 3 months after transplantation to check for inflammatory resorption (pulp necrosis). (**Fig 7-1cc**, **7-1dd**, **7-1ss**, and **7-1tt**). The transplanted tooth usually shows an EPT(+) response at 6 months. After 6 months, pulp canal calcification/obliteration and root development will be observed after 1, 2, and 3 years, and radiographs will be taken every few years (**Fig 7-1ee** to **7-1mm**, and **7-1vv** to **7-1bbb**).

Case1. Transplantation of immature third molars to sites of congenitally missing mandibular second premolars

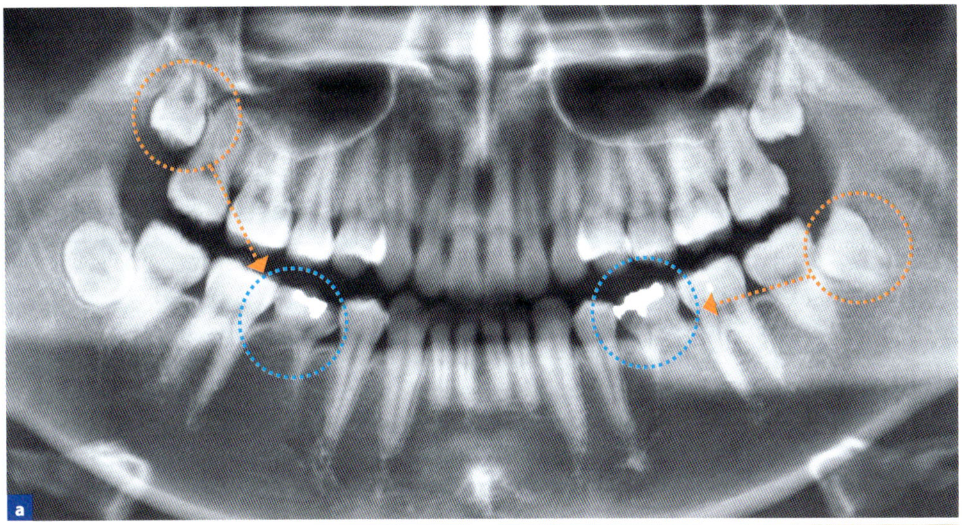

Fig 7-1a Panoramic radiograph before transplantation of a 19-year-old male whose mandibular second molars are congenitally missing. Impacted immature third molars (#18 and #38) were available and decision was made to perform transplantation.

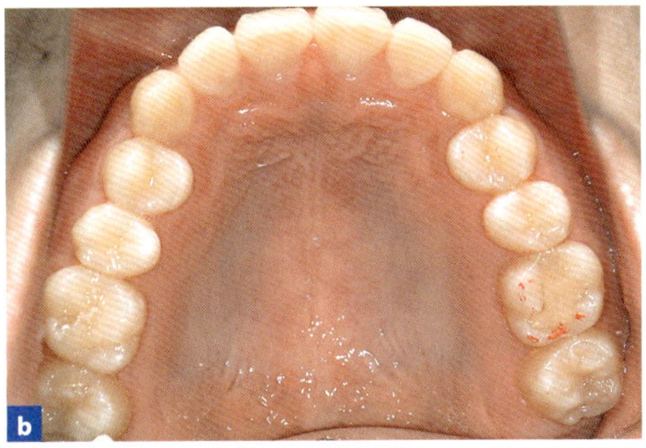

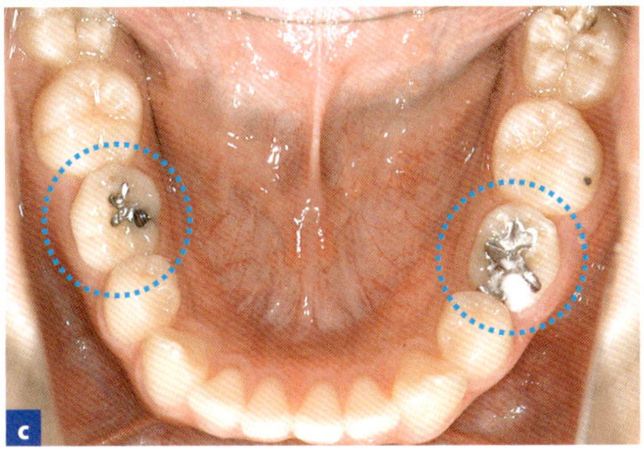

Fig 7-1b and 7-1c Views of the upper and lower occlusal surfaces before surgery.

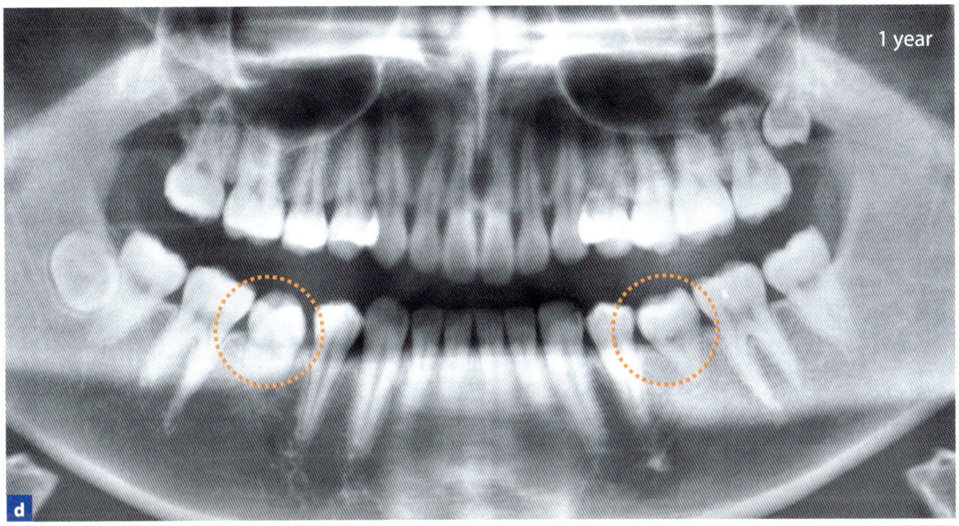

Fig 7-1d Panoramic radiograph 1 year after transplantation of #38 to #35 and 3 months after transplantation of #18 to #45.

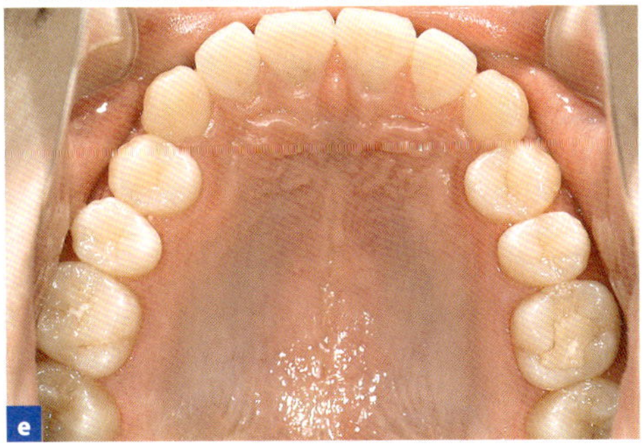

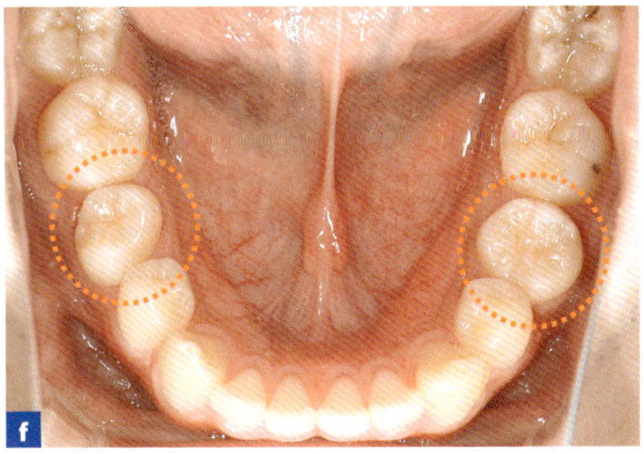

Fig 7-1e and 7-1f Views of the upper and lower occlusal surfaces on the same day as **Fig 7-1d**.

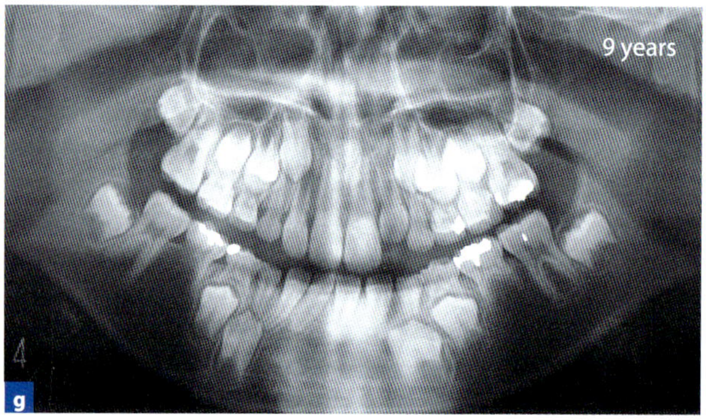

Fig 7-1g Panoramic radiograph at the age of 9. #35 and #45 were confirmed to be congenitally missing.

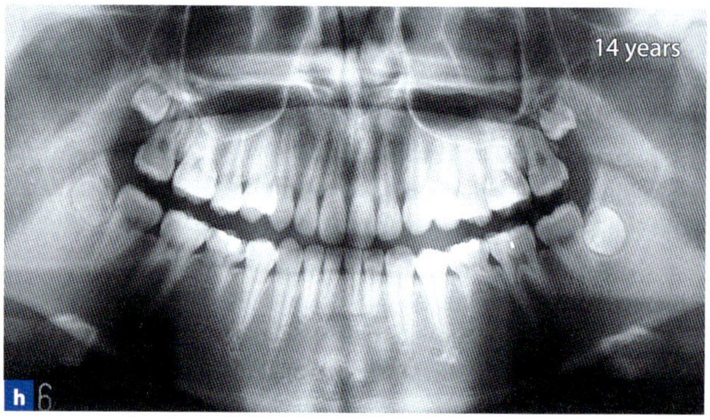

Fig 7-1h Panoramic radiograph at the age of 14. The presence of the third molars (donor teeth) was confirmed, but the developmental stage was not ideal for transplantation.

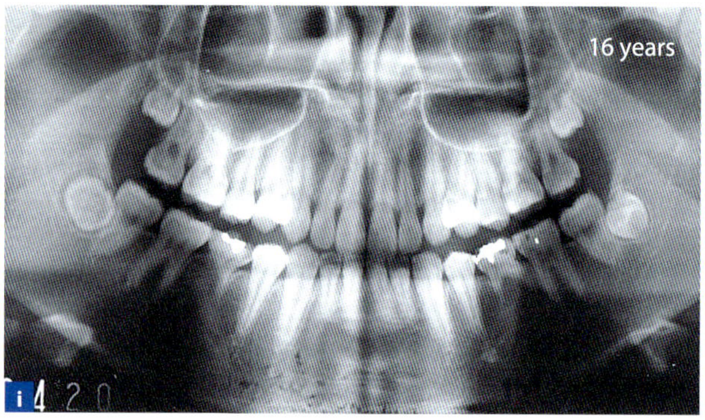

Fig 7-1i Panoramic radiograph at the age of 16. The developmental stage of the donor teeth has still not yet reached the indication for transplantation.

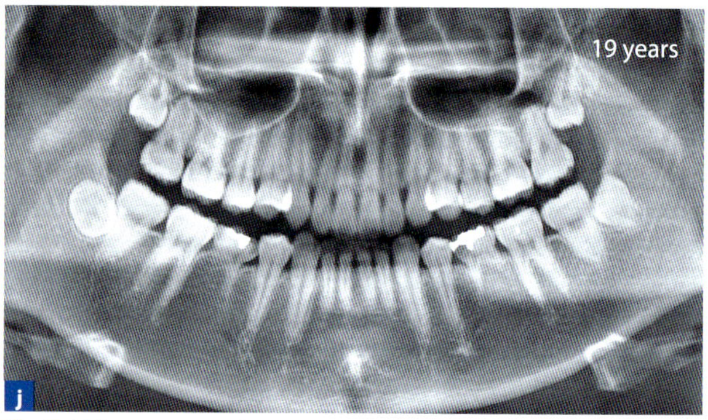

Fig 7-1j Panoramic radiograph at the age of 19. The developmental stage of the donor teeth is slightly past the ideal stage 4-5, so transplantation was advised.

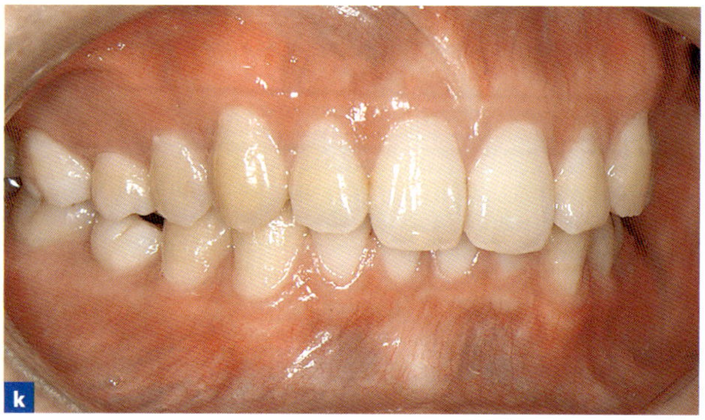

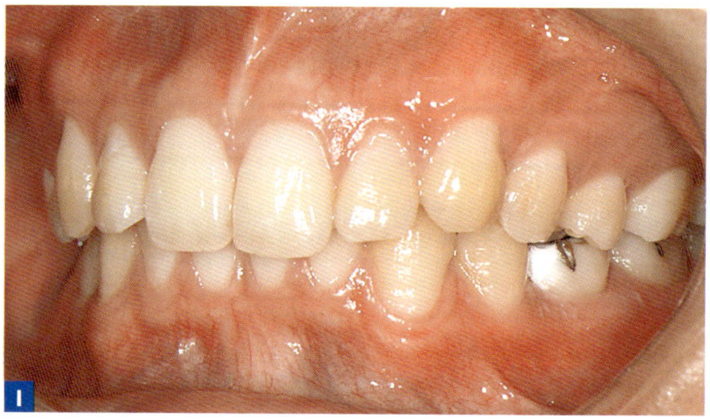

Fig 7-1k and 7-1l Lateral views before surgery (at the age of 19).

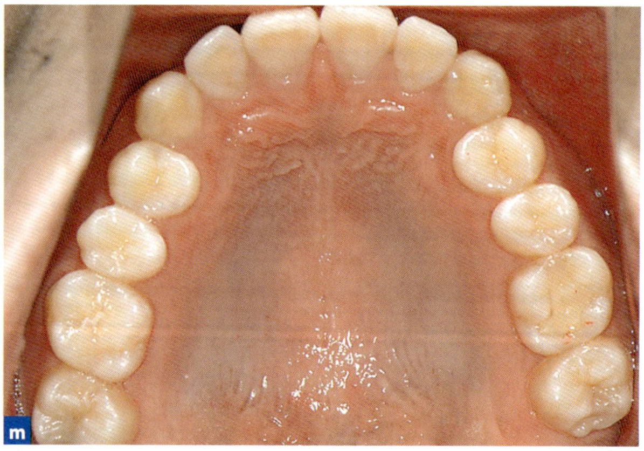

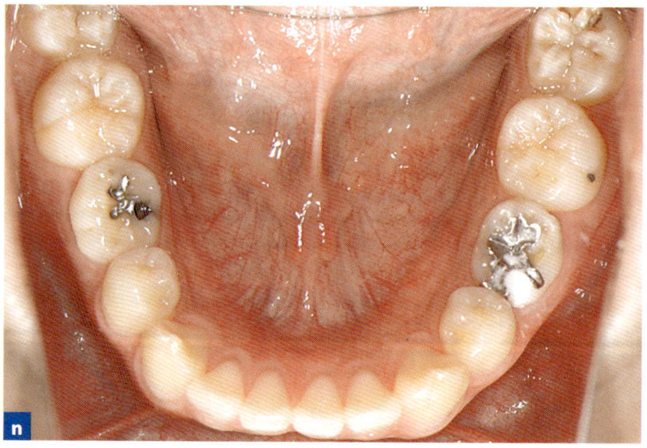

Fig 7-1m and 7-1n Occlusal views before surgery.

Transplantation of the left side

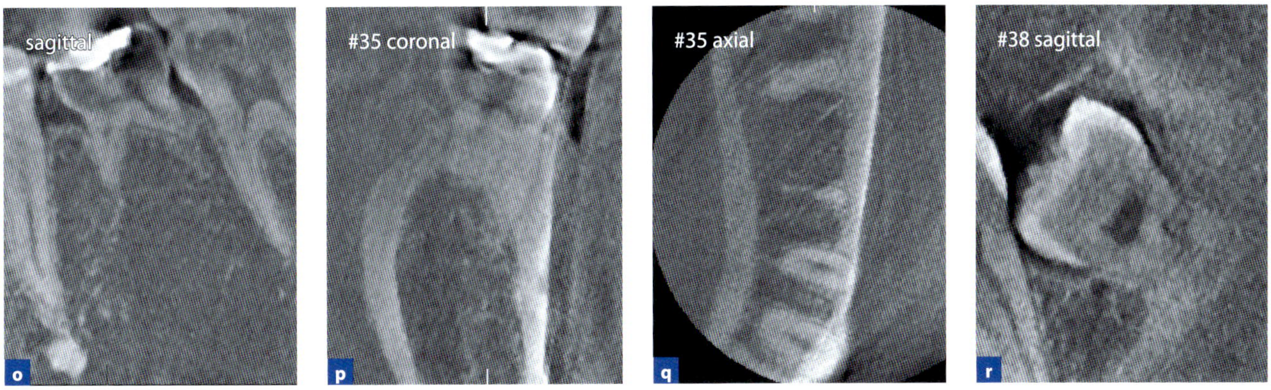

Fig 7-1o to 7-1q Preoperative CBCT images of the left recipient site. Sufficient bone width exists at the recipient site.

Fig 7-1r CBCT image of the donor tooth. The developmental stage appears to be near completion but the apex appears to still be open (wider than 1 mm).

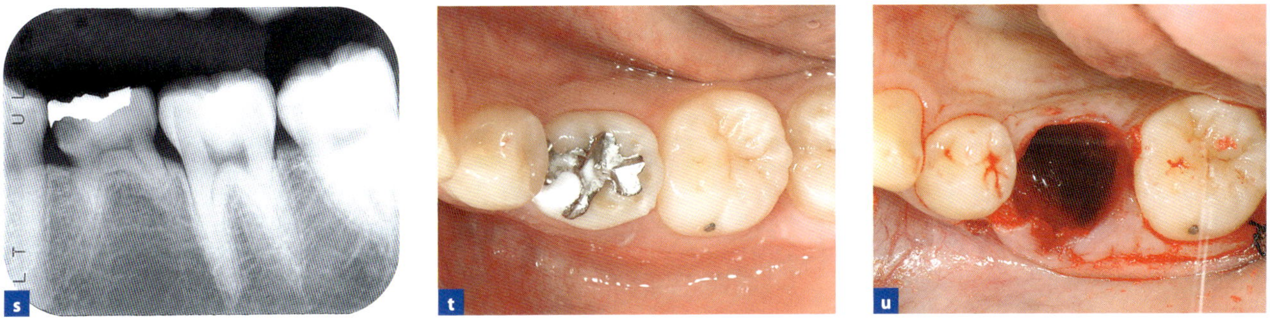

Fig 7-1s and 7-1t Views of the recipient site before transplantation.

Fig 7-1u Immediately after extraction of the deciduous tooth in the recipient site.

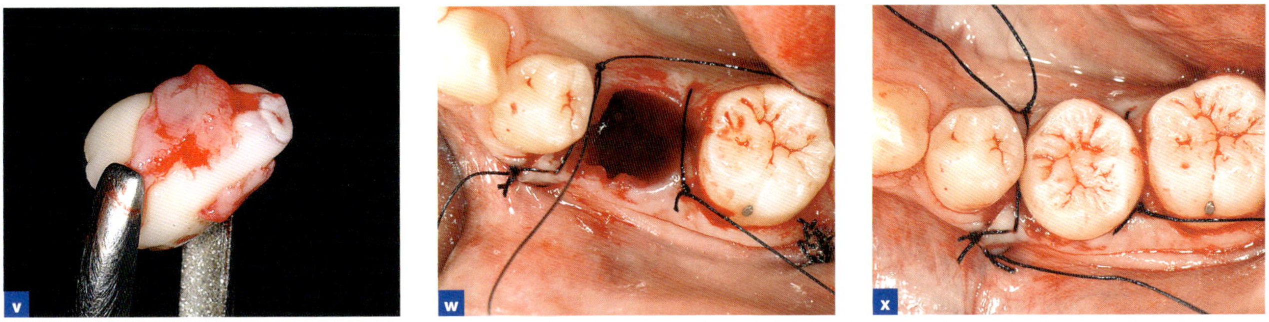

Fig 7-1v The donor tooth. The root formation is almost complete, but Hertwig's epithelial sheath can be observed at the apex. Part of the peri odontal ligament seems to be detached from the root surface, but this will rarely cause a problem in transplantation of immature teeth unless the pulp becomes infected.

Fig 7-1w Gingival flap is sutured after try-in without placing the donor tooth in the formed socket.

Fig 7-1x Placing the donor tooth.

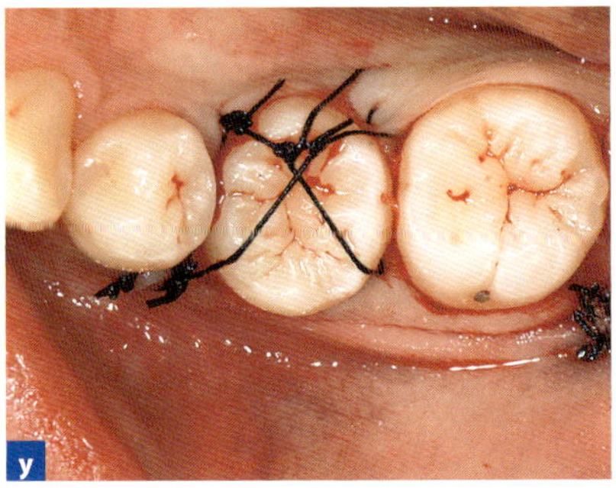

Fig 7-1y Fixation of the transplant with sutures.

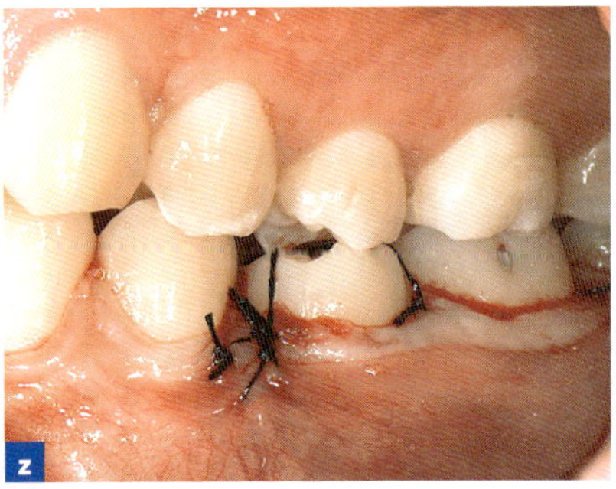

Fig 7-1z Lateral view immediately after transplantation. Note there is slight interocclusal space to the opposing teeth.

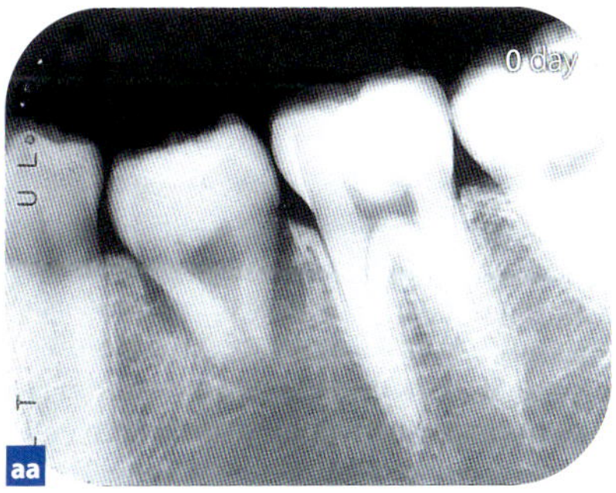

Fig 7-1aa Radiograph immediately after transplantation. Note that the apical foramen appears wider than 1 mm.

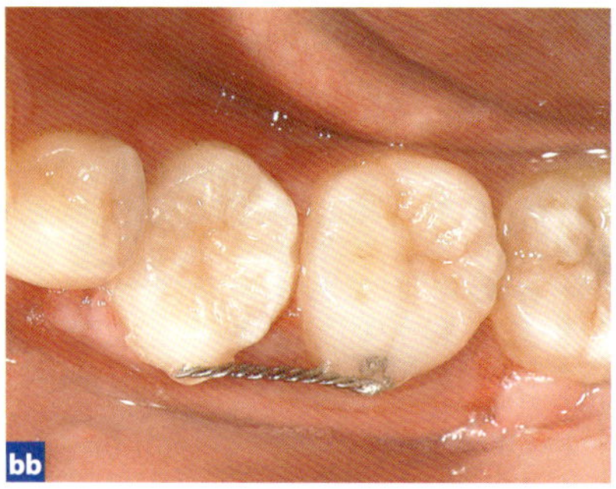

Fig 7-1bb One week after transplantation. Due to the higher mobility of the tooth, a bonded wire splint was placed.

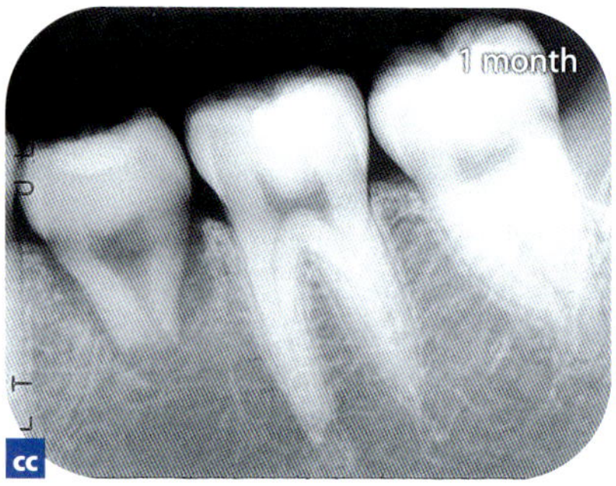

Fig 7-1cc One month after transplantation. No apparent abnormalities are observed.

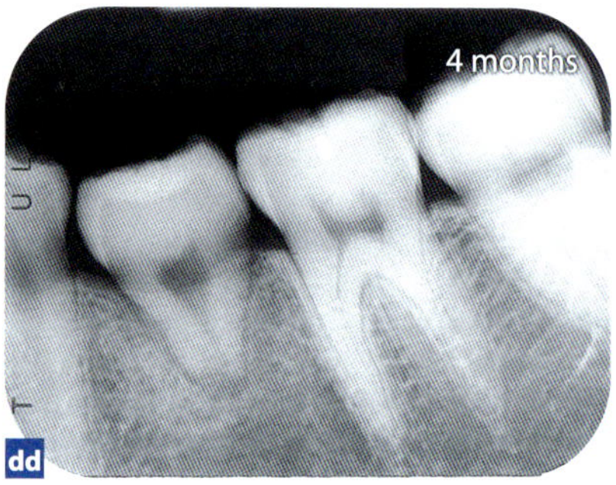

Fig 7-1dd Four months after transplantation. The root apex appears to have grown slightly.

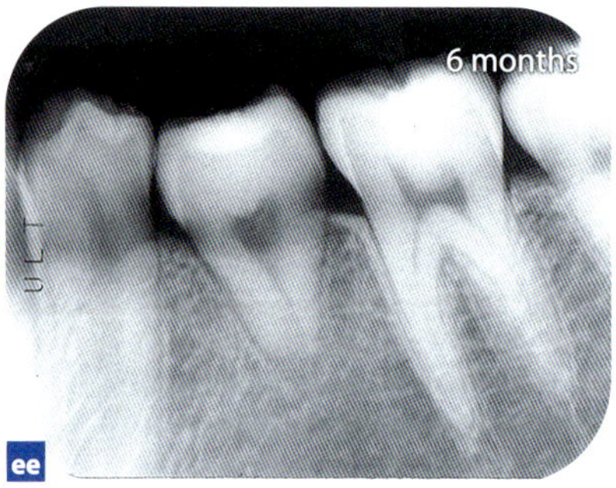

Fig 7-1ee Six months after transplantation. Pulp canal obliteration is observed, and the root is slightly more developed. The tooth responds EPT(+).

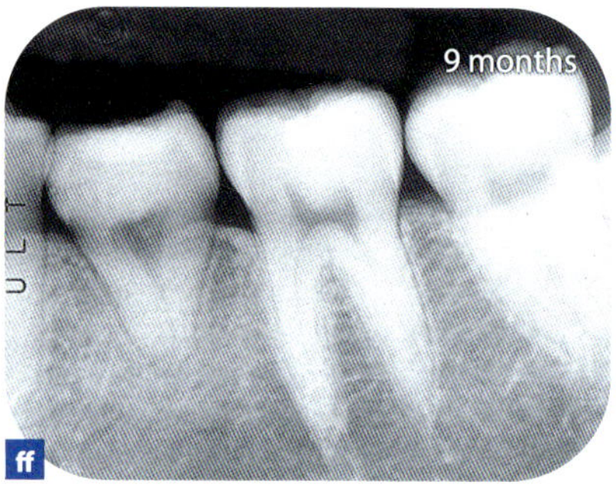

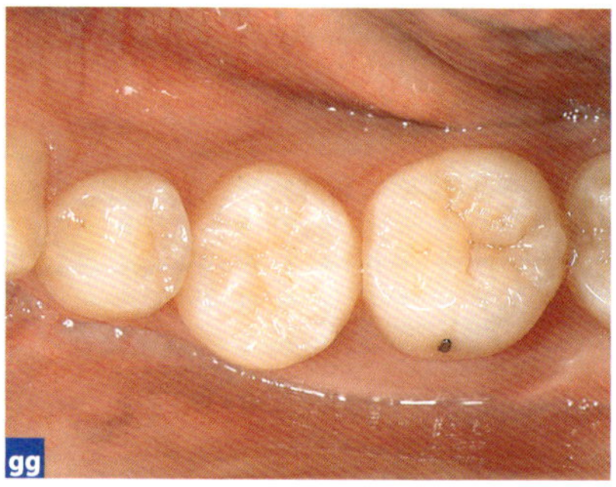

Fig 7-1ff to 7-1gg Nine months after transplantation. Pulp canal obliteration is progressing.

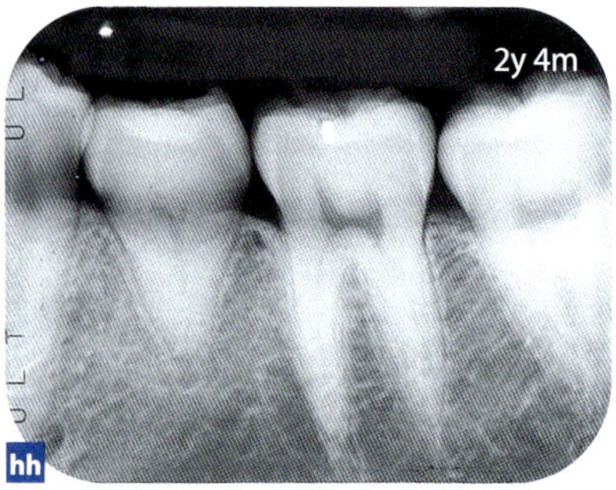

Fig 7-1hh Radiograph after 2 years and 4 months. The tooth responds EPT(+). A uniform periodontal ligament space is observed, and no problems such as root resorption are observed.

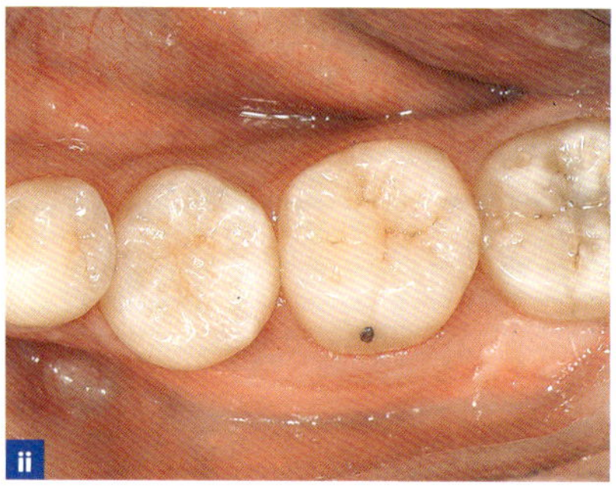

Fig 7-1ii Occlusal view after 2 years and 4 months.

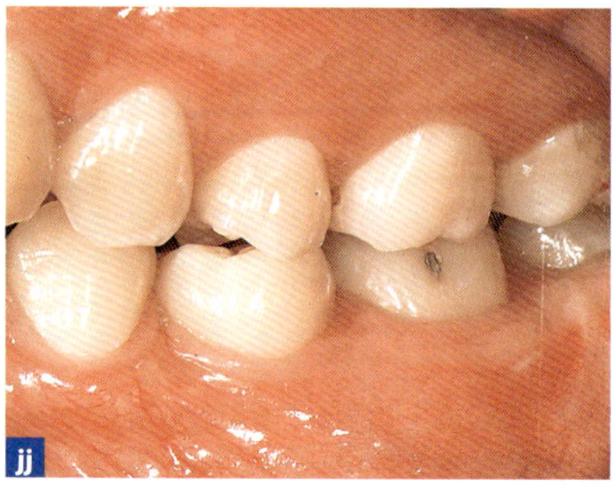

Fig 7-1jj Lateral view after 2 years and 4 months. Appropriate occlusal relationship is obtained with natural extrusion of the transplant.

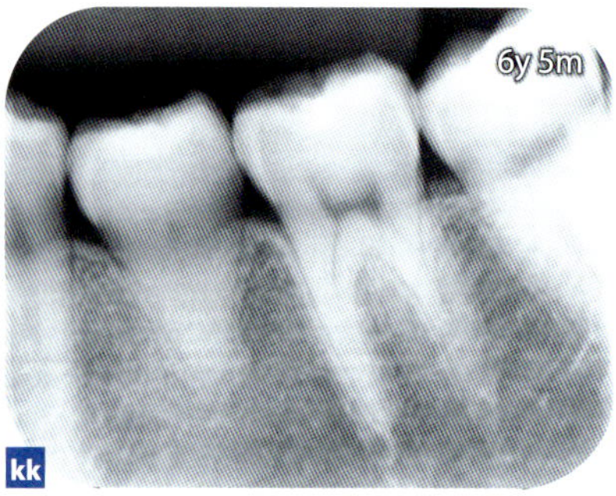

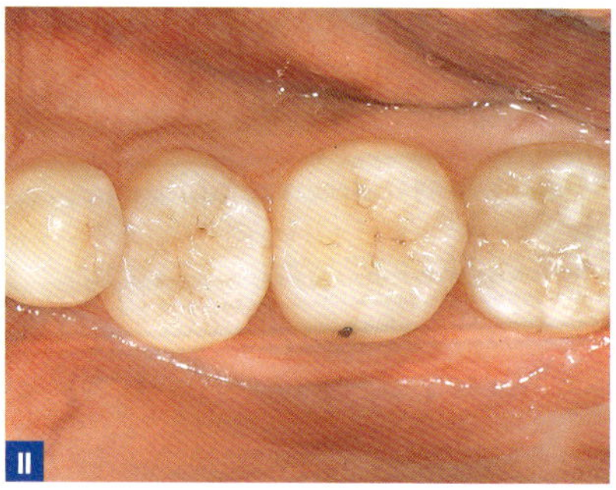

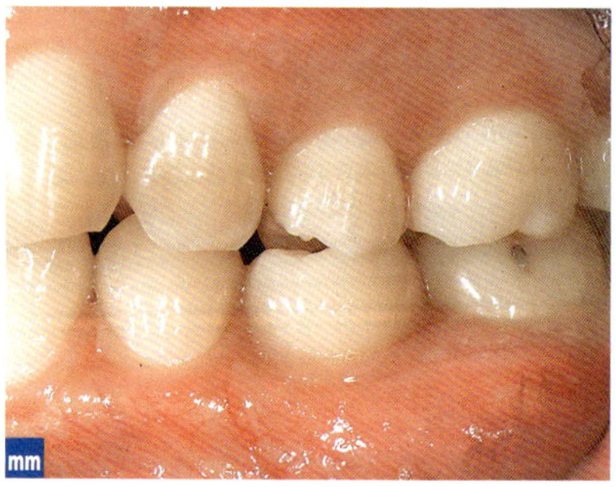

Fig 7-1kk to 7-1mm Six years and 5 months postop. No problems are observed.

Transplantation of the right side

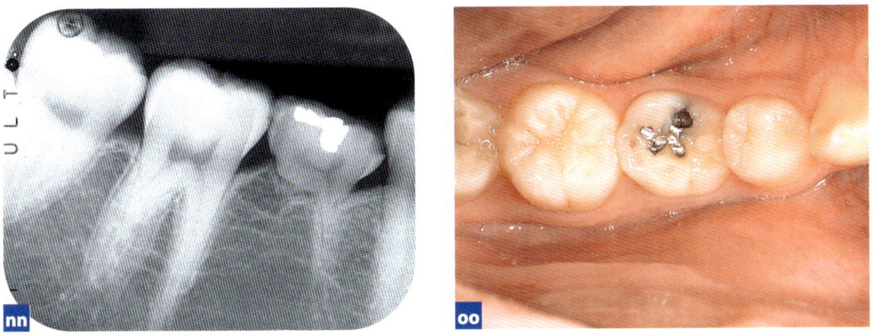

Fig 7-1nn and 7-1oo Views of the contralateral recipient site 9 months after the initial transplantation on the left site.

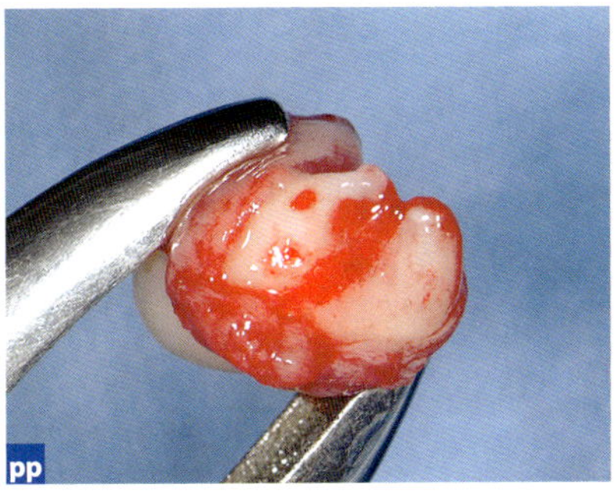

Fig 7-1pp Donor tooth. Root development is almost complete, but some remnant of Hertwig's epithelial root sheath can be observed.

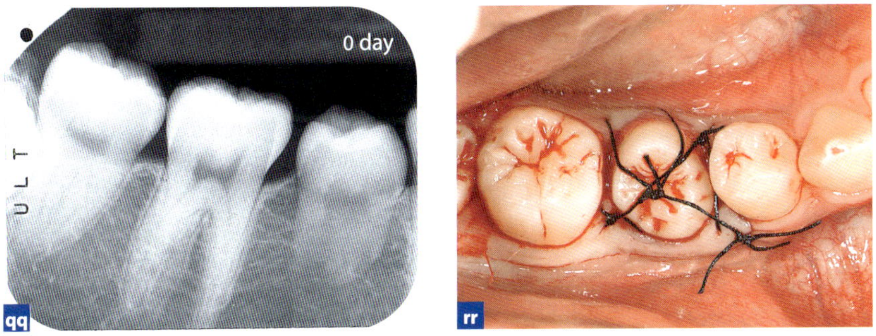

Fig 7-1qq and 7-1rr Immediately after transplantation.

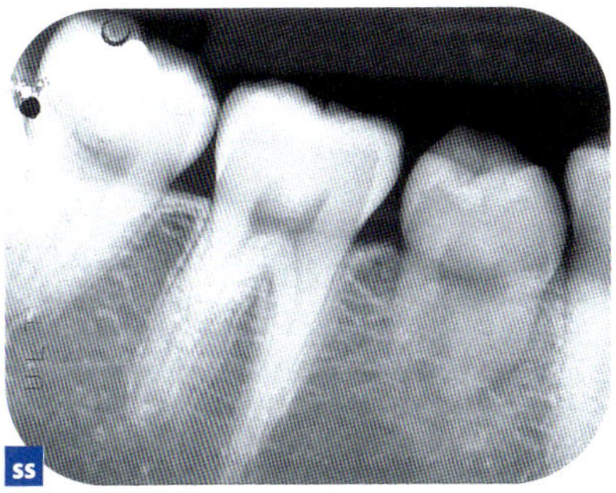

Fig 7-1ss One month after transplantation.

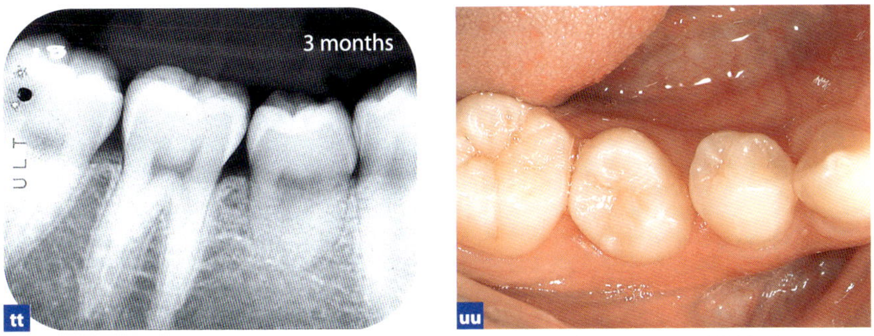

Fig 7-1tt and 7-1uu Three months after transplantation. Tooth response is EPT (−).

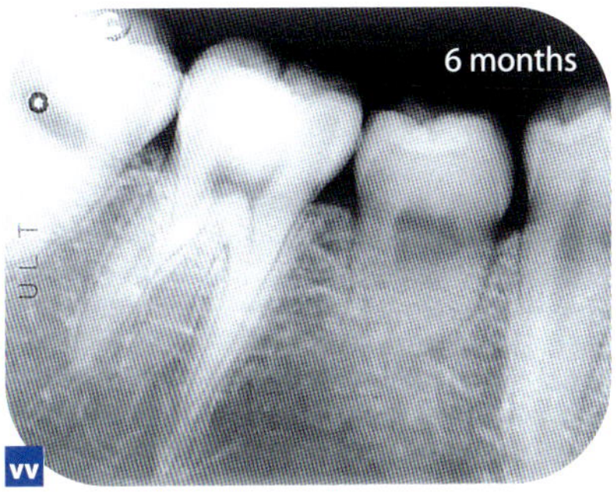

Fig 7-1vv Six months after transplantation. Tooth responds EPT(+).

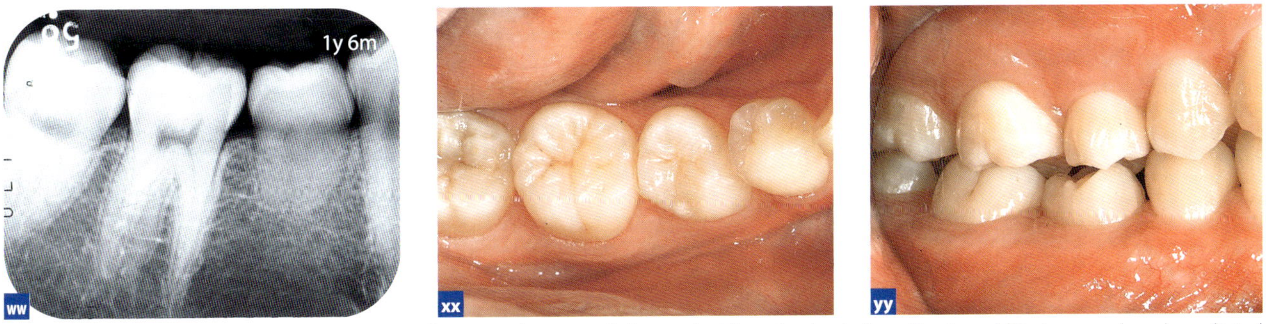

Fig 7-1ww to 7-1yy One year and 6 months after transplantation. Pulp canal obliteration is obvious. Tooth mobility is normal, and no clinical or radiographic problems are observed.

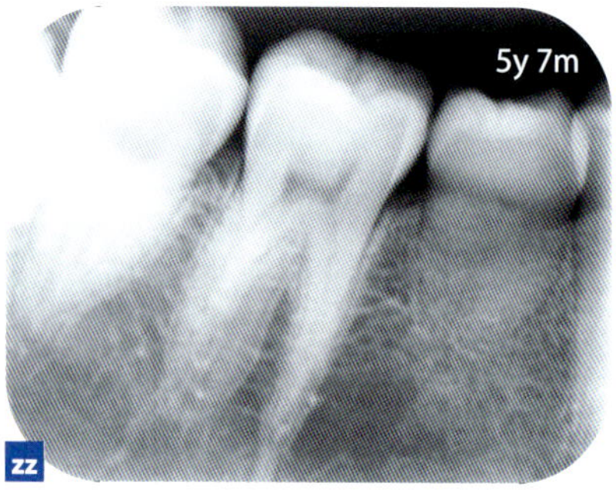

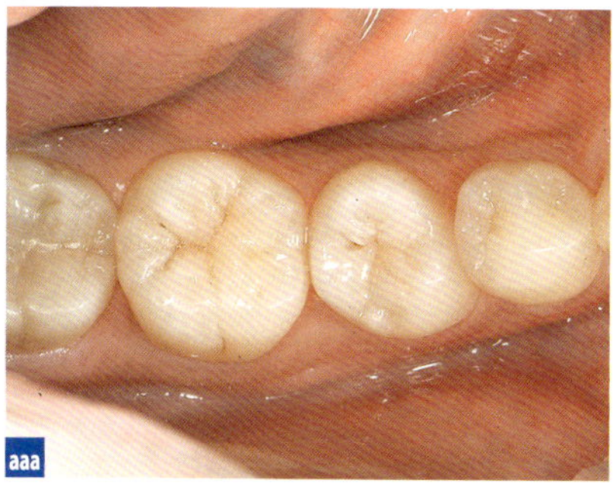

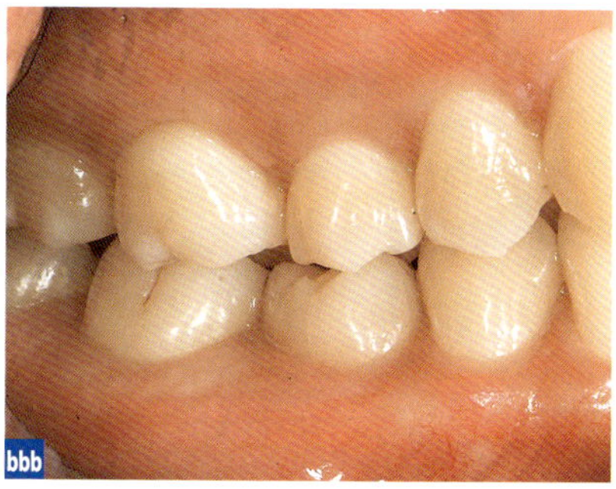

Fig 7-1zz to 7-1bbb Five years and 7 months after transplantation. A functional occlusal relationship is obtained.

Case 2. Transplantation of immature third molars to congenitally missing mandibular second premolars sites

Fig 7-2 is a case in which two second premolars are congenitally missing as in **Case 1**. Interesting differences from **Case 1** are that the donor teeth have developed slower than typically seen and that there are only two donor teeth (lower third molars) available for transplantation for the two congenitally missing teeth (**Fig 7-2a**). This patient had smaller third molars (**Fig 7-2i** and **7-2ff**) with favorable morphology and developmental stages, which helped the transplantation procedure to be carried out smoothly (**Fig 7-2g** to **7-2m**, and **7-2z** to **7-2hh**).

In this case the transplanted tooth on the left side developed pulpal necrosis after the roots developed (**Fig 7-2t**, and **7-2u**). It is suspected that this occurred due to microbial infection that entered through pit/fissures on the occlusal surface. Thus, proper maintenance and long-term follow-up are important.

This case also shows that not all cases can be completed based at an optimal or ideal time of root development. The transplantation on the right side was performed at a very early stage of root development of the donor tooth (**Fig 7-2aa** to **7-2hh**) because the patient wanted to have all the treatment completed before graduating from university. As a result, root development (length) was not ideal (**Fig 7-2kk**) but it does not seem to have negatively affected the survival of the transplant. Thus the timing of transplantation is not decided only by the doctor and the scientific knowledge but also by the personal and social desires of the individual patient.

Cases 3 to 5. Problems which may develop during the observation period up to performing transplantation

Given the time needed for donor teeth to develop enough for transplantation, it is common that 7 years or more of observation are required from the time congenitally missing teeth are typically discovered until transplantation can be performed. If the deciduous teeth continue to erupt in the same manner as the adjacent permanent teeth, usually no problems will occur. But as seen in **Fig 7-3** to **7-5**, partial ankylosis may occur and eruption of the deciduous teeth may be arrested. The problem in these cases is that both adjacent permanent teeth will likely tilt toward the deciduous tooth, reducing the space to accommodate a donor tooth (**Fig 7-3a** to **7-3c**, **7-4a**, and **7-5a** to **7-5e**).

In cases where the above mentioned problems are likely to occur, it can be of benefit to change the crown morphology of the primary teeth with composite resin (CR) at an early stage (**Fig 7-4a** and **7-4b**). Adding CR to the primary teeth can help prevent the tipping in of the adjacent teeth.

Fig 7-5 is a case in which the primary tooth showed ankylosis at the first visit, and the adjacent teeth were tilted (**Fig 7-5a** to **7-5e**). Since it was still too early for transplantation, the tilted teeth were up-righted by limited orthodontic treatment to regain the space for transplantation (**Fig 7-5f** to **7-5h**). After up-righting, the crown of the deciduous tooth was restored with CR to prevent the adjacent teeth from tilting (**Fig 7-5i**). Follow-up was continued and transplantation was performed several years later when the stage of development of the donor tooth was appropriate (**Fig 7-5j** to **7-5w**).

Case2. Transplantation of immature third molars to sites of congenitally missing mandibular second premolars

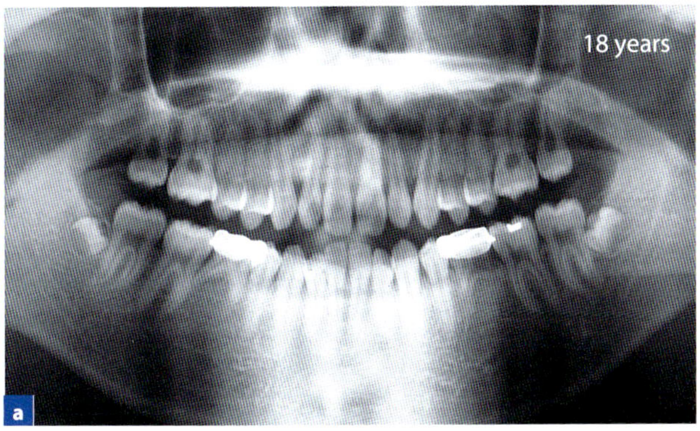

Fig 7-2a Panoramic radiograph of an 18-year-old male patient. The stages of root development of the third molars (#38 and #48) are earlier than the optimal condition for transplantation. The patient has been seen at the clinic since the age of 5, and the congenitally missing teeth were discovered at the age of 10.

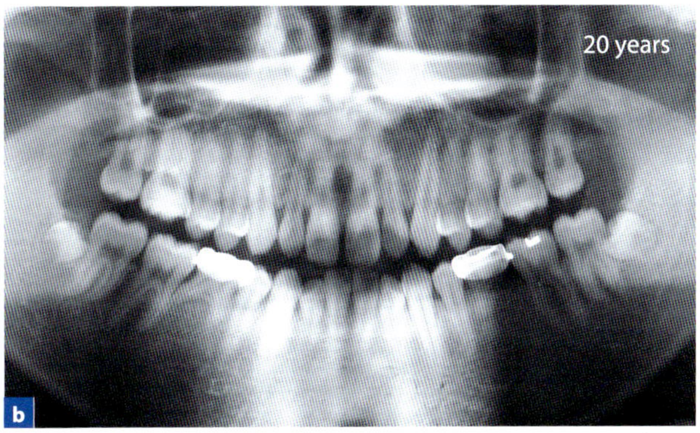

Fig 7-2b Panoramic radiograph at the age of 20. The stages of root development of the donor teeth are still earlier than the optimal condition. However, the patient strongly asked for the earlier treatment because he had graduated the university and about to start working. Thus transplantation was performed.

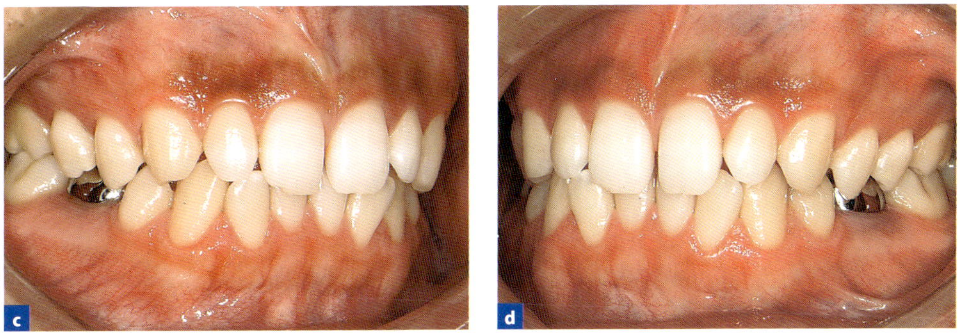

Fig 7-2c and 7-2d Preoperative lateral views.

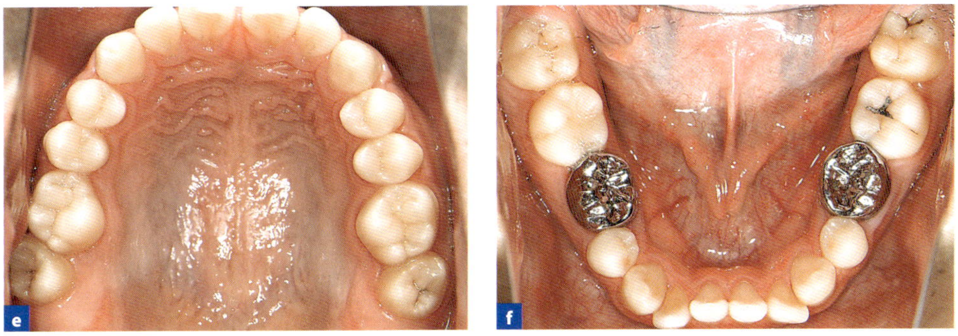

Fig 7-2e and 7-2f Occlusal views before surgery.

Transplantation of the left side

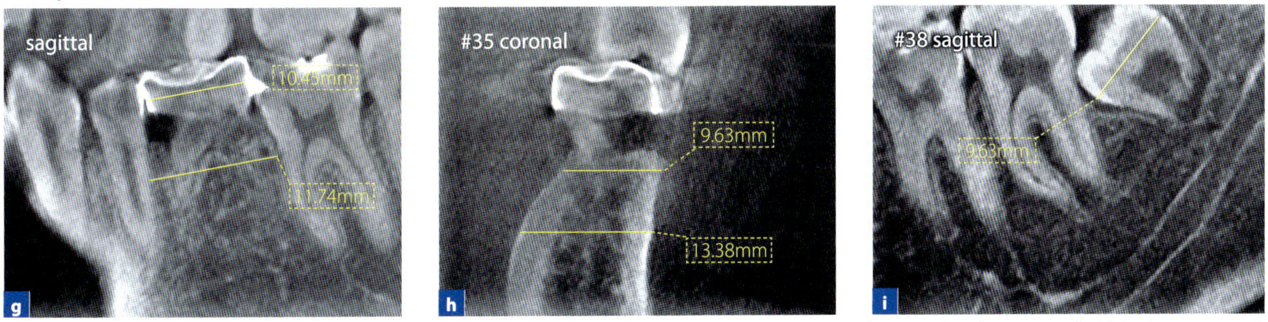

Fig 7-2g to 7-2i Preoperative analysis of the recipient and the donor tooth using CBCT images. The root development of #38 is about stage 3, a little early for transplantation. However, the direction of eruption of the donor tooth is inclined mesially and it may shift toward horizontal impaction.

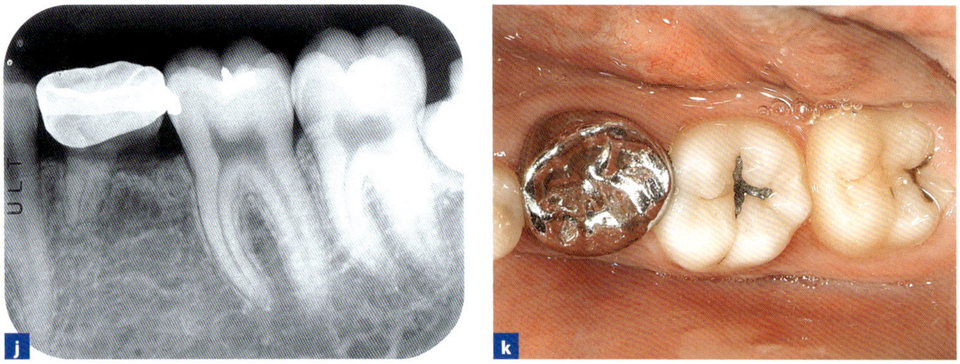

Fig 7-2j and 7-2k Views of the recipient site before transplantation.

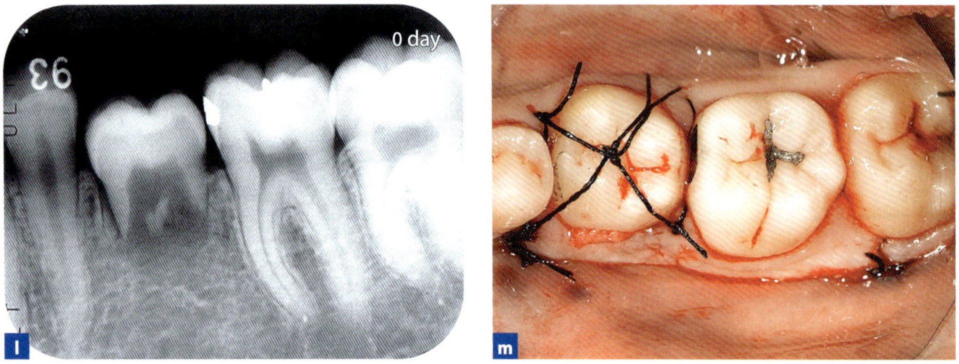

Fig 7-2l and 7-2m Immediately after transplantation.

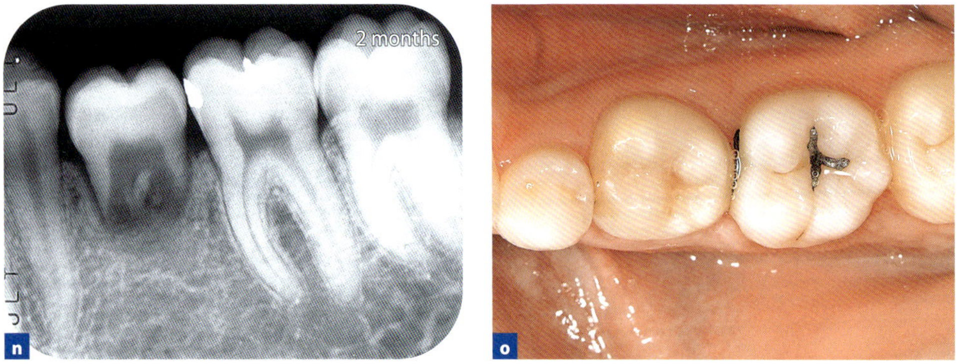

Fig 7-2n and 7-2o Two months postoperative.

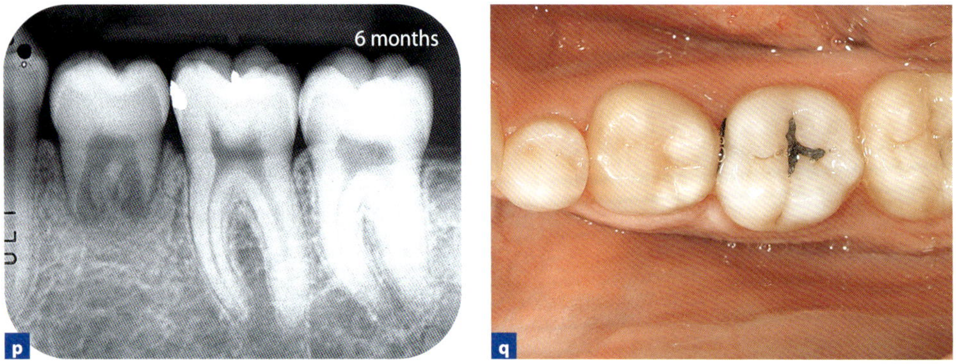

Fig 7-2p and 7-2q Six months postoperative. Root canal obliteration and root development appear to be starting. The tooth responds EPT(+).

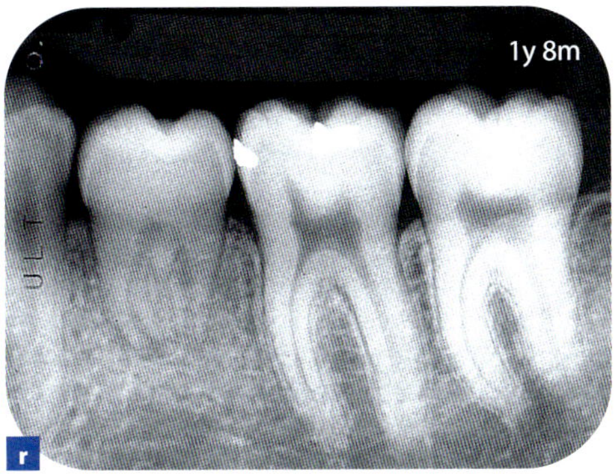

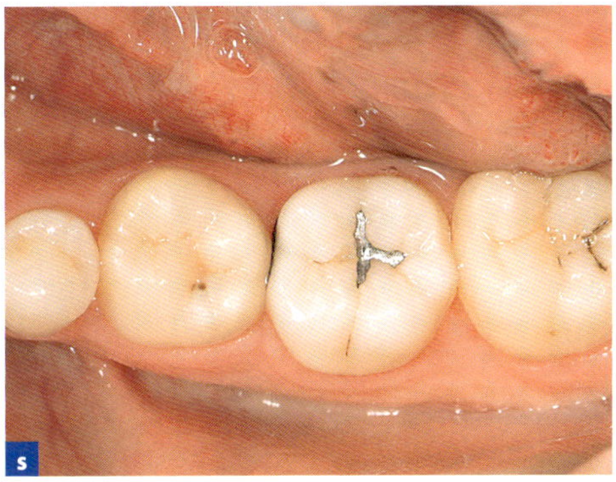

Fig 7-2r Radiograph after 1 year and 8 months. The root has developed to almost the ideal length, and intact lamina dura can be observed along the root surface. Pulp healing and root development are progressing. The tooth responds EPT(+).
Fig 7-2s Occlusal view after 1 year and 8 months.

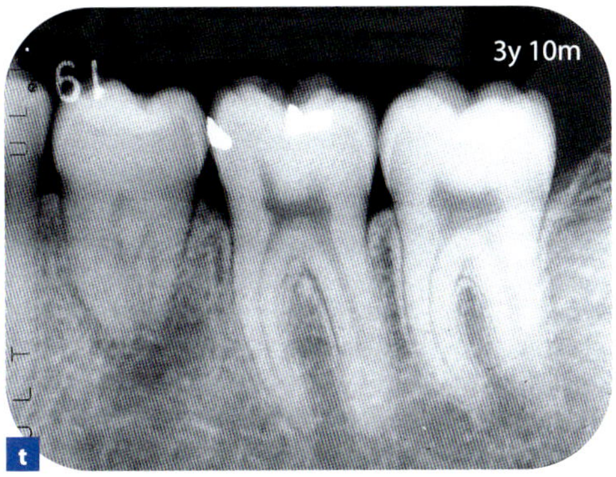

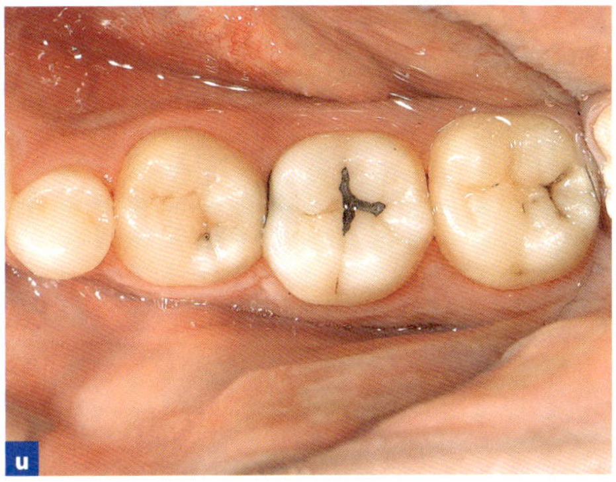

Fig 7-2t and 7-2u Three years and 10 months postoperative. There is now a PARL finding consistent with pulp necrosis.

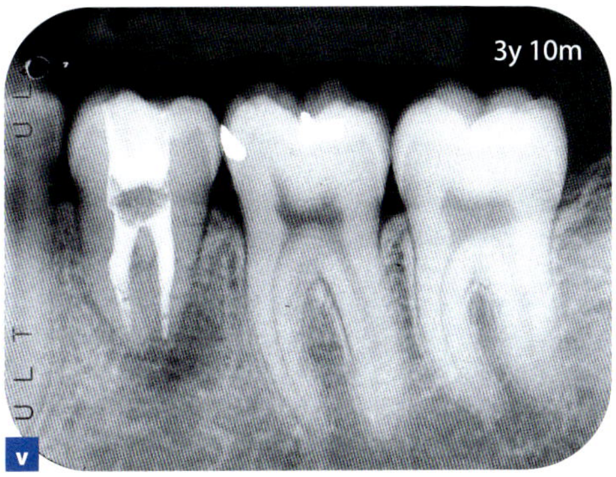

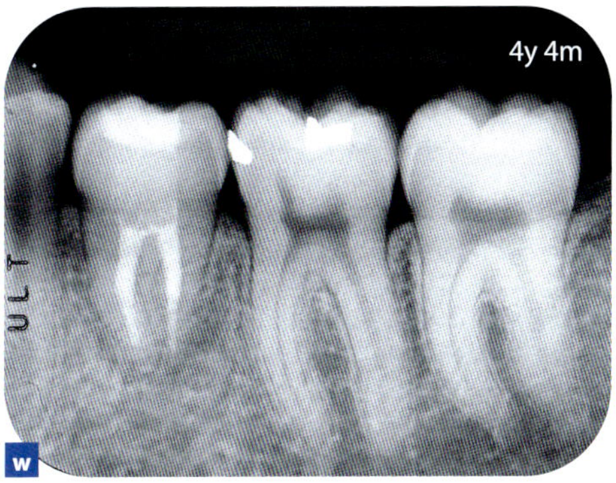

Fig 7-2v Radiograph after root canal treatment. Same day as **Fig 7-2u**. Intracanal medicament was placed using a calcium hydroxide preparation "Vitapex" (NEO DENTAL CHEMICAL PRODUCTS CO., LTD, Japan).
Fig 7-2w Four years and 4 months later. After final root canal filling with sealer and gutta-percha and crown restoration with CR.

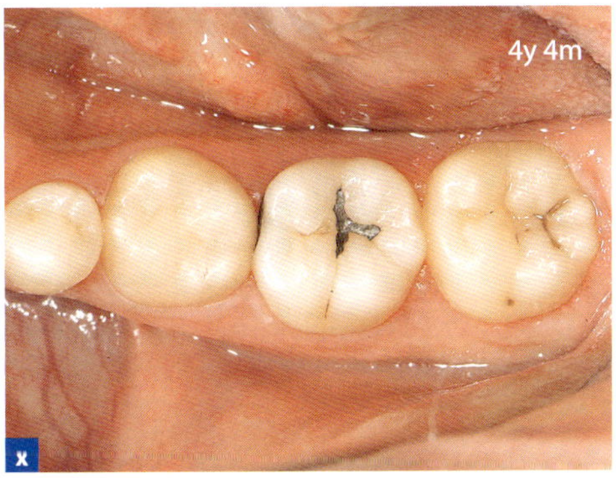

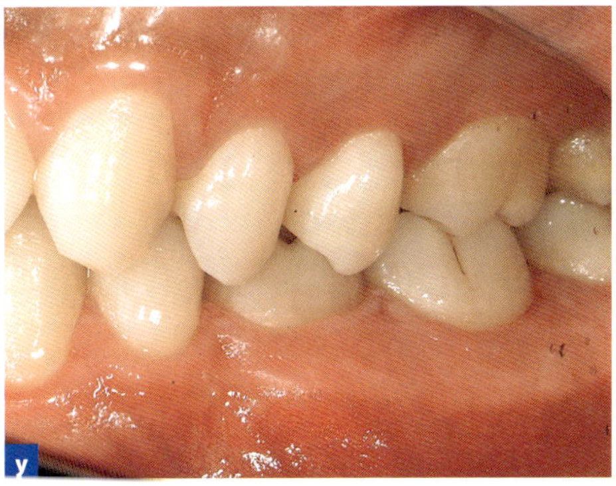

Fig 7-2x and 7-2y Clinical views after 4 years and 4 months.

Transplantation of the right side

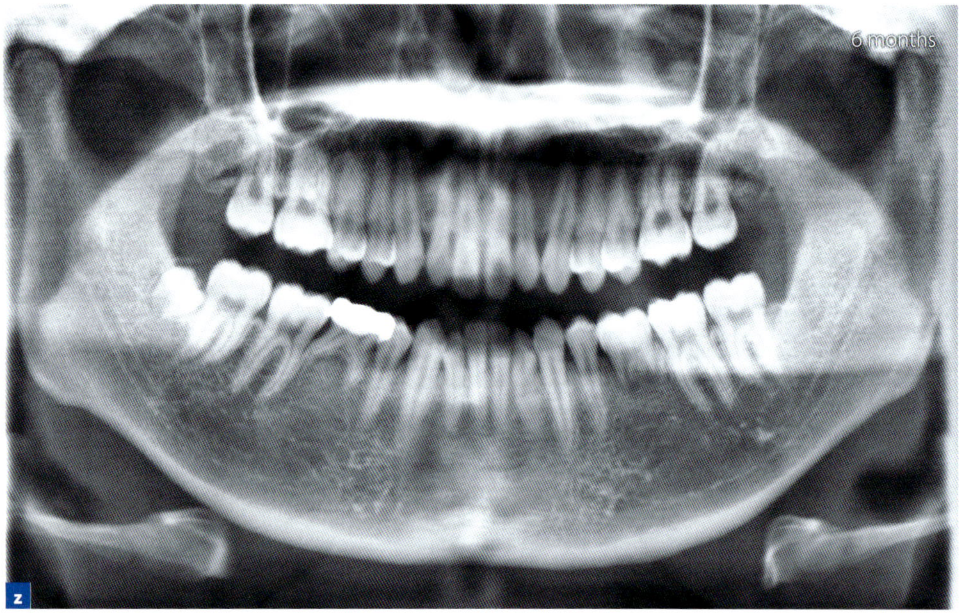

Fig 7-2z Panoramic radiograph 8 months after the first transplantation on the left site.

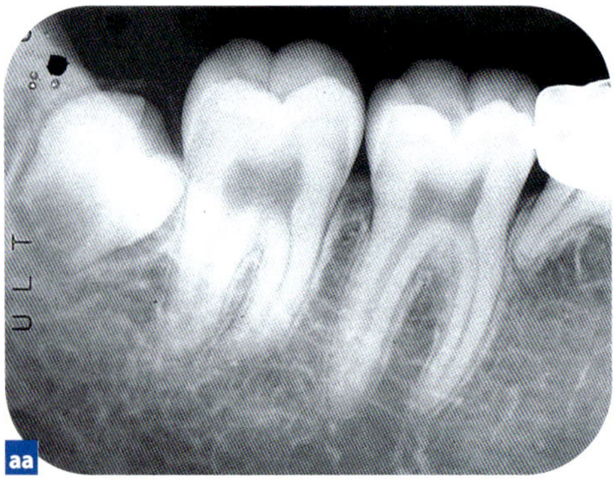

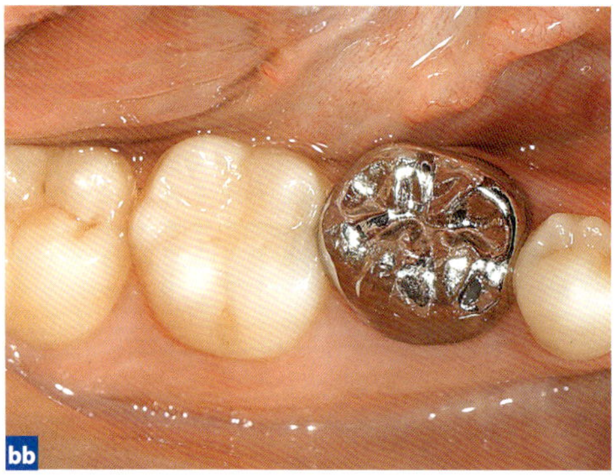

Fig 7-2aa Radiograph of #48, 8 months after the fist transplantation. Although the stage of root development was very early, transplantation was performed because of the patient's request. **Fig 7-2bb** Recipient site before transplantation.

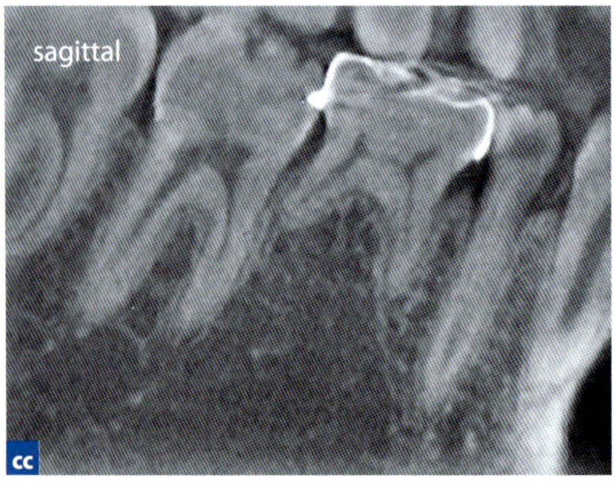

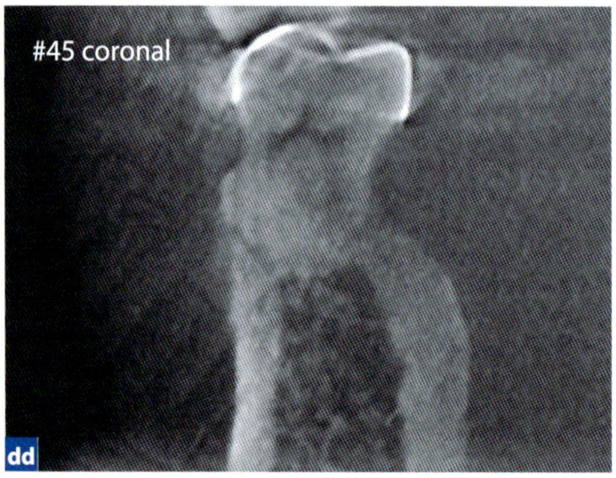

Fig 7-2cc and 7-2dd Preoperative analysis of the recipient site by CBCT.

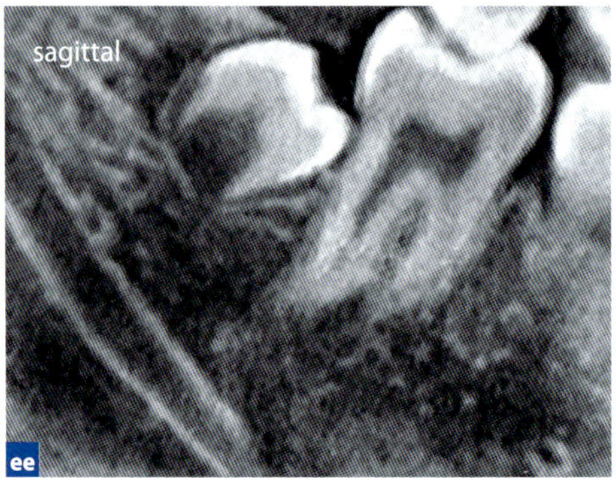

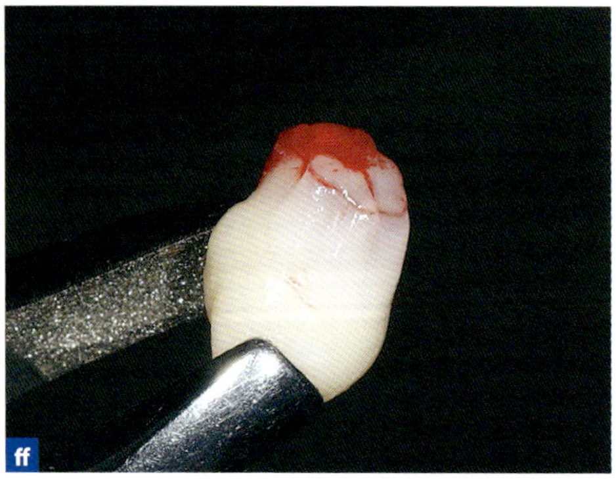

Fig 7-2ee Preoperative analysis of the donor tooth (#48) by CBCT. **Fig 7-2ff** Donor tooth.

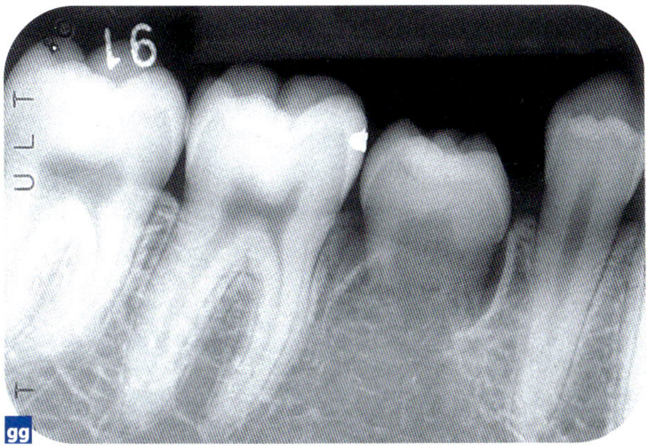

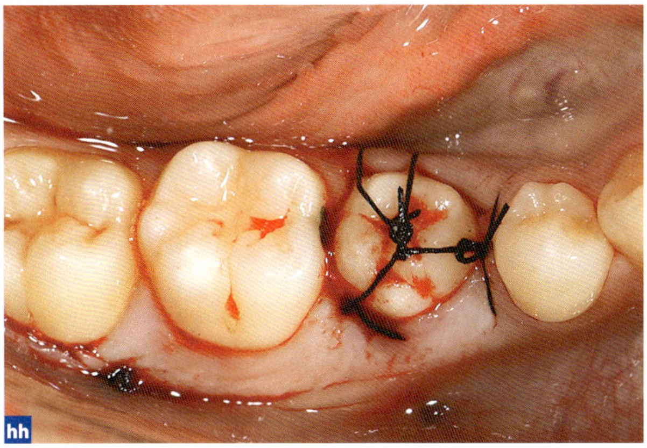

Fig 7-2gg and 7-2hh Immediately after transplantation.

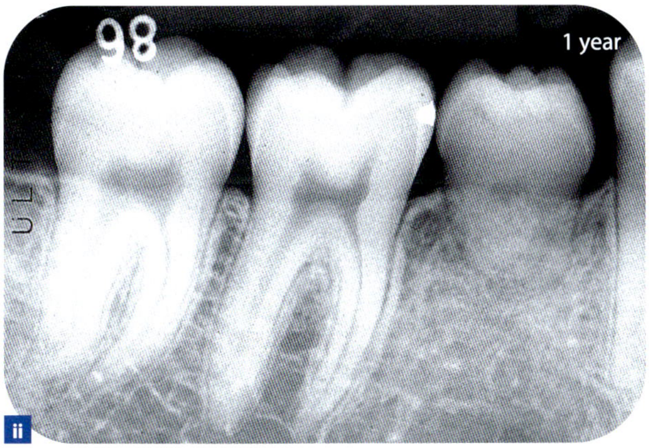

Fig 7-2ii Radiograph 1 year after transplantation. Intact lamina dura is observed. Pulp canal obliteration is progressing and the transplant responds EPT(+) but there is not much root development development.

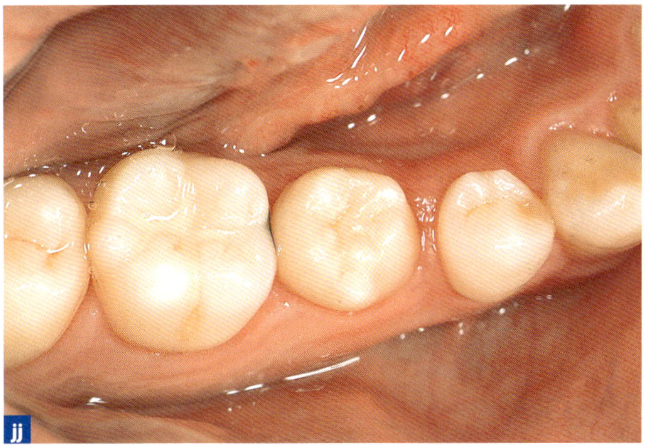

Fig7-2jj Occlusal view 1 year after transplantation. It seems that the mesial interproximal space is closing naturally.

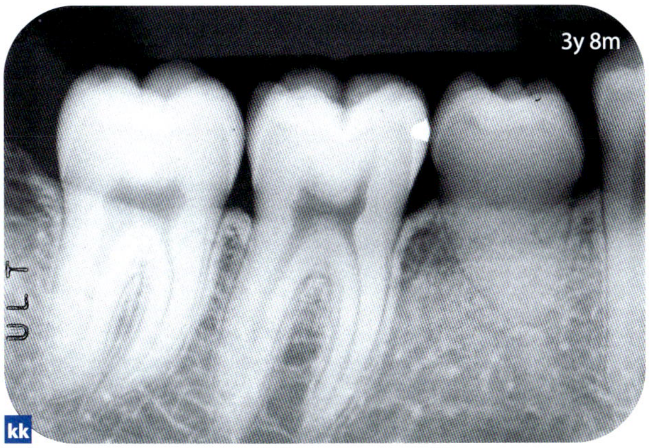

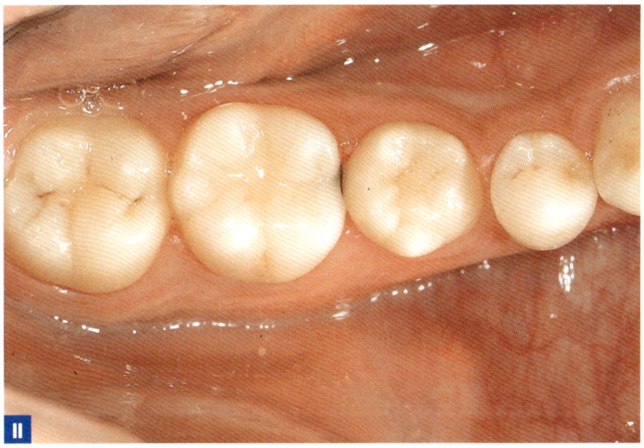

Fig 7-2kk and 7-2ll Three years and 8 months after transplantation. The root is still developing. The interproximal space is decreasing slightly.

Follow-up results 4 years and 4 months after the first transplantation

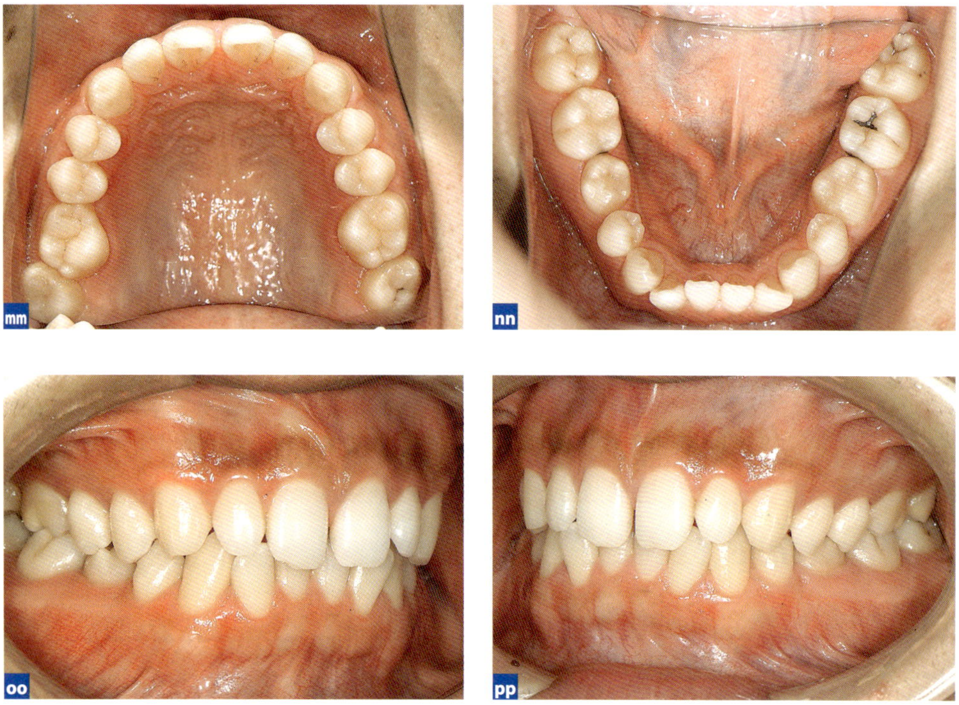

Fig 7-2mm to 7-2pp Clinical views 4 years and 4 months after the first transplantation.

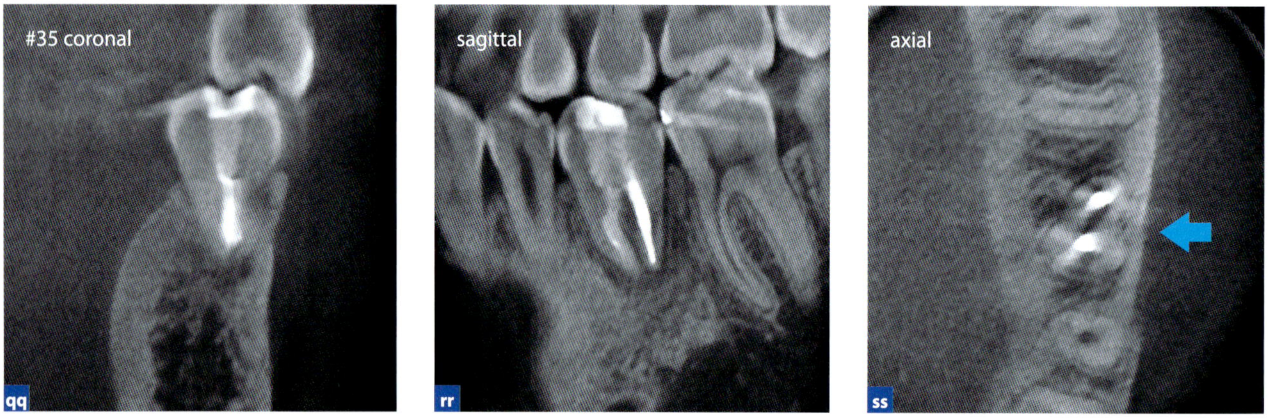

Fig 7-2qq to 7-2ss CBCT images 4 years and 4 months after transplantation of the left side.

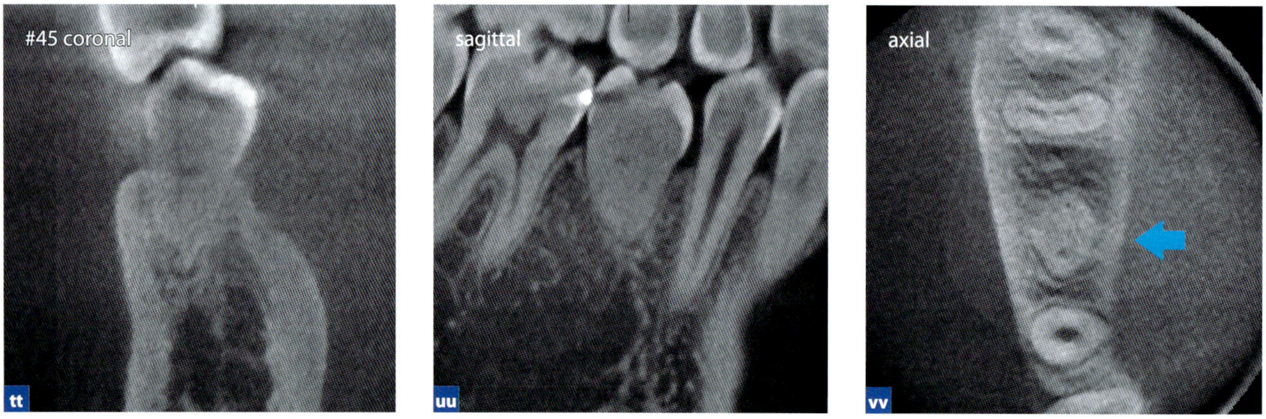

Fig 7-2tt to 7-2vv CBCT images 3 years and 8 months after transplantation of the right side.

Case3. Problems during the observation period leading up to performing transplantation

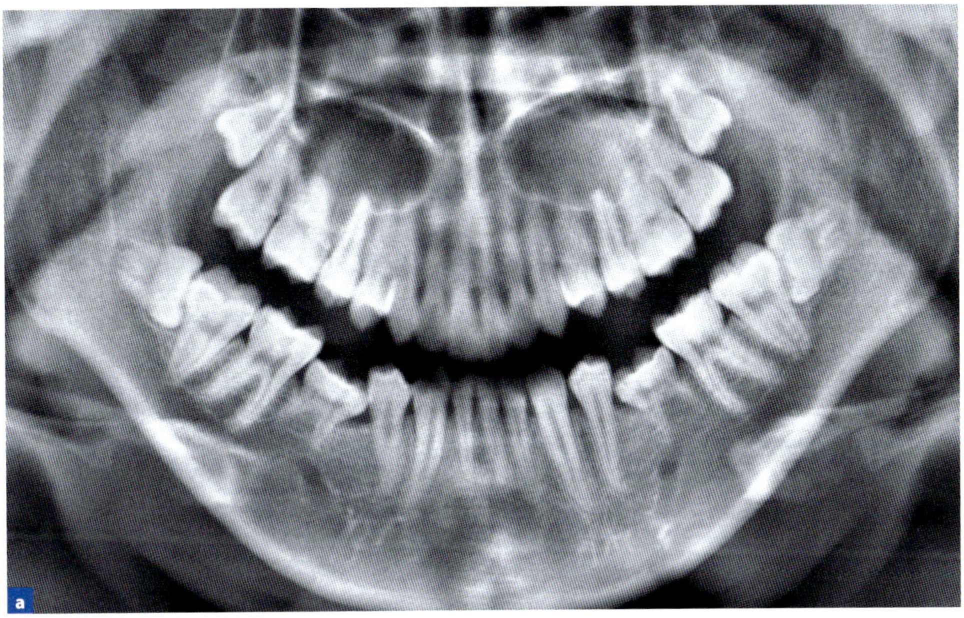

Fig 7-3a Panoramic radiograph of a 18-year-old male. #35 and #45 are congenitally missing, and the primary teeth, #75 and #85 were considered to have partial ankylosis. As ankylosis causes tooth eruption to stop, the adjacent teeth erupt but start tilting toward the ankylosed tooth, which cause the space of recipient sites to decrease and makes transplantation difficult.

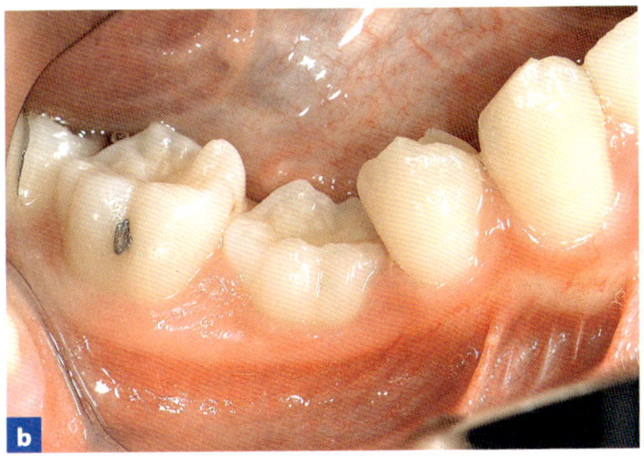

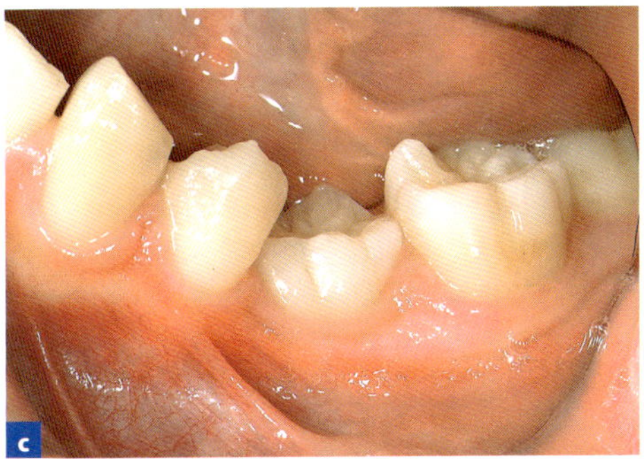

Fig 7-3b Lateral view of the right side.
Fig 7-3c Lateral view of the left side.

Case4. Problems during the observation period leading up to performing transplantation and case management ①

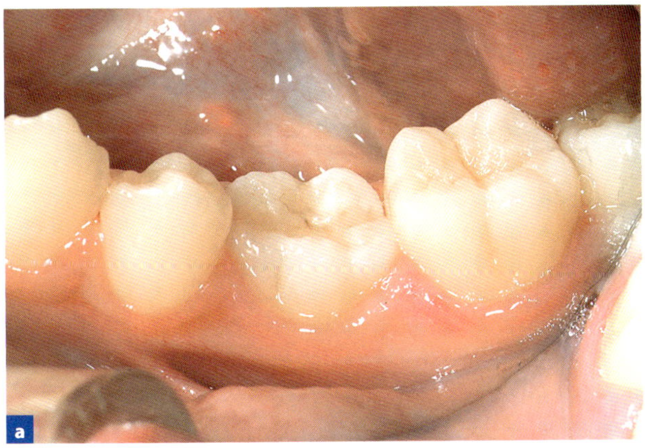

Fig 7-4a Early stage of ankylosis of the primary tooth #75.

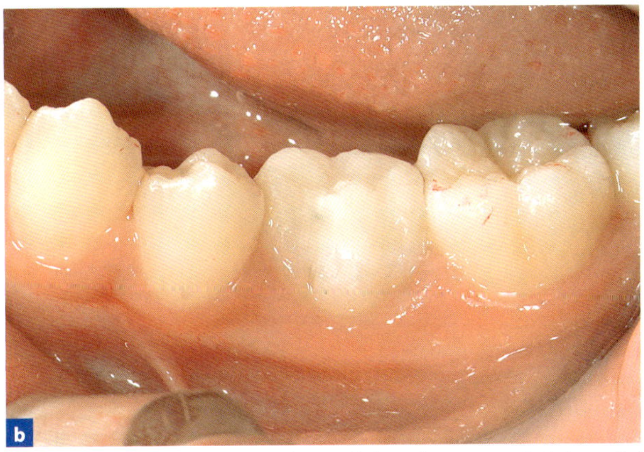

Fig 7-4b In order to prevent tilting of the adjacent teeth, it is useful to build up composite resin (CR) on the primary tooth.

Case5. Problems during the observation period leading up to performing transplantation and case management ②

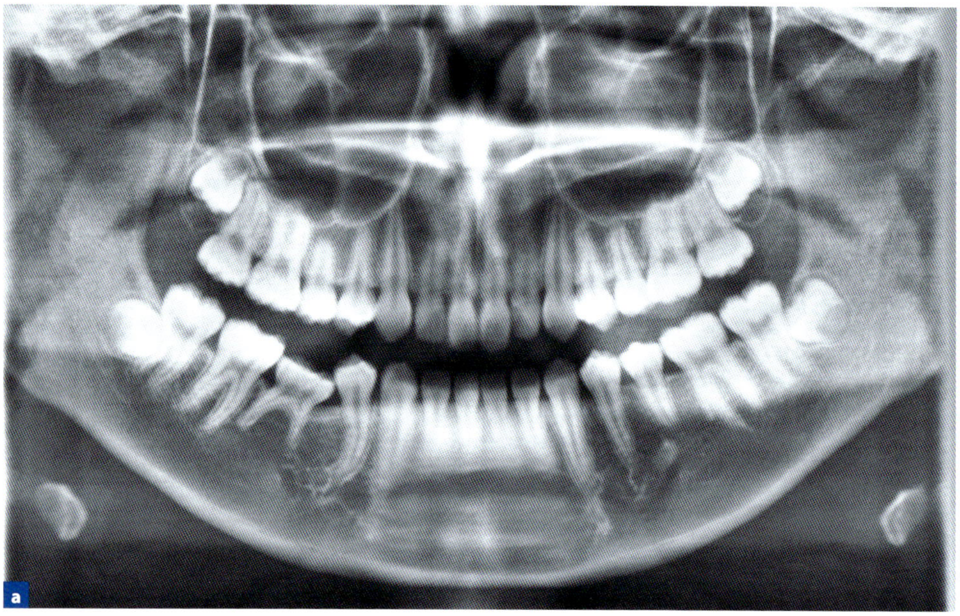

Fig 7-5a to 7-5c Panoramic radiograph of a 14-year-old female. #45 is congenitally missing and intra-occlusion of #85 has occurred and led to tilting in of the adjacent teeth. In preparation for future transplantation, regaining the space and prevention of further inclination of the adjacent teeth are important.

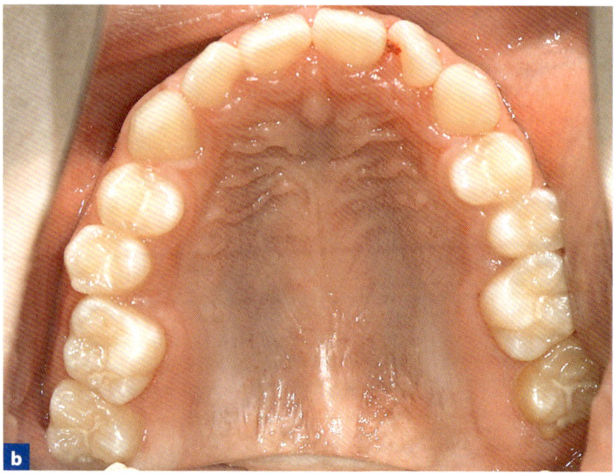

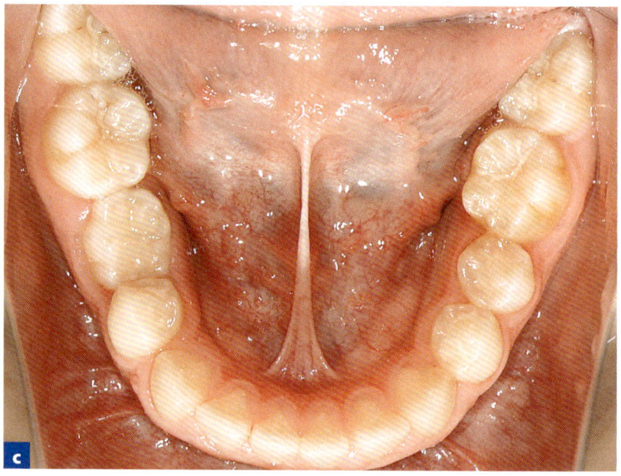

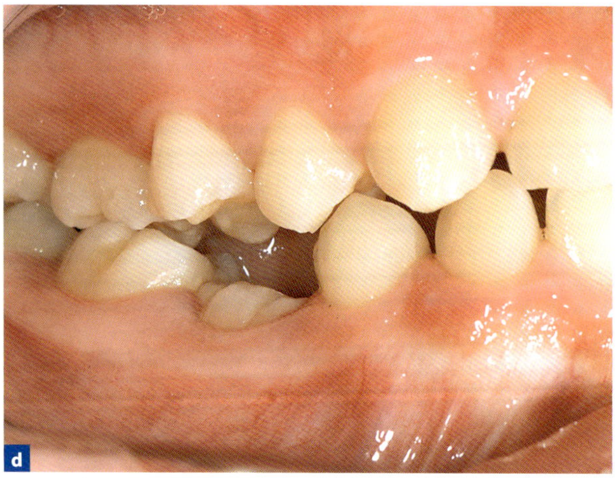

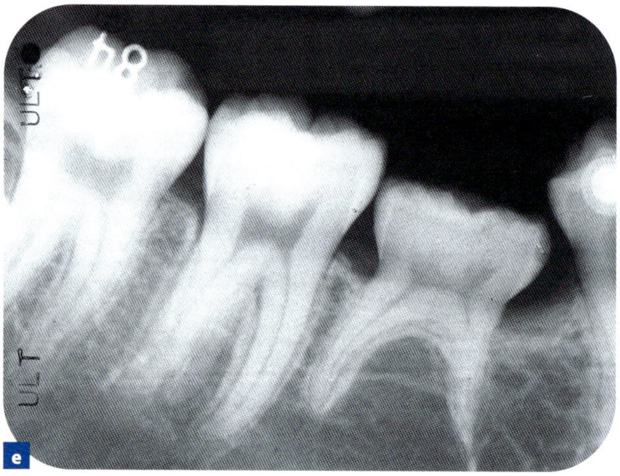

Fig 7-5d and 7-5e Views before LOT (up-righting).

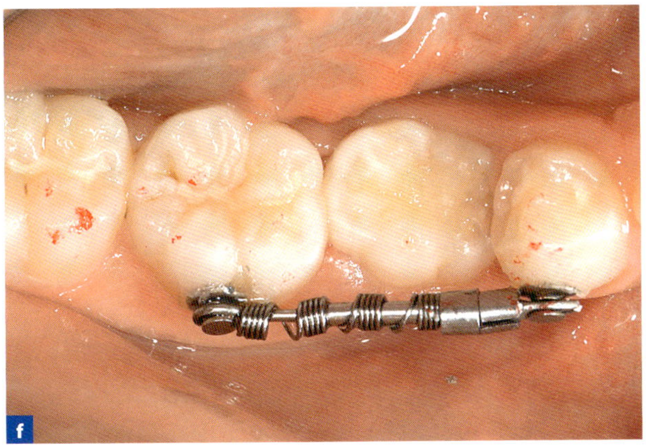

Fig 7-5f Up-righting the inclined teeth using a simple appliance.

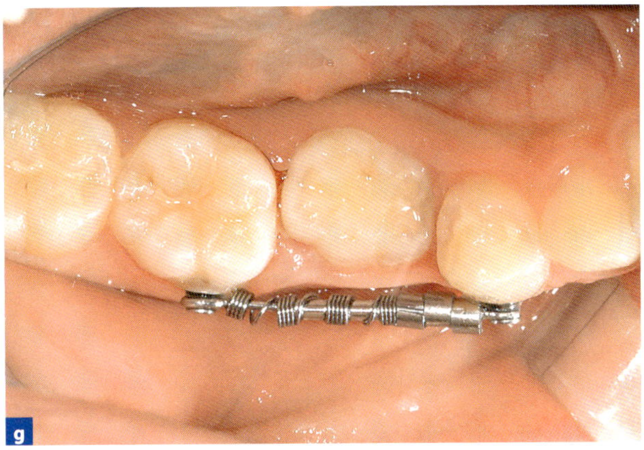

Fig 7-5g One and a half months after starting LOT. Sufficient space has already been regained.

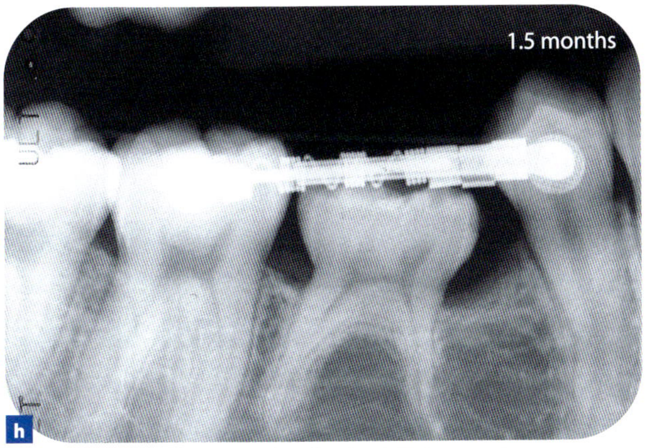

Fig 7-5h Radiograph immediately after LOT is complete.

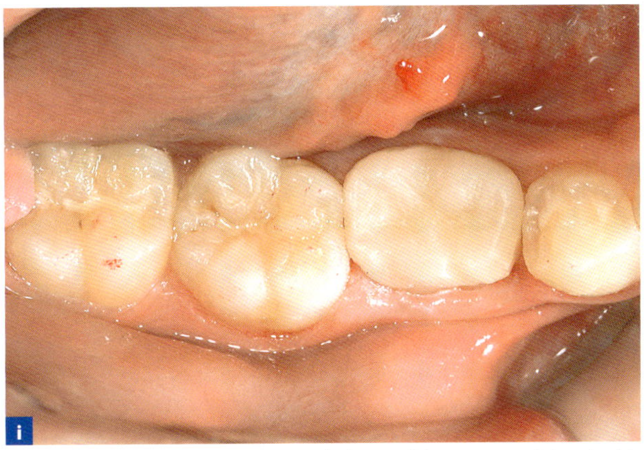

Fig 7-5i After changing the morphology of the crown of the deciduous tooth with CR.

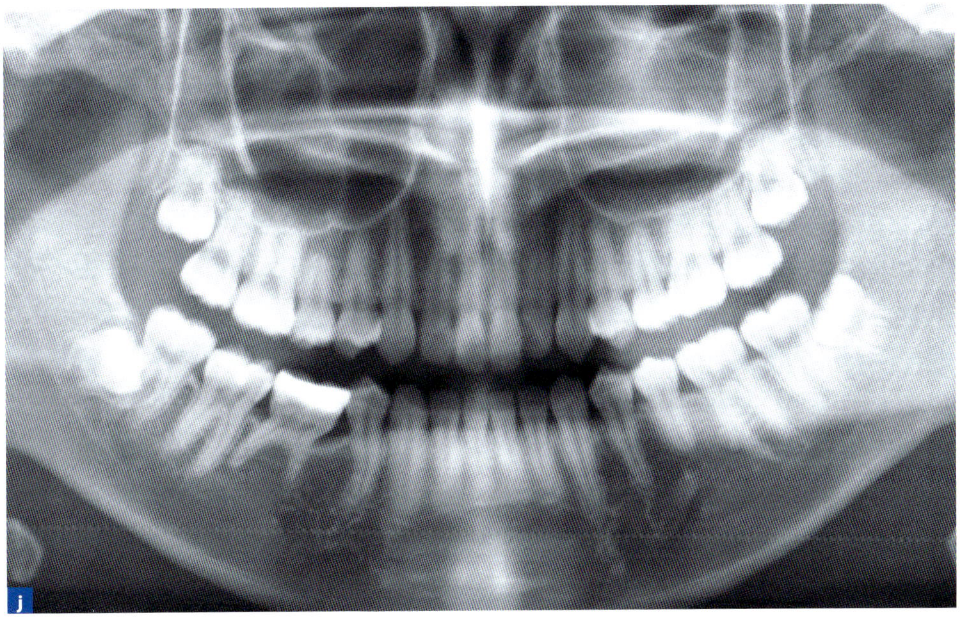

Fig 7-5j Panoramic radiograph 3 years after the first examination and immediately before transplantation. The patient is now 17-years-old. #18 is the donor tooth.

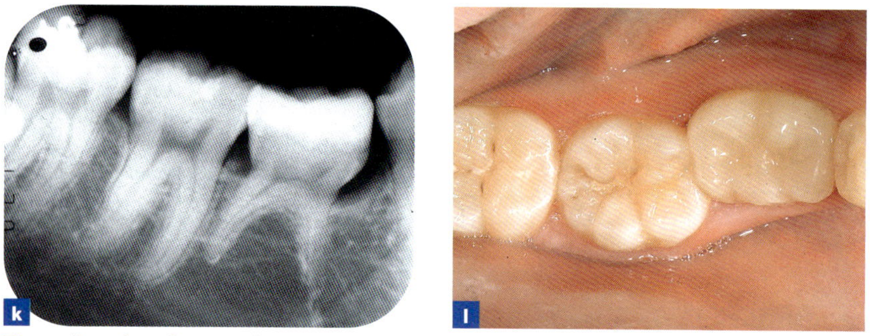

Fig 7-5k and 7-5l Views of the recipient site before surgery. The space is maintained by CR.

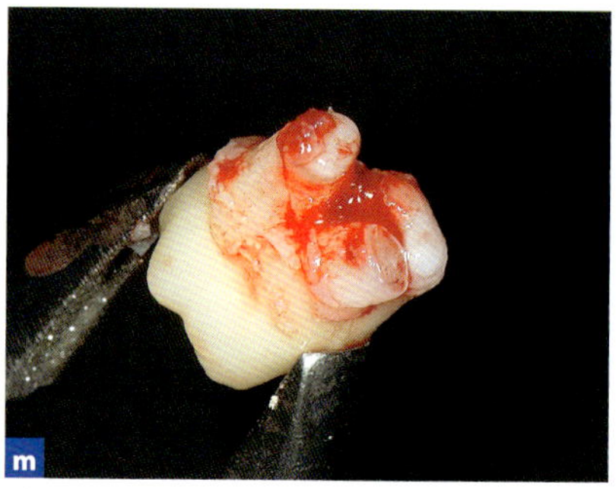

Fig 7-5m The donor tooth (#18). The stage of root development appears optimal.

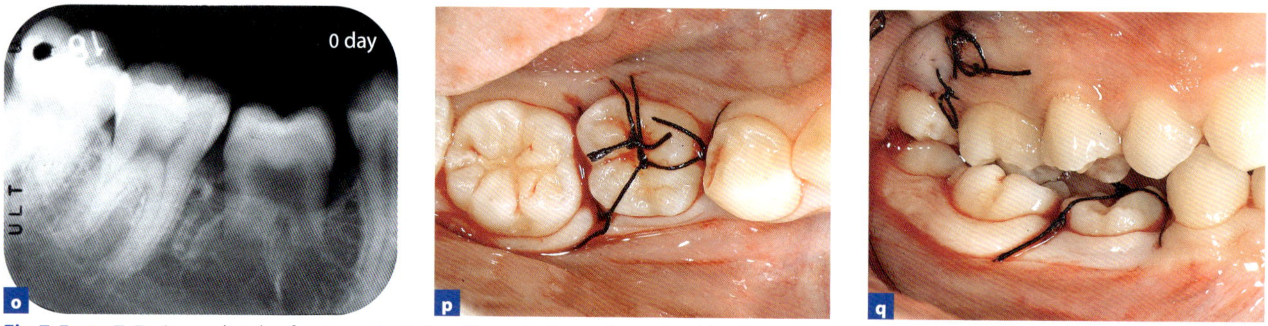

Fig 7-5o to 7-5q Immediately after transplantation. Since the buccolingual width of the alveolar ridge of the recipient site is narrow, the donor tooth is rotated 90 degrees.

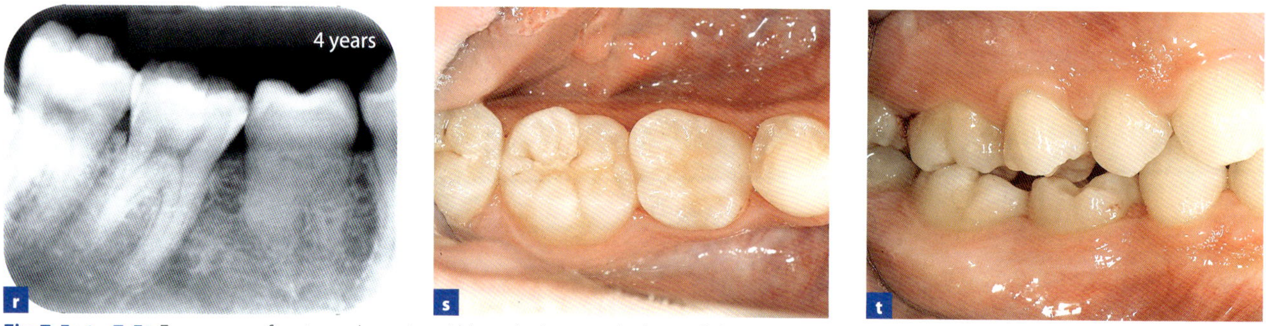

Fig 7-5r to 7-5t Four years after transplantation. Although the morphology of the crown of the transplant is not ideal, optimal healing after transplanting an immature tooth has been achieved.

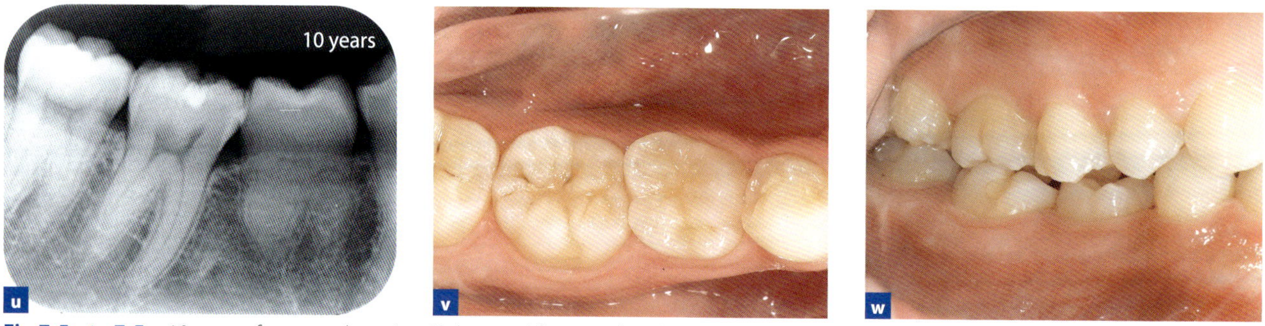

Fig 7-5u to 7-5w 10 years after transplantation. Tighter and functional occlusion has been achieved.

Case 6. Transplantation of an ectopically erupted premolar to a site of a congenitally missing tooth

Ectopically erupted premolars may be a donor tooth for congenitally missing second premolar sites (**Fig 7-6a** and **7-6b**). In such a case, it is possible to perform transplantation at a younger age, not having to wait for the third molars to develop.

When transplanting a maxillary premolar to a mandibular premolar site, it is noted that the root of the maxillary premolar may be frequently too wide buccolingually to be accommodated into the mandibular premolar site (**Fig 7-6h** to **7-6m**). In such a case, the transplant can be rotated 45 to 90 degrees to fit in the recipient site (**Fig 7-6n** to **7-6z**).

Case6. Transplantation of an ectopically erupted premolar to the site of a congenitally missing tooth

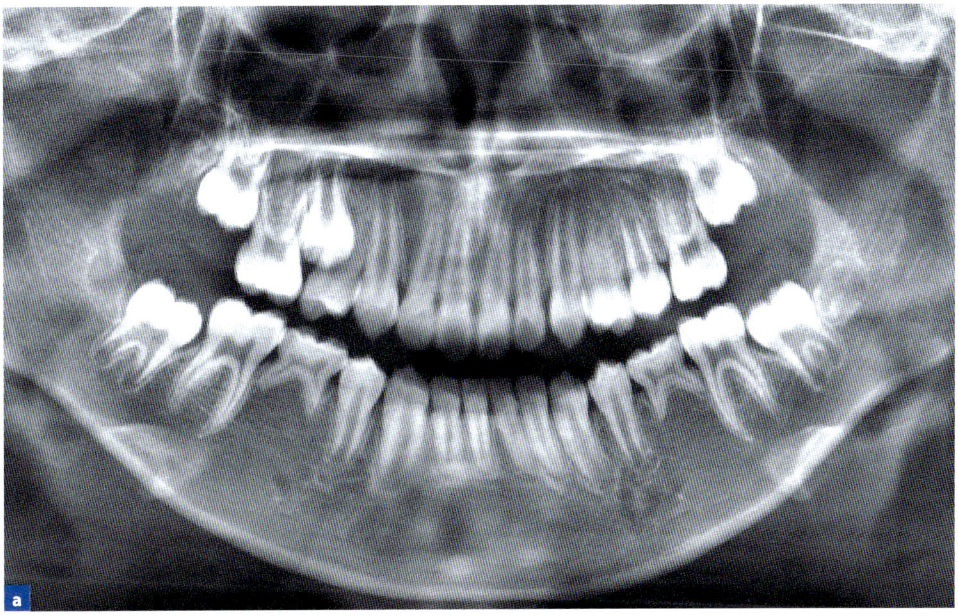

Fig 7-6a Panoramic radiograph of a 10-year and 11-month-old male. #15 has erupted ectopically on the palatal aspect and #35 and #45 are congenitally missing. Transplantation of #15 to #45 site is planned.

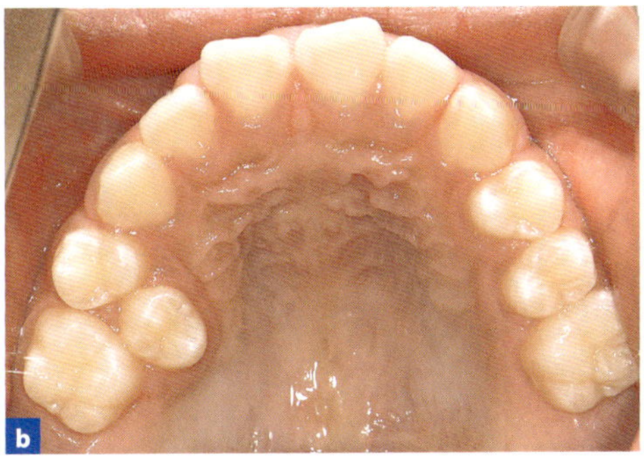

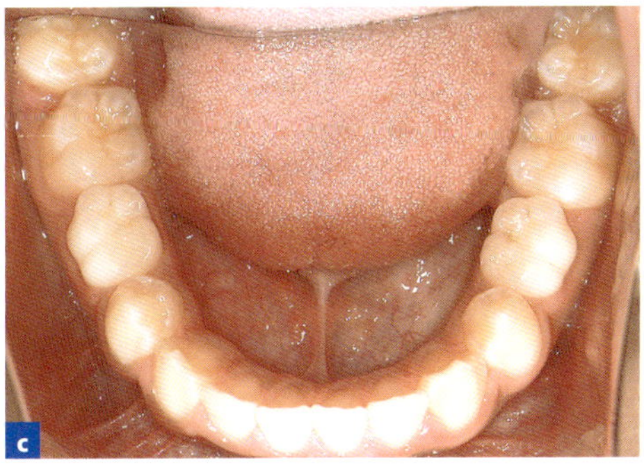

Fig 7-6b and 7-6c Occlusal views before surgery.

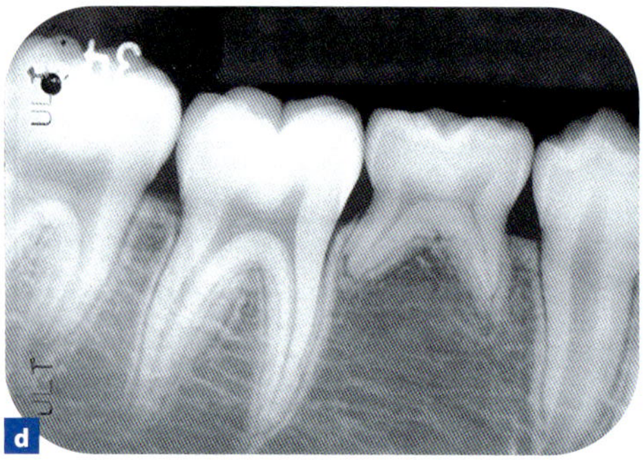

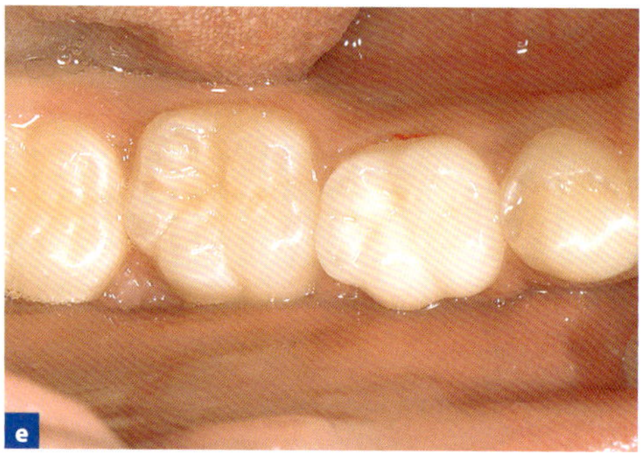

Fig 7-6d Preoperative radiograph of the recipient site.
Fig 7-6e Clinical view before surgery.

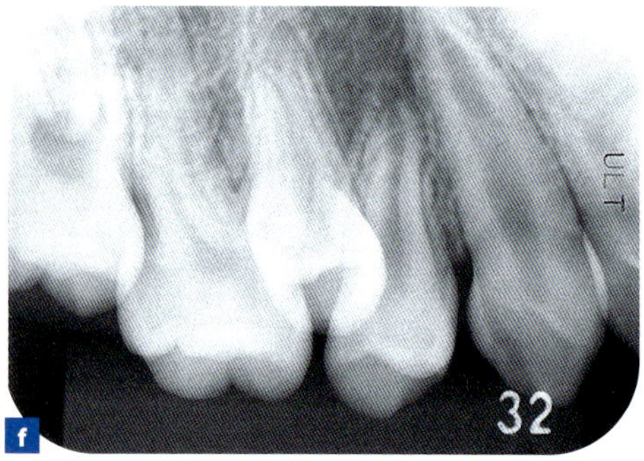

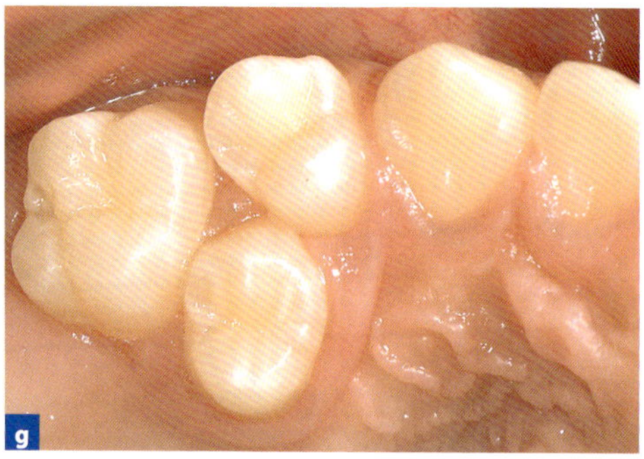

Fig 7-6f Radiograph of the donor tooth. The apex is open.
Fig 7-6g Clinical view of the donor tooth before surgery. If such crowding is left untreated, there will be high risk of caries in the future involving all of the adjacent teeth.

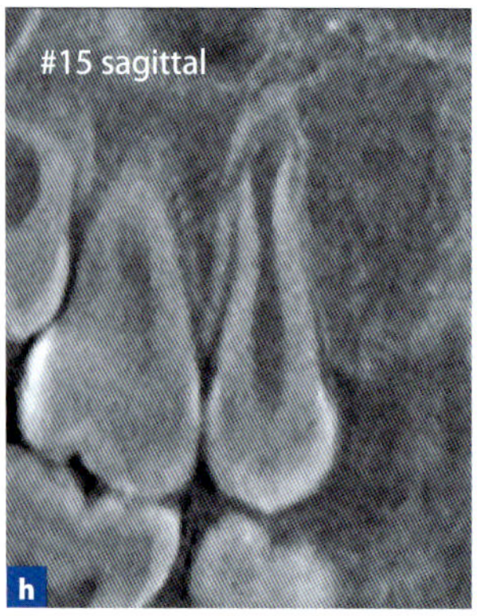

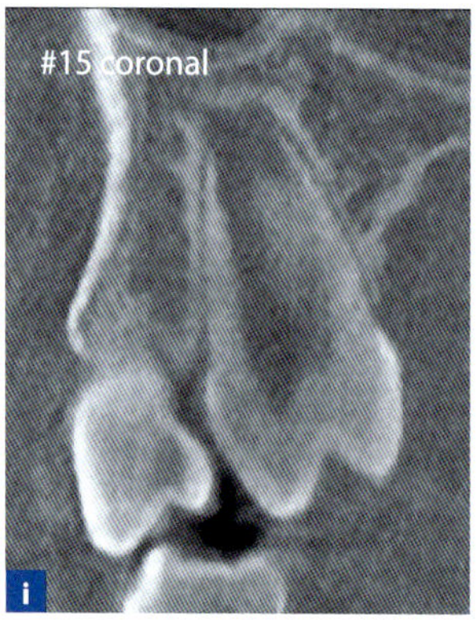

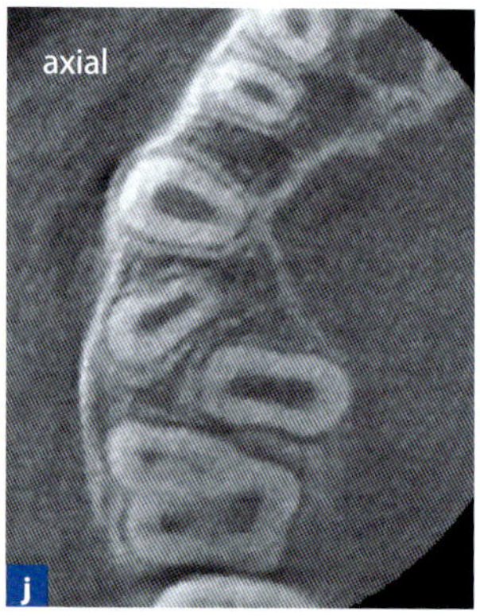

Fig 7-6h to 7-6j CBCT images of the donor tooth. The stage of the root development is good but the root morphology is wider buccolingually.

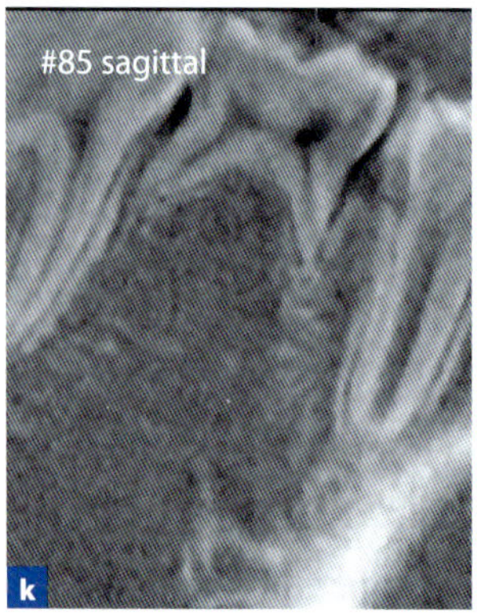

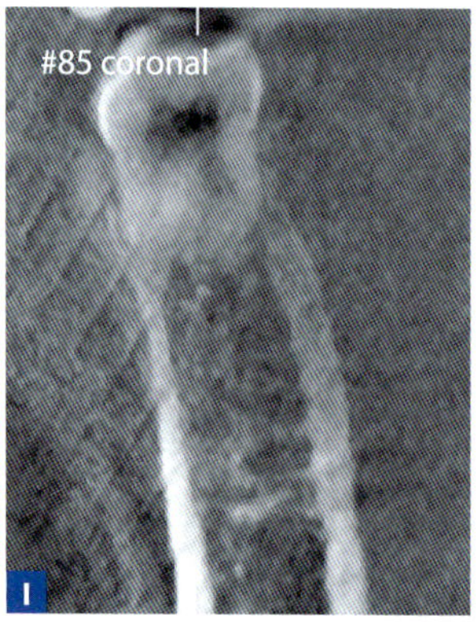

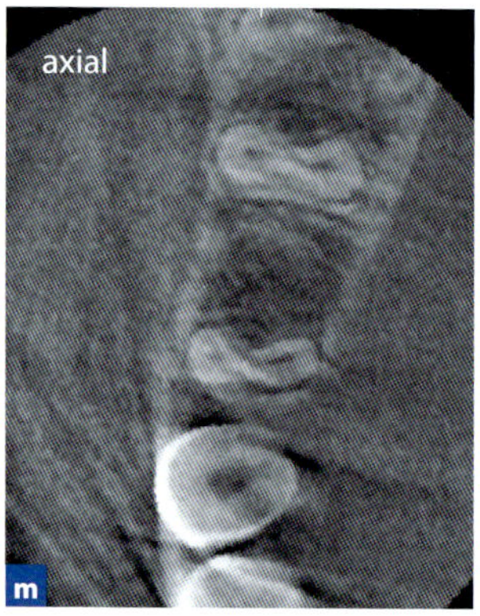

Fig 7-6k to 7-6m CBCT images of the recipient site. The imaging shows that the buccolingual width of the ridge is narrower than the buccolingual width of the donor tooth. In such a case, it is advised to rotate the donor tooth by 45 degrees.

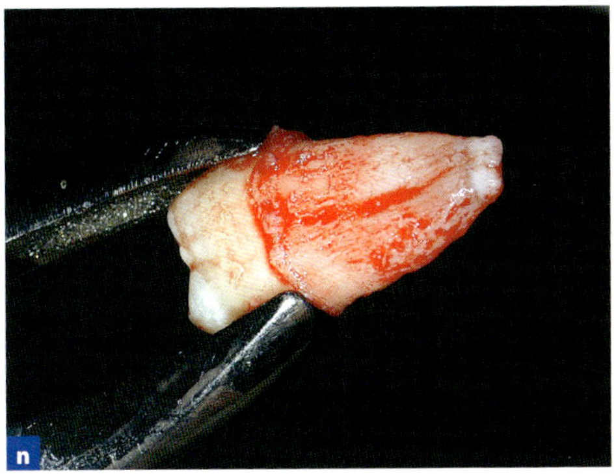

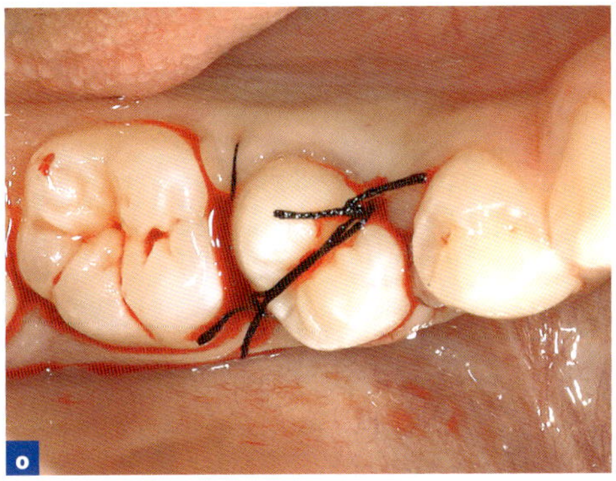

Fig 7-6n Donor tooth. Hertwig's epithelial sheath is attached around the apex.

Fig 7-6o Immediately after transplantation. The tooth is placed intentionally at 45 degrees.

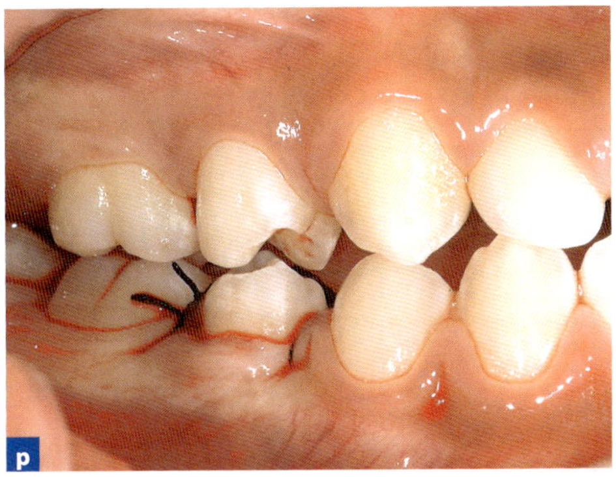

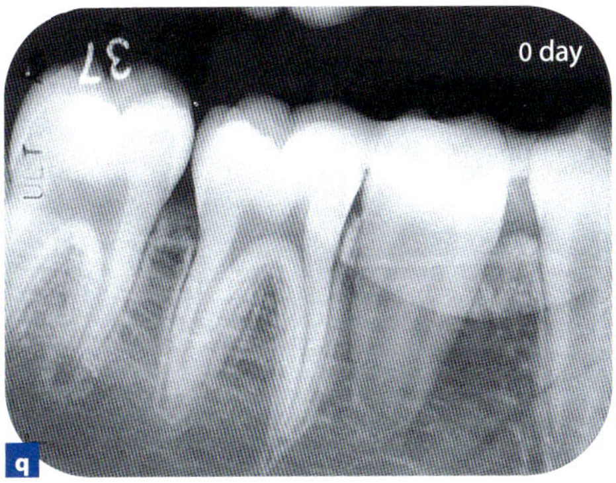

Fig 7-6p Occlusal relationship immediately after transplantation.

Fig 7-6q Radiograph immediately after transplantation.

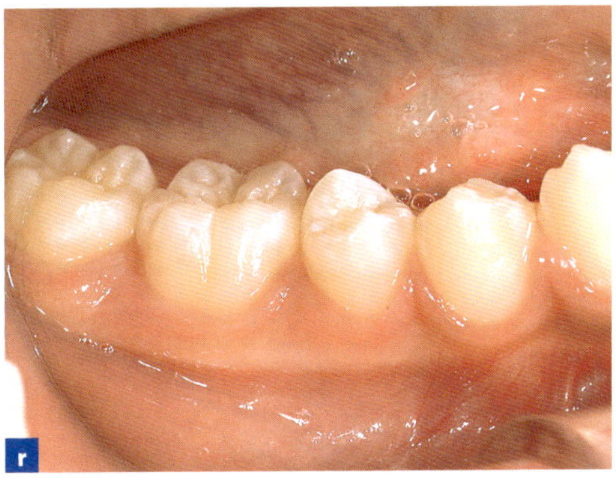

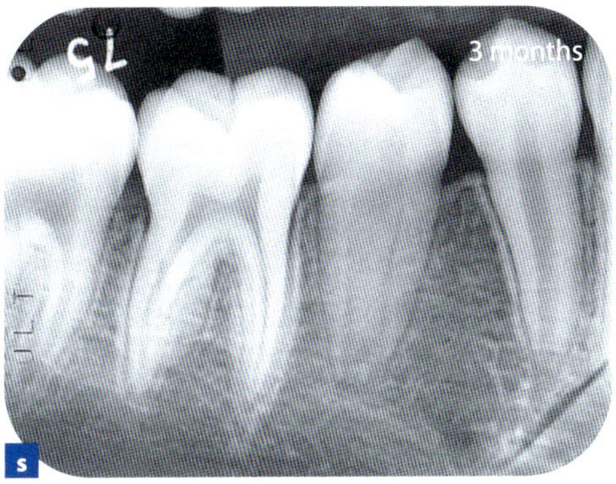

Fig 7-6r Clinical view 3 months after transplantation. No gingival inflammation is observed.

Fig 7-6s Radiograph 3 months after transplantation. Pulp canal obliteration appears to be initiating.

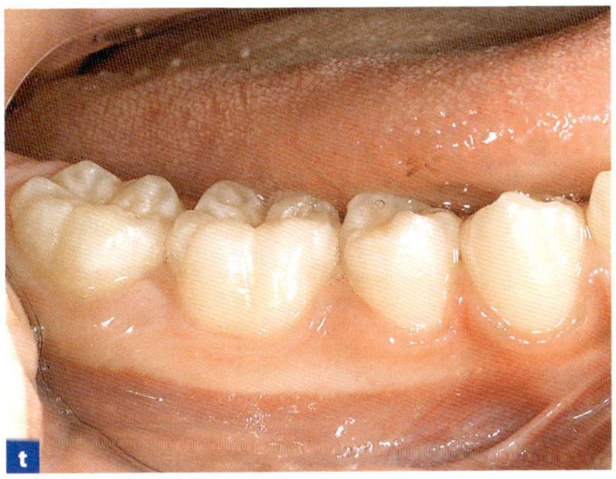

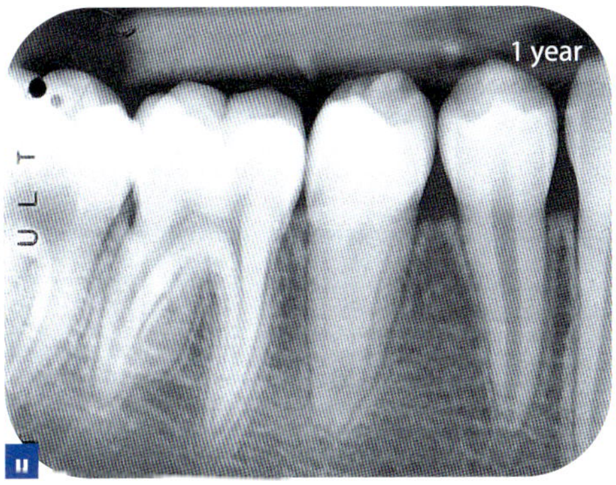

Fig 7-6t and 7-6u One year postoperative. Pulp canal obliteration is progressing and the transplant responds EPT (+).

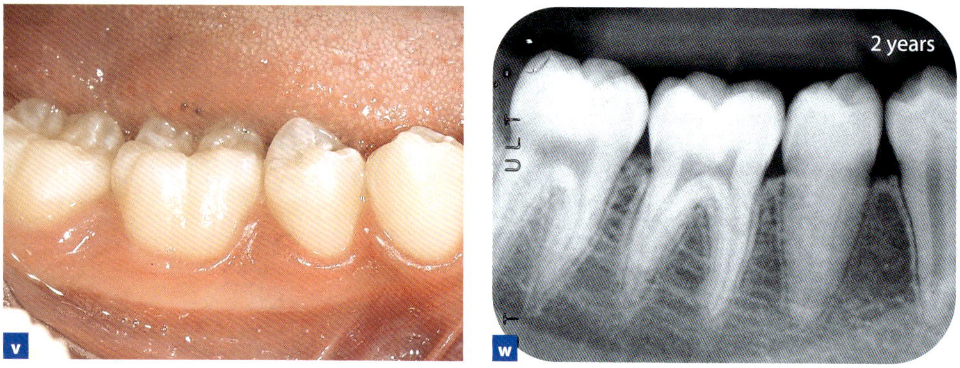

Fig 7-6v and 7-6w Two years after transplantation. The root development appears complete.

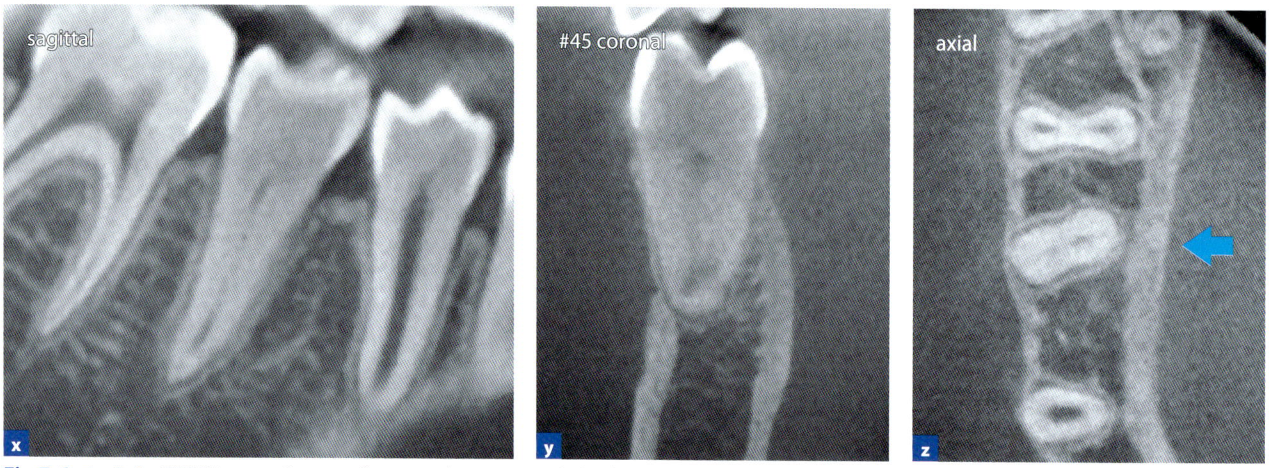

Fig 7-6x to 7-6z CBCT images 2 years after transplantation. Pulp healing and root development are observed.

There are other options in the treatment for congenitally missing teeth, such as fixed bridge, removal denture, implant and orthodontic space closure. If there is an appropriate donor tooth available, transplantation should be the first treatment of choice due to the high benefit and less invasive nature of the intervention.

CHAPTER 8

Autotransplantation of teeth in anterior regions

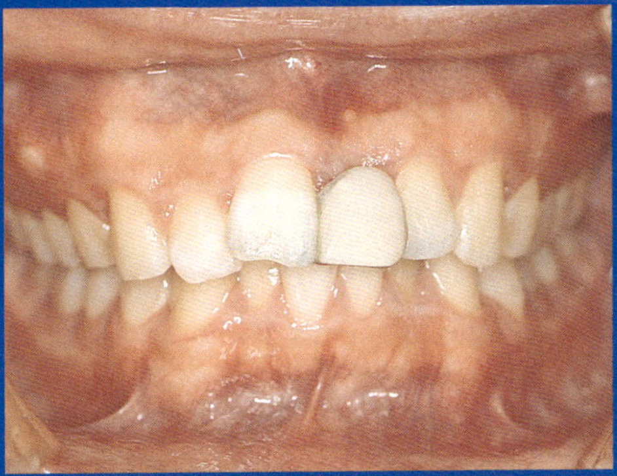

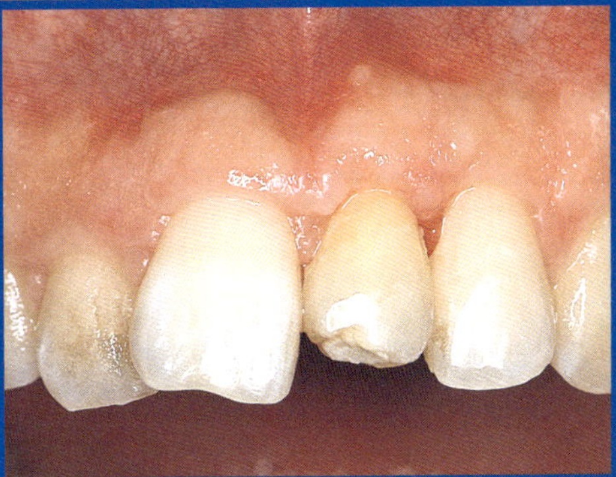

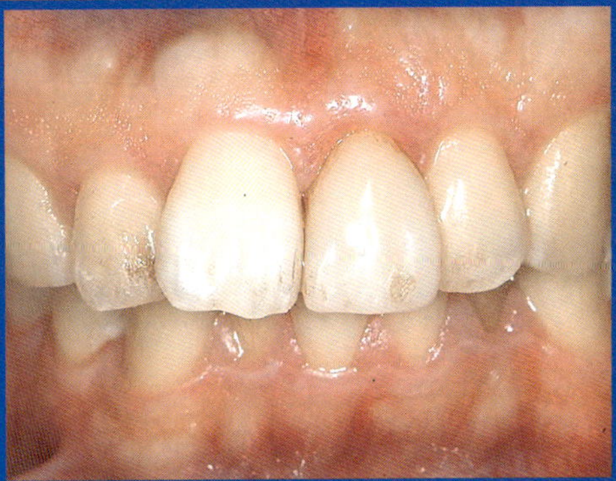

Indications for performing transplantation in anterior regions are more limited. The reason is that having a suitable donor tooth that will fit in the anterior regions are not commonly available. Potential donor teeth for anterior regions include smaller wisdom teeth, displaced premolars, and teeth extracted strategically for orthodontic treatment. Indications for transplantation and orthodontic treatment are discussed in **Chapter 9**.

Case 1. Transplantation of a supernumerary premolar to the anterior region

Fig 8-1 shows a case of a 21-year-old male who presented with interest in implant treatment in anterior region. When he was about 10 years old, #21 was avulsed and lost due to trauma. The area was restored with a Maryland bridge (**Fig 8-1a** to **8-1e**), and he hoped to have a more esthetics and functional treatment with an implant supported crown as he turned 20 years old. However, upon close examination of the oral cavity, a supernumerary impacted premolar (third premolar) was found on the right side of the mandible (**Fig 8-1a**, **8-1f**, **8-1g** and **8-1h**).

It is not always easy to esthetically restore one missing maxillary central incisor with implant treatment. In particular, when the alveolar ridge is resorbed, there are elevated risks such as soft and hard tissue management. There is also higher cost and time involved, as well as risks of long-term complications that can occur if the implant is placed too early in life. If there is an appropriate donor tooth available for transplantation, the patient can benefit from having their own natural tooth that is healthy, functional, and esthetically pleasing and can save time and cost. After discussing the advantages and disadvantages, the patient chose to pursue transplantation.

When the flap was raised, it was evident that the alveolar ridge was resorbed more than expected (**Fig 8-1i** and **8-1j**). At the time of this treatment, there was no dental cone-beam CT (CBCT) available yet, so the condition of the alveolar ridge was only accurately determined during surgery. When the alveolar ridge has been resorbed, transplantation has more advantages over implant. One of them is bone induction by the periodontal ligament of the transplant. In this case, the buccal cortical plate was removed (**Fig 8-1k** and **8-1l**), the recipient socket was formed, and the plate was placed back onto the root surface of the transplant (**Fig 8-1m** to **8-1o**). As discussed in **Chapter 3**, since the periodontal ligament of the transplant has osteoinductive ability (regenerative ability), it is uncertain whether placing the cortical bone plate over the transplant was necessary, but it may have helped to maintain the space for bone regeneration. The postoperative examination with CBCT (**Fig 8-1cc** and **8-1gg**) showed the transplant has been covered by bone on the buccal aspect.

The authors usually restore the crown of transplanted teeth with composite resin (CR) (**Fig 8-1t** to **8-1x**) because it helps preserve tooth structure, making future re-restoration easier if needed, and reduces time and cost. If the shade of the crown of the transplant is darker and the root development is completed (i.e. endodontic treatment is necessary), we recommend to perform internal bleaching before CR restoration (**Fig 8-1t**, **8-1u**, and see **Fig 8-4**).

Case 1. Transplantation of a supernumerary premolar to the anterior region

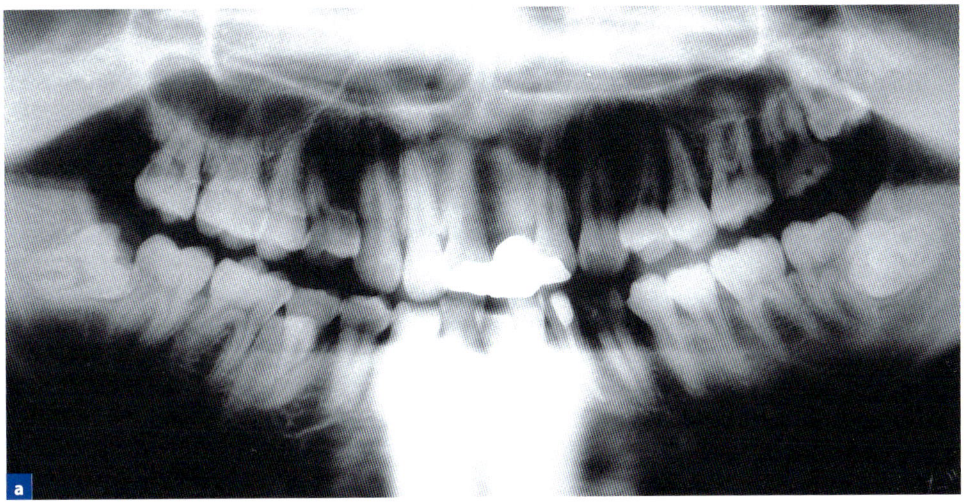

Fig 8-1a Panoramic radiograph at the first visit of a 21-year-old male. The patient desired to have an implant to #21 site which was lost due to avulsion when he was around the age of 10. However, a supernumerary tooth (premolar) on the right side of the mandible was available and thought to be a good candidate for transplantation to #21 site instead of implant supported treatment.

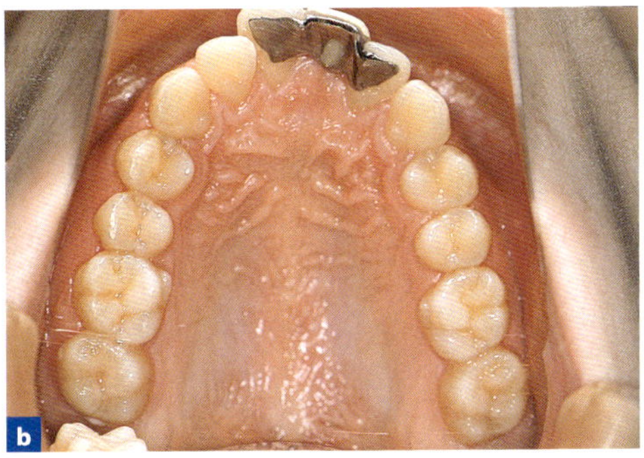

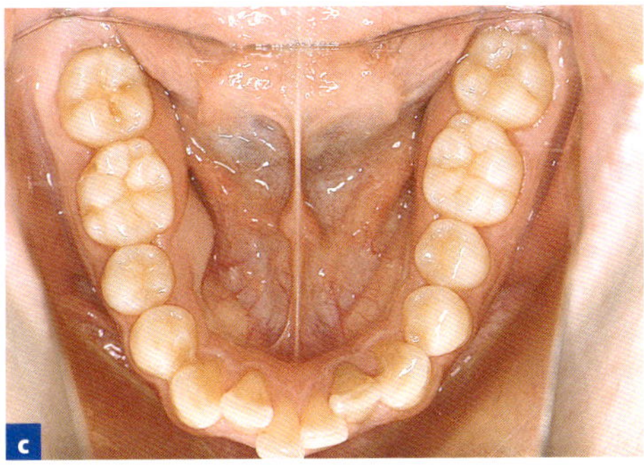

Fig 8-1b and 8-1c Preoperative occlusal views.

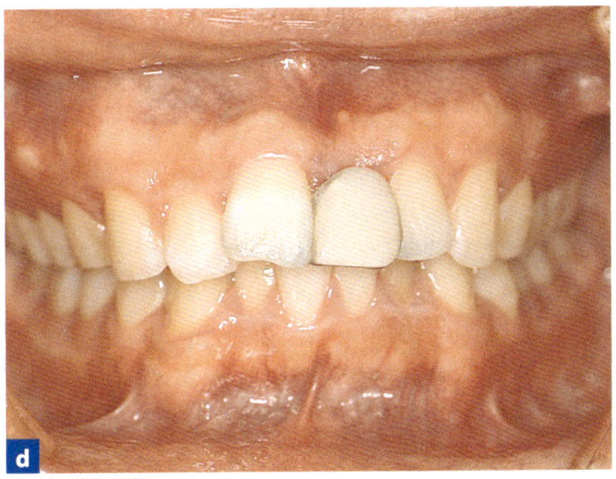

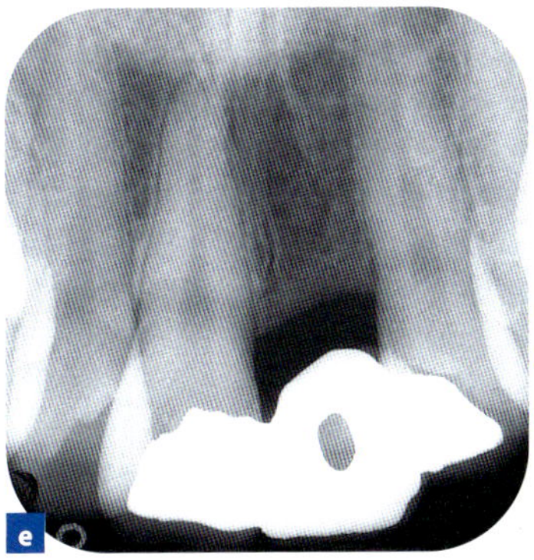

Fig 8-1d Frontal view at the first visit.
Fig 8-1e Radiograph of the recipient site at the first visit.

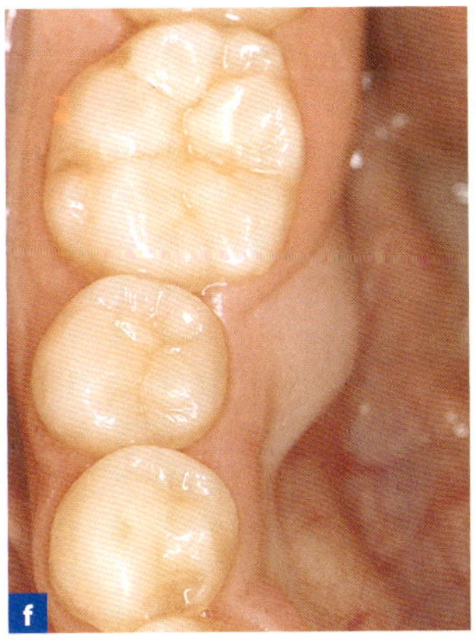

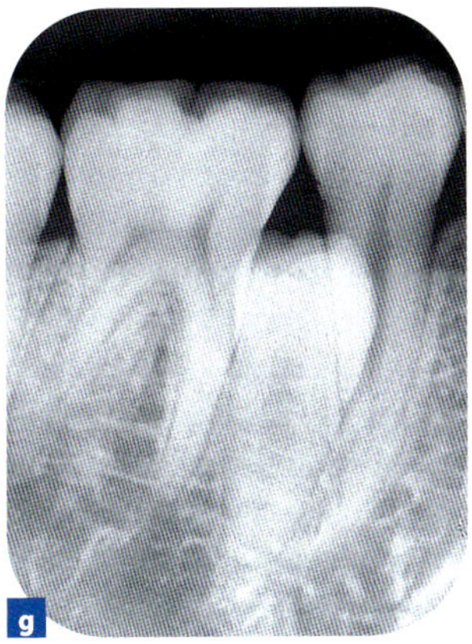

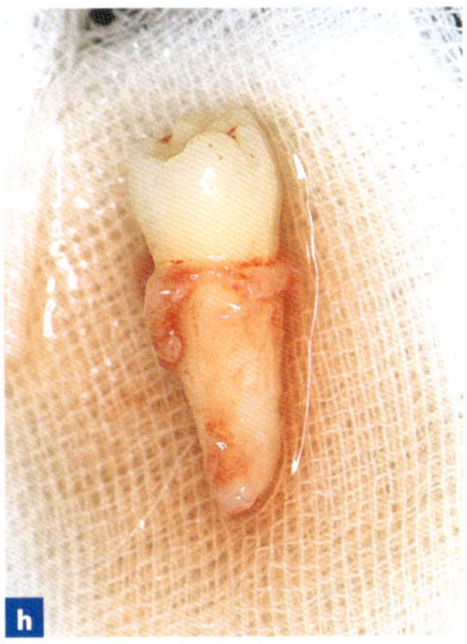

Fig 8-1f and 8-1g Donor tooth before surgery.
Fig 8-1h Extracted donor tooth. After measuring the morphology, the tooth was stored in physiological saline.

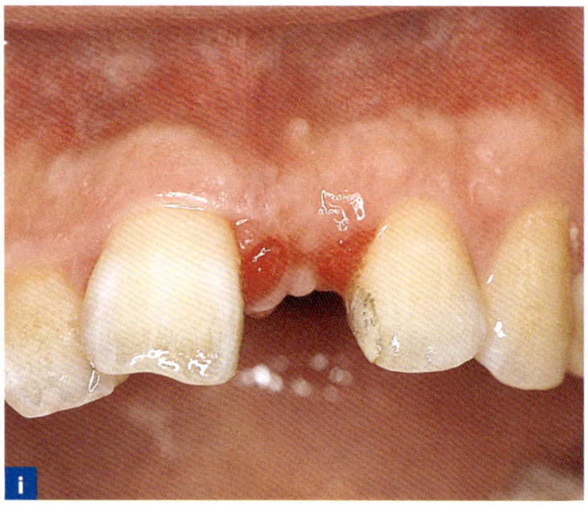

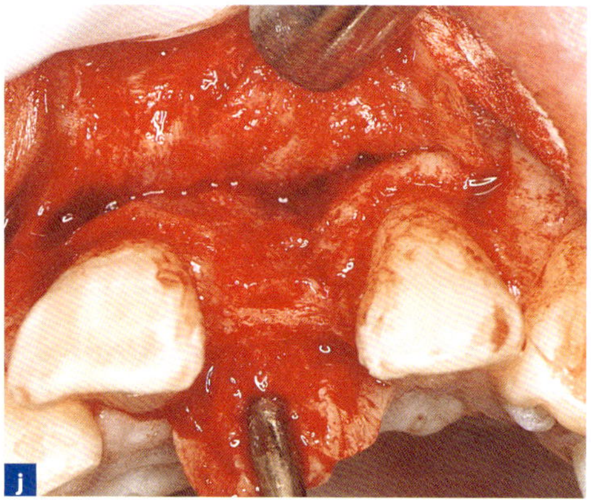

Fig 8-1i After removal of the Maryland bridge.
Fig 8-1j When the gingival flap was raised, there was evident resorption of the alveolar ridge.

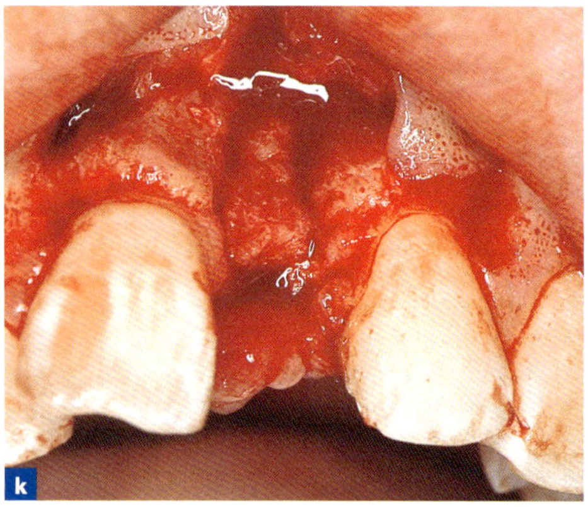

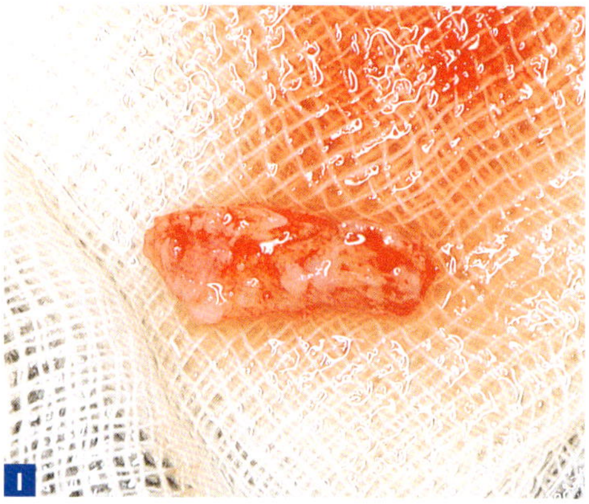

Fig 8-1k Making incision lines on the cortical bone on the buccal surface with a surgical fissure bur, the thin buccal cortical plate was removed using a chisel.
Fig 8-1l Removed cortical bone plate used as a bone graft material.

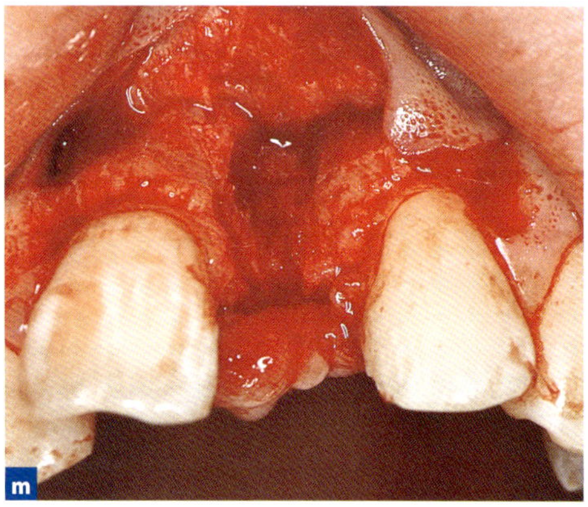

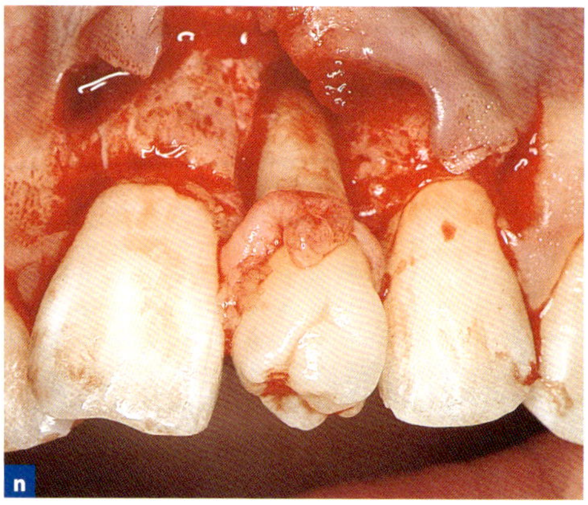

Fig 8-1m Prepared recipient socket.
Fig 8-1n Try-in of the donor tooth to the socket.

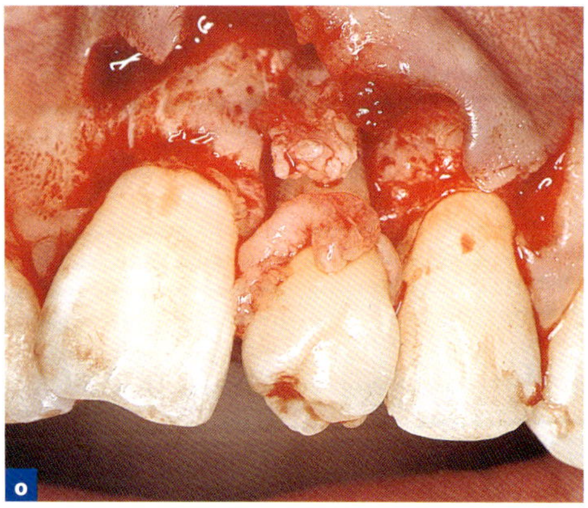

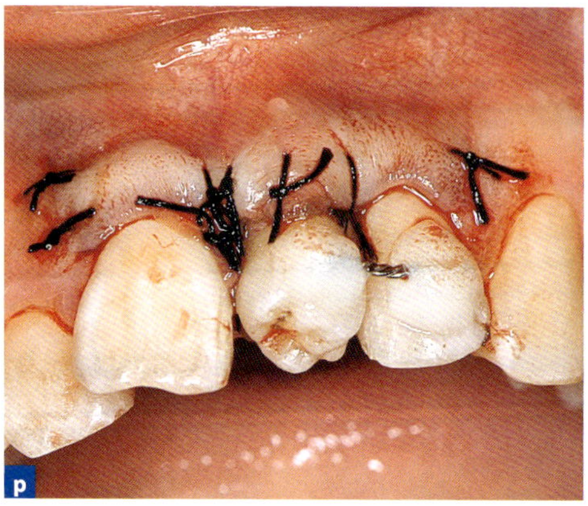

Fig 8-1o Placement of the cortical bone plate over the buccal surface of the transplant.
Fig 8-1p Suture of the gingival flap and wire splinting.

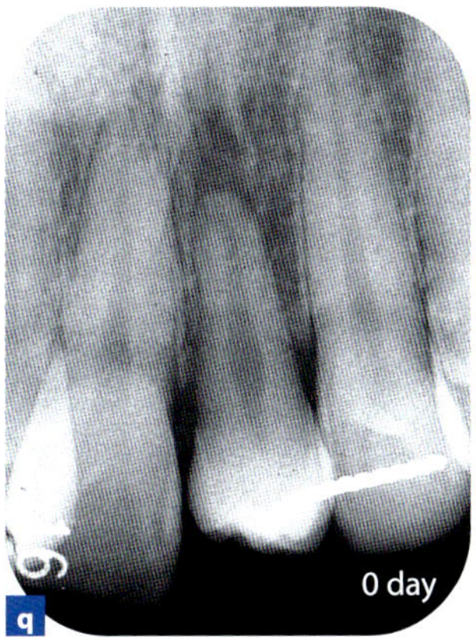

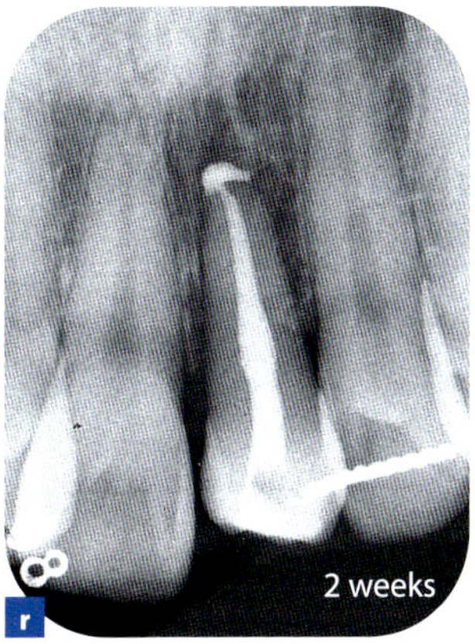

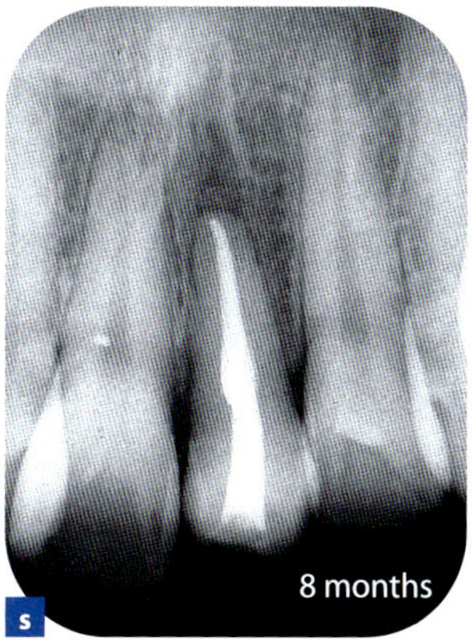

Fig 8-1q Radiograph immediately after transplantation.
Fig 8-1r Two weeks after transplantation. Root canal treatment was initiated and the canal was filled with a calcium hydroxide preparation temporarily.
Fig 8-1s Eight months after transplantation and immediately after root canal filling with sealer and gutta-percha.

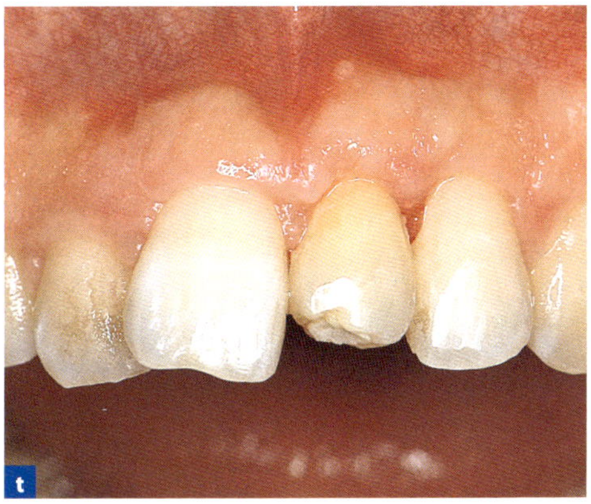

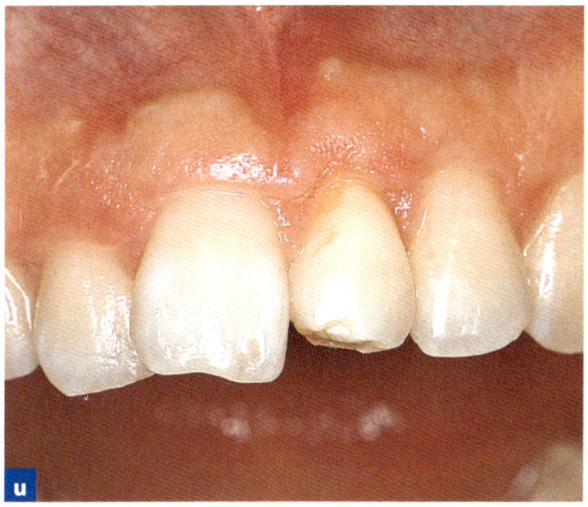

Fig 8-1t Nine months after transplantation and before walking bleach of the transplant.
Fig 8-1u After bleaching. The bleaching method is shown in **Fig 8-4** "Internal Bleaching of a crown of a non-vital tooth"(walking bleach).

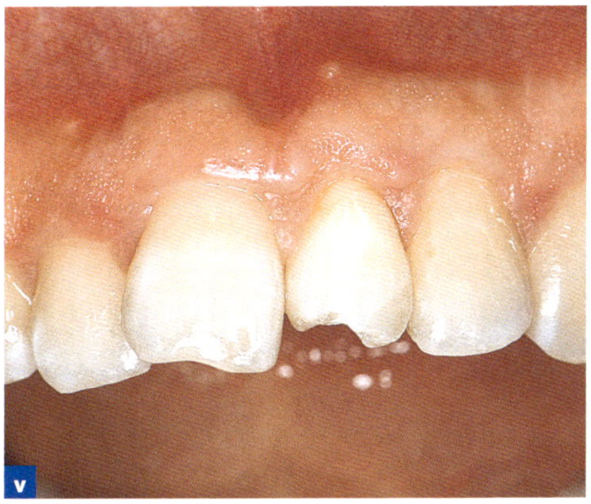

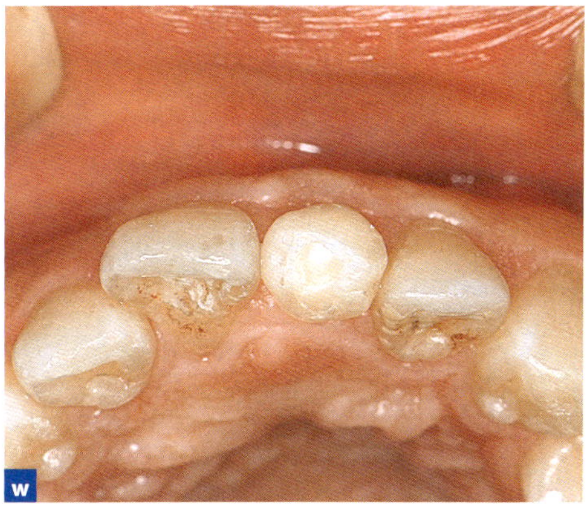

Fig 8-1v and 8-1w Morphology of the crown is modified using direct method of composite resin (CR) restoration.

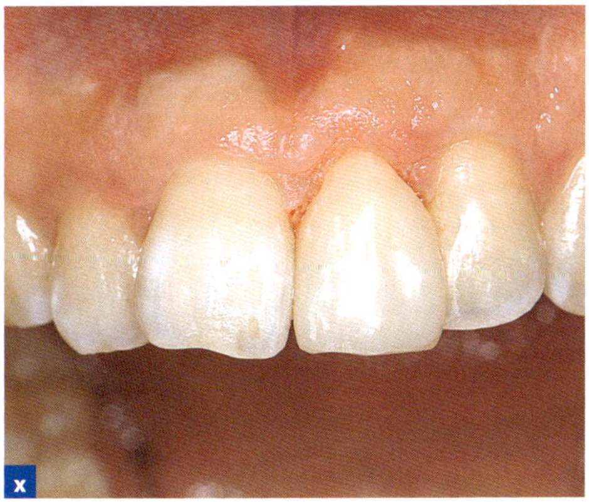

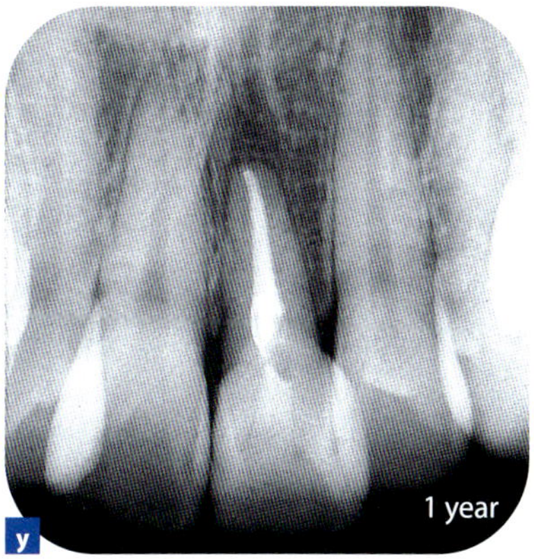

Fig 8-1x The premolar was restored to shape of a central incisor with CR.
Fig 8-1y Radiograph 1 year after surgery.

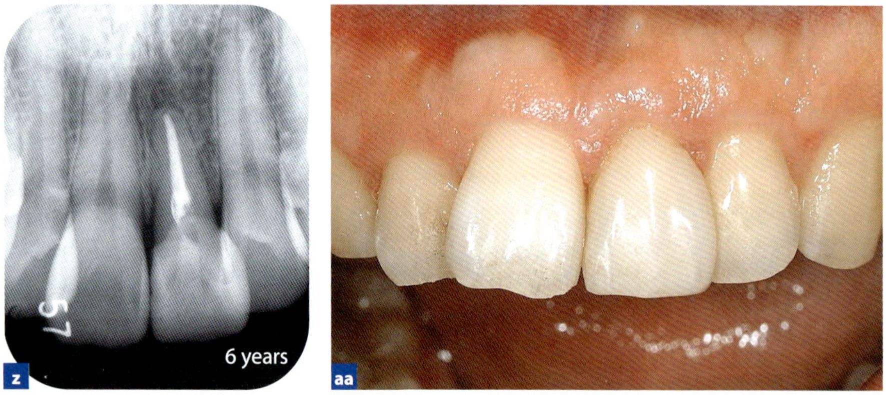

Fig 8-1z and 8-1aa Six years after transplantation. There are no evident problems.

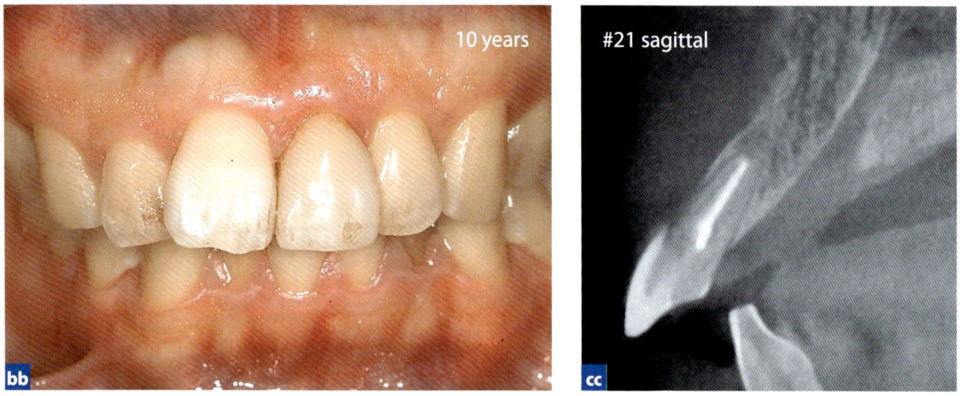

Fig 8-1bb and 8-1cc 10 years after transplantation. No root resorption is observed and newly formed bone on the buccal aspect is evident. The patient is satisfied with the esthetics and function.

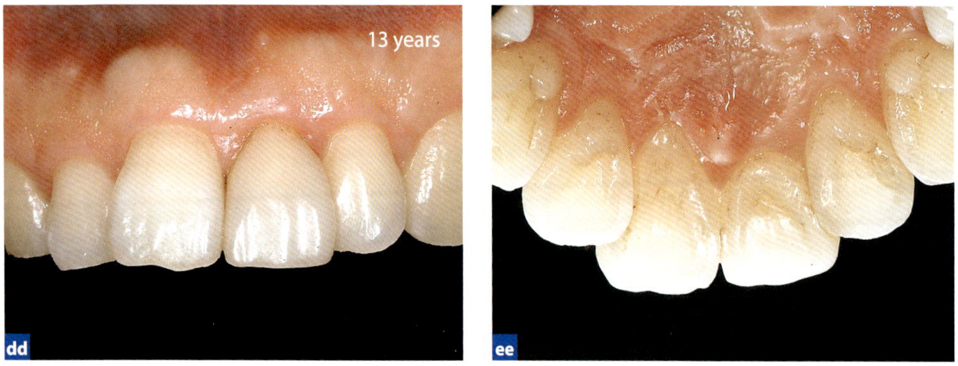

Fig 8-1dd and 8-1ee 13 years after transplantation. Esthetics and function are maintained.

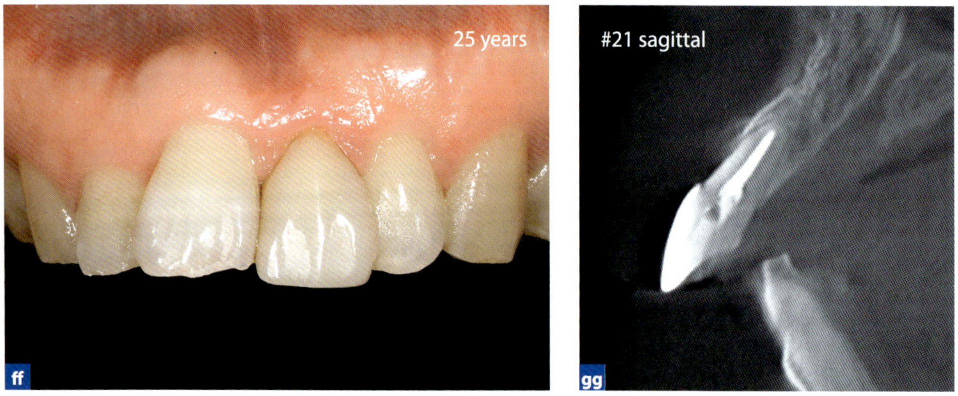

Fig 8-1ff and 8-1gg 25 years after transplantation. There was no root resorption and the buccal bone is maintained.

Case 2. Transplantation of an ectopically erupted premolar to the anterior region

Fig 8-2 shows a case of a 50-year-old male who presented with the chief complaint of pain to #12 that developed a root fracture (**Fig 8-2a** to **8-2e**). The tooth was hopeless and extracted (**Fig 8-2i**). The patient had an ectopically erupted tooth #35 (**Fig 8-2f** and **8-2g**), and there was little effect on occlusion and function even if extracted. As a treatment option after the extraction of #12, the patient chose transplantation, which has

Case 2. Transplantation of an ectopically erupted premolar to the anterior region

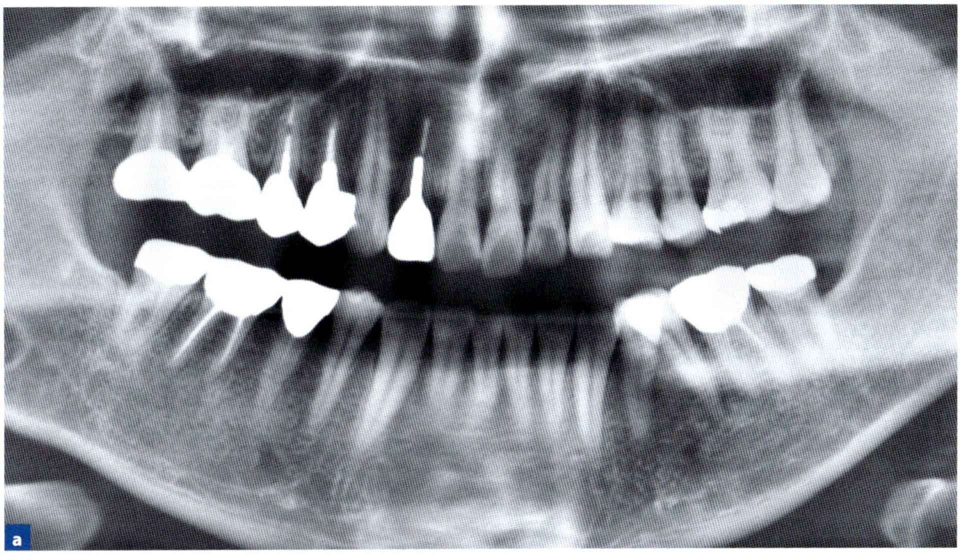

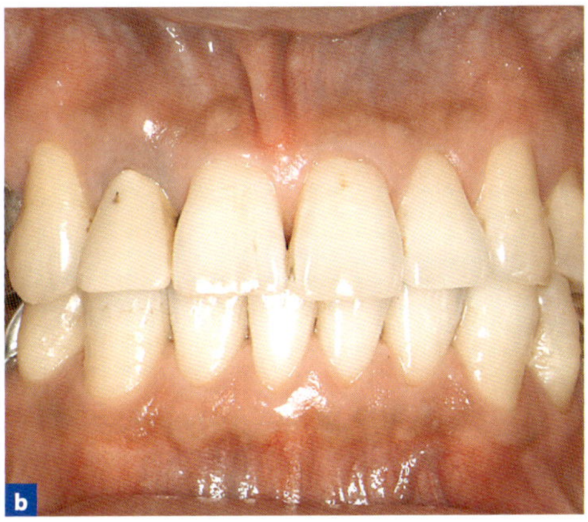

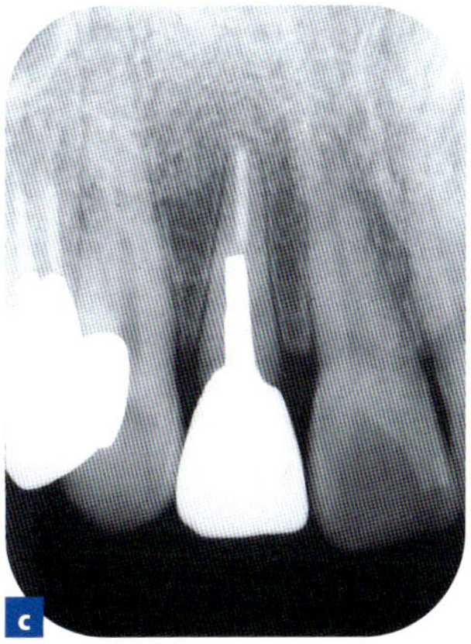

Fig 8-2a to 8-2c Views of the first visit of a 50-year-old male who presented with pain to #12 due to vertical root fracture. The patient preferred transplantation using the ectopically erupted #35 to other options that were available.

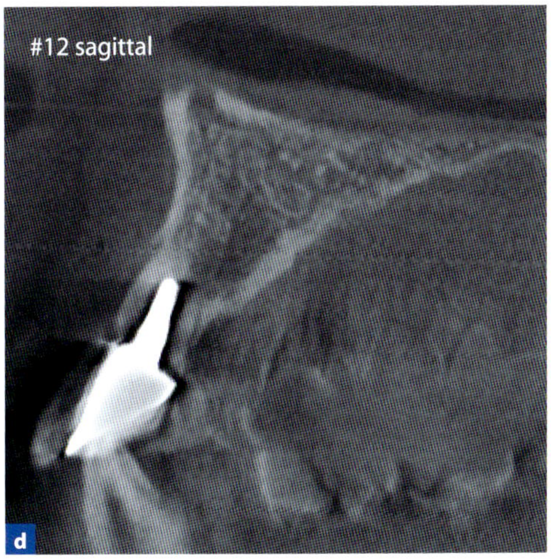

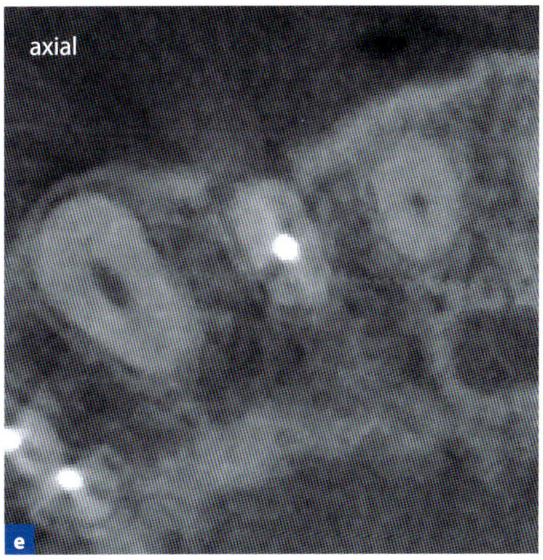

Fig 8-2d and 8-2e Preoperative CBCT images of #12. The bone on the labial side has been resorbed.

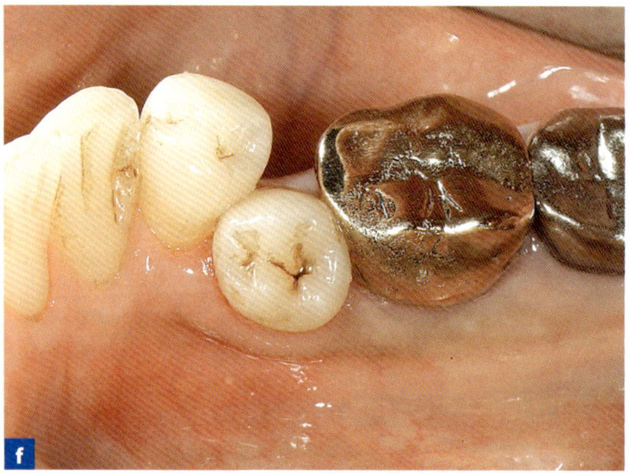

Fig 8-2f Donor tooth before extraction. The space between #34 and #36 will be closed by replacing the crown of #36 after extraction.

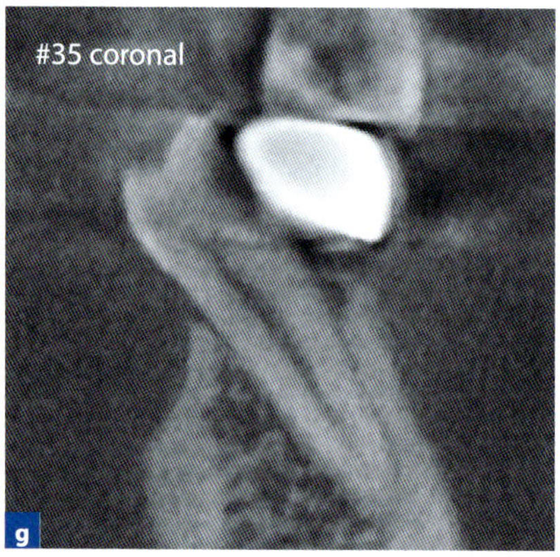

Fig 8-2g CBCT image of the donor tooth before surgery. There are no morphological problems.

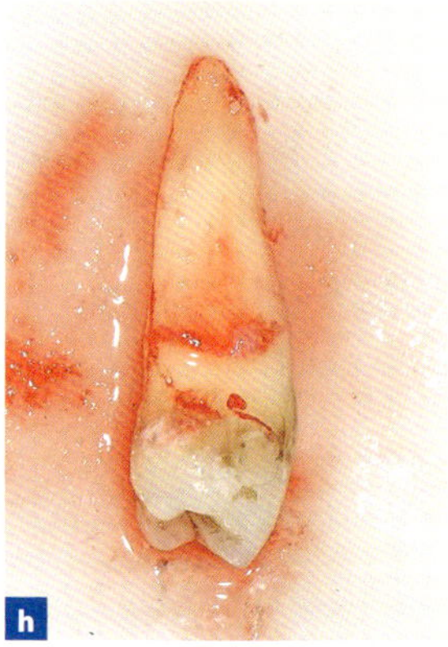

Fig 8-2h Extracted donor tooth.

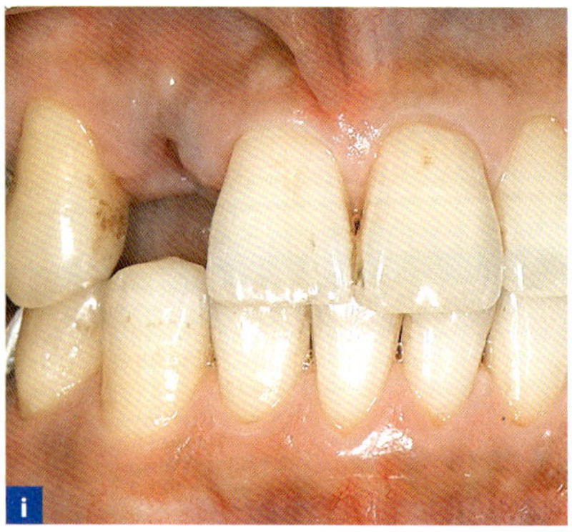

Fig 8-2i Recipient site before surgery where #12 was extracted 2 weeks before.

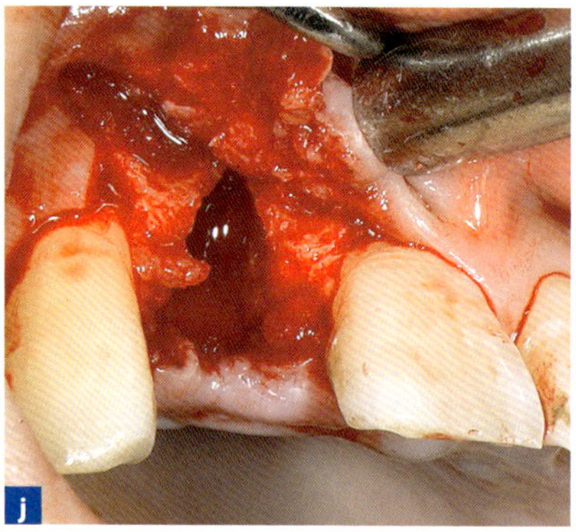

Fig 8-2j View when gingival flap was raised. Loss of buccal bone is observed.

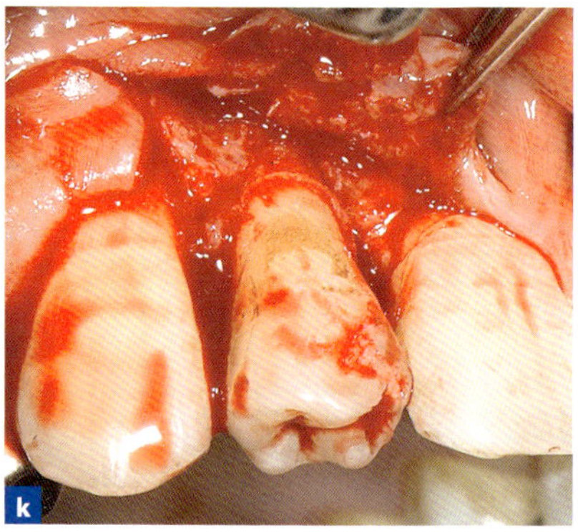

Fig 8-2k After placement of the donor tooth. The root was exposed out of the socket, but no bone graft material was used.

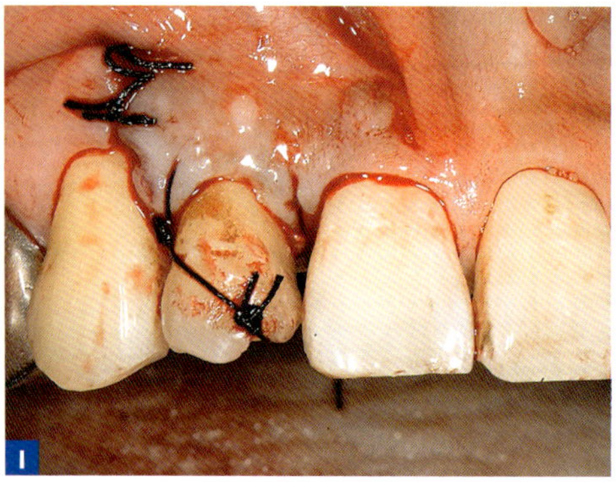

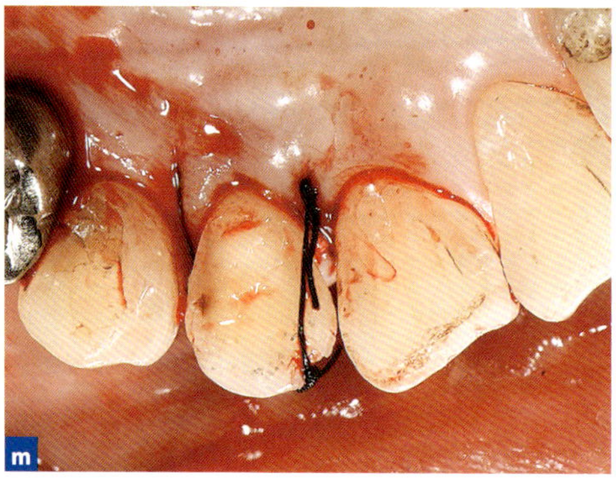

Fig 8-2l and 8-2m Immediately after suture.

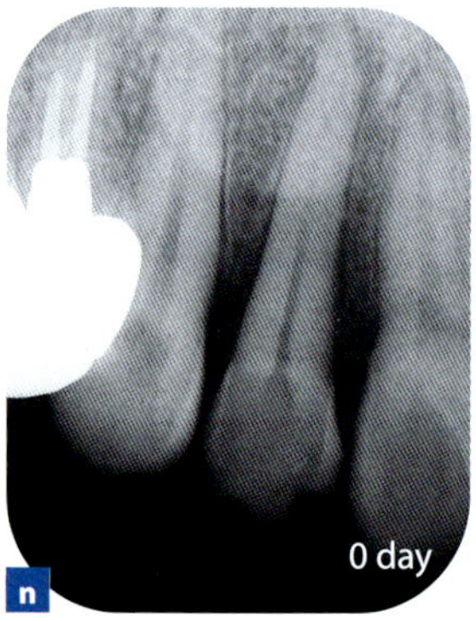

Fig 8-2n Radiograph immediate after surgery.

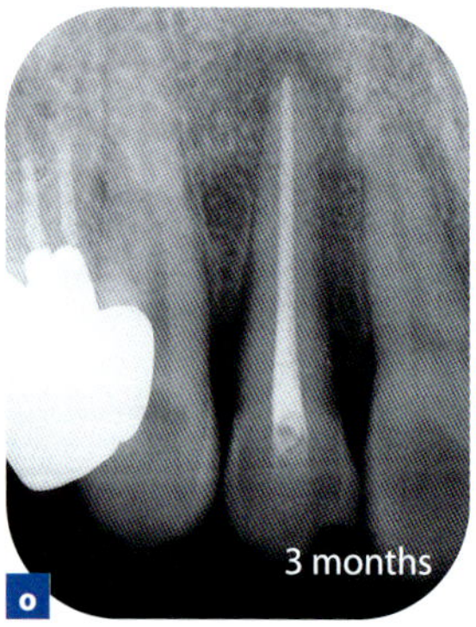

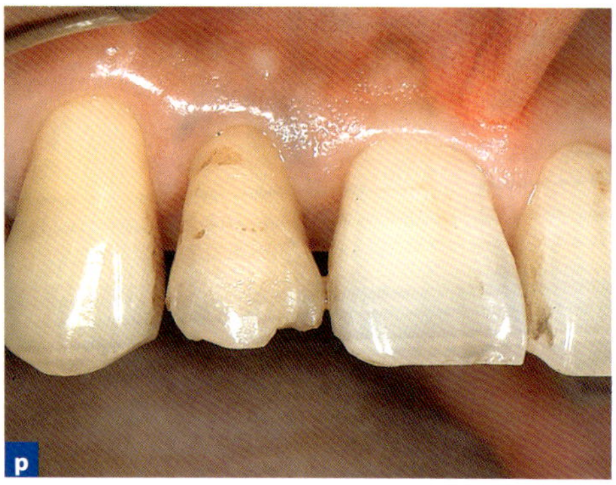

Fig 8-2o to 8-2p Three months after transplantation and before restoration of the crown.

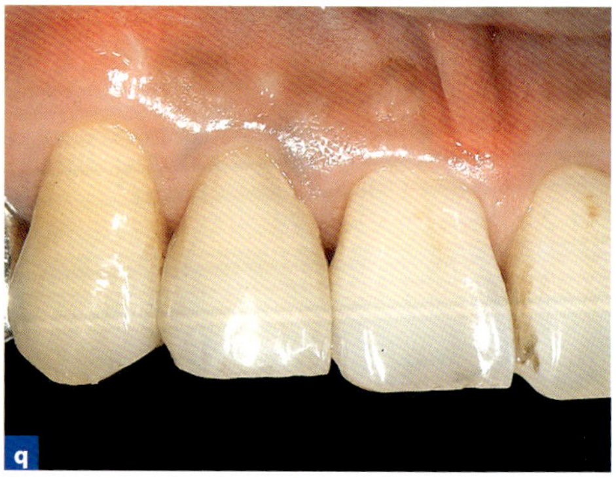

Fig 8-2q Immediately after CR restoration of the transplant.

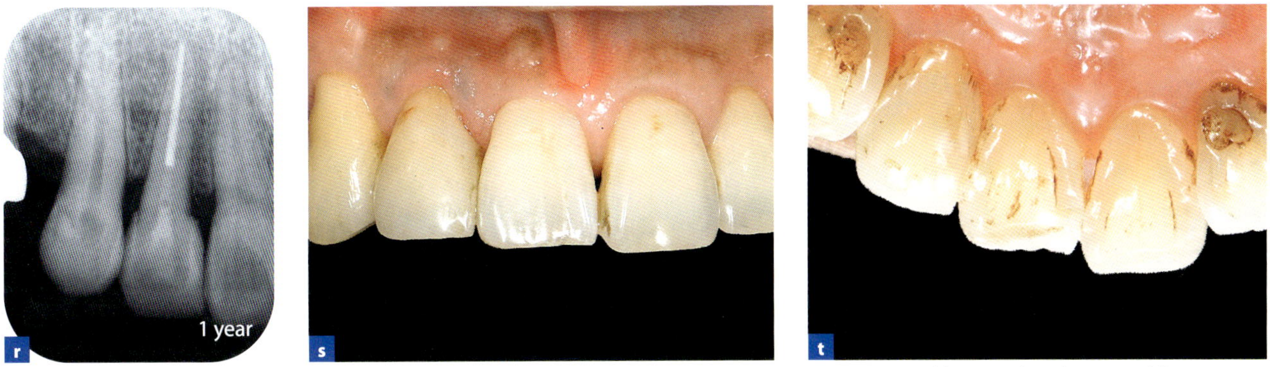

Fig 8-2r to 8-2t One year after transplantation. No root resorption was observed, and there were no problems with esthetics and function.

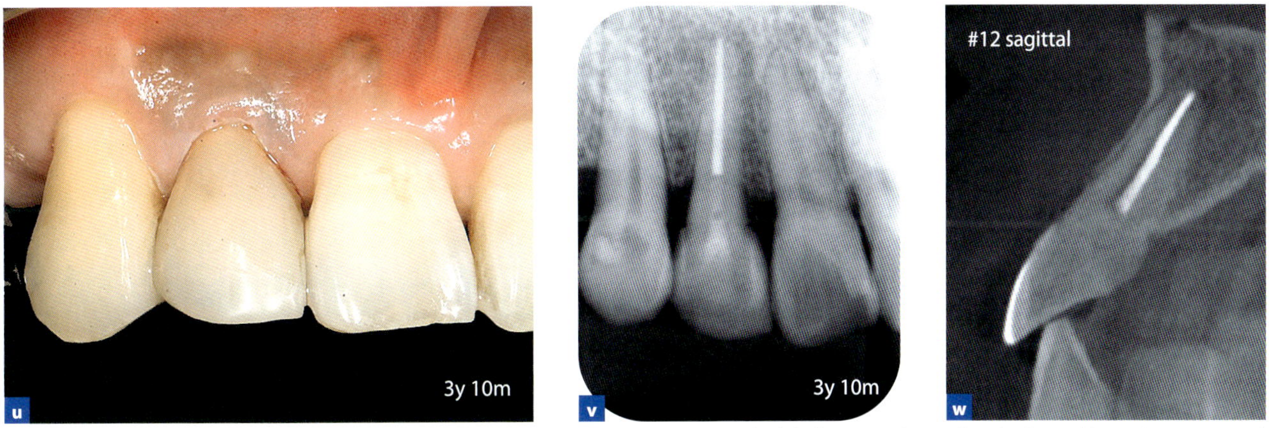

Fig 8-2u to 8-2w Three years and 10 months after transplantation. The CBCT image (right) shows evidence that the buccal bone is regenerated and maintained.

several advantages over removal denture, fixed bridge and implant supported treatment. the alveolar bone on the buccal aspect had been lost before surgery due to the root fracture, but the CBCT imaging shows evidence that it had regenerated after transplantation (**Fig 8-2w**) and the transplant was nicely restored with CR to provide esthetics and to reduce time and cost.

Case 3. Transplantation of a small third molar to the anterior region

Fig 8-3 shows a case of a 34-year-old female who presented with horizontal root fracture of #12 that was thought to be hopeless and was extracted (**Fig 8-3a** to **8-3e**). Fortunately, the patient had a small third molar on the upper jaw available (**Fig 8-3a** and **8-3f**), and she chose transplantation.

Looking at the donor tooth during the surgery, the morphology was by no means ideal (**Fig 8-3g**). In addition, the periodontal ligament was partially lost around the cervical area. Therefore, the postoperative crown-root ratio was not ideal (**Fig 8-3h** to **8-3q**). However, there were no functional or esthetic problems during follow-up period of about 25 years (**Fig 8-3r** to **8-3y**).

Case 3. Transplantation of a small third molar to the anterior region

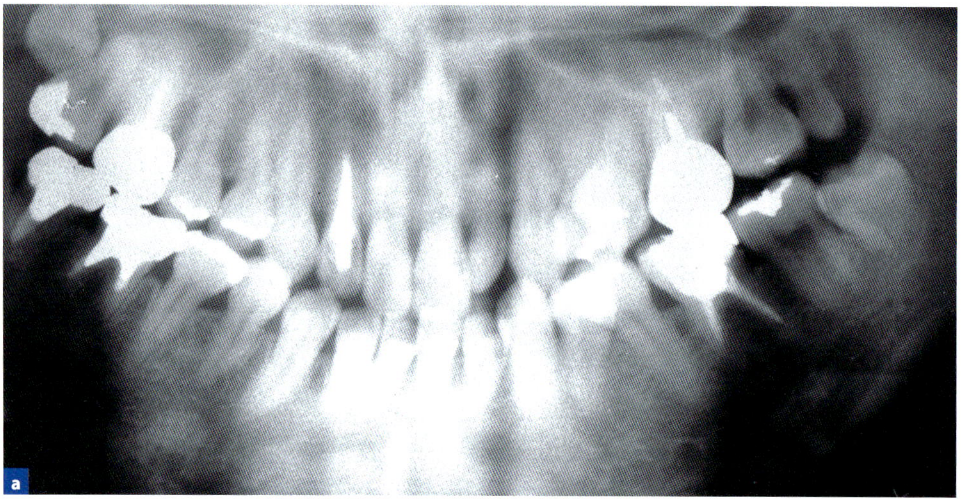

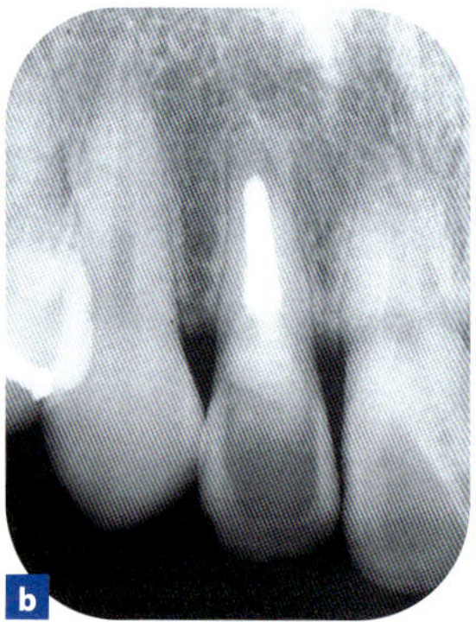

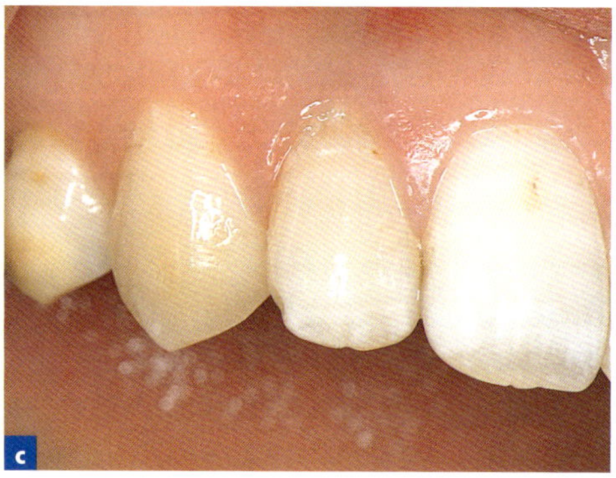

Fig 8-3a to 8-3c Views at the first visit of a 34-year-old female who presented with discomfort to #12. #12 was diagnosed with horizontal root fracture around the cervical area. The patient preserved a tiny third molar which was considered to be a good candidate as a donor tooth for transplantation to replace the hopeless #12.

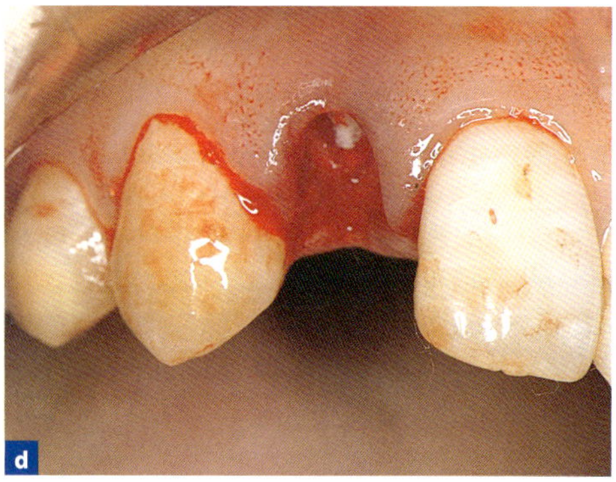

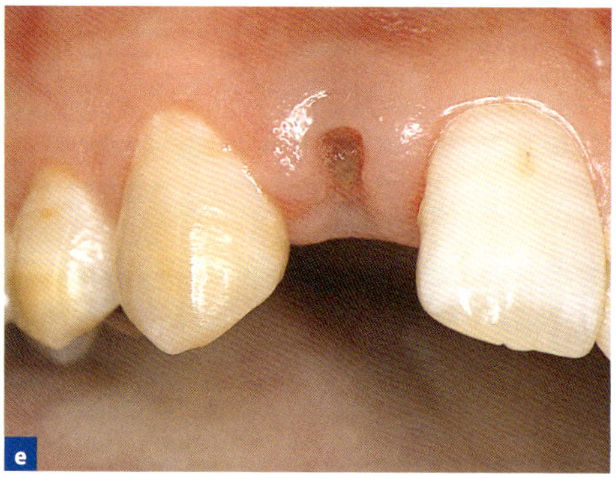

Fig 8-3d View after removing the crown fragment of #12. The tooth was extracted because the remaining root was too short and thin to preserve.
Fig 8-3e Two weeks after tooth extraction and before transplantation.

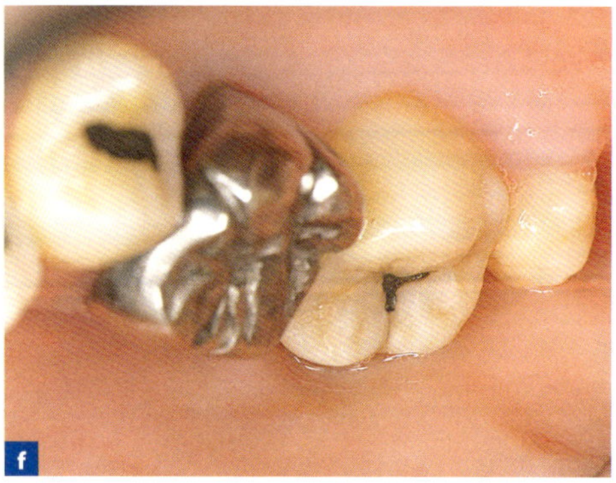

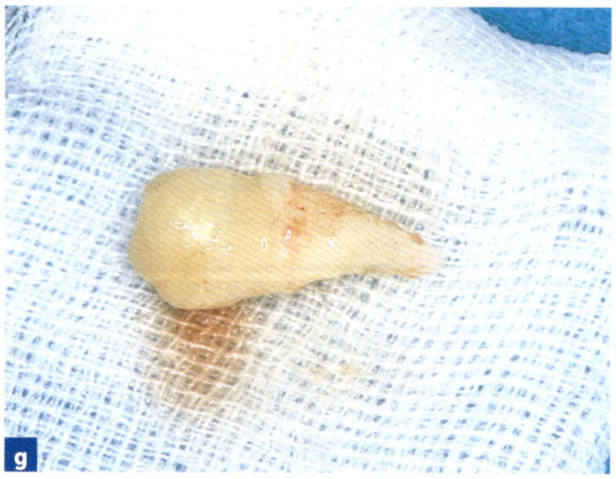

Fig 8-3f Donor tooth before surgery.
Fig 8-3g Extracted donor tooth.

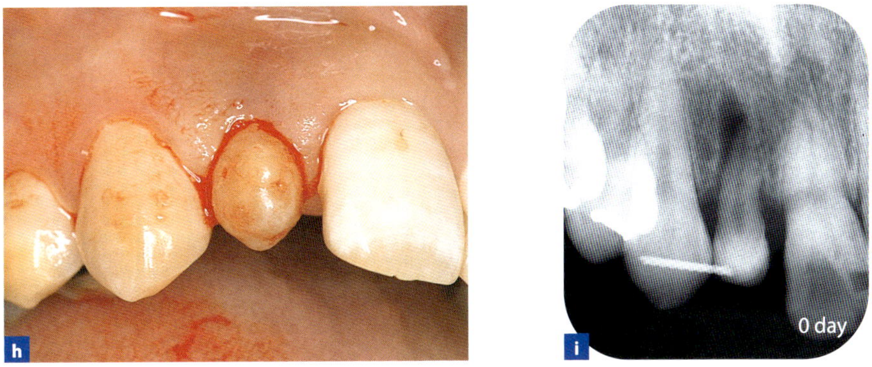

Fig 8-3h Immediate after transplantation.
Fig 8-3i Radiograph immediately after transplantation.

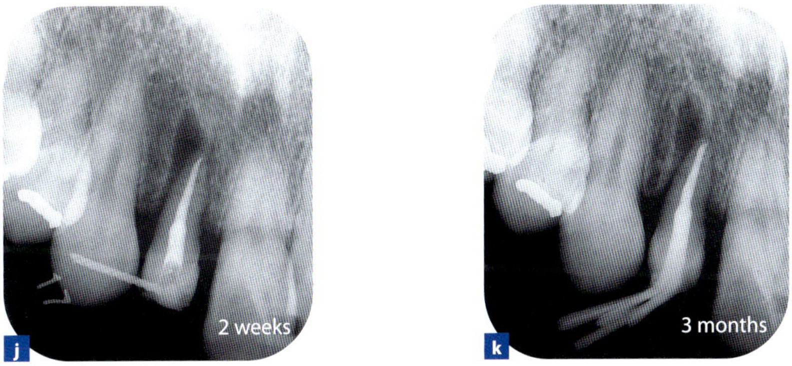

Fig 8-3j Two weeks after transplantation. Immediately after temporary root canal filling with calcium hydroxide preparation.
Fig 8-3k Three months after transplantation. Immediately after root canal filling with sealer and gutta-percha.

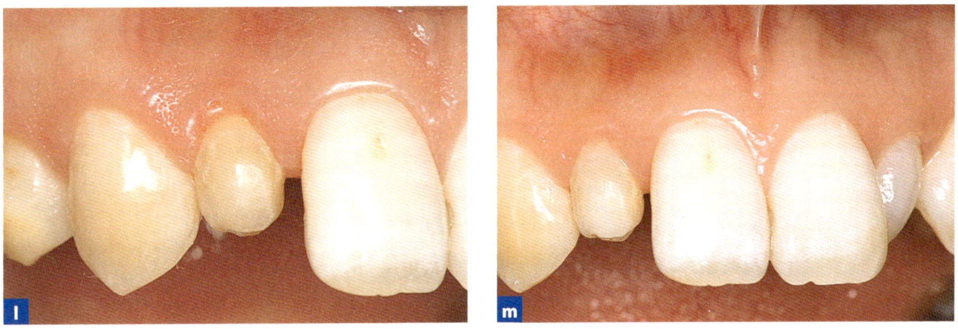

Fig 8-3l Three months after transplantation. The crown color of the transplant is slightly dark.
Fig 8-3m After internal bleaching of the crown (see **Fig 8-4** for bleaching method).

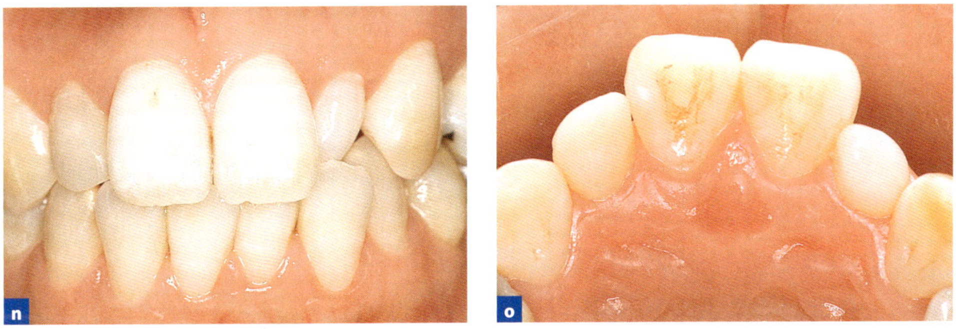

Fig 8-3n and 8-3o After restoration of the crown with CR.

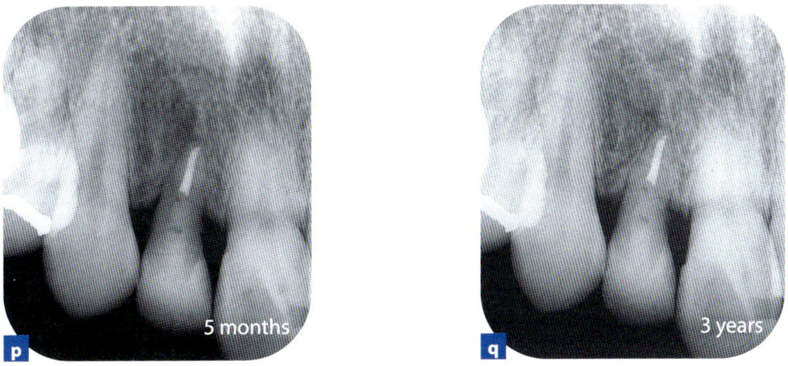

Fig 8-3p Radiograph 5 months after transplantation.
Fig 8-3q Three years after transplantation.

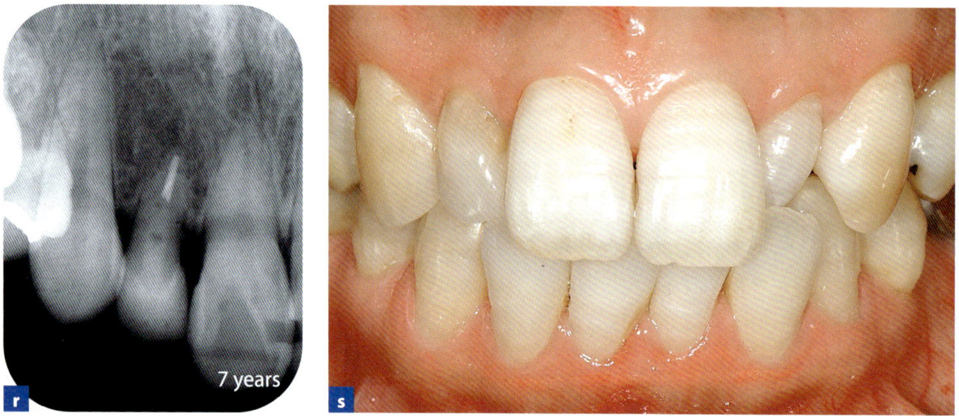

Fig 8-3r and 8-3s Seven years after transplantation.

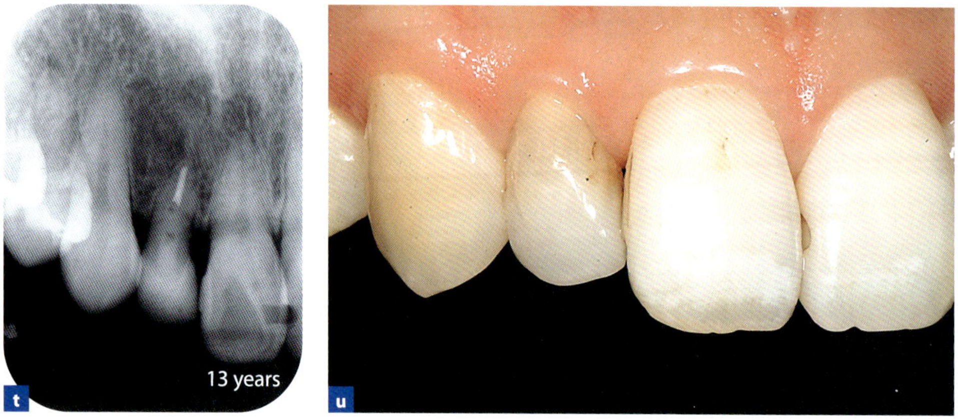

Fig 8-3t and 8-3u 13 years after transplantation. No problems were observed.

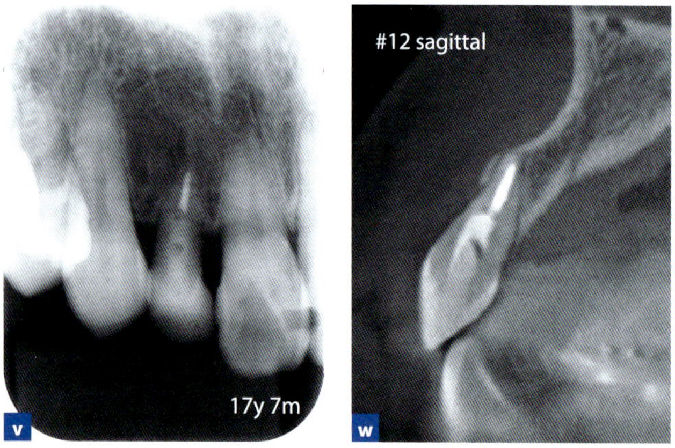

Fig 8-3v and 8-3w 17 years and 7 months after transplantation.

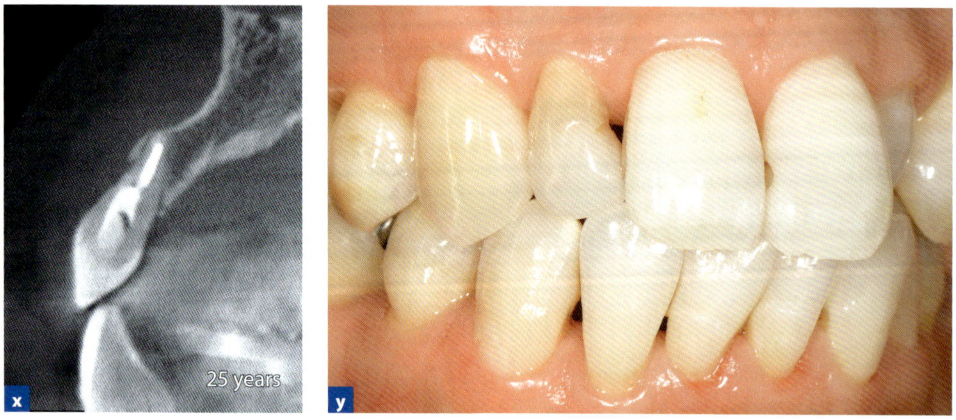

Fig 8-3x CBCT sagittal image of the transplant 25 years after transplantation. No root resorption is observed. The bone level on the labial side is lower than that on the palatal side, but the tooth mobility is normal.

Fig 8-3y Clinical view after 25 years. Slight gingival recession is observed but there are no problems with esthetics and function.

Internal bleaching of a crown of a non-vital tooth (walking bleach)

Before CR restoration of the crown of a transplant, walking bleach is useful for esthetics. It is relatively easy to bleach the crown of a discolored non-vital tooth (**Fig 8-4a** to **8-4c**). After removing the root canal filling material to an appropriate depth (**Fig 8-4d**), the cavity is etched with about 37% phosphoric acid aqueous solution for about 5 seconds to remove the smear layer. A mixture of sodium peroxoborate and 3% hydrogen peroxide solution (or water) is placed directly into the prepared cavity or by wrapping it in Japanese paper (**Fig 8-4e** to **8-4h**), and the cavity is temporarily sealed with glass ionomer cement (**Fig 8-4i**). During temporary placement, one can

Internal bleaching of a crown of a non-vital tooth (walking bleach)

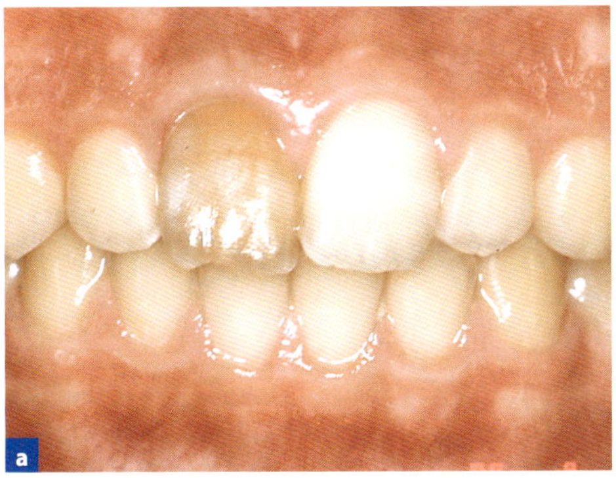

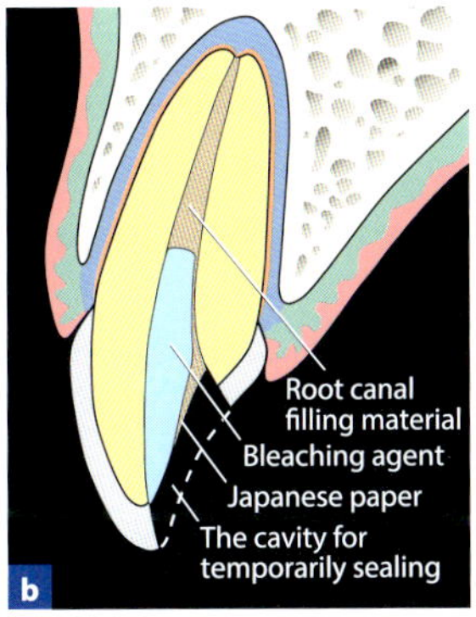

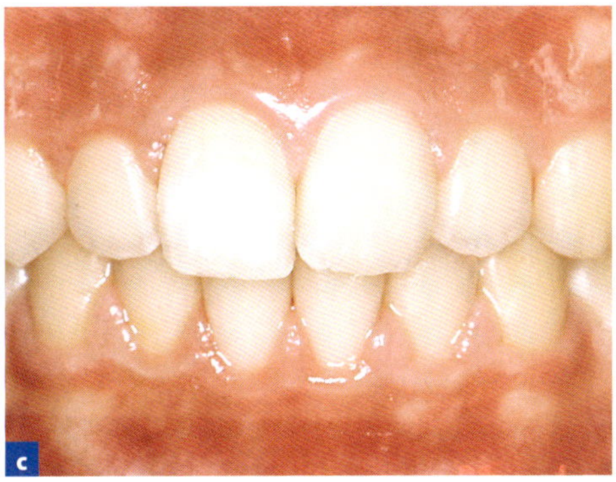

Fig 8-4a Preoperative frontal view of a 12-year-old female. There is dark discoloration of the crown of #11.
Fig 8-4b Schematic diagram showing the technique of walking bleach. Discoloration will be improved by applying bleaching agent to the canal space for 7 to 14 days. The root canal filling material should be removed to an appropriate depth.
Fig 8-4c Two weeks after bleaching. The discoloration has been improved almost to the original color.

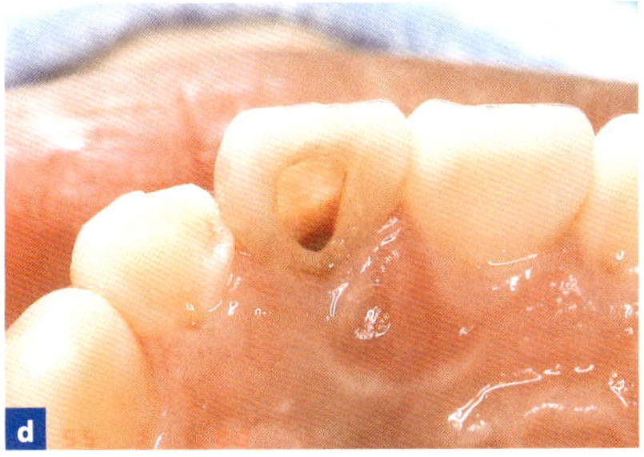

Fig 8-4d View after forming the space for the bleaching agent. The root canal filling material is removed deep enough so that bleaching effect can reach the cervical level. No soft tissue remnants must be left in the pulp horns.

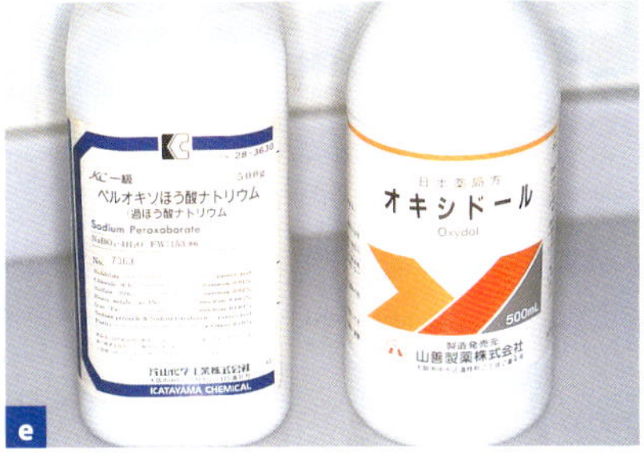

Fig 8-4e Bleaching agent. Prepare sodium peroxoborate and 3% hydrogen peroxide solution. Water can be used instead of 3% hydrogen peroxide.

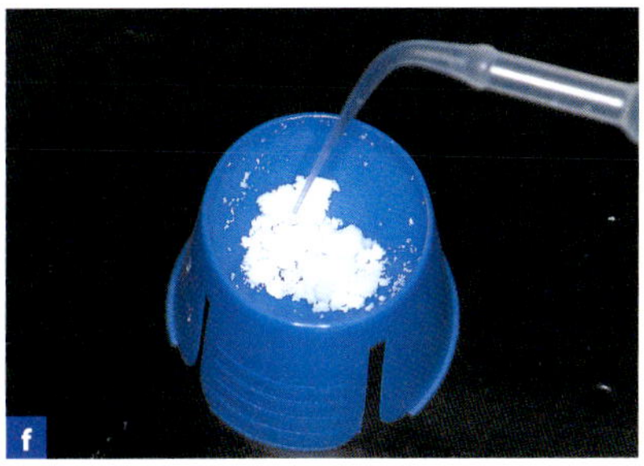

Fig 8-4f Take sodium peroxoborate in a Dappen glass and add an appropriate amount of 3% hydrogen peroxide solution (or water) to make a paste.

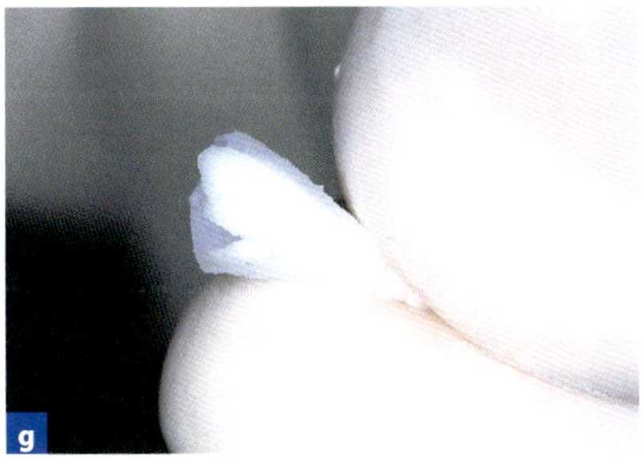

Fig 8-4g Roll an appropriate amount of the paste into Japanese paper.

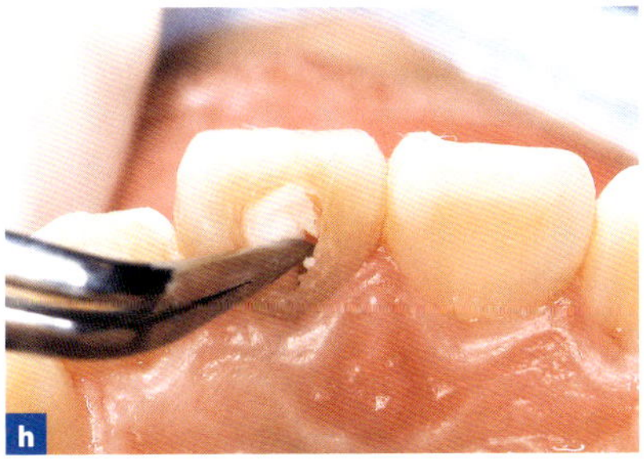

Fig 8-4h Delivery of the paste into the root canal. The paste wrapped in Japanese paper is put into the root canal. It is preferable to cover the inner surface of the canal of the buccal aspect with the paper.

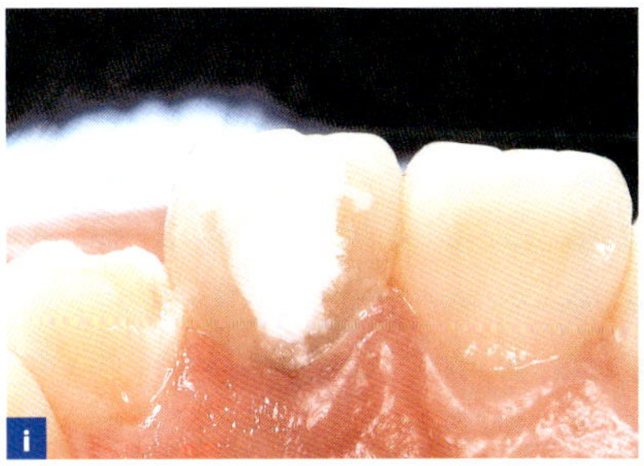

Fig 8-4i Sealing the access hole. The access hole is sealed with conventional glass ionomer cement. It is recommended to hold it with a gloved fingers coated with Vaseline until the glass ionomer cement sets.

achieve a good seal by holding the cavity area firmly with your fingers until the temporary sealing material sets. The bleaching effect usually appears in 7 to 14 days, but if improvement is not obtained, repeat the same procedure until the desired result is achieved.

Looking back on the 3 cases discussed above, transplantation cases to anterior regions may be a more rare occurrence. Several things have to be in place at the right time for this treatment option to be available, but if it is and the clinician has the knowledge and skill to perform the transplantation, results can be of such great benefit to the patient.

CHAPTER 9

Autotransplantation of teeth in orthodontic treatment

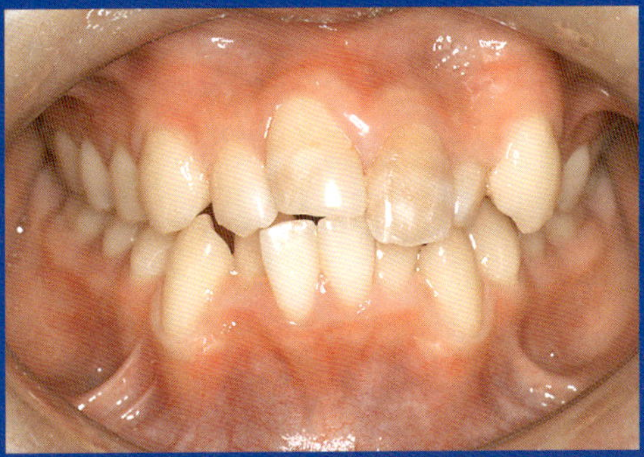

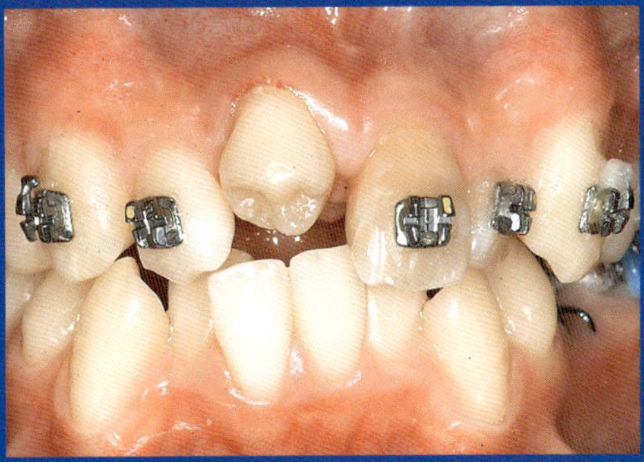

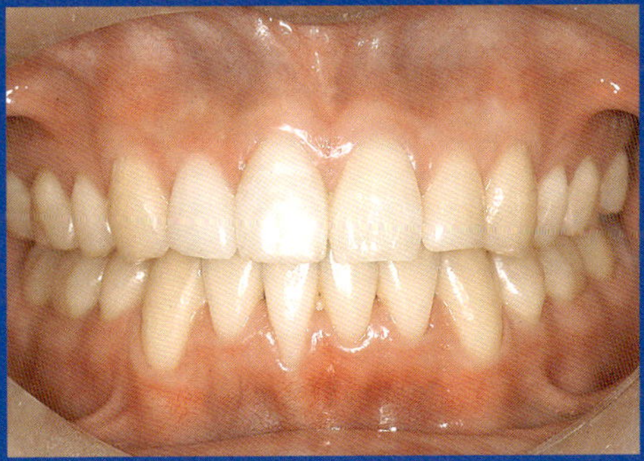

The following are reasons why there is an important role of transplantation in orthodontic treatment:

(1) Some orthodontic patients have malocclusion caused by congenitally missing teeth.

(2) There are cases in which premolar teeth are extracted strategically as part of the orthodontic treatment plan, and these teeth can be suitable for transplantation to the anterior and premolar regions as donor teeth.

(3) Since transplanted teeth respond to orthodontic tooth movement in the same way as other natural teeth, transplantation can be performed even in young patients undergoing growth and development of bodies and jaws, etc.

Also, in adult orthodontics, if there are root canal treated teeth for which long-term prognosis is doubtful, transplantation should be considered in treatment planning by replacing them with preserved third molars or strategically extracted teeth.

This chapter mainly discusses the usefulness of transplantation in orthodontic treatment for patients who suffer congenital missing teeth and those who have lost teeth due to trauma.

Case 1. Orthodontic treatment for a patient with congenitally missing teeth

Fig 9-1 shows a case of a 12-year-old female who presented with the chief complaint of spaces in the arch due to congenitally missing teeth. As can be seen in the panoramic radiographs, #15, #12, #22, #25 were congenitally missing, while the mandibular dentition was intact (**Fig 9-1a** and **9-1b**). In this case, it was considered appropriate to transplant two second premolars in the mandible to the maxillary second premolar sites in conjunction with orthodontic treatment.

In orthodontic treatment which may benefit from strategic extractions, the first premolar is often chosen. However, based on the author's long-term experience, the morphology of the roots of the second premolars is typically much more suitable for transplantation than the first premolars. In this case as well, the mandibular second premolars were chosen as donor teeth from not only a morphological but also from a developmental stage viewpoint. At the initial examination, the root development of the first premolars were almost complete and it was less likely to expect pulpal healing. Furthermore, considering that extraction of immature teeth can be more easily carried out with less risk of damage to the periodontal ligament, the second premolars were chosen as the donor teeth.

There are some points to note in cases where second primary molars are extracted and premolars are transplanted:

1. It is necessary to avoid immediate transplantation on the same day as extraction of the recipient site. The reason is that the width of the socket of primary second molars is wider than that of the root diameter of permanent premolars, making it difficult to close transplanted teeth tightly with the gingival flap. Therefore, as was done in this case, it is better to perform transplantation 2-3 weeks after extraction of primary teeth (**Fig 9-1c** to **9-1u**). This increases the amount of keratinized gingiva and makes it easier to achieve a tighter closure of the gingival flap around the transplanted teeth.

2. The floor of the maxillary sinus is often located coronally and in close proximity to the socket of the extracted teeth (**Fig 9-1f** to **9-1i**). If the sinus floor is too close, then a maxillary sinus floor elevation will be necessary at the time of the transplantation. Maxillary sinus elevation surgery for transplantation is relatively easier than with implant related treatment (**Fig 9-1j** to **9-1u**) and the procedure is explained in **Chapter 5 Fig 5-5**).

There are some questions that come up about if and when transplanted teeth can undergo orthodontic movement. Theoretically, it is best to wait until the periodontal ligament has completely healed, so in young patients who heal quickly, orthodontic tooth movement can be performed around 3 months after transplantation. But in transplantation of very immature teeth, there will be less risk if one can wait for orthodontic movement until the root development has completed to some extent because the roots may be affected by movement (i.e. curvature formation of the root). If the desired movement is in the extrusive direction only, the transplant can be moved one month after surgery because the periodontal ligament is not undergoing compressive forces.

By taking the above discussions into consideration, transplanted teeth can be expected to heal (periodontal ligament healing, bone healing, pulp healing, and root development) while achieving the goals of orthodontic treatment. (**Fig 9-1v** to **9-1ll**).

Case 1. Orthodontic treatment for a patient with congenitally missing teeth

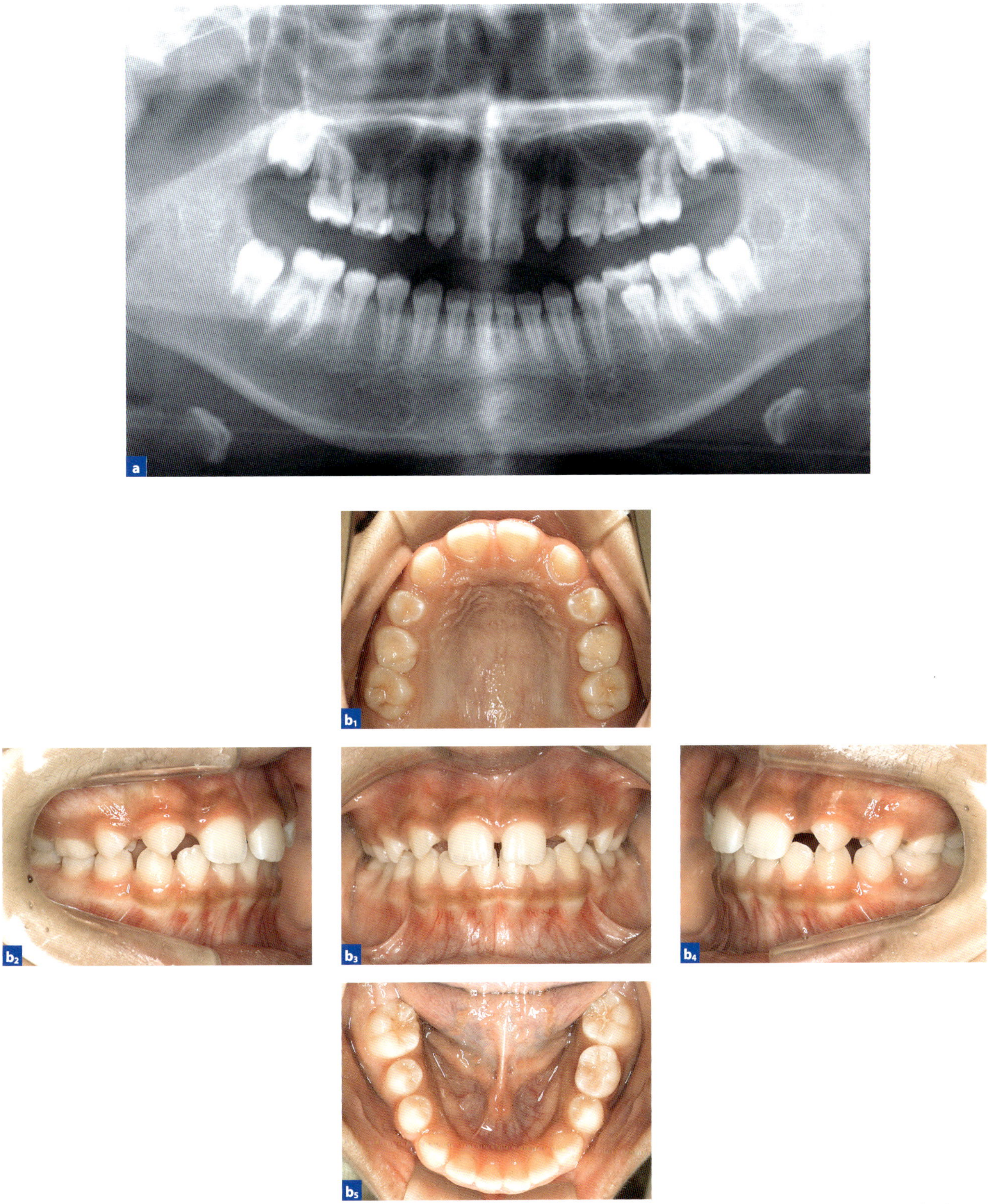

Fig 9-1a and 9-1b Preoperative panoramic radiograph and intraoral photographs of a 12-year-old female. She presented with the chief complaint of spacing between her teeth and wished to pursue orthodontic treatment. #15, #12, #22 and #25 in the maxilla were congenitally missing and there were no missing teeth in the mandibular arch. After analysis and diagnosis of the case, it was decided to transplant the lower second premolars to the upper sites.

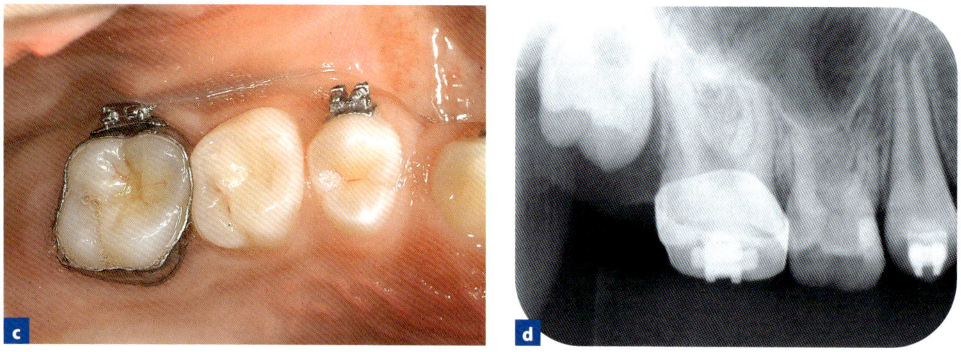

Fig 9-1c and 9-1d Views of the preoperative maxillary right recipient site. Since #55 has wider cross-section of the root than that of #45, it is more favorable to perform delayed transplantation.

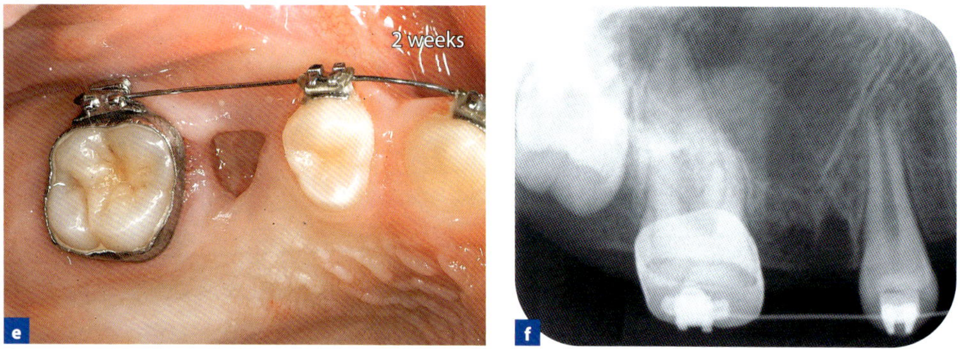

Fig 9-1e and 9-1f Two weeks after #55 extraction. Sufficient amount of keratinized gingiva is now available to obtain good closure around the transplanted tooth.

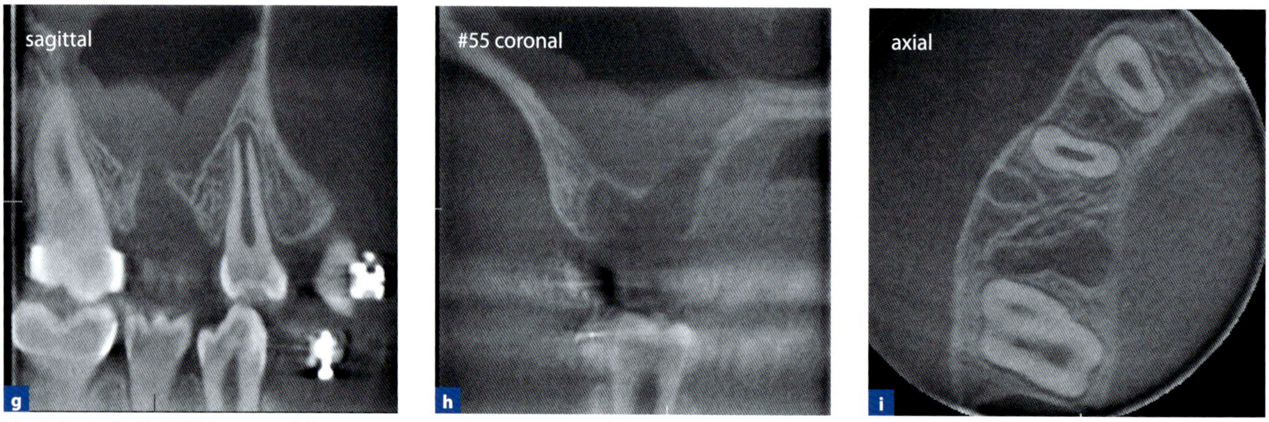

Fig 9-1g to 9-1i CBCT images of the recipient site after extraction of #55. The extraction socket and the floor of the maxillary sinus are separated only by a thin layer of bone. Therefore, maxillary sinus elevation surgery was necessary at the time of transplantation.

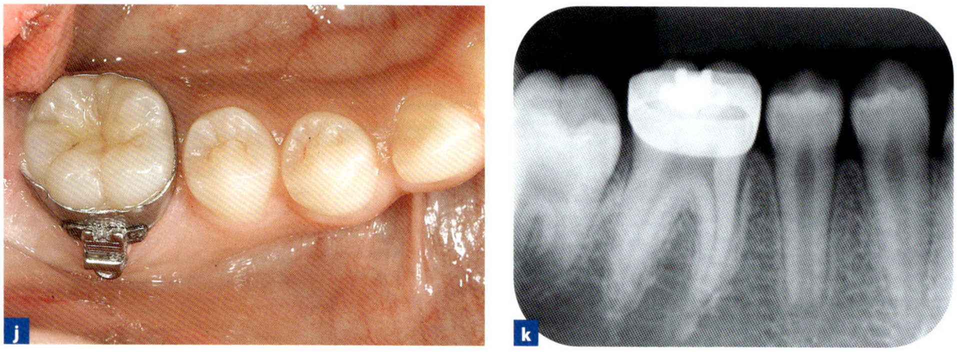

Fig 9-1j and 9-1k Donor tooth before surgery. The root formation appears to be four-fifths complete, but the apex was still wide open.

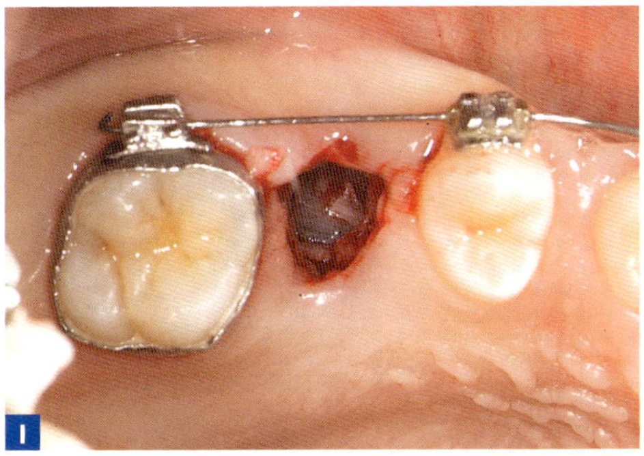

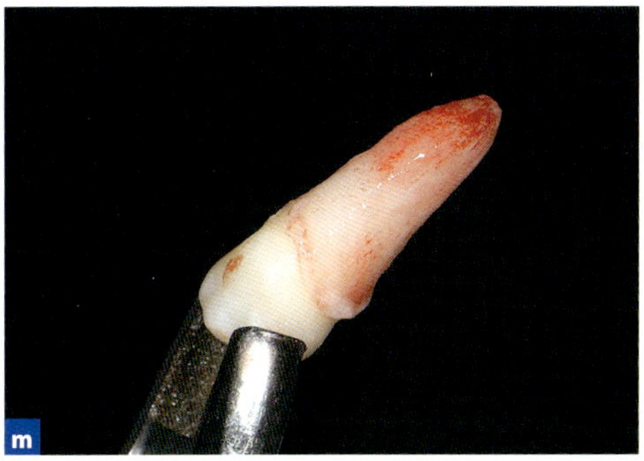

Fig 9-1l View after sinus floor elevation (crestal approach).
Fig 9-1m Extracted donor tooth.

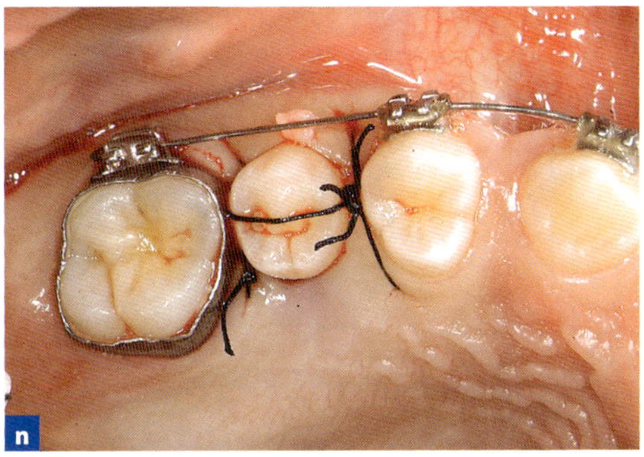

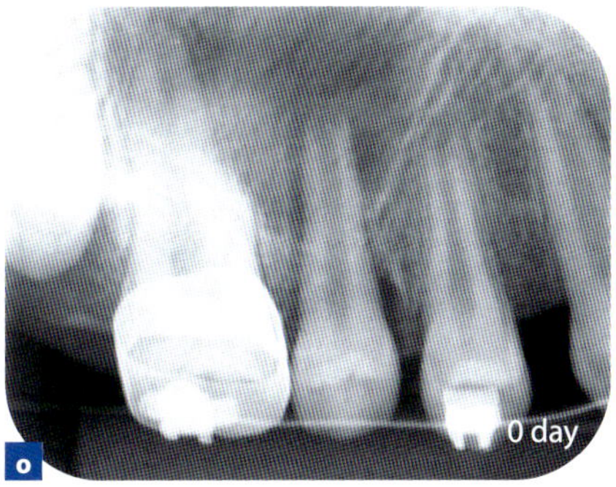

Fig 9-1n and 9-1o Immediately after transplantation. The transplant was deeply placed in the maxillary sinus. No bone graft material was used.

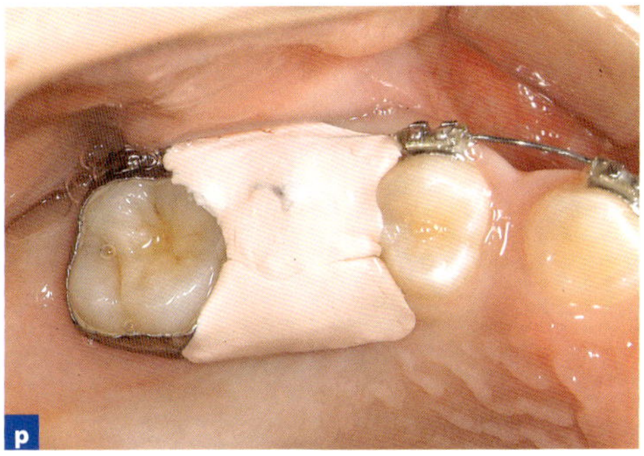

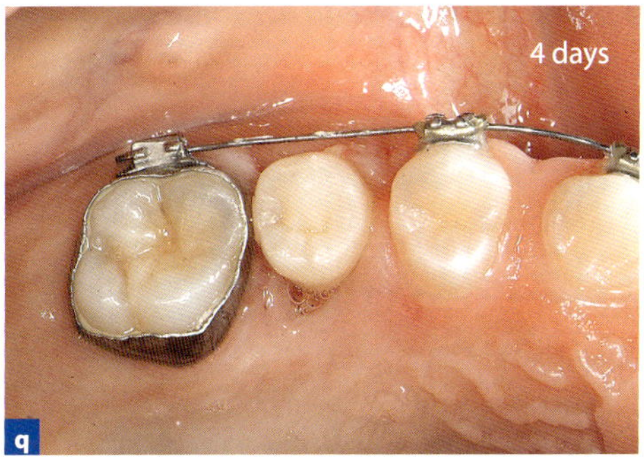

Fig 9-1p Coverage and protection of the wound site by surgical dressing.
Fig 9-1q Four days after surgery. Immediately after surgical dressing and suture removal. Since the transplant was stable (low tooth mobility), wire and resin splinting was not applied.

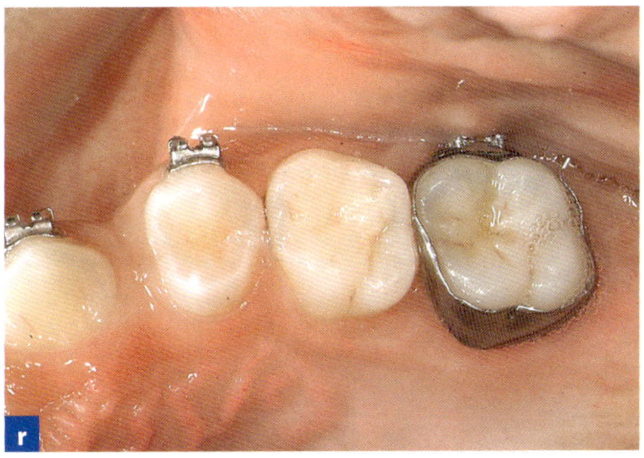

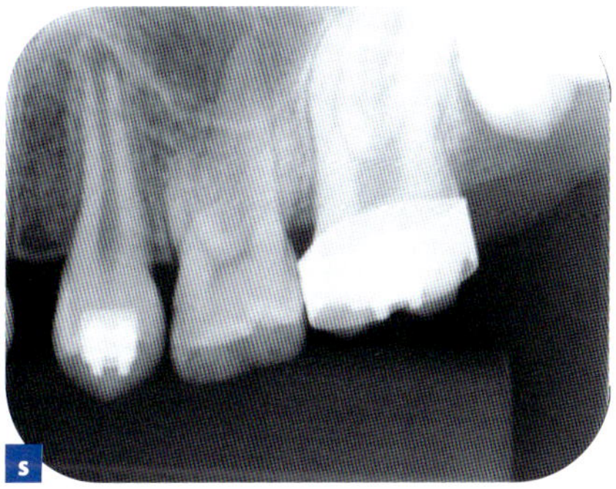

Fig 9-1r and 9-1s Views of the maxillary left recipient site before transplantation. One month after the first transplantation, the contralateral transplantation was performed.

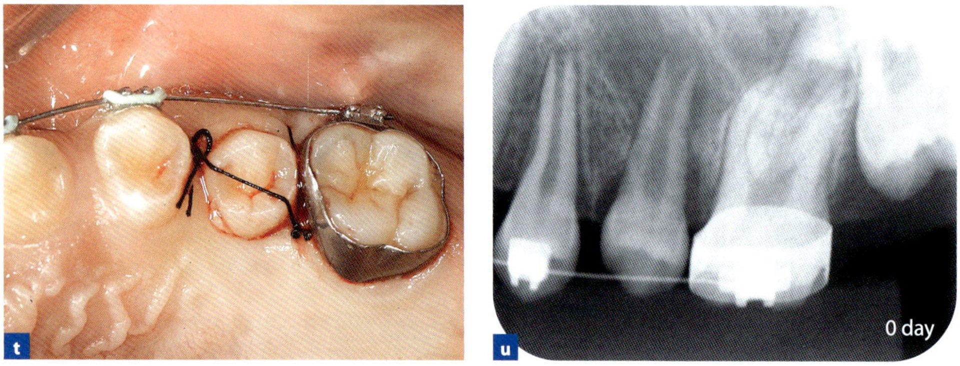

Fig 9-1t and 9-1u Immediately after transplantation. In the same way as the right side, the transplantation was performed with sinus elevation.

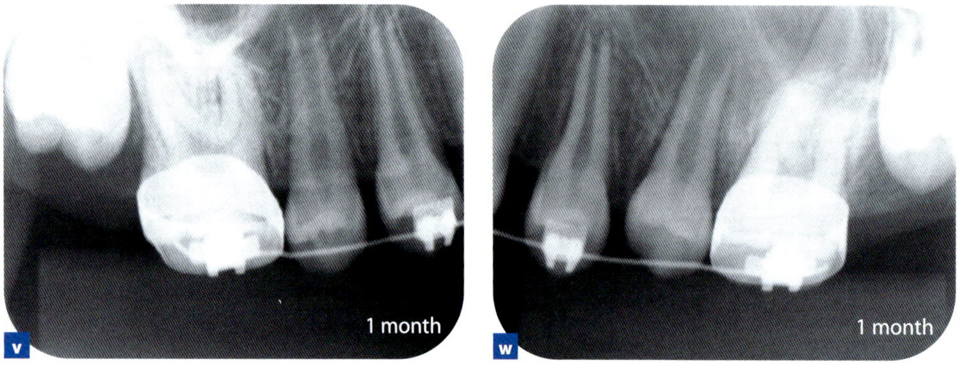

Fig 9-1v and 9-1w Radiographs 1 month after transplantation. It seems that bone regeneration is already occurring around the transplants.

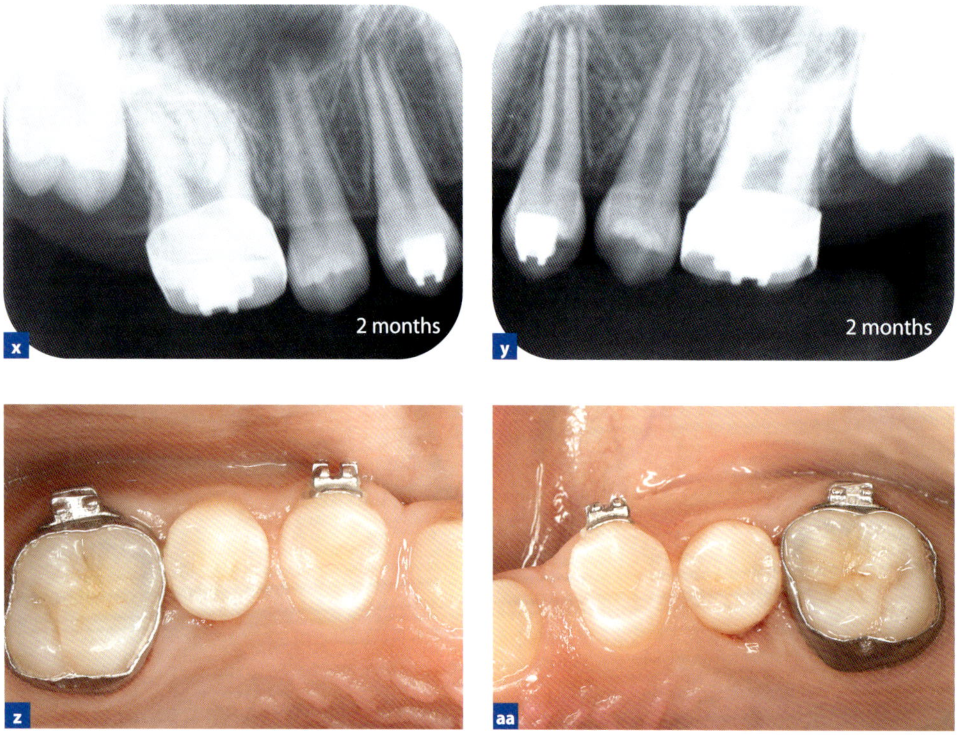

Fig 9-1x to 9-1aa Two months postop. Normal healing appears to be occurring.

Fig 9-1bb Seven months postop on the right side. The transplant responded EPT(+). The root appears to be surrounded by new bone.

Fig 9-1cc Six months postop on the left side. The transplant responded EPT(+). The root appears to be surrounded by new bone.

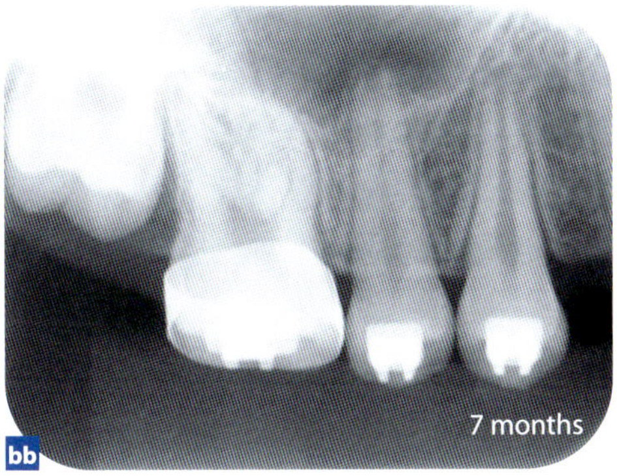

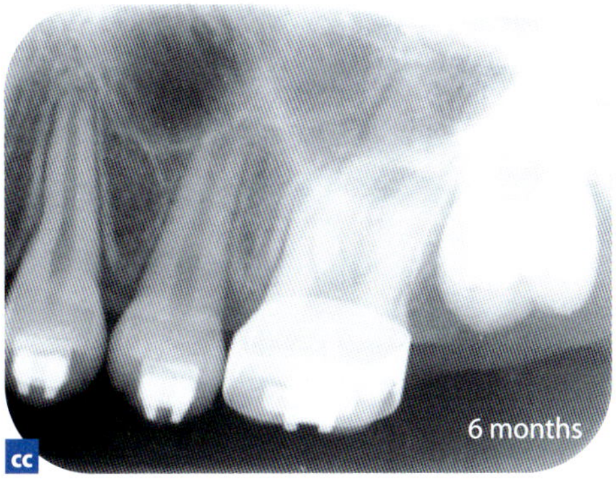

Fig 9-1dd Radiograph 1 year and 7 months after transplantation on the right side. Pulp canal obliteration of the transplant (a sign of pulp healing) and root development were observed.

Fig 9-1ee Radiograph 1 year and 6 months after transplantation on the left side. Pulp canal obliteration of the transplant and root development were observed.

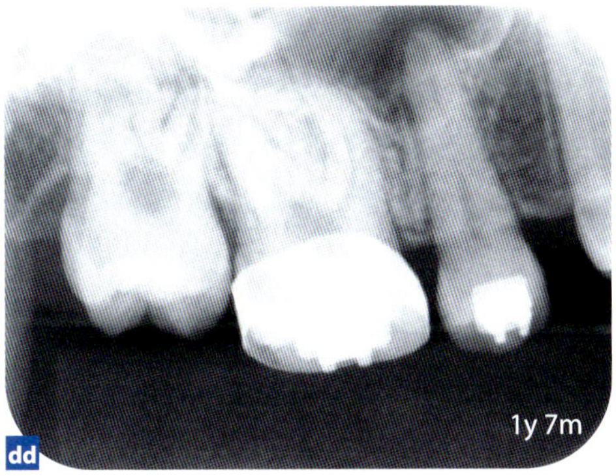

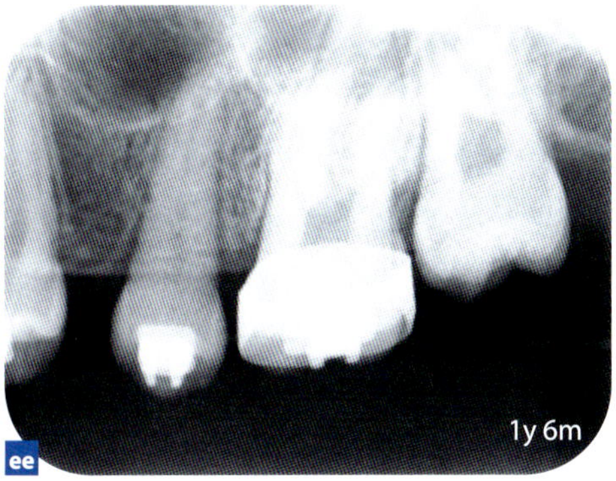

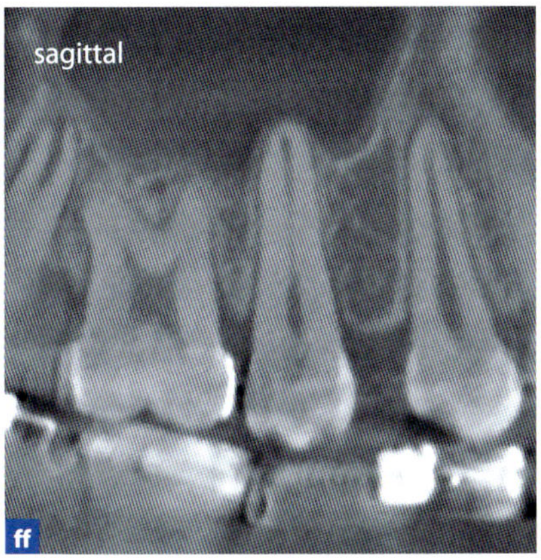

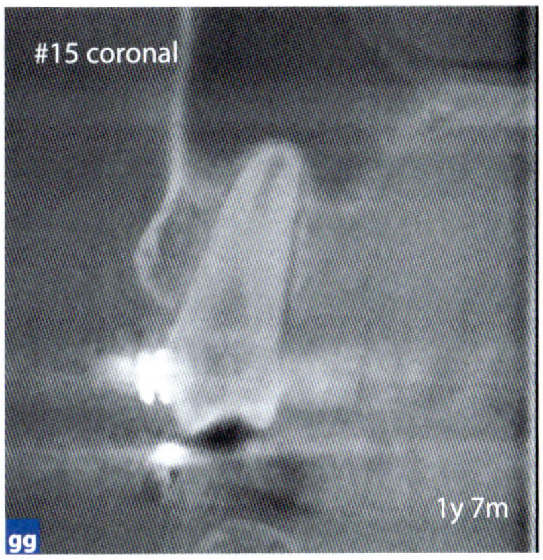

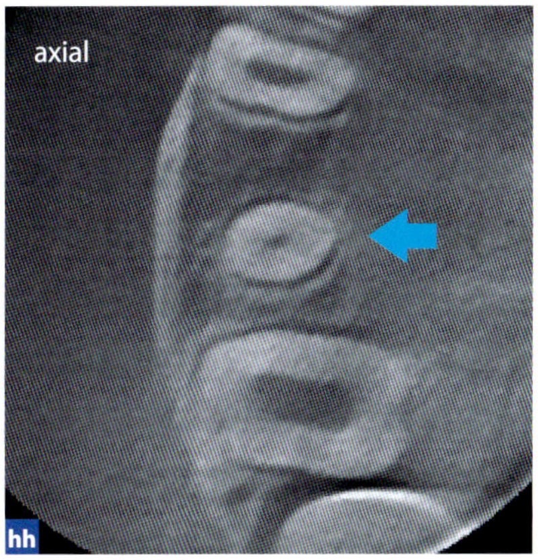

Fig 9-1ff to 9-1hh CBCT images 1 year and 7 months after transplantation on the right side. Pulp canal obliteration and new bone formation around the root were observed.

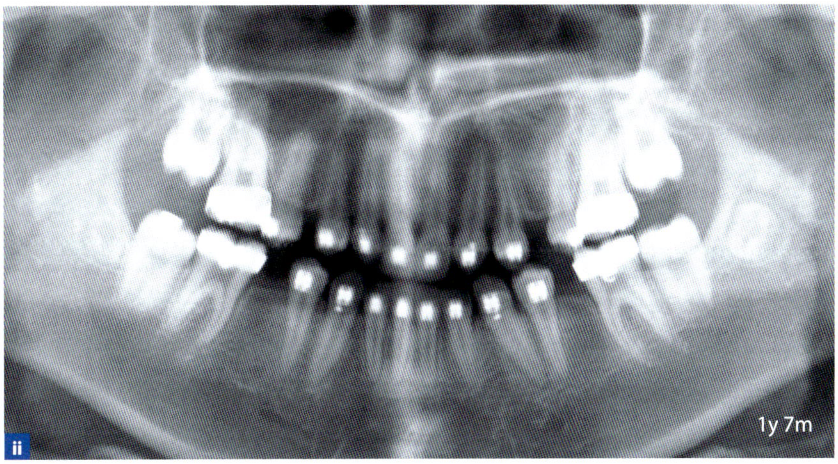

Fig 9-1ii Panoramic radiograph 1 year and 7 months after the first transplantation.

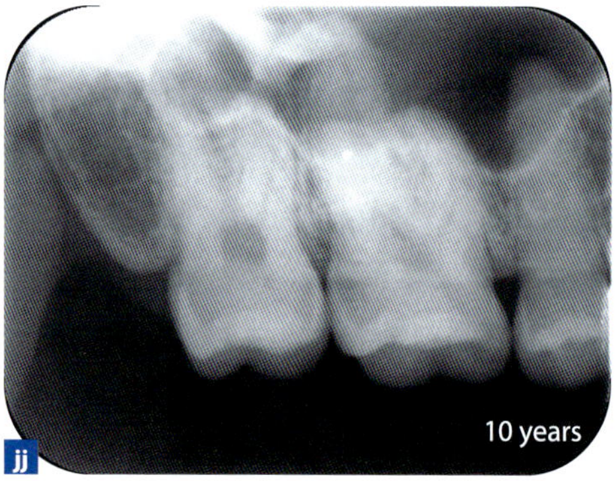

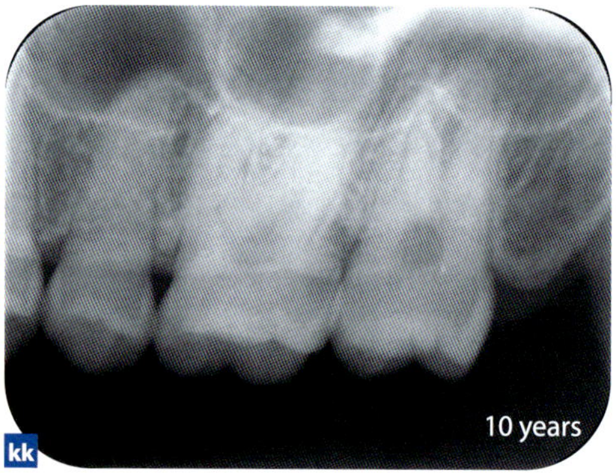

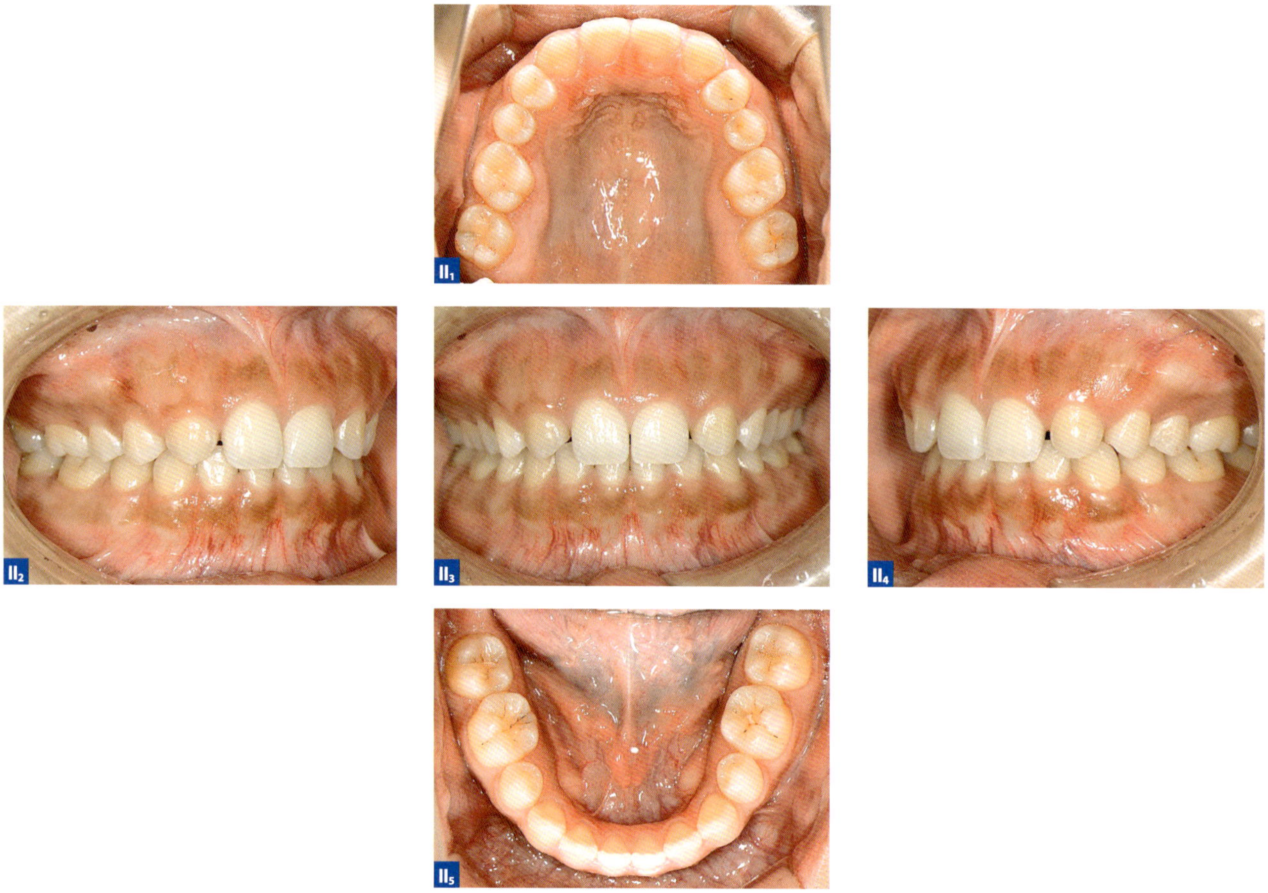

Fig 9-1jj and 9-1kk Radiographs 10 years after transplantation. Both transplants responded EPT(+).
Fig 9-1ll Views 10 years after transplantation.

Case 2. Orthodontic treatment for a patient involved in an ankylosed central incisor due to trauma

Fig 9-2 shows a case of a 13-year and 10-month-old male, who presented with the desire for orthodontic treatment for crowding (**Fig 9-2a** and **9-2b**). The patient had a history of trauma to the maxillary central incisors when he was 10 years and 3 months old, with subluxation of #21 and avulsion of #11 (information provided from the referring dentist). Unfortunately, #11 had already developed replacement root resorption and infra-occlusion due to ankylosis (**Fig 9-2c** to **9-2g**), so this tooth would not respond to orthodontic treatment and thus extraction was advised.

Going over the strategy for orthodontic treatment, it was decided that four premolars on the left and right sides of the upper and lower jaws would be extracted. Therefore, replacement of the ankylosed tooth with one of the extracted premolars was proposed and the patient and his family agreed. Initially, it was planned to use #34 as a donor tooth, but cone beam CT (CBCT) analysis suggested #35 had a more favorable root morphology.

In this case, it was decided to pursue immediate transplantation of #35 to replace #11. Fabricating a replica was not available at this time, so the morphology of the recipient socket and donor tooth (cross-sectional morphology, root length, etc.) were measured by CBCT in advance (Fig 9-2h to 9-2m).

In order to minimize extra-oral time of a donor tooth during surgery, it is preferred to fabricate a replica of the donor tooth prior to surgery and use it as a try-in before transplanting the actual donor tooth (Fig 9-2q to 9-2s).

Case 2. Orthodontic treatment for a patient involved in an ankylosed central incisor due to trauma

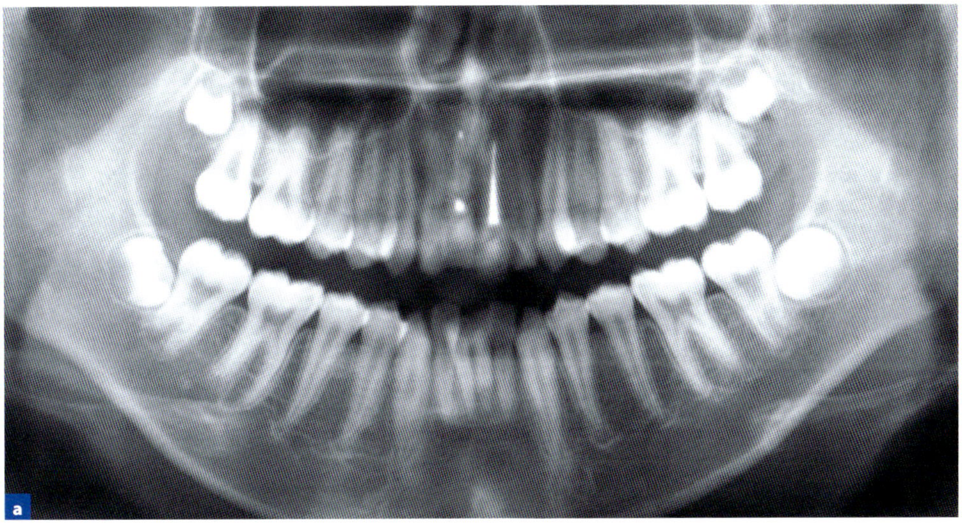

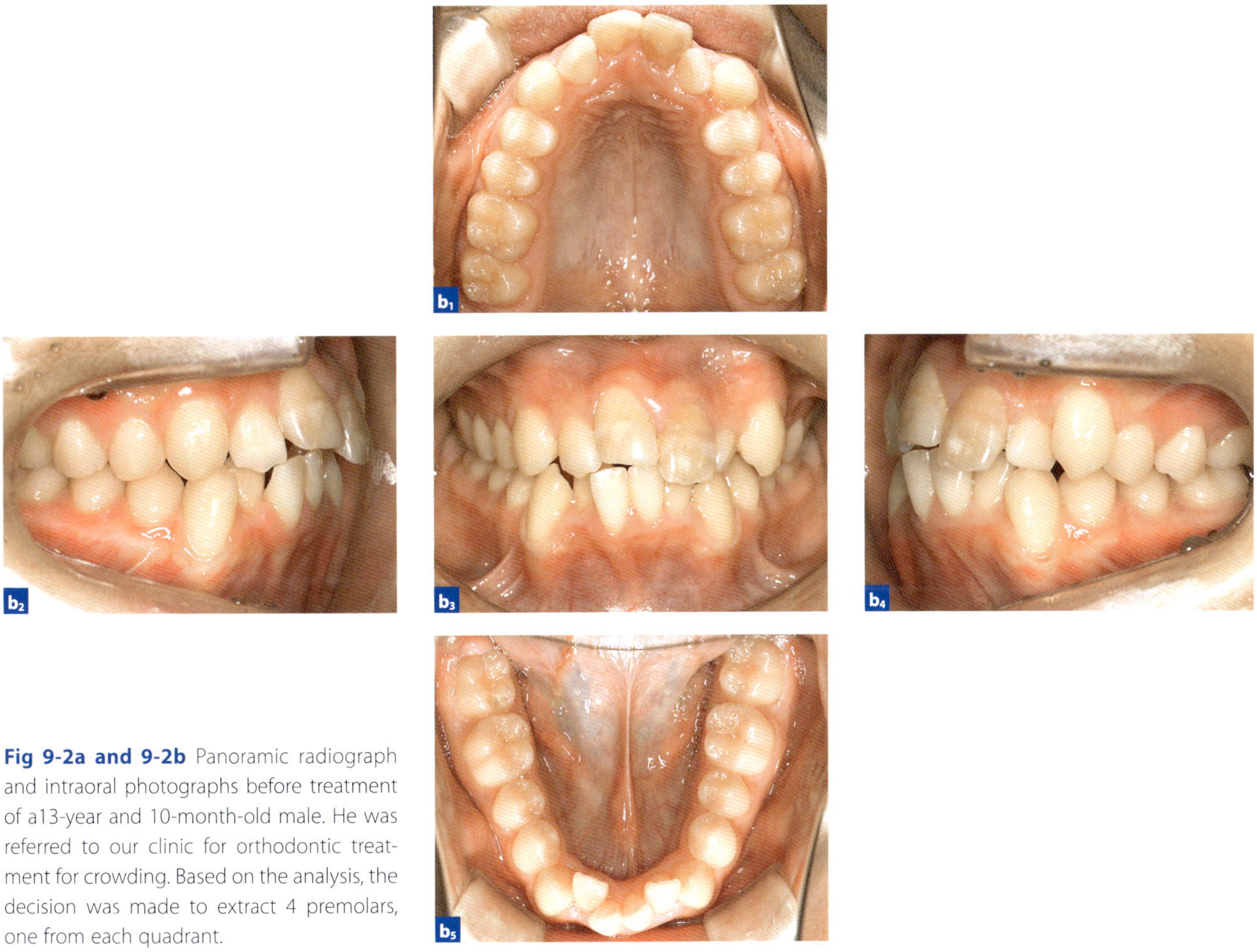

Fig 9-2a and 9-2b Panoramic radiograph and intraoral photographs before treatment of a13-year and 10-month-old male. He was referred to our clinic for orthodontic treatment for crowding. Based on the analysis, the decision was made to extract 4 premolars, one from each quadrant.

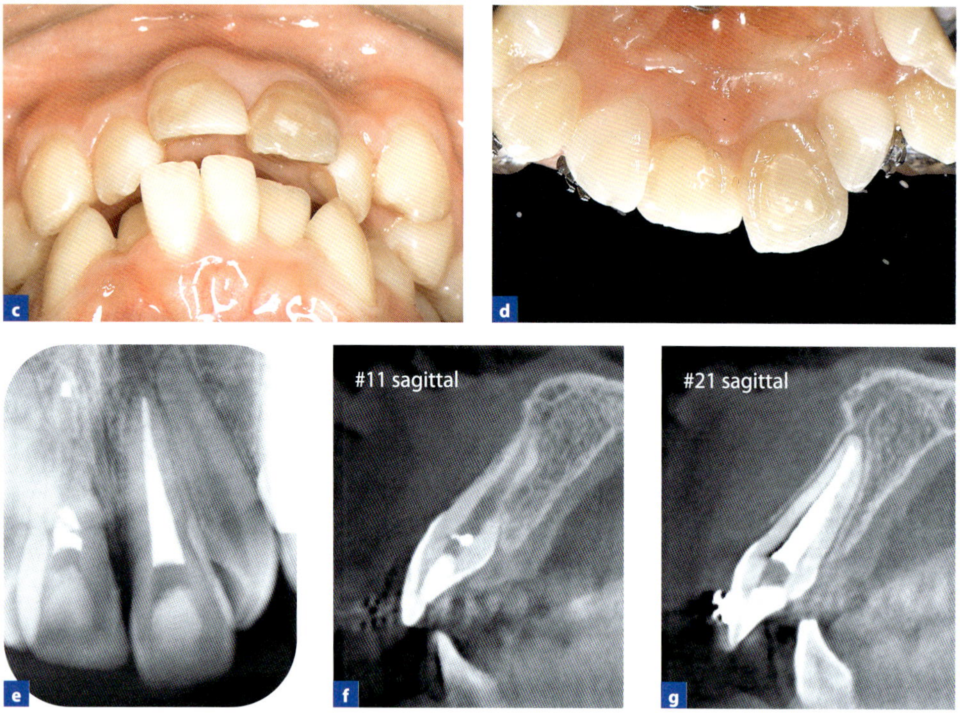

Fig 9-2c to 9-2g Views of the maxillary anterior region before treatment. At the age of 10 years and 3 months, the patient suffered trauma to the maxillary central incisors. #21 was involved in subluxation and #11 was avulsed and replanted. Appropriate treatments for traumatized teeth were performed at that time by the referring dentist, but #11 developed root resorption and infra-occlusion due to ankylosis. Thus, transplantation using one of the extracted premolar teeth as a donor was planned. Based on the CBCT examination, #35 was diagnosed to be suitable as a donor.

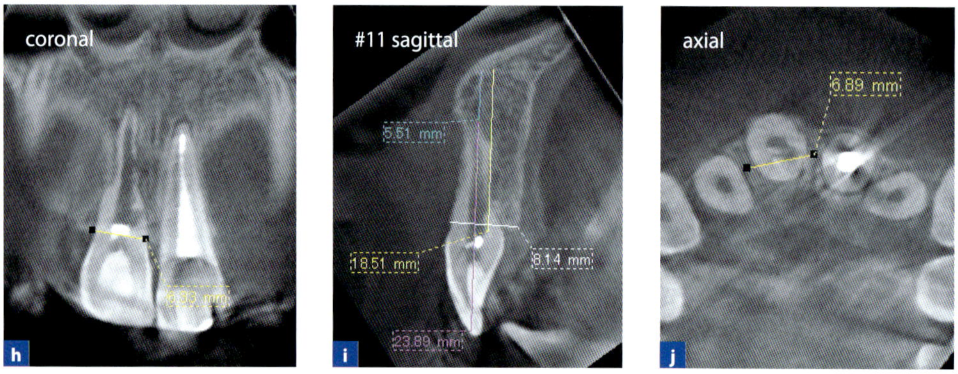

Fig 9-2h to 9-2j Measurement of recipient site by CBCT.

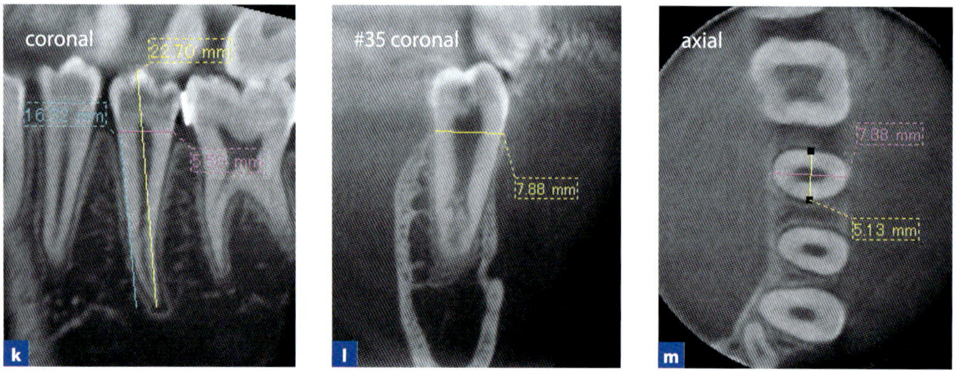

Fig 9-2k to 9-2m Analysis of the donor tooth, #35 by CBCT.

When transplanting a premolar to a maxillary central incisor site in which ankylosis has occurred and there is a discrepancy in the gingival level and thinner buccal cortical plate, the transplant should be placed deeply and labially so that there is more root submergence (**Fig 9-2v** to **9-2z**). The crown of the transplant will protrude labially and the cervical line positioned apically (**Fig 9-2y**). However, this issue can be resolved with orthodontic treatment which can be initiated 3 months after surgery. Orthodontic movement can align the cervical line of the transplant with the adjacent teeth (**Fig 9-2bb** to **9-2kk**).

If a tooth with complete or near complete root formation is used as the donor tooth, root canal treatment should be performed about 2 weeks (**Fig 9-2aa**) later. If the apex is slightly open but pulp necrosis will be highly likely, apexification can

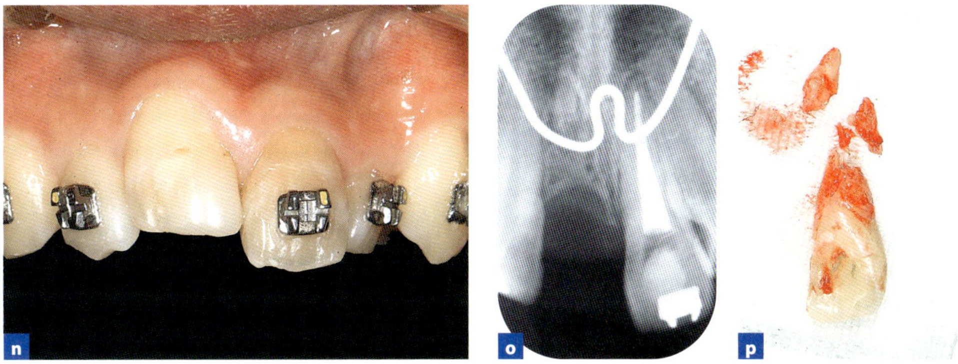

Fig 9-2n Recipient site just before immediate transplantation. **Fig 9-2o** Radiograph during extraction of #11. The root has not been removed completely yet. **Fig 9-2p** All of the fragments of extracted #11.

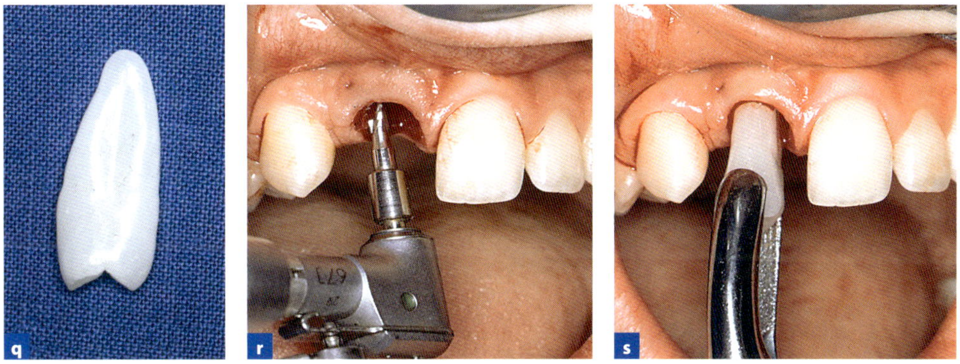

Fig 9-2q to 9-2s Example of preparation of a recipient socket (courtesy of Dr. Jens O. Andreasen). A plastic 3D replica of the same shape as a donor tooth is prepared. A recipient socket of appropriate size is prepared in advance by try-in with the replica before extracting the donor tooth. Extra-oral time and risk of damage to the PDL can be reduced significantly this way.

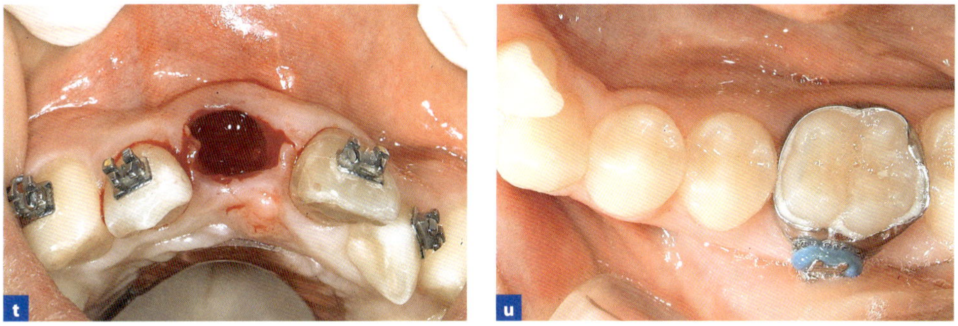

Fig 9-2t After preparation of the recipient socket. In this case, a replica was not available because the case was performed years before the availability of fabricating replicas. But if possible, using a replica is strongly recommended.
Fig 9-2u Donor tooth (#35) before extraction.

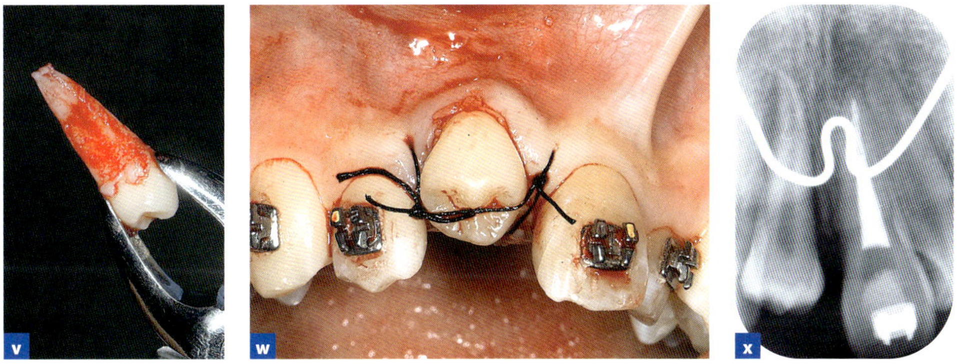

Fig 9-2v Extracted donor tooth.
Fig 9-2w and 9-2x Immediately after transplantation.

be performed (longer-term temporary root canal filling with calcium hydroxide preparation), and after the apex area has healed and created a barrier with cementum, final root canal filling with sealer and gutta-percha is performed (**Fig 9-2hh** to **9-2jj**).

This type of treatment is never aesthetically pleasing immediately after transplantation. The crown morphology of premolars are completely different from that of central incisors, which may cause some patients to experience social anxiety. Therefore, it is desirable to perform temporary morphological correction with composite resin (CR) at an early stage (**Fig 9-2bb** to **9-2ee**).

When transplanted or traumatized teeth are moved orthodontically, it is desirable to perform radiographic examinations every 6 months and CBCT examinations every year, if possible.

There is risk of developing invasive cervical resorption[1-8] (**Fig 9-2kk** to **9-2pp**). Root resorption is more likely to occur on the compressed side, so it is important to closely monitor the palatal side. This type of root resorption can often be detected only by CBCT imaging (**Fig 9-2mm** to **9-2pp**). If invasive cervical resorption is discovered, surgical access can be performed, invasive resorptive tissue cleaned and restored with composite resin, glass ionomer cement or MTA cement. Invasive cervical resorption can be treated and arrested up to a Class 3 progression[9-12] and so active monitoring and early detection can be of

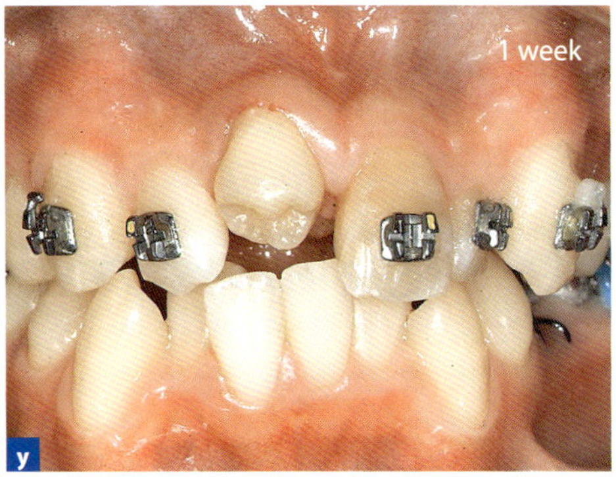

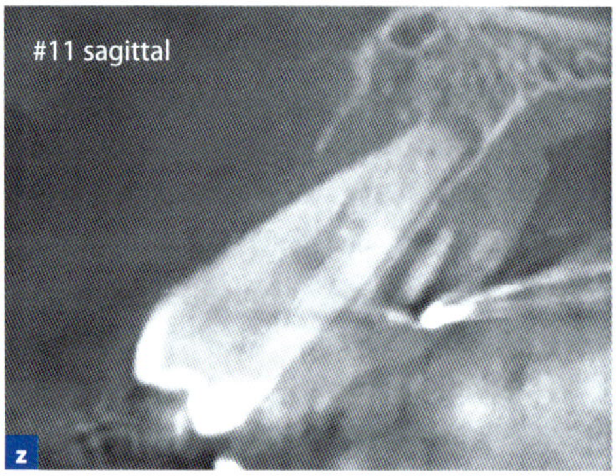

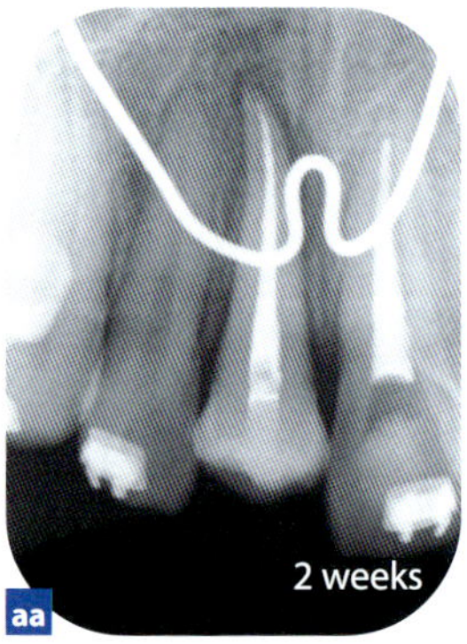

Fig 9-2y One week postop.
Fig 9-2z Sagittal CBCT image after 1 week. Note the absence of bone on the labial side of the transplant. No bone graft material was used.
Fig 9-2aa Two weeks postop. Immediately after root canal treatment of the transplant and temporary canal filling with calcium hydroxide preparation.

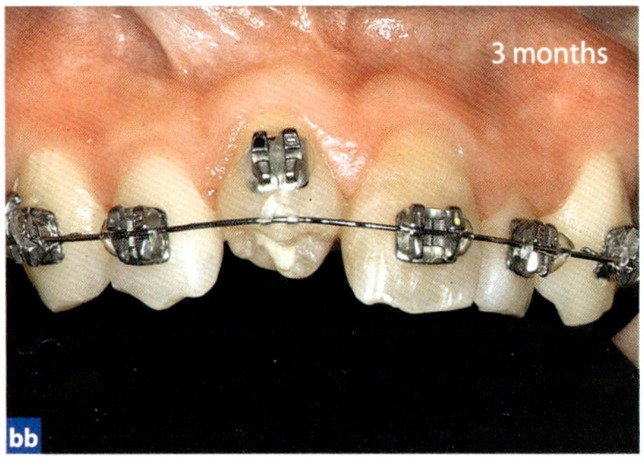

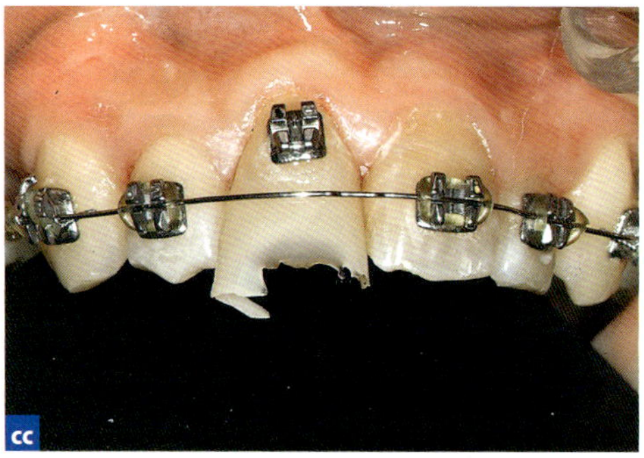

Fig 9-2bb Three months postop and immediately before the initiation of orthodontic treatment.
Fig 9-2cc The same day as **Fig 9-2bb**. The crown of the transplant is being temporarily modified with CR.

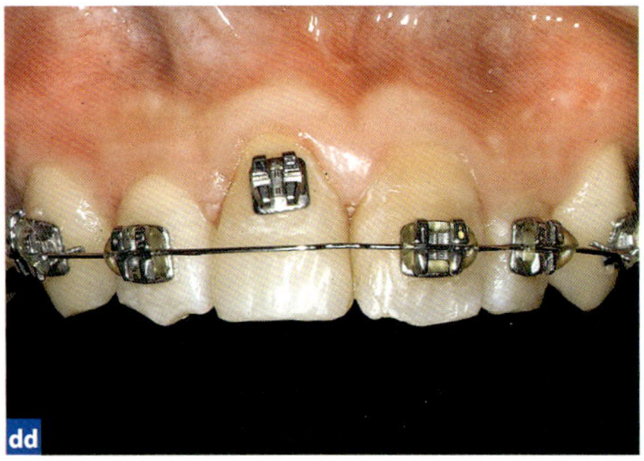

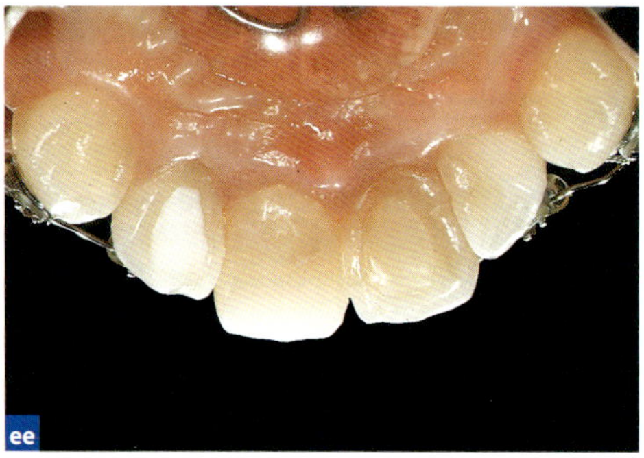

Fig 9-2dd and 9-2ee Immediately after temporary restoration with CR .

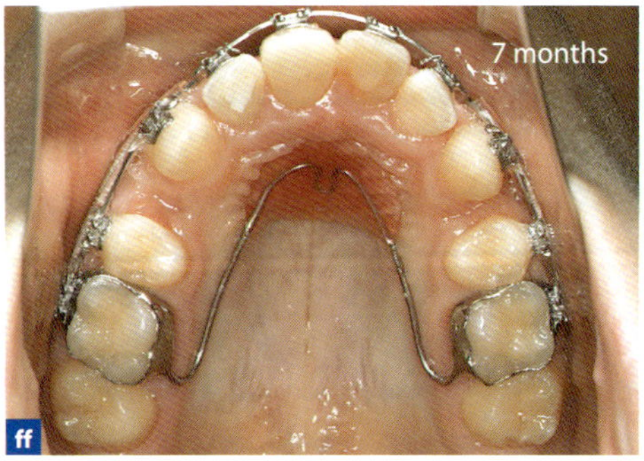

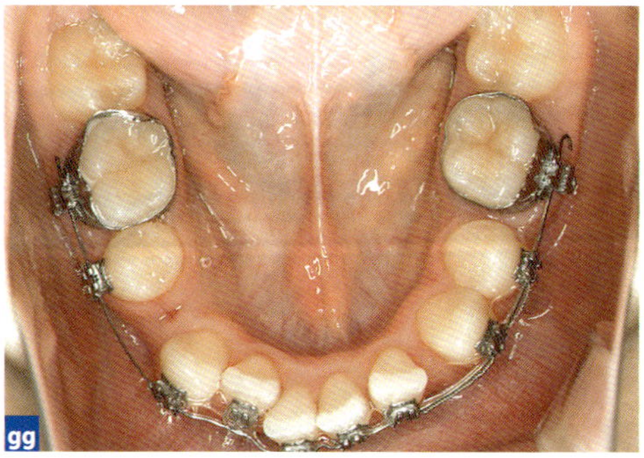

Fig 9-2ff and 9-2gg Occlusal views of the upper and lower arches after 7 months.

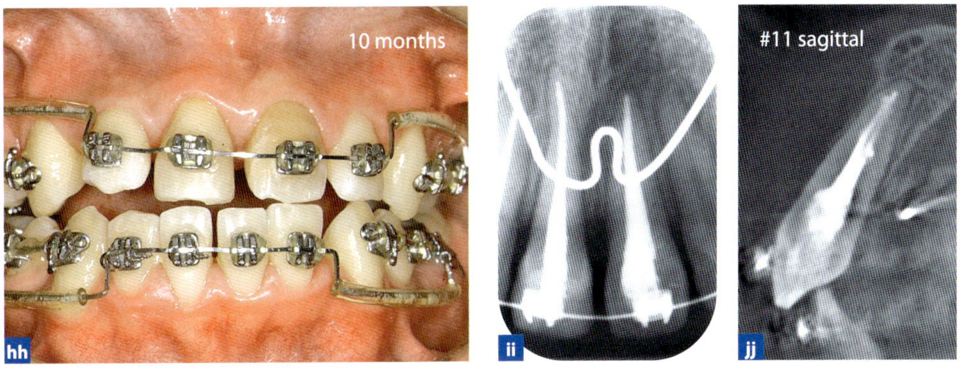

Fig 9-2hh and 9-2ii 10 months after transplantation. Immediately after root canal filling with sealer and gutta-percha.

Fig 9-2jj CBCT image of the transplant after 10 months. It can be observed that there is evidence of bone forming on the labial aspect.

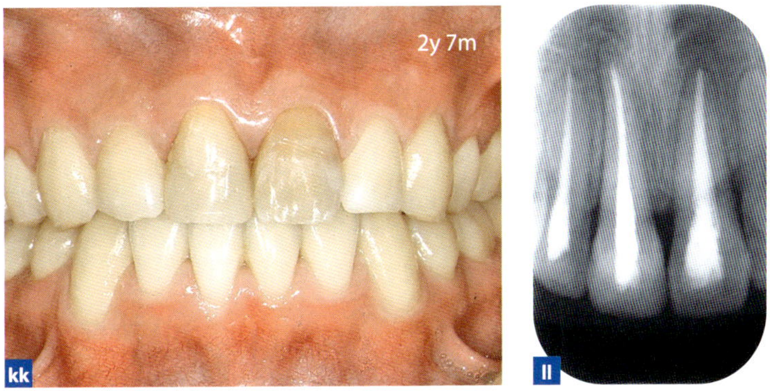

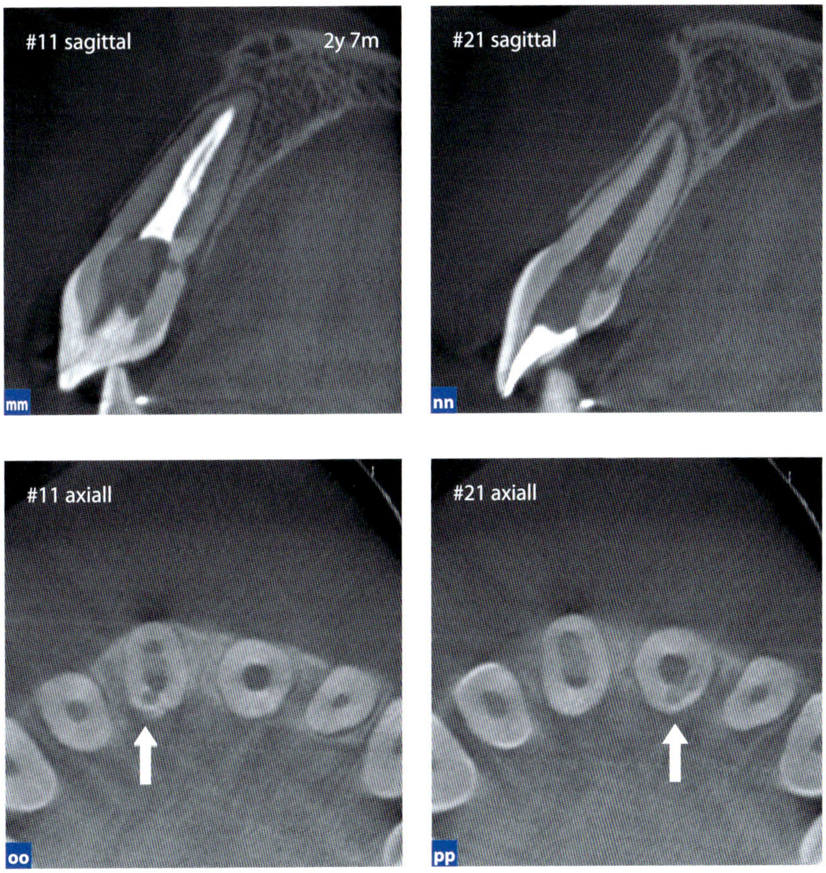

Fig 9-2kk to 9-2pp Two years and 7 months postop. Immediately after completion of orthodontic treatment. Canal filling materials were removed from the coronal parts of the crowns of #11 and #21 to correct discoloration. But when removing the gutta-percha from #21, bleeding occurred because of invasive cervical resorption (ICR). Then, #11 and #21 were analyzed with CBCT. The transplanted tooth (#11) and the subluxated tooth (#21) involved long time ago seemed to have suffered ICR during orthodontic teeth movement.

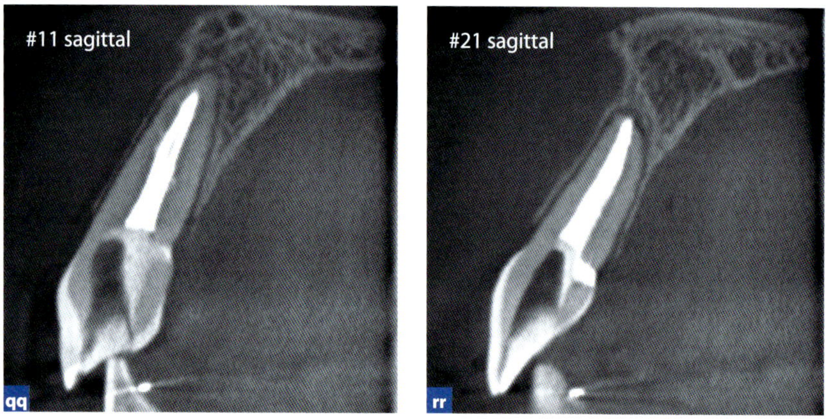

Fig 9-2qq and 9-2rr After treatment of ICR. A flap was raised and invasive granulation tissue was removed from outside of the root and internally as well. The spaces were filled with glass ionomer cement.

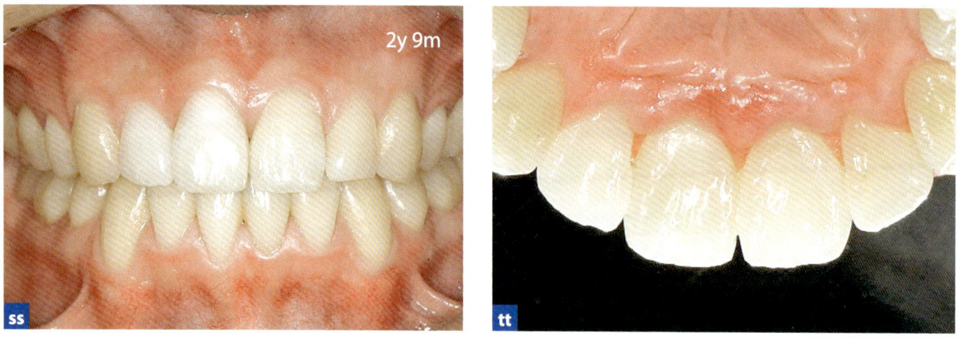

Fig 9-2ss and 9-2tt After walking bleach and restoration of the crowns of #11 and #21.

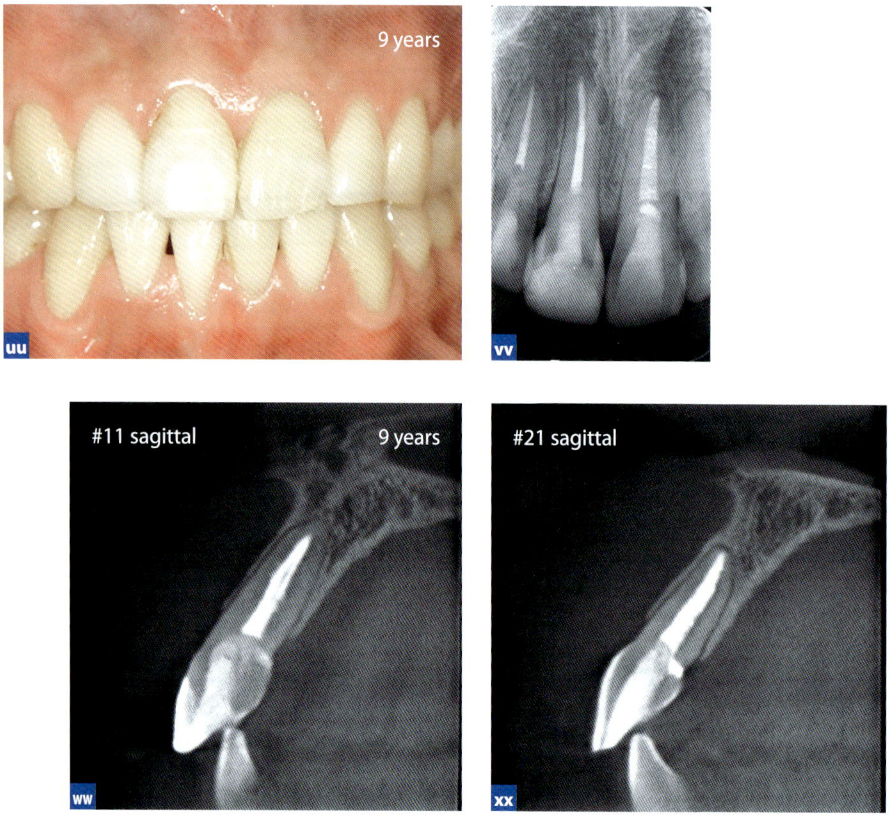

Fig 9-2uu to 9-2xx Nine years after transplantation. Note that bone on the labial aspect is maintained. and ICR is completely arrested.

great benefit (**Fig 9-2qq** and **9-2rr**).

After orthodontic treatment is completed, the final morphology of the transplant is usually shaped with CR. However, if there is discoloration of the crown, the restoration should be done after performing internal walking bleach (**Fig 9-2ss** and **9-2tt**). Though this case suffered invasive cervical resorption, it was treated and controlled nicely with long-term follow-up (**Fig 9-2uu** to **9-2xx**).

Case 3. Orthodontic treatment for an adult patient with congenitally missing teeth

Fig 9-3 shows a case of a 35-year-old female who presented with the desire to have orthodontic treatment to address the occlusion in the molars' region and crowding in the mandibular anterior region. All four premolars in the maxilla were con-

Case 3. Orthodontic treatment for an adult patient with congenitally missing teeth

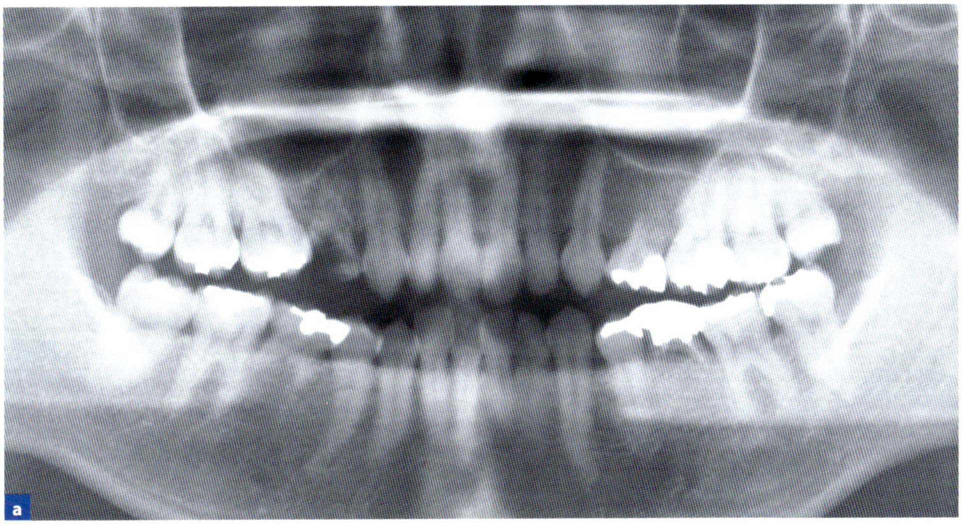

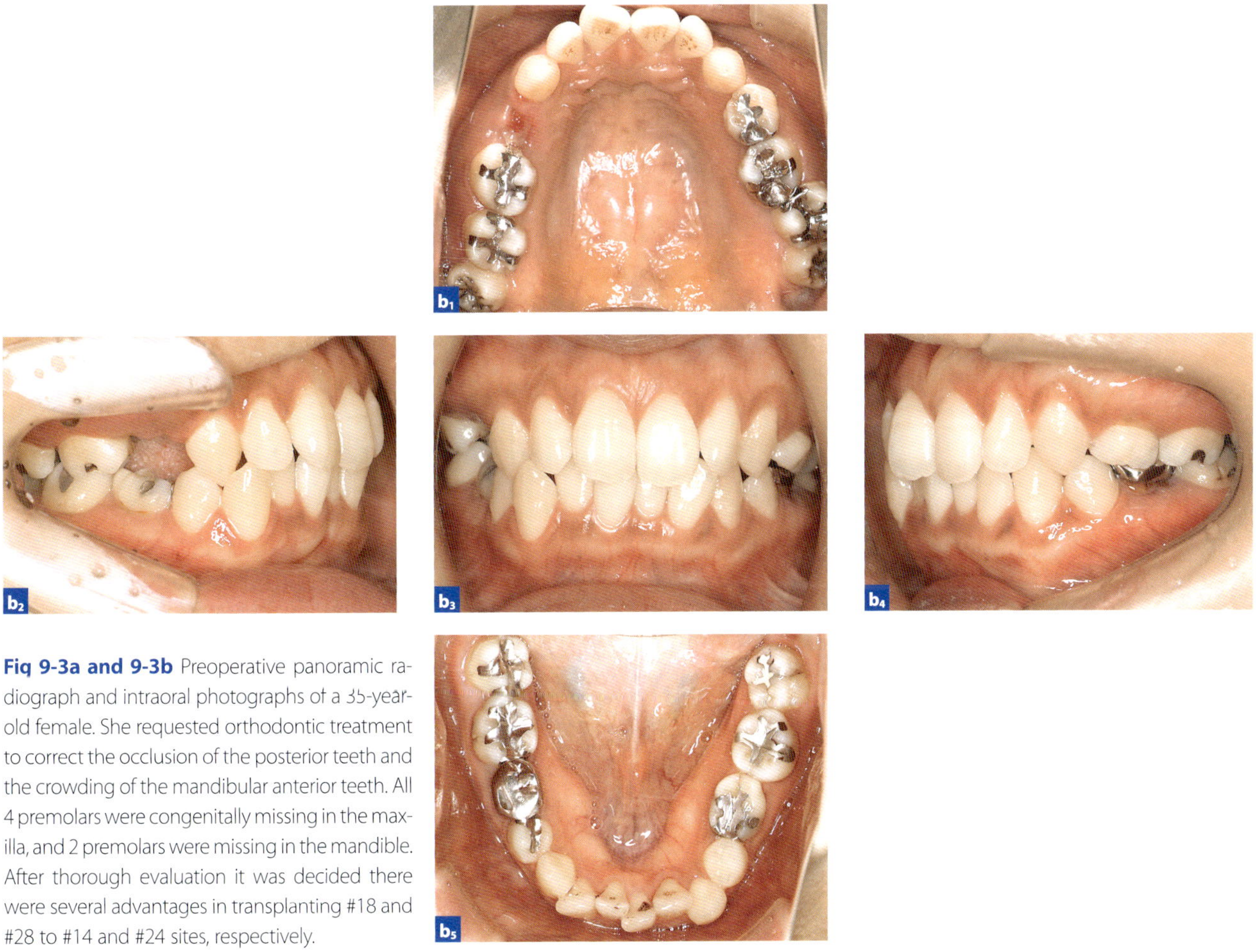

Fig 9-3a and 9-3b Preoperative panoramic radiograph and intraoral photographs of a 35-year-old female. She requested orthodontic treatment to correct the occlusion of the posterior teeth and the crowding of the mandibular anterior teeth. All 4 premolars were congenitally missing in the maxilla, and 2 premolars were missing in the mandible. After thorough evaluation it was decided there were several advantages in transplanting #18 and #28 to #14 and #24 sites, respectively.

genitally missing, and two premolars were missing in the mandible (**Fig 9-3a** and **9-3b**). Since the third molars had erupted normally in the maxilla, it was considered to extract the deciduous molars and close the spaces with orthodontic movement. However, considering the risks and difficulty of protracting all 6 maxillary molars and the esthetic problems that may develop, transplanting the smaller third molars to the first premolar sites were considered to be a better treatment strategy. From the measurements, it was found that the mesiodistal width of the recipient sites was insufficient to fit the transplants (**Fig 9-3c** to **9-3e** and **9-3m** to **9-3o**), so the recipient spaces were firstly expanded orthodontically (**Fig 9-3f ,9-3g, 9-3p** and **9-3q**),

Right-sided transplantation:

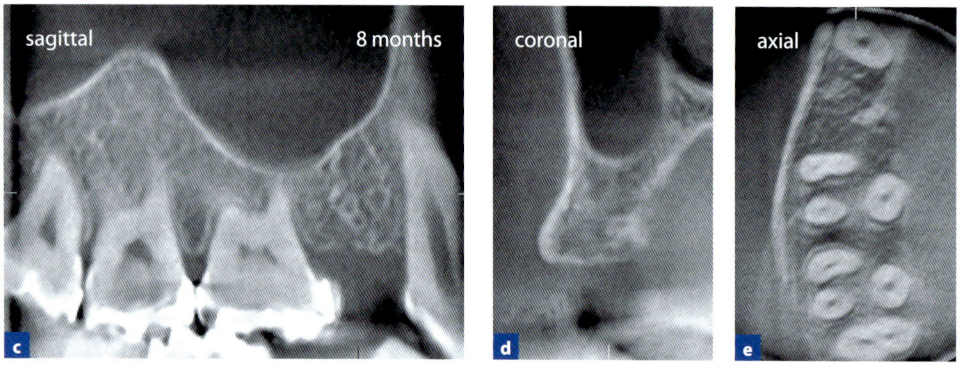

Fig 9-3c to 9-3e CBCT images of the right recipient site and the donor tooth 8 months after initiation of orthodontic treatment. Buccolingually, there is sufficient bone width on the recipient site, but the mesiodistal width is still insufficient.

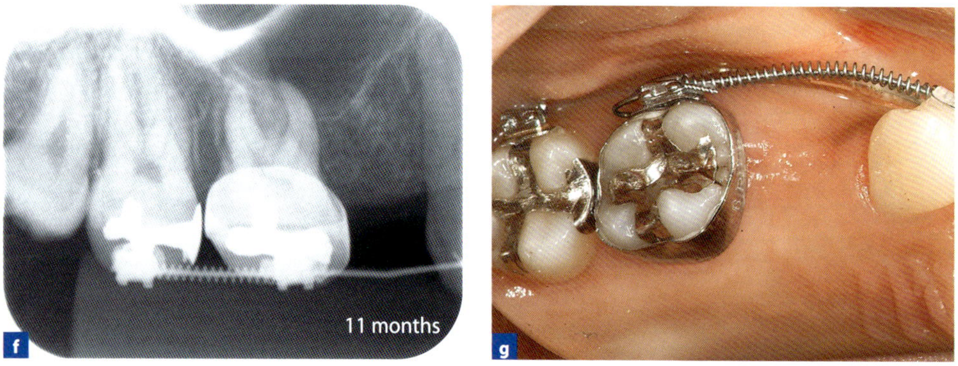

Fig 9-3f and 9-3g After 11 months of orthodontic treatment. Sufficient mesiodistal width is now gained.

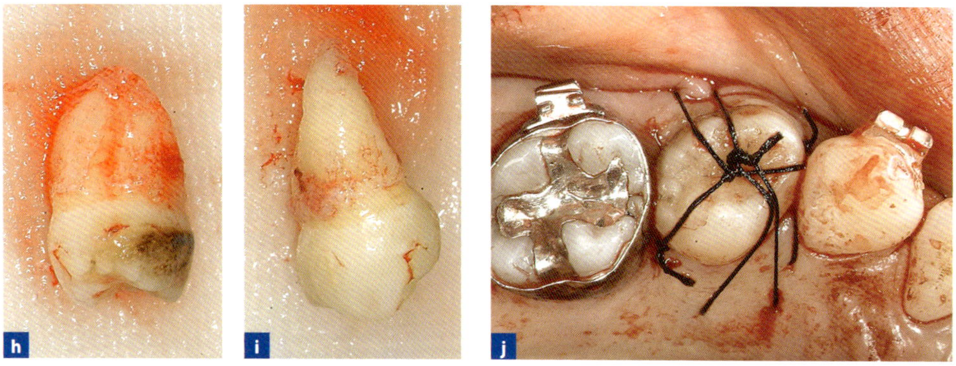

Fig 9-3h and 9-3i Extracted donor tooth. It has a simple root morphology suitable for transplantation.
Fig 9-3j View immediately after transplantation.

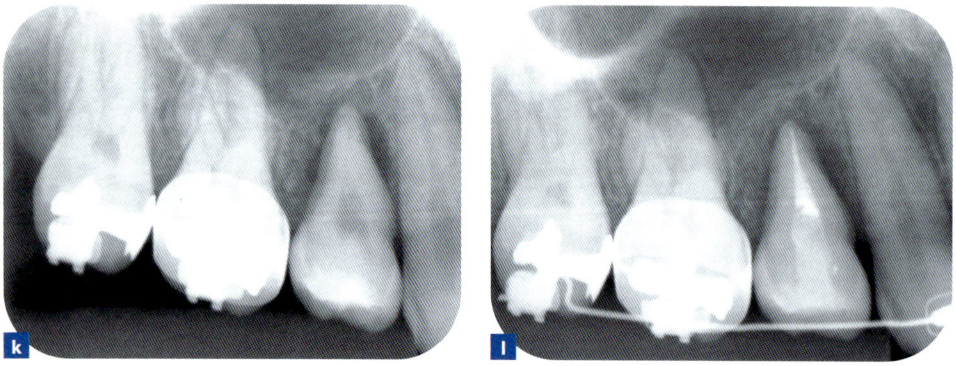

Fig 9-3k Radiograph immediately after transplantation.
Fig 9-3l One month after transplantation, immediately after root canal filling with sealer and gutta-percha.

and then #18 and #28 were transplanted (**Fig 9-3h** to **9-3k** and **9-3r to 9-3u**). Since the transplanted teeth had completed root formation, root canal treatment was started 2 weeks after surgery, and the root canal space was obturated 1 month later (**Fig 9-3l** and **9-3v**). The orthodontic treatment of the transplanted was started 3 months after the transplantation and the total orthodontic treatment was completed about 3 years after the transplantation (**Fig 9-3w** to **9-3ff**). After completion of the orthodontic treatment, the morphology of the transplanted teeth were changed with CR and the case was followed with recall examinations (**Fig 9-3gg** and **9-3hh**).

Left-sided transplantation:

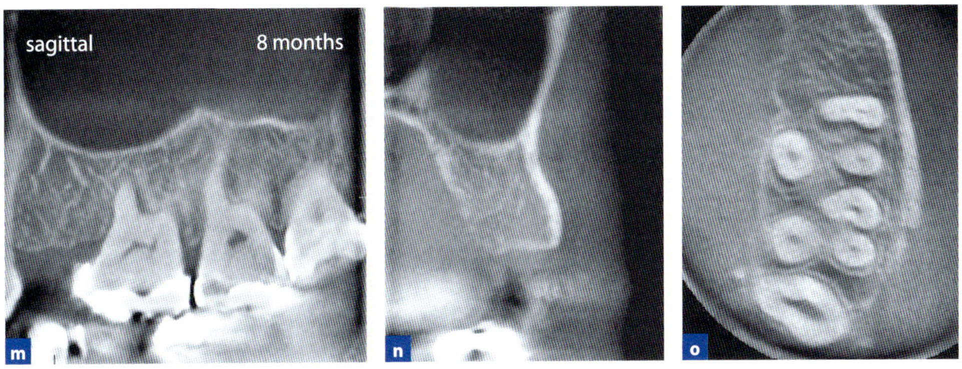

Fig 9-3m to 9-3o CBCT images of the left recipient and the donor tooth 8 months after the initiation of orthodontic treatment. Buccolingually, there is sufficient bone width on the recipient site, but the mesiodistal width is still insufficient.

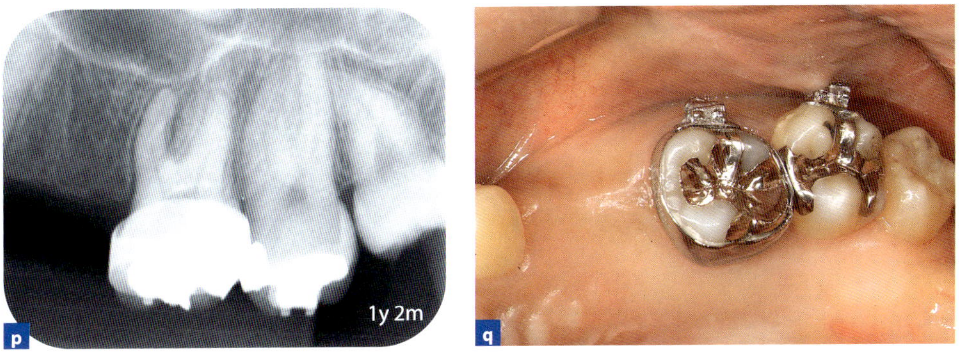

Fig 9-3p and 9-3q After 1 year and 2 months. Sufficient mesiodistal width is gained.

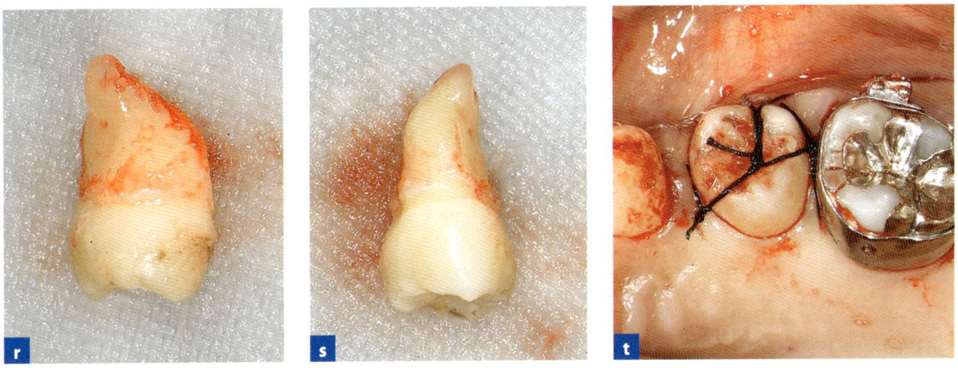

Fig 9-3r and 9-3s Extracted donor tooth. It has a simple root morphology suitable for transplantation.
Fig 9-3t Immediately after transplantation.

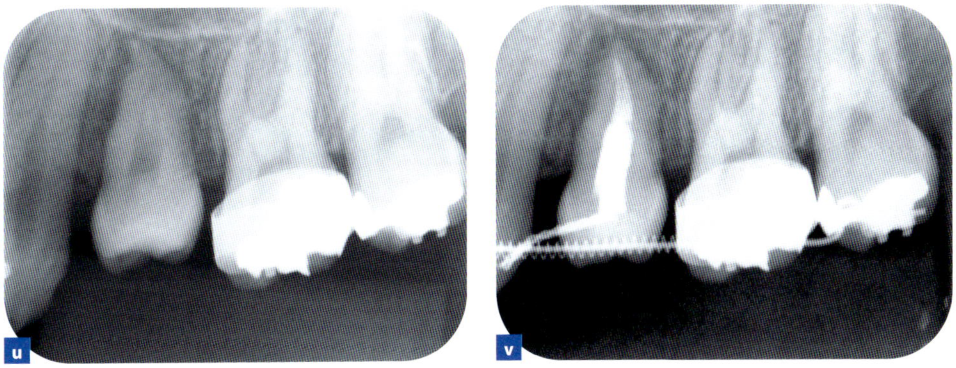

Fig 9-3u Radiograph immediately after transplantation.
Fig 9-3v One month after transplantation. Immediately after root canal filling with sealer and gutta-percha.

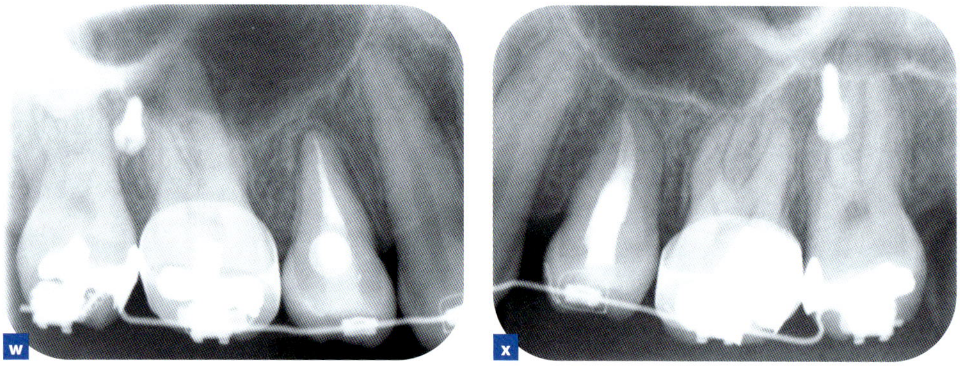

Fig 9-3w and 9-3x Radiographs 1 year and 6 months after initiation of orthodontic treatment. No abnormalities were observed in the transplanted teeth.

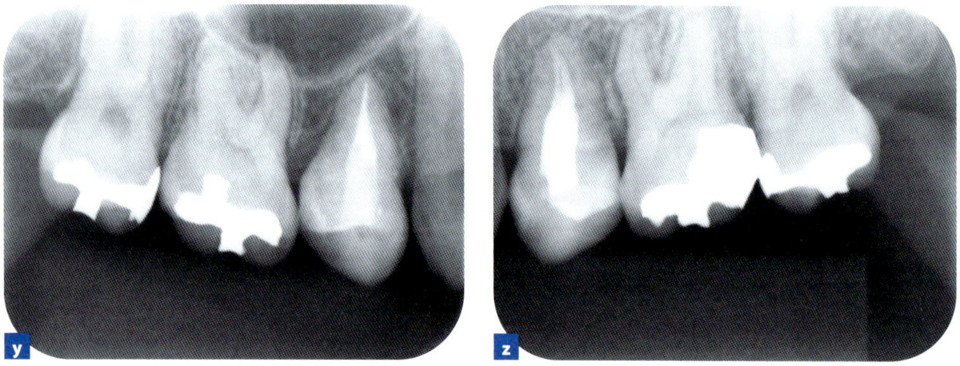

Fig 9-3y Radiograph 3 years and 2 months after transplantation on the right side.
Fig 9-3z Radiograph 2 years and 11 months after transplantation on the left side.

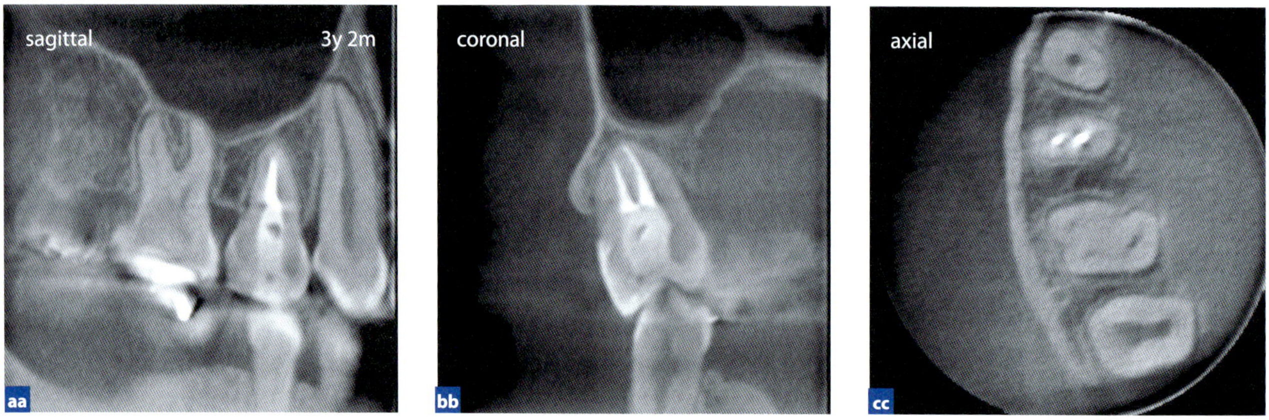

Fig 9-3aa to 9-3cc CBCT images 3 years and 2 months after transplantation on the right-side. No abnormalities were observed.

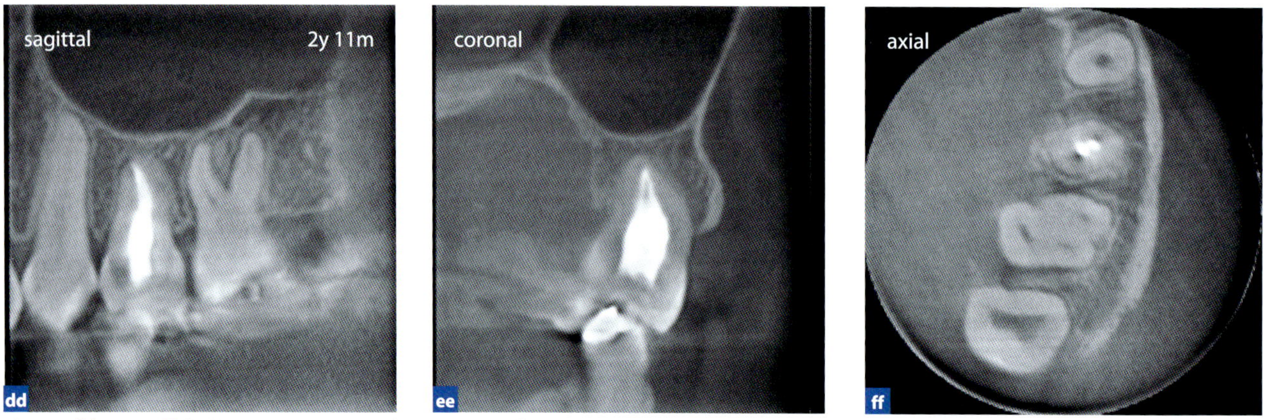

Fig 9-3dd to 9-3ff CBCT images 2 years and 11 months after transplantation on the left-side. No abnormalities were observed.

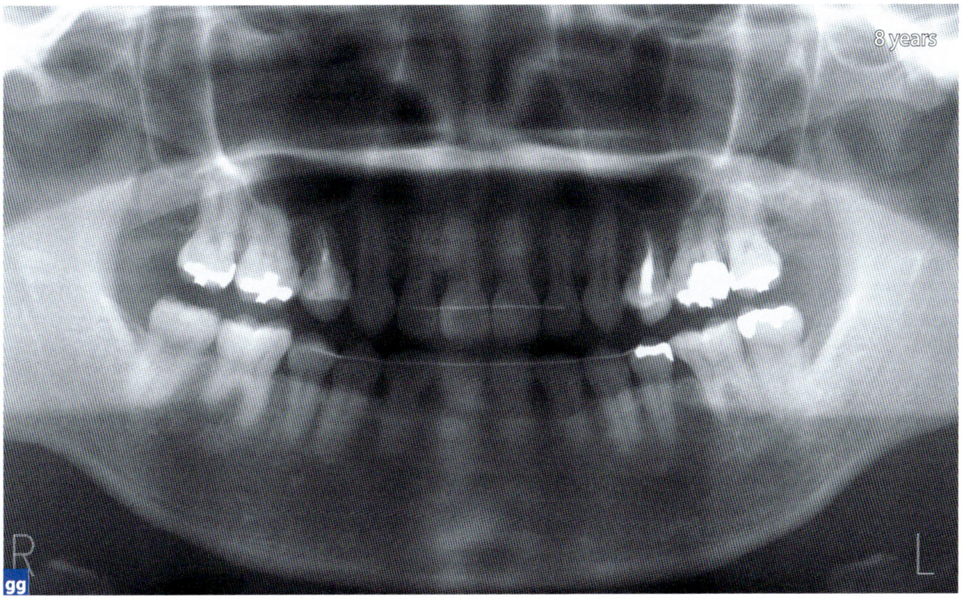

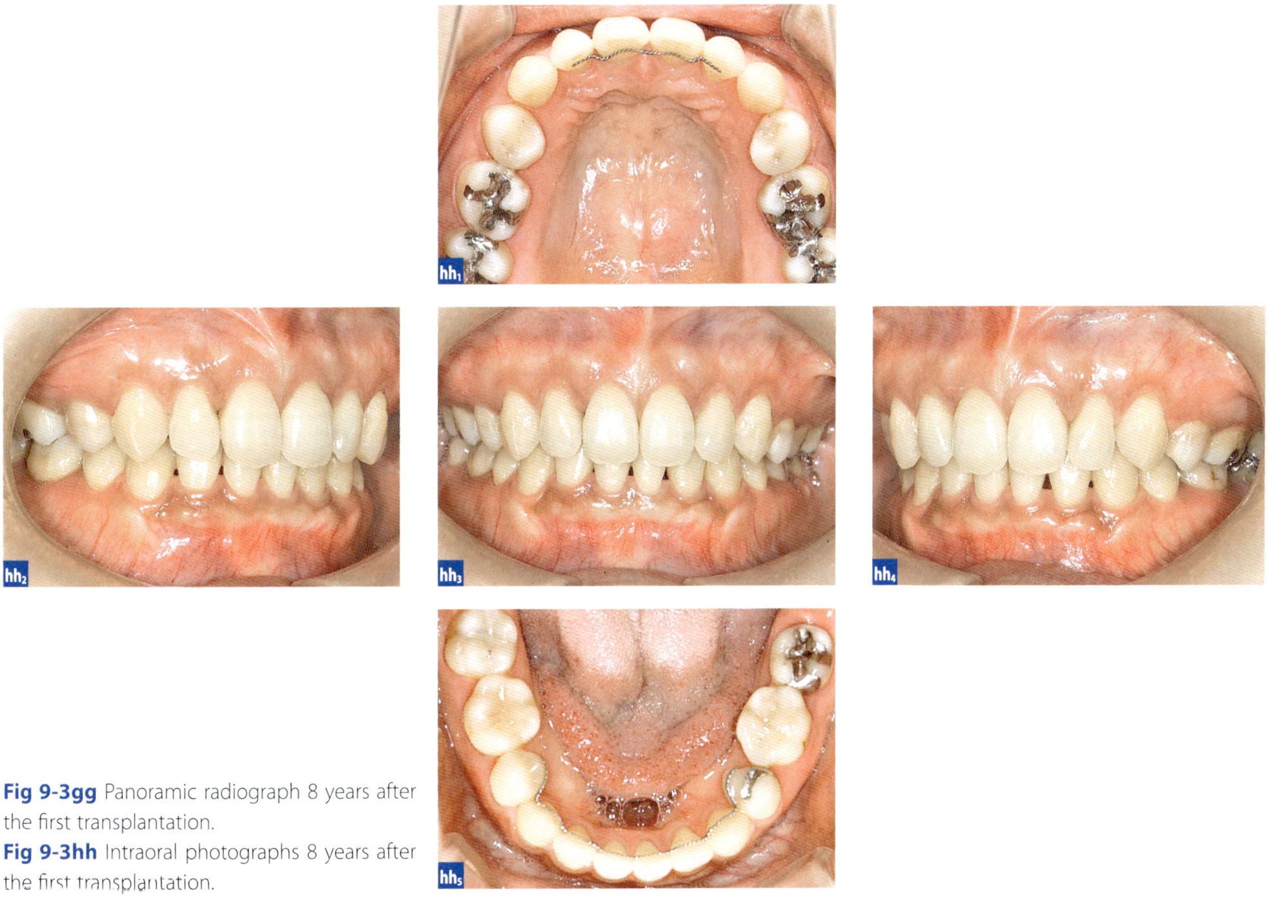

Fig 9-3gg Panoramic radiograph 8 years after the first transplantation.
Fig 9-3hh Intraoral photographs 8 years after the first transplantation.

Case 4. Orthodontic treatment for a patient who lost 3 maxillary anterior teeth due to trauma

Fig 9-4 shows a case of a 19-year-old male who lost 3 maxillary anterior teeth in a traffic accident. The accident occurred when the patient was 16 years and 10 months old. Delayed replantation was attempted but they had to be extracted 2 years later. The patient had severe crowding of his dentition, and it was considered advantageous to have orthodontic treatment to improve alignment and space closure (**Fig 9-4a** to **9-4c**). However, orthodontic tooth movement alone was not enough to accomplish the desired outcome and required a tooth in the maxillary left central incisor site. Therefore, transplantation was performed using #34 as a donor tooth, which was strategically extracted (**Fig 9-4d** to **9-4f**). It took 6 years to accomplish the treatment because of the patient's compliance, but the end goal was successfully achieved. Immediately after orthodontic treatment, the maxillary anterior teeth were morphologically modified with CR (**Fig 9-4j** to **9-4l**).

Case 5. Orthodontic treatment for a patient who lost 3 maxillary anterior teeth due to trauma soon after strategic extractions of two premolars

Fig 9-5 shows a case of a 15-year-old female who was referred to our clinic on the next day after a bicycle accident. Three anterior teeth, #13, #12 and #11 were avulsed but were not replanted by a dentist who treated her immediately after the accident (**Fig 9-5a** to **9-5b**). Unfortunately, the patient had her 2 maxillary premolars strategically extracted 2-3 weeks prior to the accident. So the patient ended up losing 5 teeth almost at once. The orthodontist who was treating her referred her for possible transplantation of the mandibular premolars to the maxilla that were planned to be strategically extracted prior to her accident. #21 was involved in a crown fracture and was already treated endodontically with pulpectomy and restoration with temporary crown but may have had a more conservative treatment with a partial pulpotomy and CR restoration.

Three days after the trauma, #35 was transplanted in #11 site, and #45 was transplanted in #14 site because the alveolar ridge had been preserved more than the other sites (**Fig 9-5c** to **9-5i**). Since root formation was almost complete, it was unlikely to expect pulpal healing. So root canal treatment of transplanted teeth was performed at an appropriate time. Orthodontic treatment began 3 months after surgery at the referring clinic. One year and 2 months after surgery, the patient was transferred to our clinic to continue her orthodontic treatment. (**Fig 9-5j** to **9-5n**).

Two years and 2 months after transplantation, orthodontic treatment was completed (**Fig 9-5l** to **9-5n**). It was decided that the edentulous site of #12 would be restored with a fixed bridge along with ridge augmentation with connective tissue graft to improve the esthetic outcome (**Fig 9-5o** to **9-5r**). Upon completion of her treatment, the process and patient-centered outcomes (esthetics and function) were reached with complete satisfaction (**Fig 9-5s** to **9-5z**).

Case 4. Orthodontic treatment for a patient who lost 3 maxillary anterior teeth due to trauma

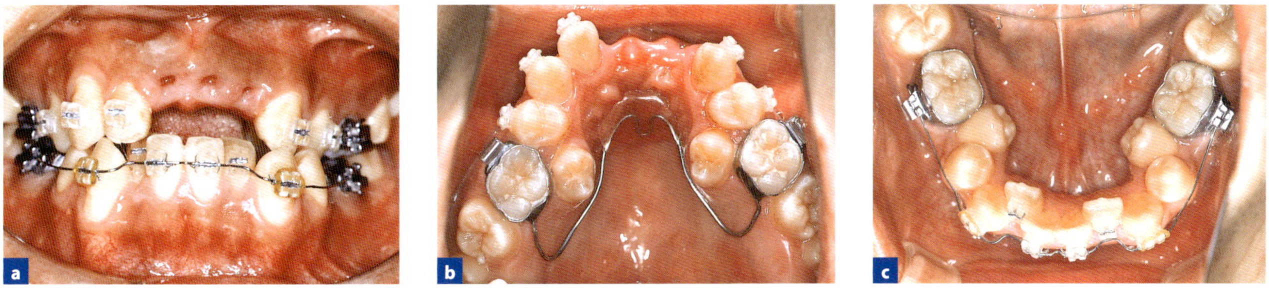

Fig 9-4a to 9-4c Views immediately after the start of orthodontic treatment of a 19-year-old male. At the age of 16 years and 10 months, he lost 3 maxillary anterior teeth due to trauma (avulsion and delayed replantation).

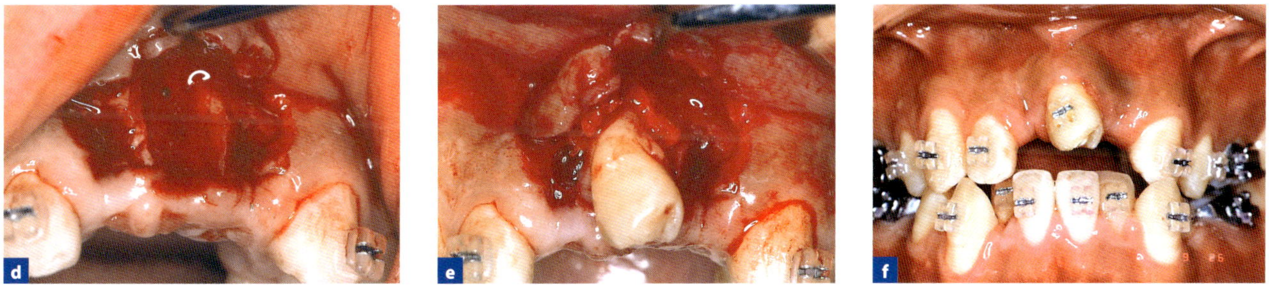

Fig 9-4d to 9-4f During surgery. #34, which was extracted strategically for orthodontic reasons, was transplanted to #11 site.

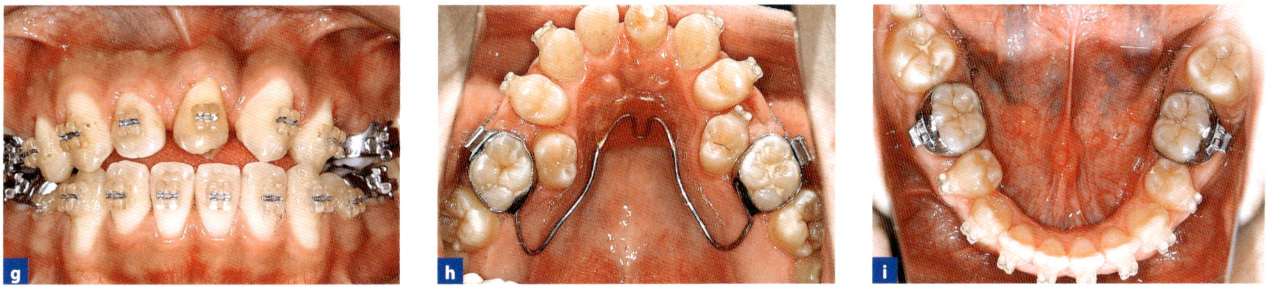

Fig 9-4g to 9-4i Two years and 3 months after transplantation.

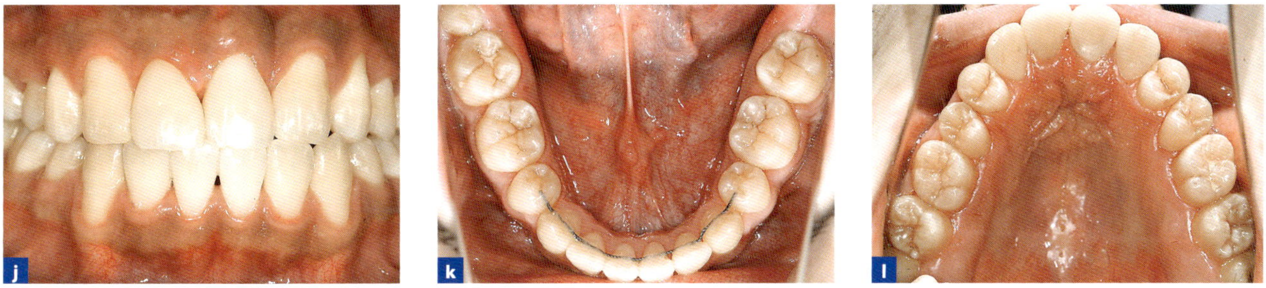

Fig 9-4j to 9-4l Six years after transplantation #12, #11, #21 and #22 were morphologically modified with CR.

Case 5. Orthodontic treatment for a patient who lost 3 maxillary anterior teeth due to trauma soon after strategic extractions of two premolars

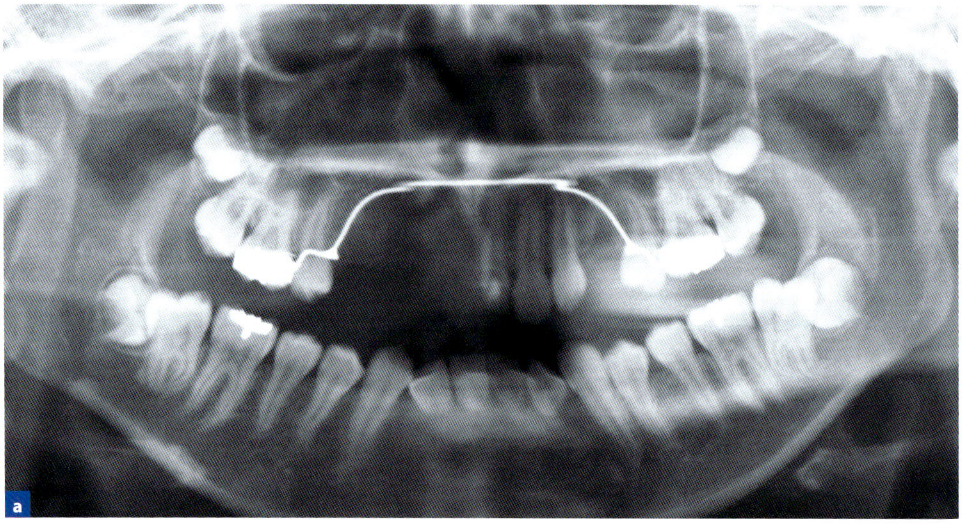

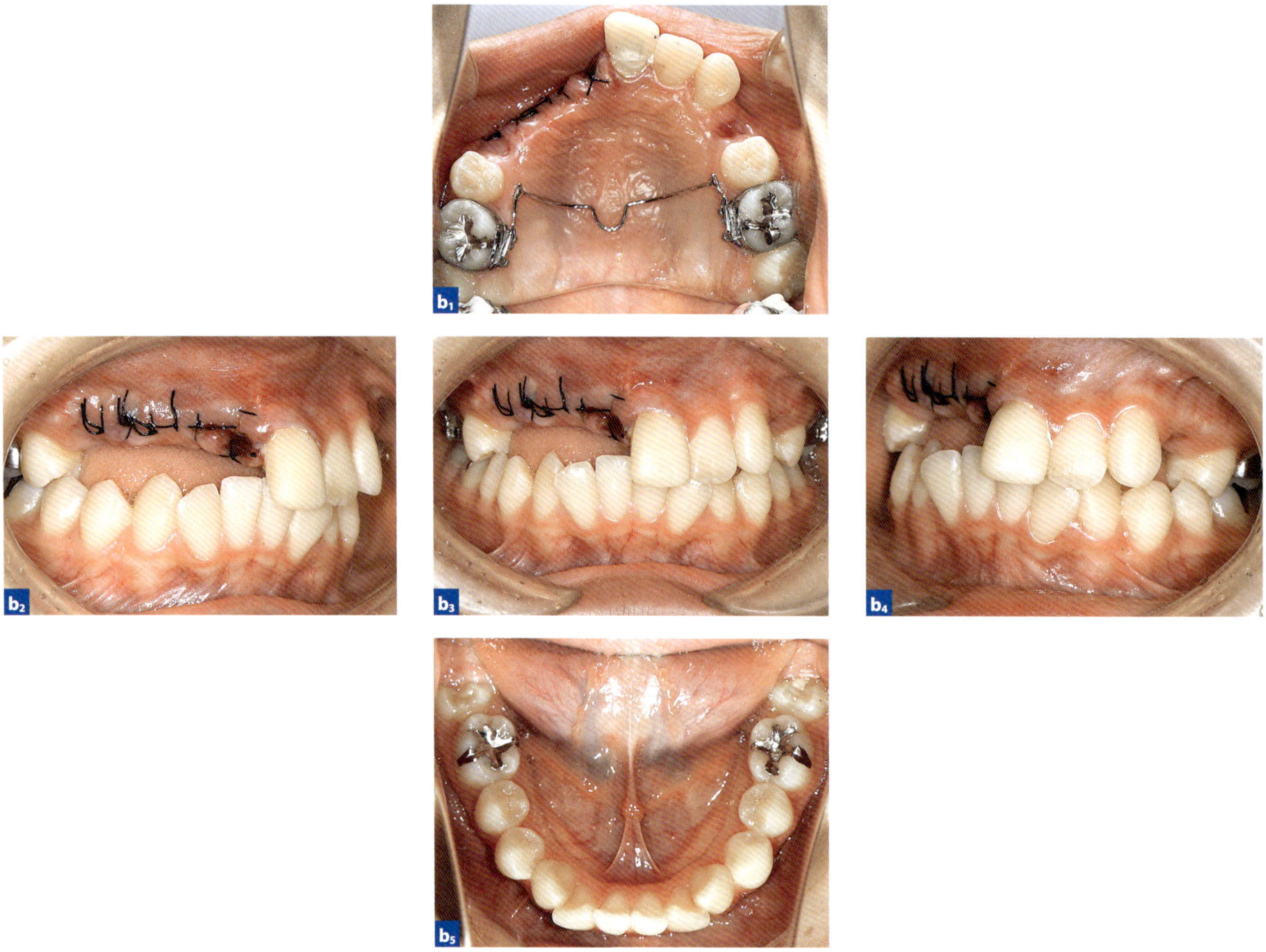

Fig 9-5a and 9-5b Panoramic radiograph and clincal Views before treatment of a 15-year-old female who was referred by an orthodontist one day after a bicycle accident. She lost 3 anterior teeth (#13, #12, #11) due to the accident and unfortunately had just had 2 maxillary premolars extracted 2 to 3 weeks earlier for orthodontic reasons. So unfortunately she lost 5 teeth almost at once. The orthodontist requested that the mandibular premolars, which were scheduled to be extracted, be transplanted to the maxillary anterior region.

Fig 9-5c Radiographs at the first visit. CBCT images of cross section at the yellow line are shown in **Fig 9-5d**.
Fig 9-5d Axial CBCT image at the first visit. Much of the buccal alveolar bone was lost. The numbers, '4', '3', '2' and '1' indicate sagittal slice planes for CBCT images of the #14, #13, #12 and #11 sites.

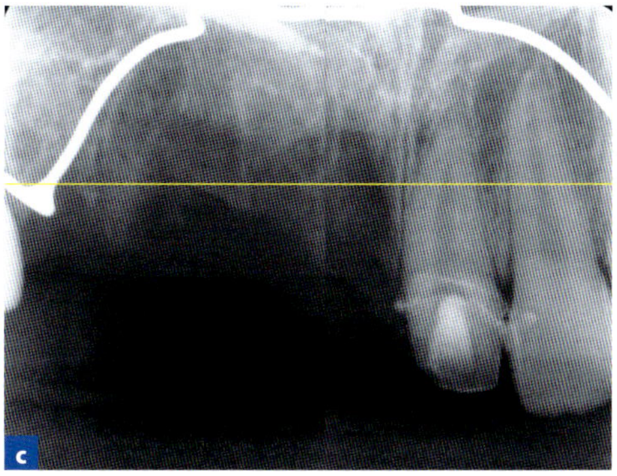

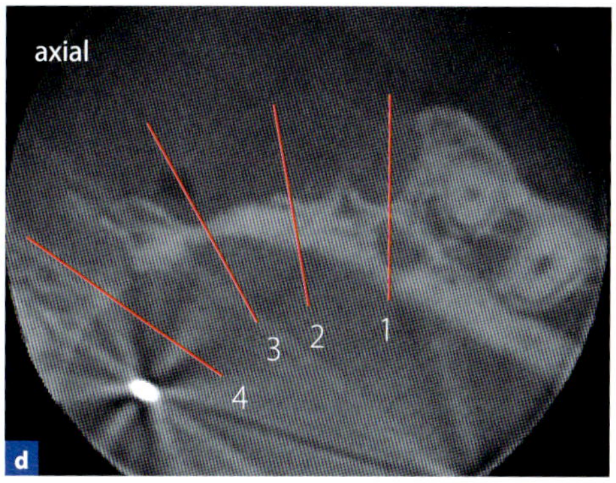

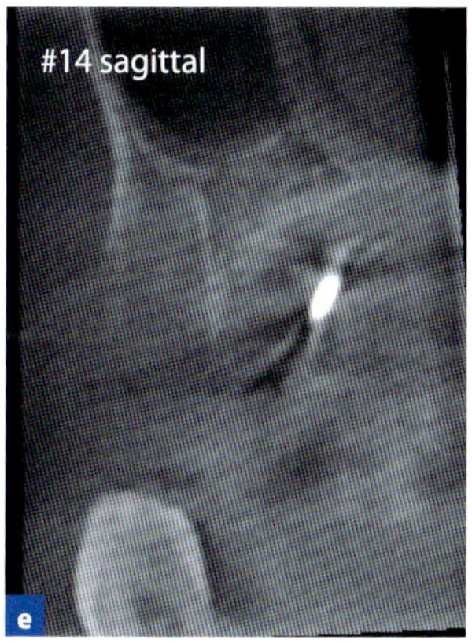

Fig 9-5e Sagittal CBCT image of #14 site.

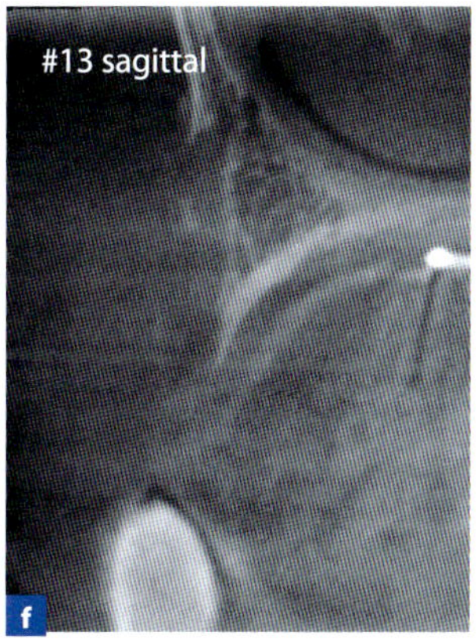

Fig 9-5f Sagittal CBCT image of #13 site.

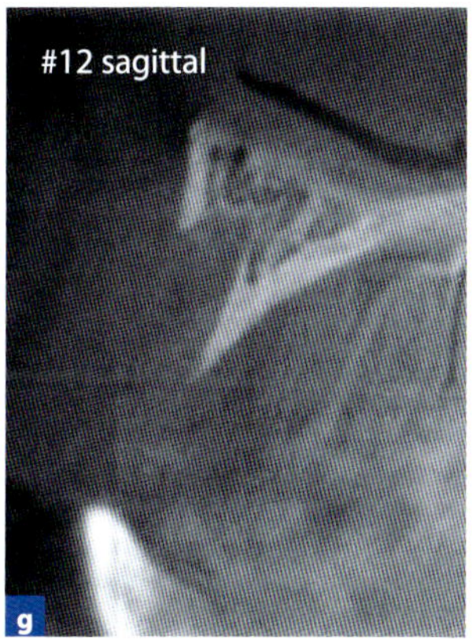

Fig 9-5g Sagittal CBCT image of #12 site.

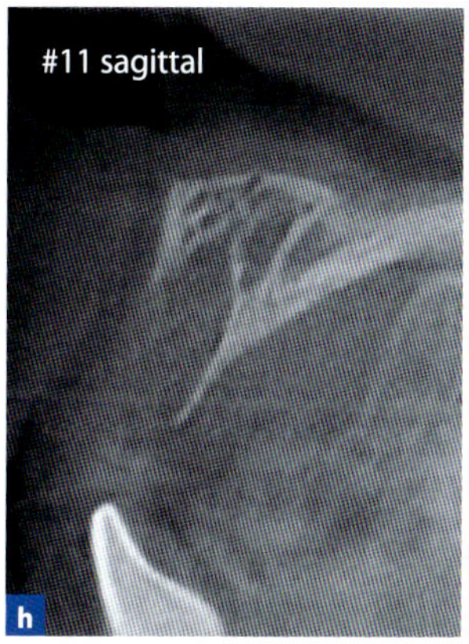

Fig 9-5h Sagittal CBCT image of #11 site.

Fig 9-5i Three months after the first visit. #35 was transplanted into the #11 site 3 days after the first visit and #45 was transplanted into the #14 site 20 days after the first surgery.
Fig 9-5j Seven months postop.

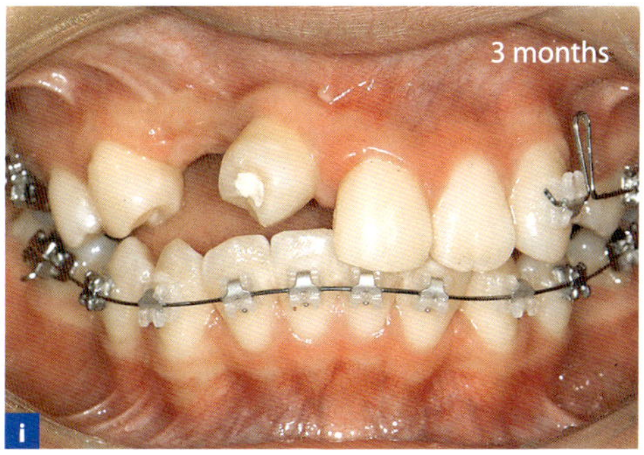

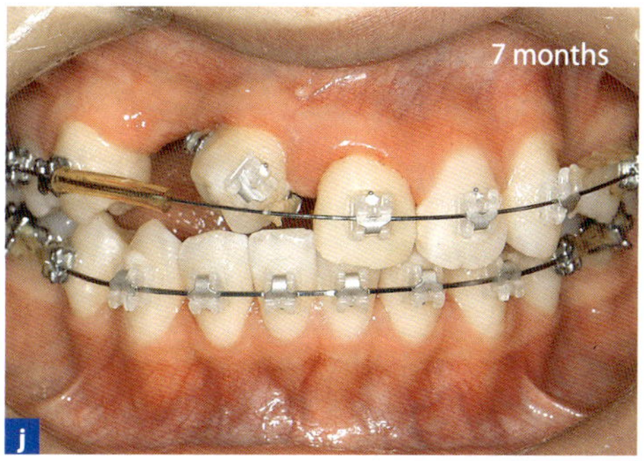

Fig 9-5k 10 months postop.
Fig 9-5l Two years and 2 months later. Orthodontic treatment was continued at our clinic for about 11 months at this time.

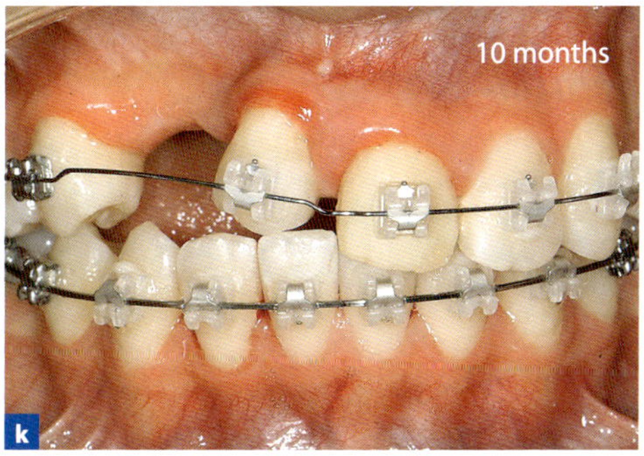

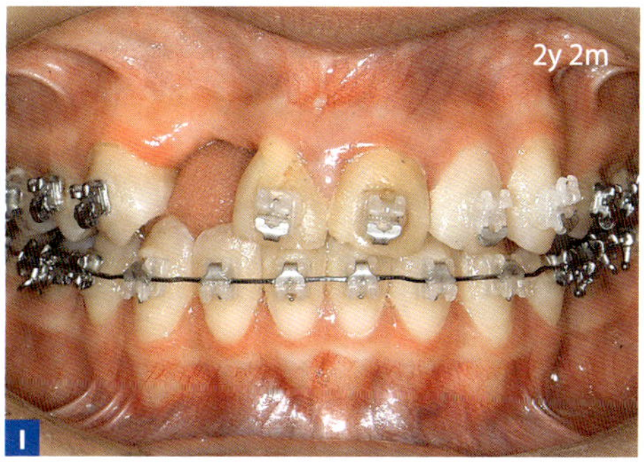

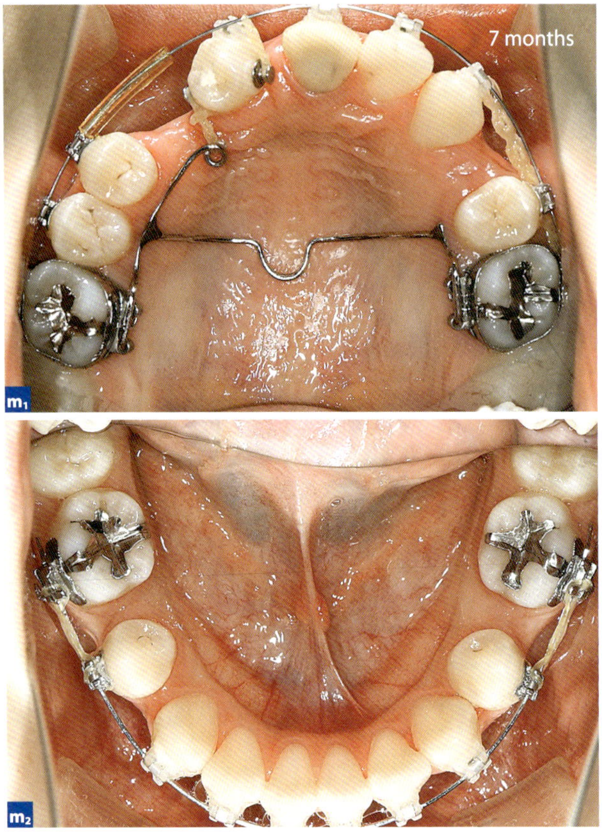

Fig 9-5m Occlusal views of the maxilla and the mandible 7 months after transplantation.

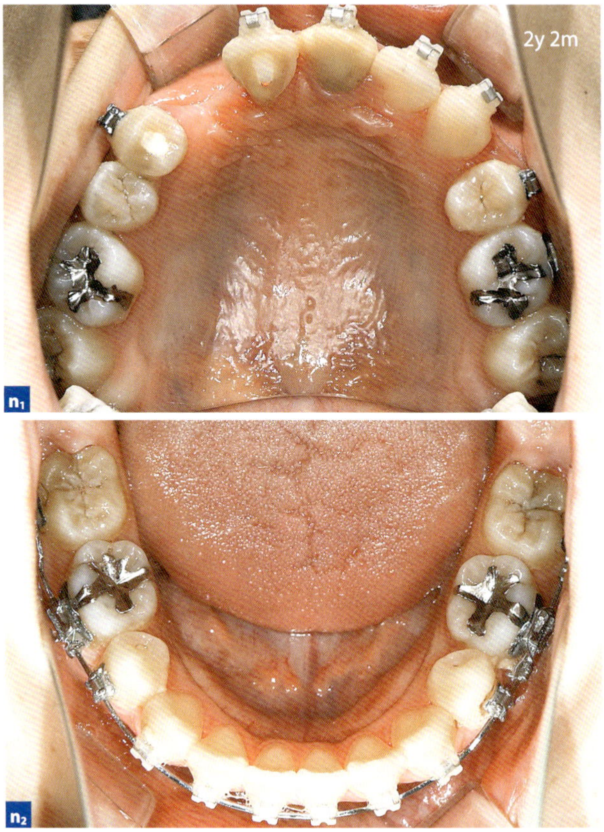

Fig 9-5n Occlusal views after 2 years and 2 months. Just before the end of orthodontic treatment.

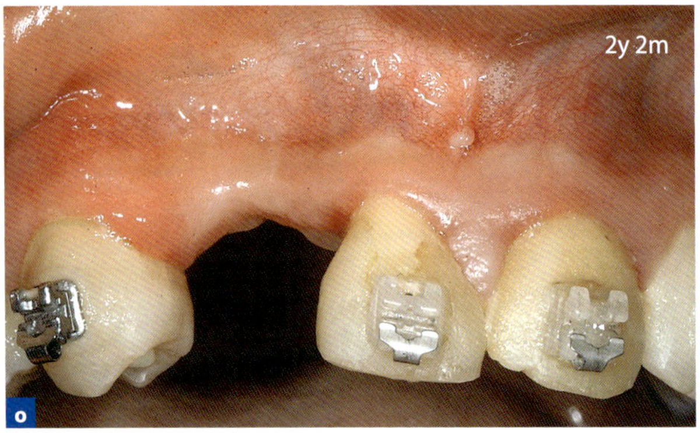

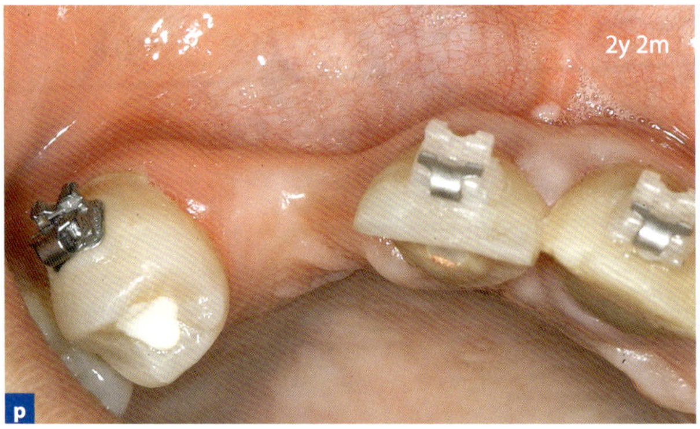

Fig 9-5o and 9-5p Views of the maxillary anterior region on the same day as **Fig 9-5n**. A larger amount of resorption of the alveolar ridge is present at the #12 site, the treatment of which is planned to have a fixed bridge. It was decided that it would be of benefit to perform ridge augmentation with a connective tissue graft (CTG).

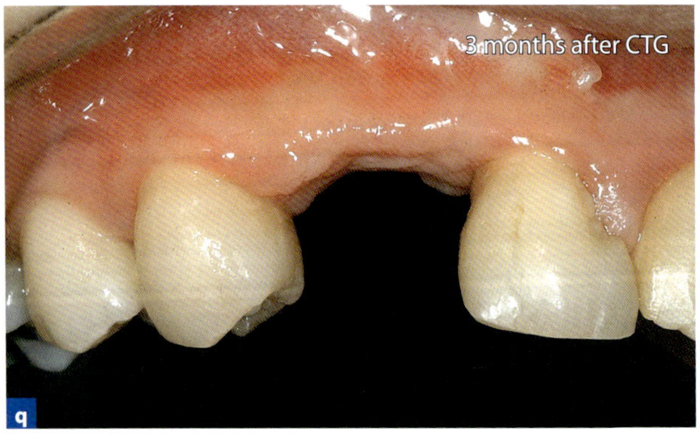

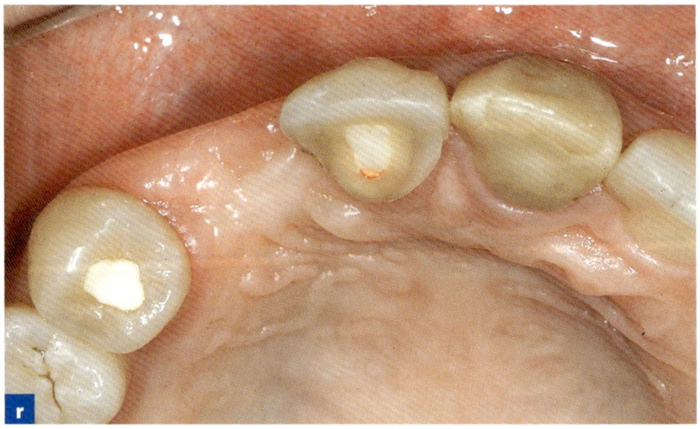

Fig 9-5q and 9-5r Three months after CTG.

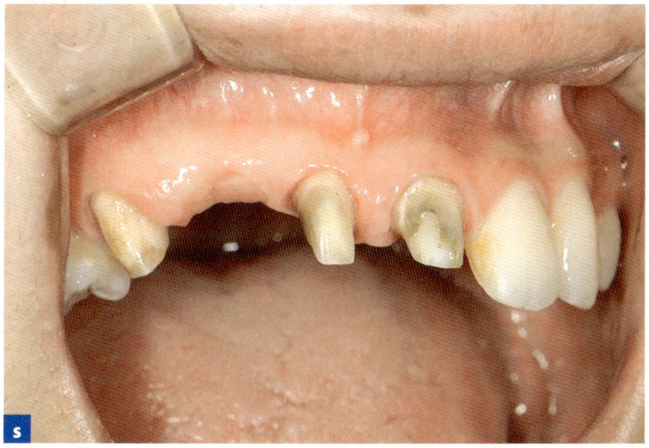

Fig 9-5s View before fabricating the fixed bridge.

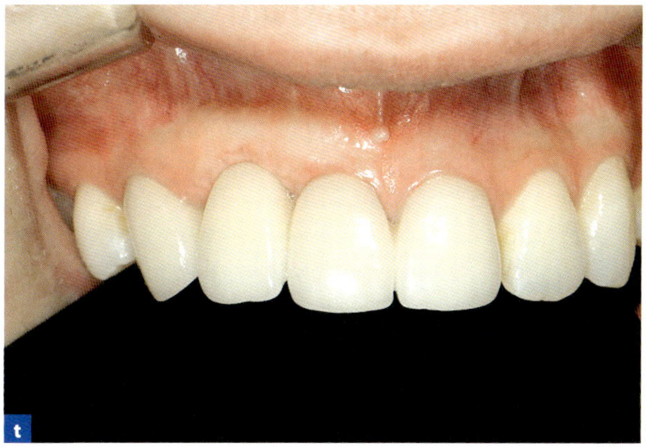

Fig 9-5t View after the prosthesis is delivered.

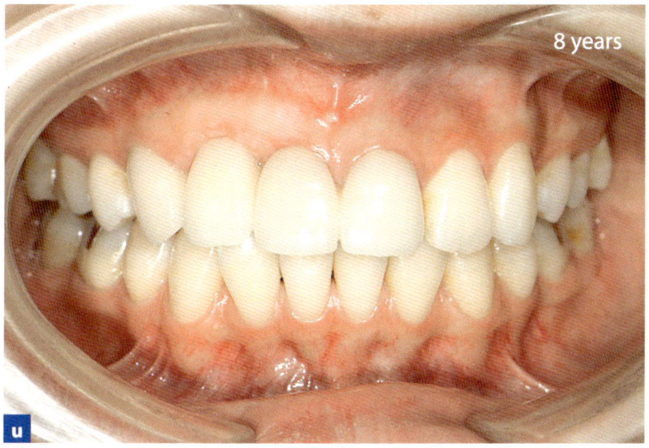

Fig 9-5u View 8 years after transplantation.

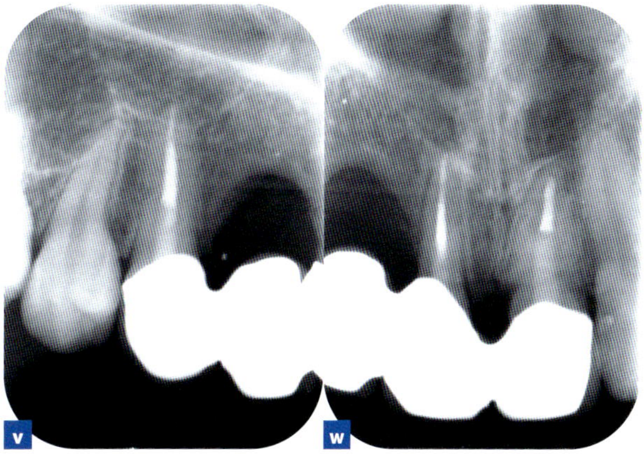

Fig 9-5v Radiograph of #13, 8 years after transplantation.
Fig 9-5w Radiograph of #11 and #21, 8 years after transplantation.

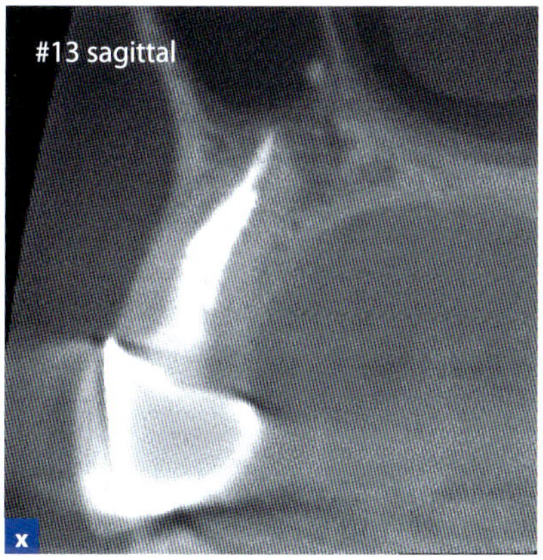

Fig 9-5x CBCT image of #13 after 8 years.

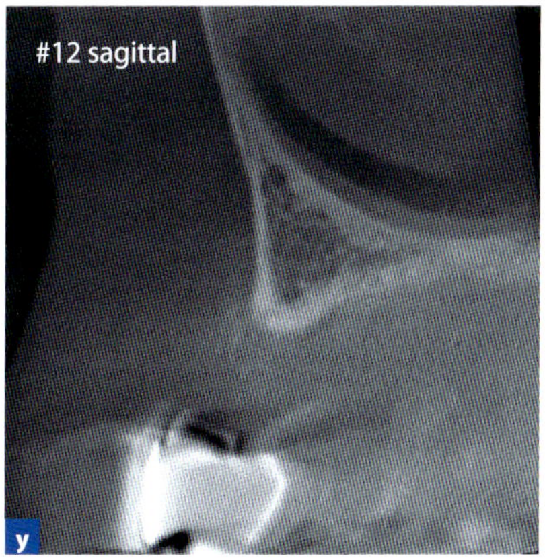

Fig 9-5y CBCT image of #12 site after 8 years.

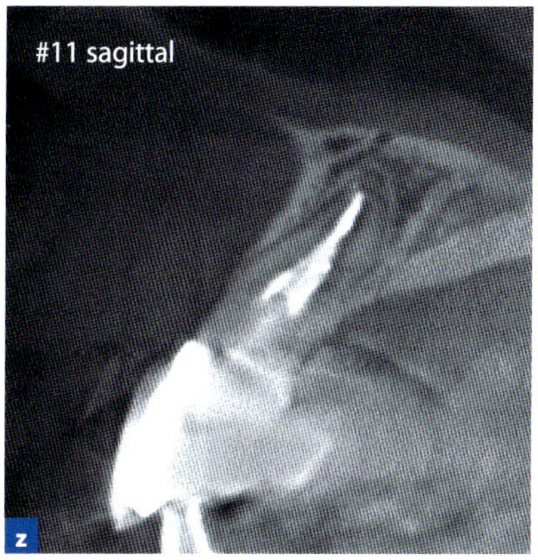

Fig 9-5z CBCT image of #11 after 8 years.

Transplantation as part of the orthodontic treatment is becoming more common due to the high success rates and outcomes that have been achieved through better understanding of the process and biological principles. Patients that may suffer from congenitally missing teeth or loss of anterior teeth due to trauma often require both transplantation and orthodontic treatment. Therefore, it is worthwhile for orthodontists to be aware of the possibility of transplantation in treatment options. There are lower risks of developing complications such as root resorption so it is important to assess each case before going through with treatment. If the risks of complications may be higher, there may be less risk through conventional orthodontic treatment such as space closure.

Some of the problems that arise after transplantation come from the delay in detection of pathology due to the lack of proper follow up and communication between the orthodontist and the dentist who performed the transplantation. Thus, in cases where orthodontic treatment and transplantation treatment are performed via different providers, it is important to have good communication and continuous monitoring of the patient during the active and recall phases of treatment.

All of the orthodontic treatment of the cases presented in this chapter (with the exception of the first part of case 5) were performed by Dr. Chie Tsukiboshi. We are grateful for her expertise and care for the patients.

References

1. Irinakis E, Aleksejuniene J, Shen Y, Haapasalo M. External Cervical Resorption: A Retrospective Case-Control Study. J Endod. 2020 Oct; 46(10): 1420-7.
2. Mavridou AM, Hauben E, Wevers M, Schepers E, Bergmans L, Lambrechts P. Understanding External Cervical Resorption in Vital Teeth. J Endod. 2016 Dec; 42(12): 1737-51.
3. European Society of Endodontology (ESE) developed by:; Patel S, Lambrechts P, Shemesh H, Mavridou A. European Society of Endodontology position statement: External Cervical Resorption. Int Endod J. 2018 Dec; 51(12): 1323-6.
4. Patel S, Mavridou AM, Lambrechts P, Saberi N. External cervical resorption-part 1 : histopathology, distribution and presentation. Int Endod J. 2018 Nov; 51(11): 1205-23.
5. Mavridou AM, Pyka G, Kerckhofs G, Wevers M, Bergmans L, Gunst V, Huybrechts B, Schepers E, Hauben E, Lambrechts P. A novel multimodular methodology to investigate external cervical tooth resorption. Int Endod J. 2016 Mar; 49(3): 287-300.
6. Heithersay GS. Invasive cervical resorption: an analysis of potential predisposing factors. Quintessence Int. 1999 Feb; 30(2): 83-95.
7. Mavridou AM, Bergmans L, Barendregt D, Lambrechts P. Descriptive Analysis of Factors Associated with External Cervical Resorption. J Endod. 2017 Oct; 43(10): 1602-10.
8. Mavridou AM, Hauben E, Wevers M, Schepers E, Bergmans L, Lambrechts P. Understanding external cervical resorption patterns in endodontically treated teeth. Int Endod J. 2017 Dec; 50(12): 1116-33.
9. Heithersay GS. Invasive cervical resorption. Endodontic Topics. 2004; 7 (1): 73-92.
10. Heithersay GS. Management of tooth resorption. Aust Dent J. 2007 Mar; 52(1 Suppl): S105-21.
11. Patel S, Foschi F, Condon R, Pimentel T, Bhuva B. External cervical resorption: part 2 - management. Int Endod J. 2018 Nov; 51(11): 1224-38.
12. Heithersay GS. Treatment of invasive cervical resorption: an analysis of results using topical application of trichloracetic acid, curettage, and restoration. Quintessence Int. 1999 Feb; 30(2): 96-110.

CHAPTER 10

Surgical extrusion and intentional replantation

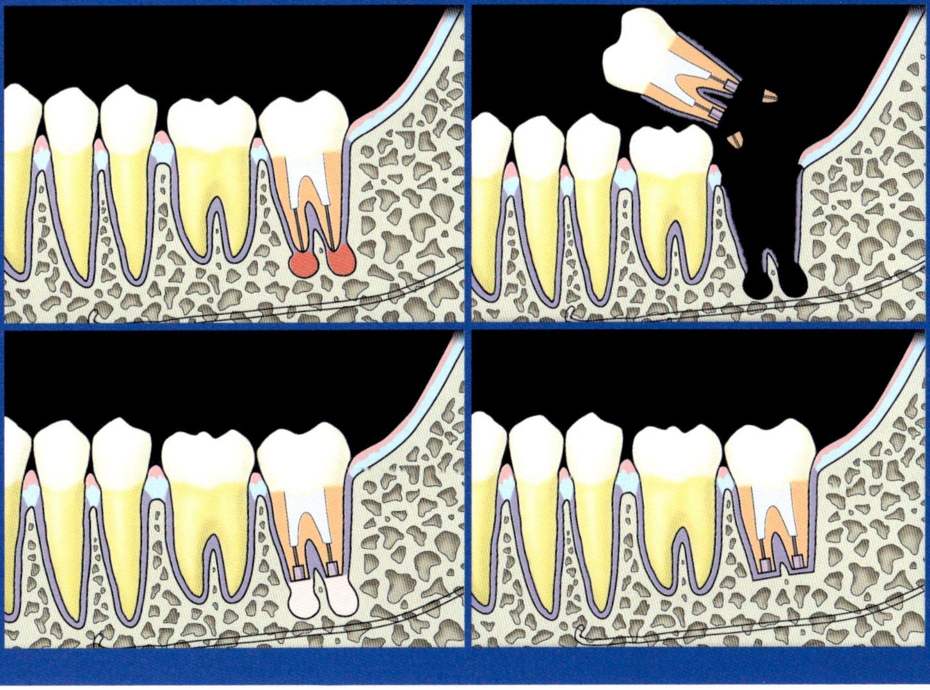

Teeth that are difficult to treat with conventional methods may be preserved by surgical extrusion or intentional replantation, which involves extracting the teeth, performing necessary procedures extraorally, and then placing them back to the same socket. Surgical extrusion and intentional replantation are basically the same but the difference is in the position and direction of the teeth when placed back into the original socket. The flow of treatment from examination/diagnosis to postoperative management does not differ significantly from conventional transplantation.

The classification and definition of surgical extrusion and intentional replantation have already been discussed in **Chapter 4**.

Surgical extrusion

When performing crown restoration of a tooth that has lost healthy dentin to or below the level of crestal bone due to trauma or caries, it is important to reestablish the biologic width and have a certain amount of intact tooth structure above the gingival margin for adequate ferrule so to increase the chances for long-term success. If the restorative margin is set below the gingival margin impinging into the biological width, it may cause gingival inflammation, and restorations with inadequate ferrule have been shown to have higher failure rates[1-9].

There are three options to achieve the above objectives: crown lengthening procedure[10,11] (apically positioned flap with bone resection), orthodontic extrusion[12,13], and surgical extrusion[14-17]. Although each method has advantages and disadvantages, surgical extrusion has several advantages for traumatized teeth (**Fig 10-1**) because of the following reasons:

(1) Most trauma occurs to the anterior incisors, which are easier to extract.
(2) Luxation may have already occurred due to trauma, and it would be easier to extract.
(3) Other root fractures or pathologies may be found during tooth extraction (a more definitive diagnosis can be made).
(4) By positioning the deepest part of the fracture on the buccal side (rotation can be performed at the same time as the extrusion), a more accessible and aesthetic restoration is possible with a minimum amount of extrusion.
(5) Coronal restoration is usually possible 1 month after surgery (i.e. overall treatment period is short). Restoration with composite resin (CR) would enable more conservative treatment in terms of time, cost, and ease of future restorative retreatment.

Criteria for choosing surgical extrusion

In terms of predictability, orthodontic extrusion will typically be the first option. However, surgical extrusion can be indicated when some of the following criteria are involved and overlapping.

- ☐ **When reestablishment of biologic width may lead to a better outcome**
- ☐ **When the shape of the tooth root is relatively easy to extract**
- ☐ **When rotation of the tooth at the same time as extrusion is preferable**
- ☐ **When definitive diagnosis during surgery is necessary**
- ☐ **When periapical pathology and deep caries are present at the same time**
- ☐ **When autotransplantation is not an option (if there is a good candidate, transplantation may be the first option)**

Procedures of surgical extrusion

Using a tooth with deep caries as an example (**Fig 10-2a** to **10-2b**), the procedural steps of surgical extrusion are as follows:

1. Anesthesia and removal of softened dentin if involved in caries
2. Resection of the inner gingival epithelium and intra-crevicular(sulcular) incision to cut periodontal ligament around the tooth
3. Raising a flap to reveal 1 to 2 mm of crestal bone
4. Extraction of the tooth
5. Extraoral root-end resection, preparation and retro filling (if periapical pathology is present)
6. Replantation of the tooth in desired position
7. Gingival flap suturing and suture fixation of the tooth
8. Surgical dressing (dressing and suture are removed in one week)
9. Restoration of the crown in about one month
10. Follow-up

1. Anesthesia and removal of softened dentin

After administering local anesthesia, the softened dentin is thoroughly removed, and the remaining intact tooth structure is checked.

2. Resection of the inner gingival epithelium and intra-crevicular incision

Gingival flap is usually raised to visualize the area around the root (often not necessary for traumatized teeth). As shown in **Fig 10-2c** to **10-2e**, the incision line is made, passing through the gingival sulcus and mesiodistally along alveolar crest of the adjacent tooth, and through the free gingiva of the tooth to be extruded. Make an incision line in the gingival sulcus of the adjacent teeth, and take care not to remove interproximal gingiva. An incision line is made around the extruding tooth to remove the inner marginal epithelium but to preserve as much gingiva as possible for esthetics. The inner epithelium must be removed so that reattachment at cervical area can occur smoothly immediately after replantation.

Purposes and procedures of surgical extrusion for a traumatized tooth

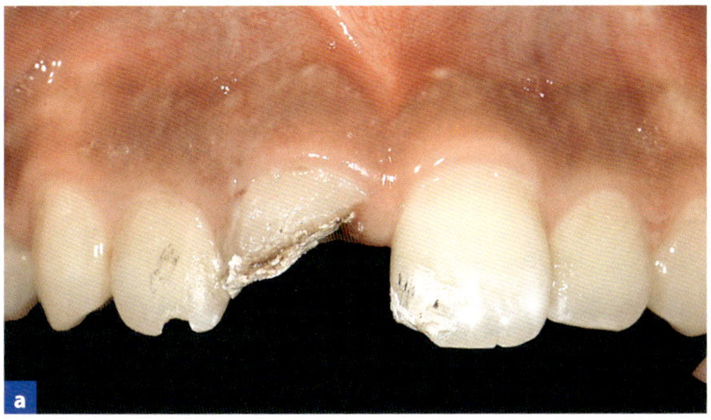

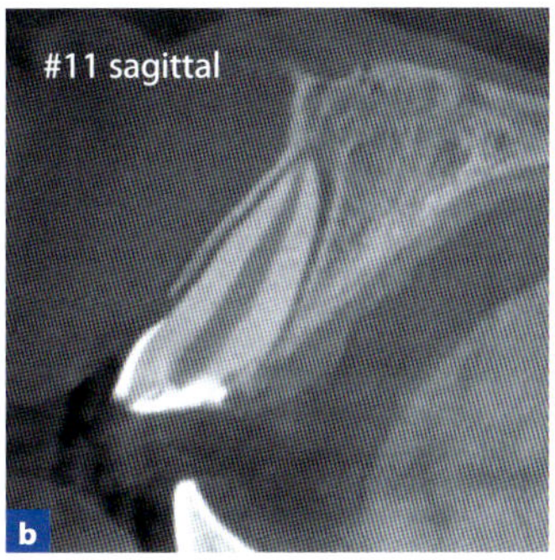

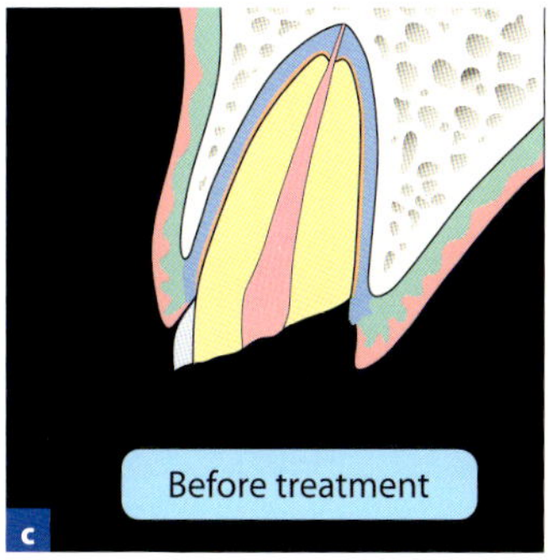

Fig 10-1a Preoperative view of a 12-year-old male who suffered crown-root fracture of #11.
Fig 10-1b Preoperative CBCT sagittal image. The findings show evidence that the fracture extends to the bony ridge on the palatal side.
Fig 10-1c Schematic diagram showing the preoperative state.

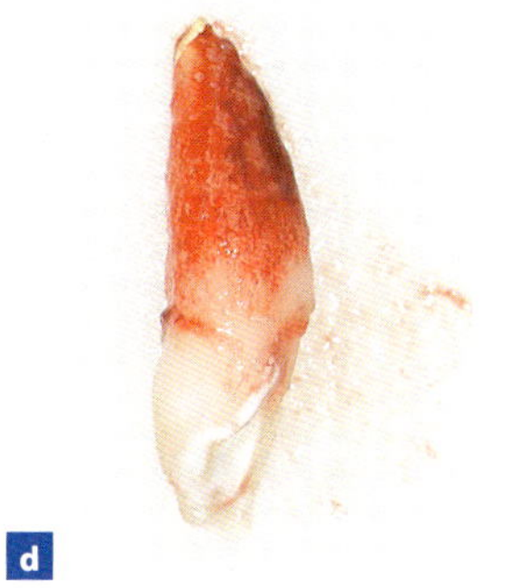

Fig 10-1d Extracted #11 for surgical extrusion.

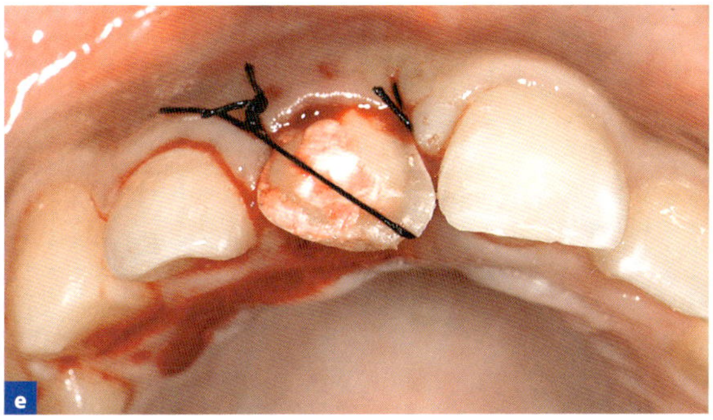

Fig 10-1e Immediately after surgical extrusion. The tooth has been rotated 180 degrees.

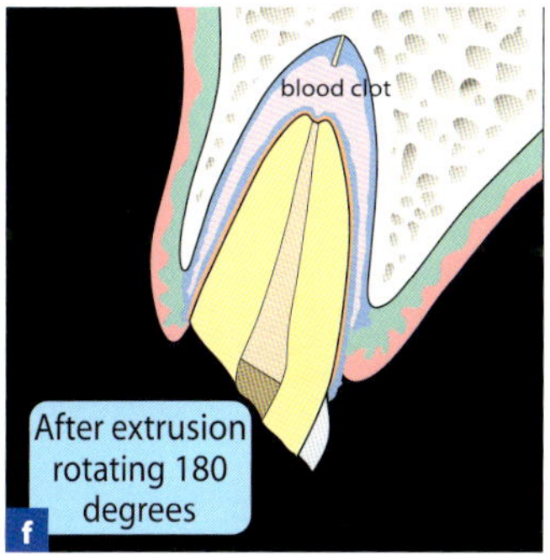

Fig 10-1f Schematic diagram after repositioning with surgical extursion.

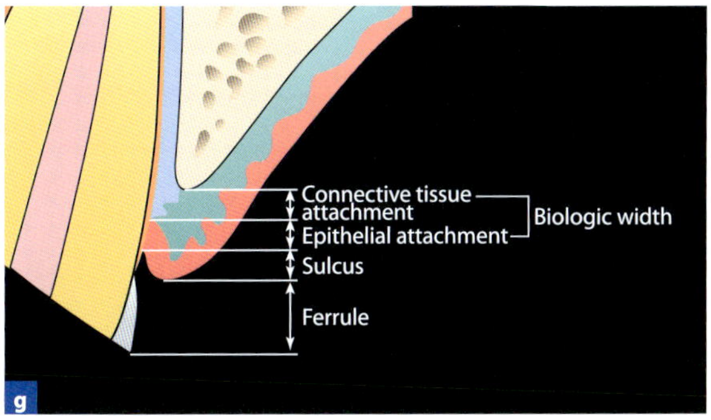

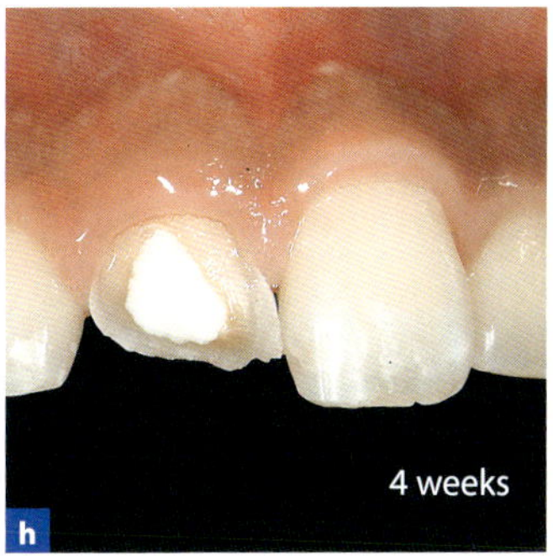

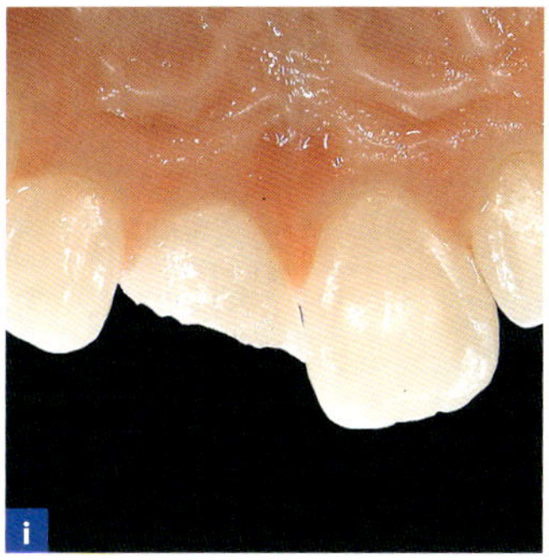

Fig 10-1g Purposes of surgical extrusion are to reestablish the biologic width of 2 mm and to secure a certain amount of intact tooth structure above the gingival margin for ferrule (more than 1 mm if possible). This would provide about 4 mm of intact tooth structure above the crestal margin of bone.
Fig 10-1h and 10-1i Clinical views after 4 weeks.

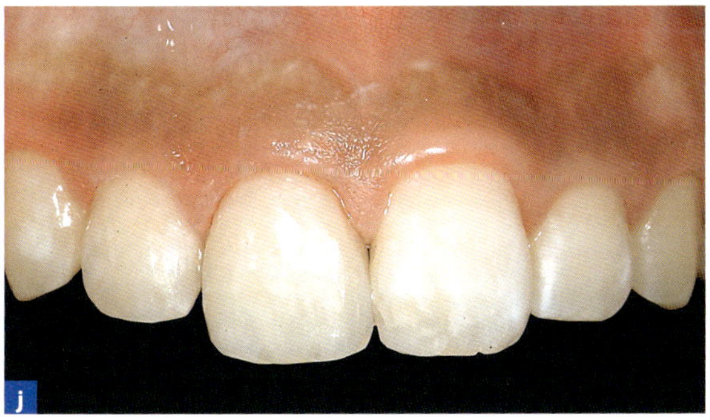

Fig 10-1j Crown restoration with composite resin (CR).

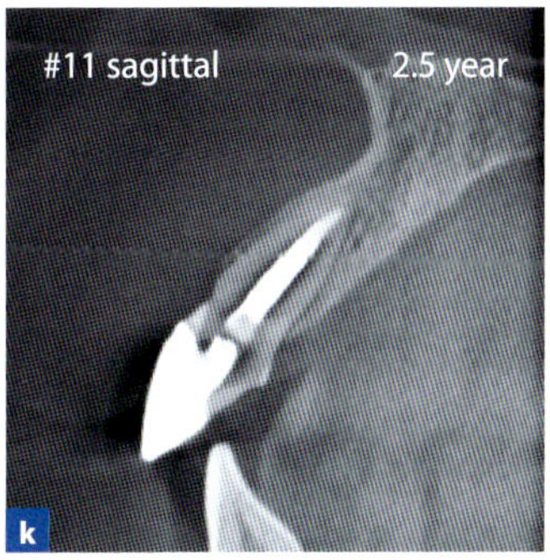

Fig 10-1k CBCT sagittal image 2 and a half years after surgery.

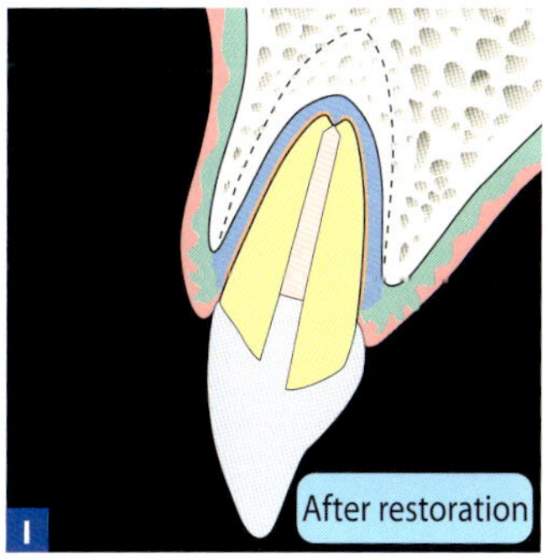

Fig 10-1l Schematic diagram after completion of the treatment.

Procedures of surgical extrusion

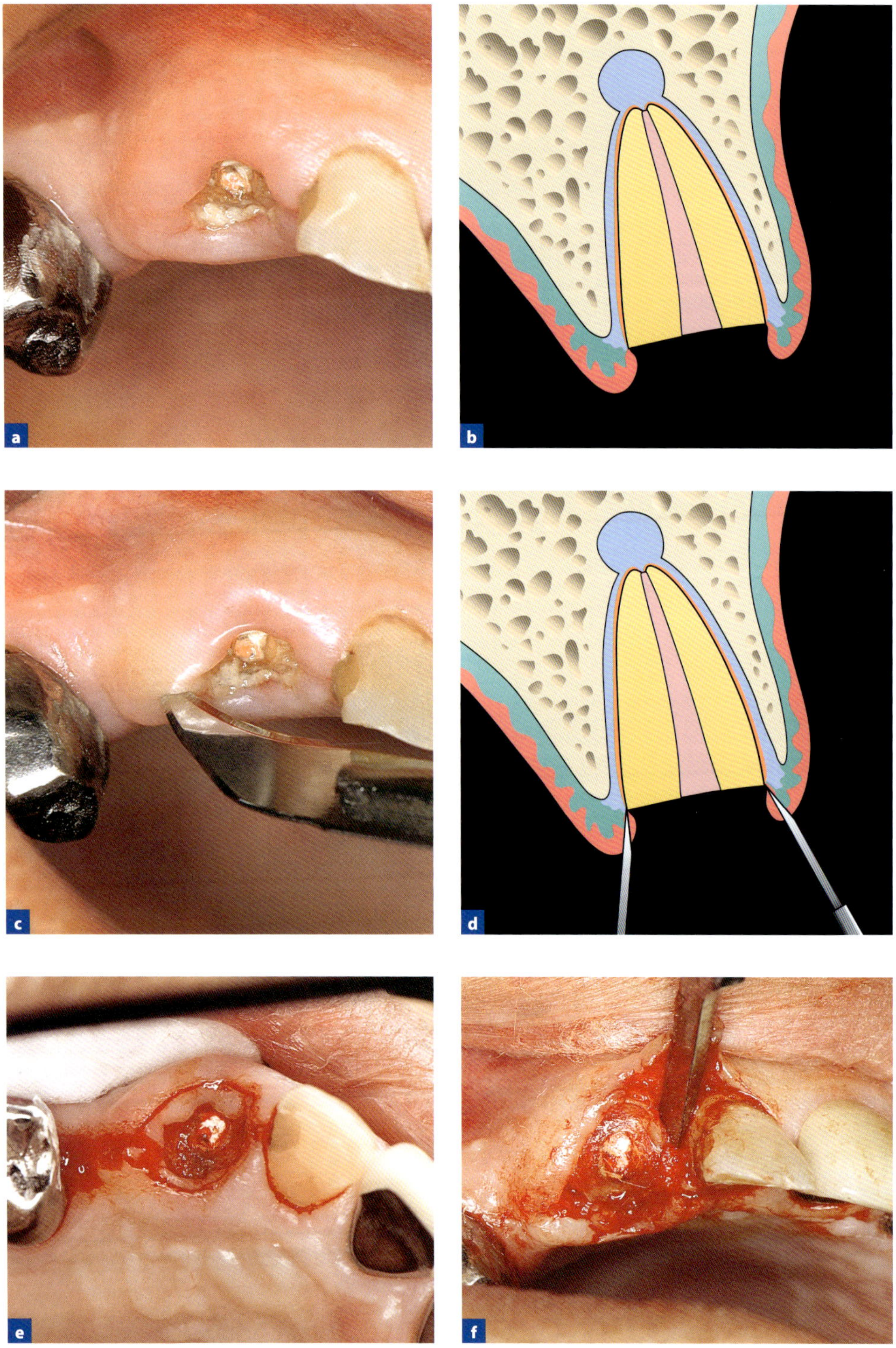

Fig 10-2a and 10-2b Preoperative examination and diagnosis. Evaluate the root shape (ideally the root is round and tapered or cone shaped), that there is sufficient root length available after extrusion, and whether or not there is an apical lesion.

Fig 10-2c to 10-2e How to make incisions.

After local anesthesia, incisions are made so that it passes through the gingival sulcus and alveolar crest of the adjacent teeth, and through the free gingiva of the extruded tooth. Remove inner epithelium around the extruded tooth but preserve interdental papilla as much as possible.

Fig 10-2f Luxation of the tooth. After slightly raising the gingival flap, a thin and narrow elevator with a narrow tip is inserted into the periodontal space at an angle of about 45 to 70 degrees to the tooth axis and pressure is applied in a twisting motion. Once the tooth is luxated, extract it with forceps and place it in saline. Then, remove any granulation tissue without scraping the intact socket walls.

3. Raising the flap

Raise the flap to expose the bony crest around the tooth to be extruded. It is enough to raise the gingival flap so that about 2 mm of bone is exposed (**Fig 10-2f**).

4. Extraction of the tooth and removal of granulation tissue

After raising the flap the tooth is luxated (extracted). If the coronal portion has collapsed and is not able to be grasped by forceps, use a thin and narrow elevator with a narrow tip, insert it at angle of about 45 to 70 degrees to the tooth axis, and rotate it to luxate it out (**Fig 10-2f** to **10-2h**). The periodontal ligament is mechanically damaged to some extent, but this part of the periodontal ligament will extruded out of the socket after extrusion. The extracted tooth is kept in saline. Then, granulation tissue is thoroughly removed from the periapical lesion area but don't scrape the intact socket walls so to preserve periodontal ligament.

5. Extraoral root resection and retro canal filling (only if necessary)

The luxated tooth is taken out and checked for fractures, apical lesion tissue, root resorption, etc (**Fig 10-2h**).

For a tooth with a periapical lesion, open apex, or a case where root canal filling cannot be obturated and sealed well due to a ledge or blockages, apicoectomy and retro canal filling is performed extraorally (**Fig 10-2i** to **10-2j**). While treating the root area extraorally, it is important to protect the root surface with gauze soaked in saline to minimize damage to the periodontal ligament from drying, and to refrain from using tap water cooling. Even a tooth that have been well obturated with sealer and gutta-percha but has an apical lesion should undergo retro canal filling after resection of the root apex to help prevent micro-leakage. Extraoral root resection usually does not need to be performed for a tooth that does not have an apical lesion and adequate root filling. In a young patient with an open apex, retro canal filling may decrease the healing period and help prevent possible future endodontic problems.

6. Replanting the tooth

Replant the extracted tooth back in the original socket. It would be ideal to position the tooth having at least 4 mm of healthy dentin above the crestal bone level (**Fig 10-2k**). If there is a deep oblique fracture, caries or resorption the tooth can be rotated 90 to180 degrees to make that part of the root surface face labially and position it to have at least 2.5 mm of intact tooth structure above the crestal bone level. This will provide as much root structure as possible back into the socket and can make it easier to restore the tooth (see **Fig 10-1**). Even with 2.5mm of root structure above the crestal bone level, the restoration of the crown can be performed with adequate biological width and esthetic outcome (see **Fig 10-1**).

7. Gingival flap suturing and suture fixation of the tooth

In surgical extrusion, the treatment time can be shortened by suturing the gingival flap and fixing the tooth with suture string at the same time. Because the shape of the socket and the root are same, there is good initial stability of the tooth after replantation. In addition, healing can occur more quickly than with conventional transplantation because periodontal ligament exists on the socket walls.

For tooth fixation with sutures, an interrupted suture is first made on the mesial (or distal) part of gingival flap (**Fig 10-2l**). At that time, the knot should be positioned on the lingual (or buccal) side. Cut the string leaving about 4 cm of one of the ends of the string. Next, the distal (or mesial) part of the gingival flap is sutured. Place the knot on the buccal (or lingual) side (**Fig 10-2m** and **10-2n**). Then, without cutting the string, wrap the longer thread around the tooth twice, and then tie the knot again (**Fig 10-2o** to **10-2q**). This will create some extrusive forces on the tooth; then by adding a cross-suture with the remaining 4 cm mesial string, the tooth is pressed down and fixed at the intended position (**Fig 10-2r**). This method is very simple, easy and convenient.

8. Surgical dressing

In order to protect the area and allow for healing (reattachment), cover the surgical site with sterilized aluminum foil and surgical dressing to protect the wound surface, prevent infection, and preserve the blood clot (**Fig 10-2s** and **10-2t**). The surgical dressing and sutures are removed about 7 days after surgery (**Fig 10-2u**). Early reattachment is achieved at the cervical area, and the risk of detachment of the replanted tooth is rare. Care should be taken not to apply excessive occlusal force to the extruded tooth for 3 weeks after surgery.

9. Restoration of the crown

Restoration of the crown of the surgically extruded tooth can be started about 1 month after surgery (**Fig 10-2v**). However, if tooth mobility is still high, then wait longer for the tooth to become more stable. The authors usually perform the restoration with the direct method using CR (see **Fig 10-1**, **10-4**, and **10-5**). Depending on the situation, indirect prosthetic treatment is performed after fabricating a post and core.

10. Follow-up

Maintain the tooth to prevent caries and periodontal disease as part of the normal routine. If increasing mobility of the treated tooth is observed, occlusal adjustment can be performed to stabilize the tooth and surrounding periodontal tissue. The tooth is followed up with radiographs taken at 3 months, 6 months, 1 year and thereafter every 2 to 3 years.

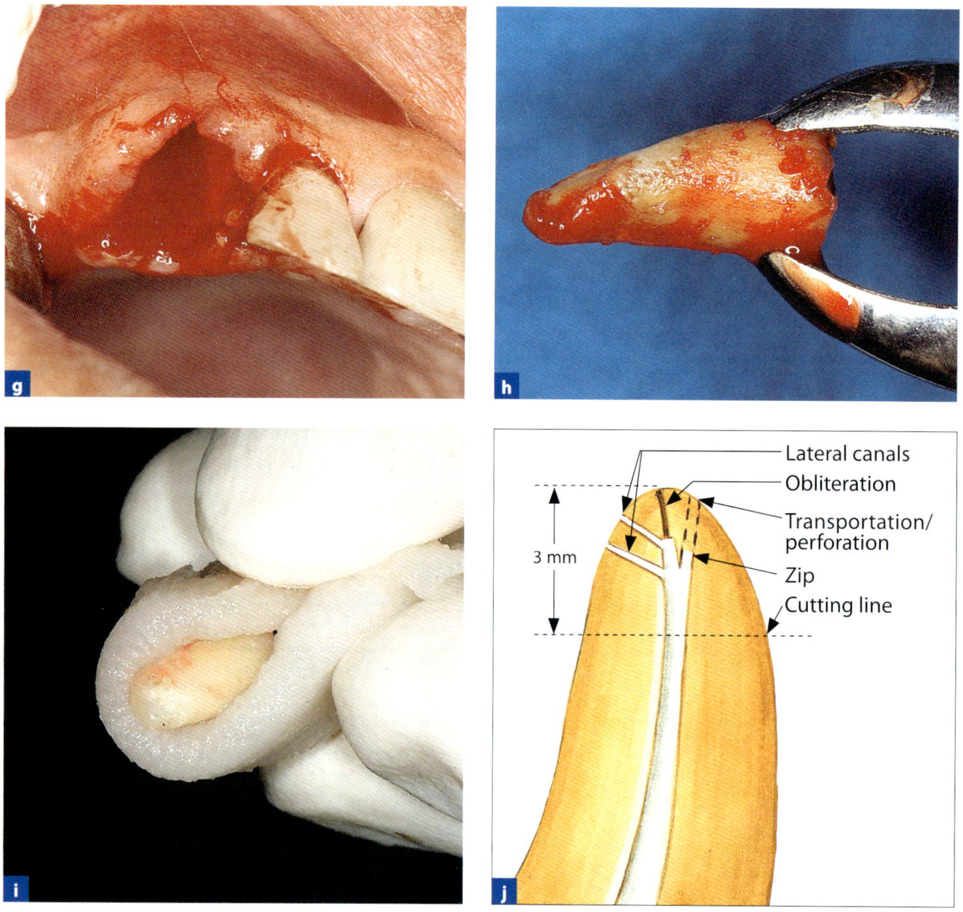

Fig 10-2g to 10-2j Observation of the extracted tooth, root apex resection, retro canal filling if necessary.

Check for cracks and apical lesion. For a tooth with apical lesion, it is advised to perform extraoral apicoectomy with retro canal filling because endo problems which cannot be resolved by conventional root canal treatment such as lateral canals, isthmuses, fins, transportations and perforation caused by the previous treatment may be present. Usually 3 mm of apex is resected. Retro filling material such as MTA is placed.

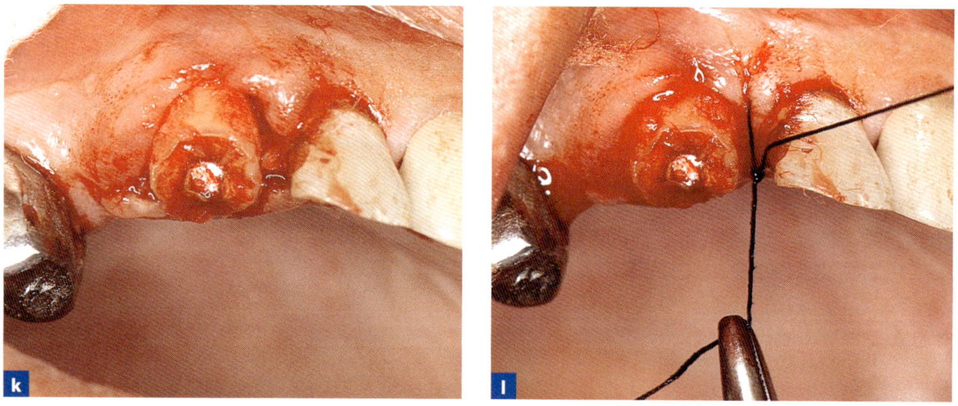

Fig 10-2k to 10-2l Suture of gingival flap and fixation of the tooth with suture string.

Ideally, the tooth is placed to a position where there is 4mm or more of intact dentin above the bone crest, and the tooth is fixed with suture string at the same time the gingival flap is sutured. First, the mesial aspect of the gingival flap is sutured with a simple interrupted suture. The knot should be placed on the palatal side (or labial). Cut the suture leaving about 4 cm of one of the ends.

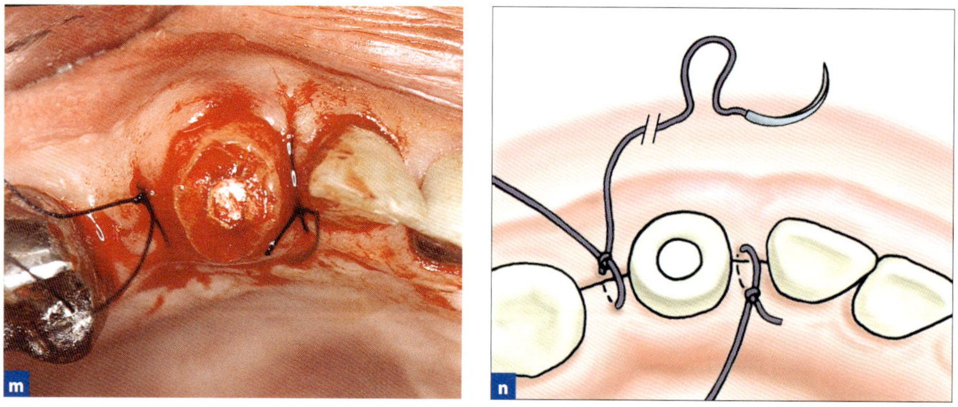

Fig 10-2m and 10-2n Suture the distal aspect of the gingival flap. The knot is placed diagonally to the mesial knot (labial or palatal side).

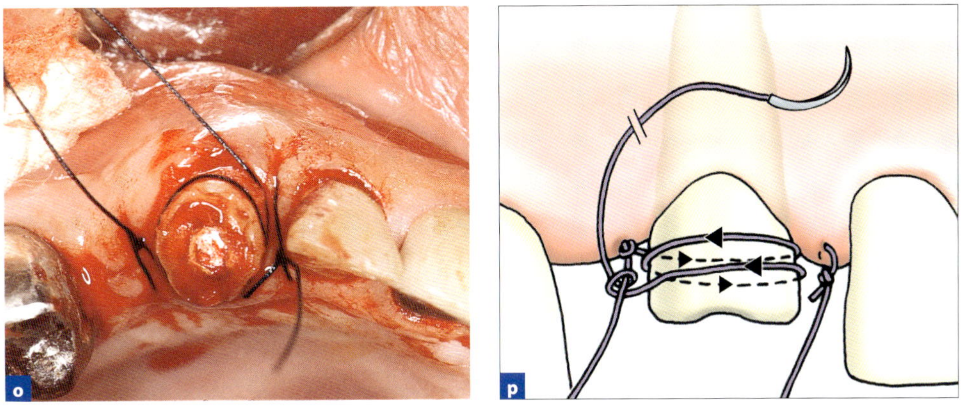

Fig 10-2o and 10-2p The longer end of the distal suture thread is wrapped around the extruded root twice, and then tied back to the distal end with a knot.

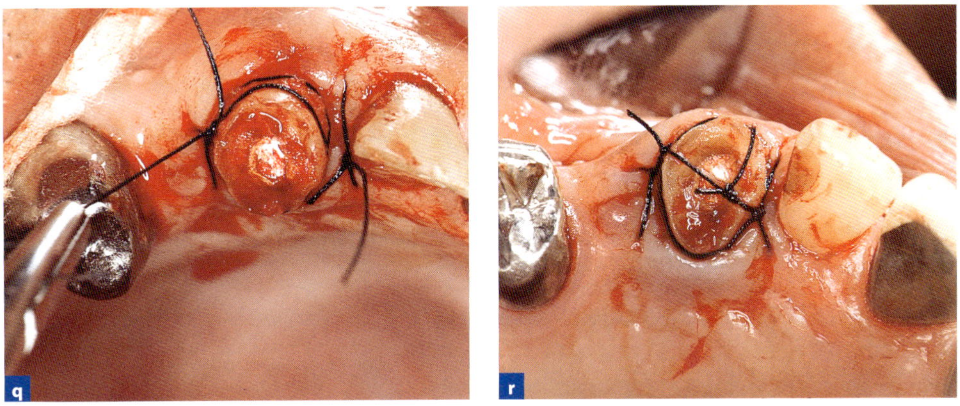

Fig 10-2q and 10-2r Wrapping the thread around the root twice will create some extrusive force, So, then a cross suture using the thread left on the mesial aspect is placed on the occlusal aspect root surface to hold down the tooth in place. This allows the tooth to be easily fixed at the given position.

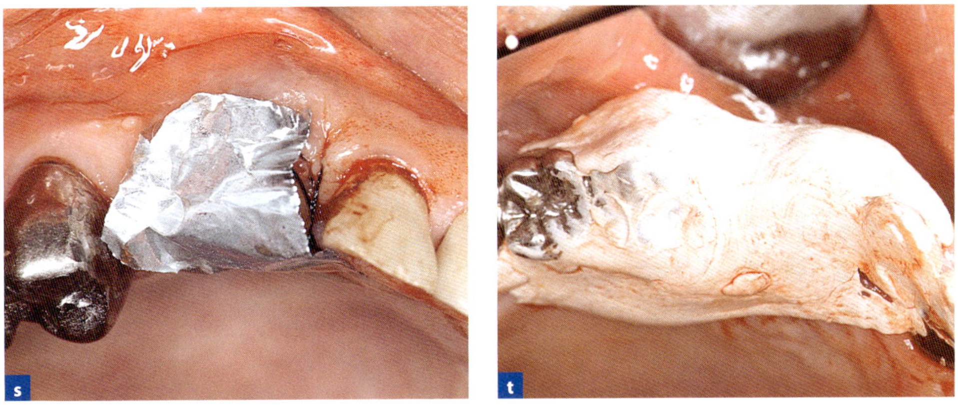

Fig 10-2s and 10-2t Protect the wound and prevent infection with aluminum foil and surgical dressing.

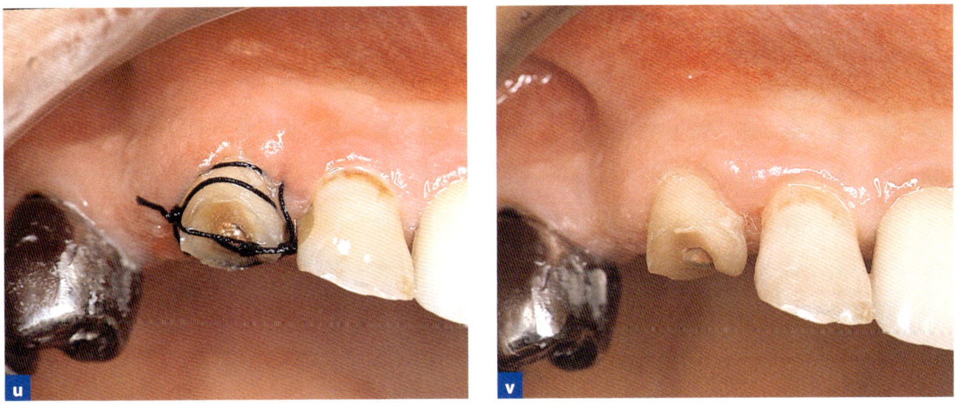

Fig 10-2u Seven days after surgery. Surgical dressing and suture are removed.
Fig 10-2v One to 3 months after surgery. After confirmation of healing, the tooth is restored appropriately.

Case presentations of Surgical Extrusion

Surgical extrusion of a tooth involved in crown-root fracture due to trauma (Fig 10-3)

Fig 10-3 shows a case of a 12-year-old male whose #21 was involved in crown-root fracture due to trauma (Fig 10-3a to 10-3d). The treatment goal for crown-root fracture due to trauma is to restore the crown through reestablishing the biologic width and obtaining a certain amount of ferrule above the crestal bone level either by surgical or orthodontic extrusion. As discussed previously, central incisors have rounded and tapered roots, making them easy to extract, which can result in high success rates for surgical extrusion.

Advantages of surgical extrusion over orthodontic extrusion include being able to make a definitive diagnosis at the time of extraction, the flexibility to fleely rotate and reposition the tooth, and shorter treatment time (see Fig 10-1). Usually, crown restoration can be performed 3 to 4 weeks after surgical extrusion. In this case, the enamel shell (Fig 10-3n) which was created from his own crown fragment was adhered to the original tooth with composite (Fig 10-3o to 10-3r). Restoration with using the patient's own tooth is considered to be the most aesthetic and functional (Fig 10-3s to 10-3x).

Surgical extrusion of a tooth with external resorption ① (Fig 10-4)

Fig 10-4 shows a case of a 20-year-old male whose #21was involved in external root resorption (Fig 10-4a to 10-4c). As can be seen in CBCT images (Fig 10-4d and 10-4e), external root resorption had progressed deep into the dentin from the palatal cervical region, and a relatively large periapical radiolucency is observed at the apex (Fig 10-4e). As is discussed in Fig 10-3, it was considered that surgical extrusion had more advantages over orthodontic extrusion for this case (Fig 10-4f to 10-4k). Crown restoration with CR was completed 3 weeks after the surgery (Fig 10-4l to 10-4n). It seemed that the treatment was more conservative, and the burden on the patient was reduced in terms of both time and cost. Another advantage of CR is that it is easy to modify its shape by adding or subtracting it in the future.

In the CBCT images 1 year and 6 years after surgical extrusion, there is no evidence of root resorption, a uniform periodontal ligament space can be observed around the entire root surface and the alveolar bone on the labial side is maintained (Fig 10-4o to 10-4w).

Surgical extrusion of a tooth involved in crown-root fracture due to trauma ①

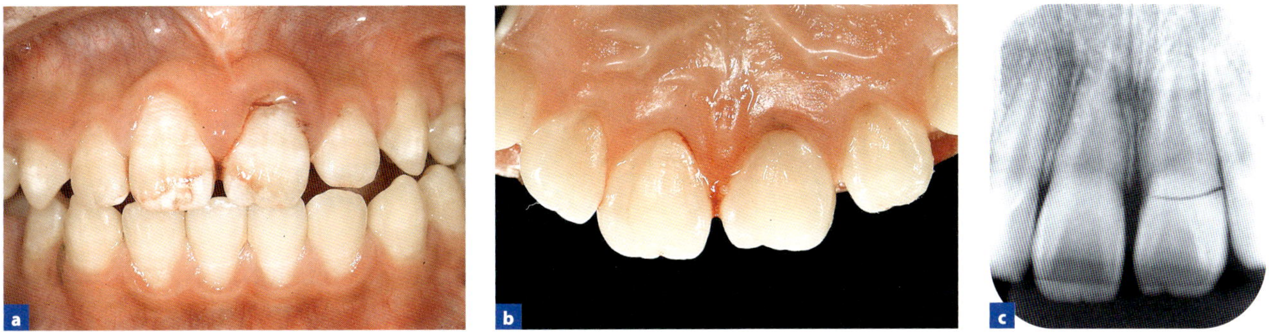

Fig 10-3a to 10-3c Views at the first visit of a 12-year-old male who suffered crown-root fracture of #21.

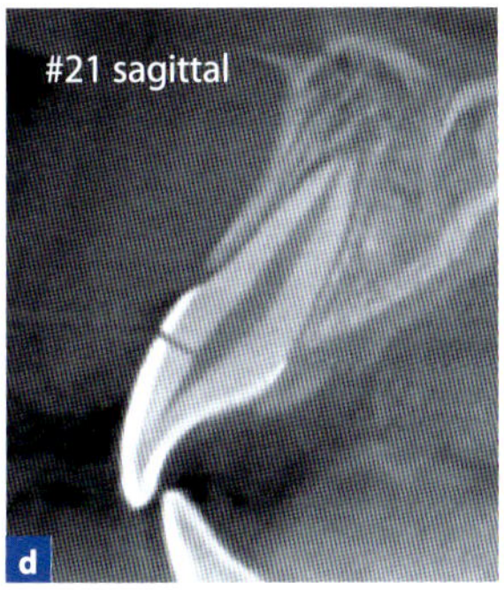

Fig 10-3d CBCT sagittal image of #21. The findings appear to show that the fracture reaches below the bone crest on the palatal side.

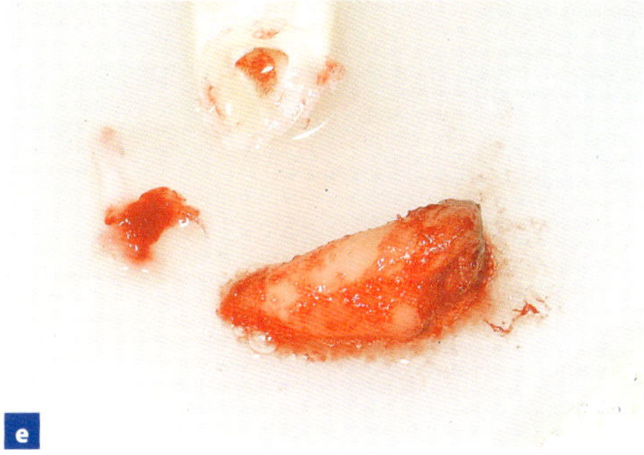

Fig 10-3e Tooth was extracted for surgical extrusion. The tooth was actually fractured into three fragments.

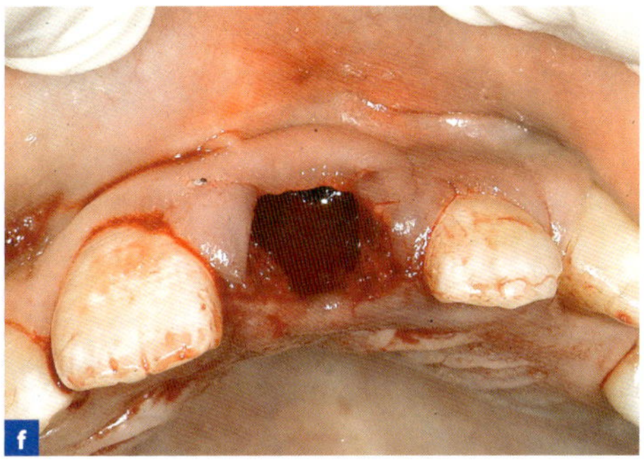

Fig 10-3f Extraction socket.

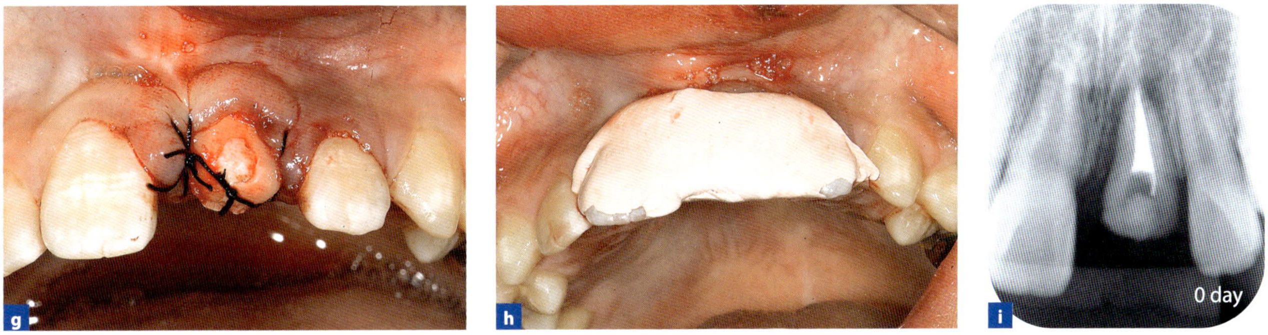

Fig 10-3g Immediately after surgical extrusion. The root was rotated 180 degrees.
Fig 10-3h Wound protection by surgical dressing.
Fig 10-3i Radiograph immediately after surgery. Prior to tooth extraction, the root canal was temporarily filled with calcium hydroxide preparation, 'Vitapex (NEO DENTAL CHEMICAL PRODUCTS CO., LTD, Japan)'.

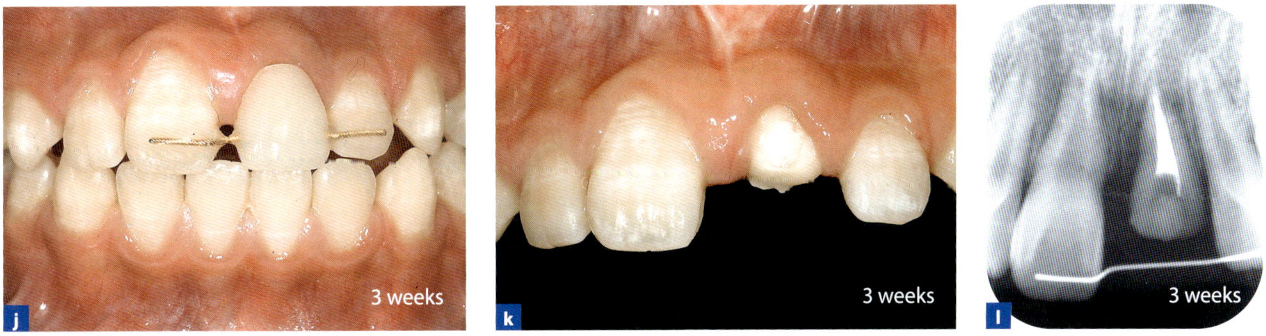

Fig 10-3j to 10-3l Views after 3 weeks. The suture was removed 7 days after surgery, and the provisional crown was fixed to the adjacent teeth concurrently after surgery. The temporary crown was removed in 3 weeks and the calcium hydroxide preparation was replaced with sealer and gutta-percha and then the crown was restored on the same day.

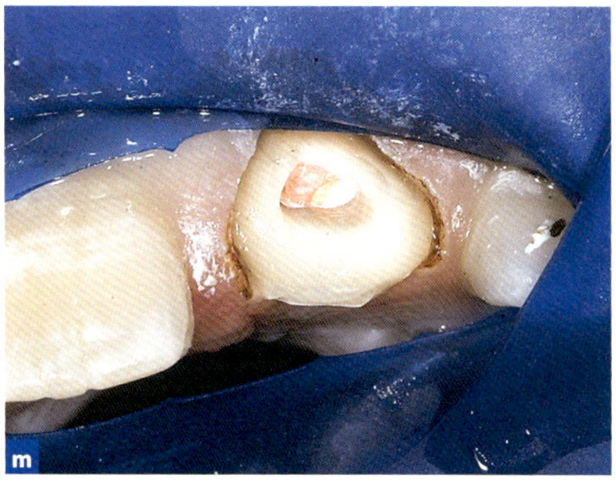

Fig 10-3m Immediately after root canal filling with sealer and gutta-percha. the same day as **Fig 10-3j** to **10-3l**.

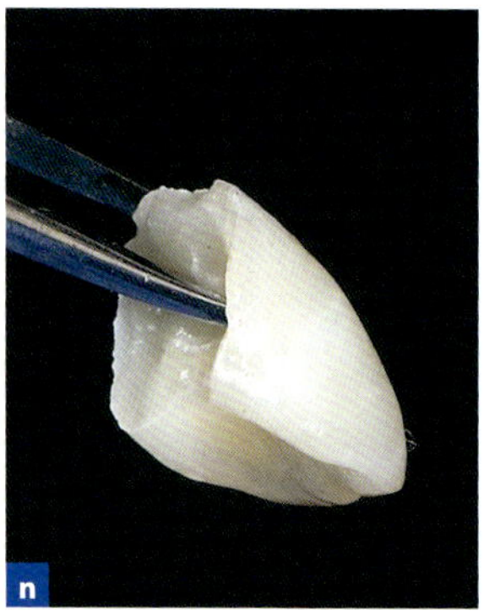

Fig 10-3n Enamel shell was made from the patient's own tooth.

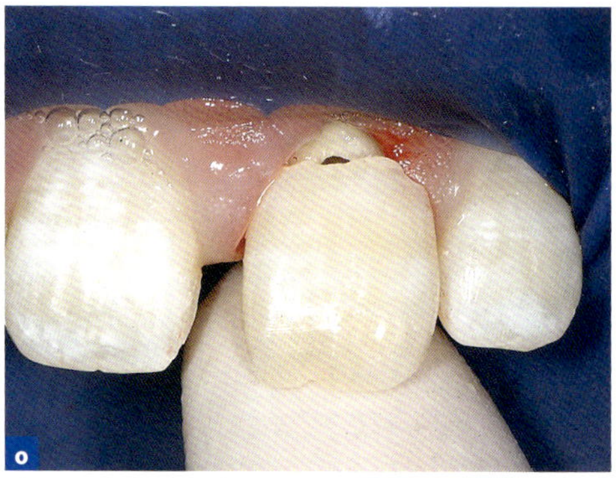

Fig 10-3o Try-in of the enamel shell.

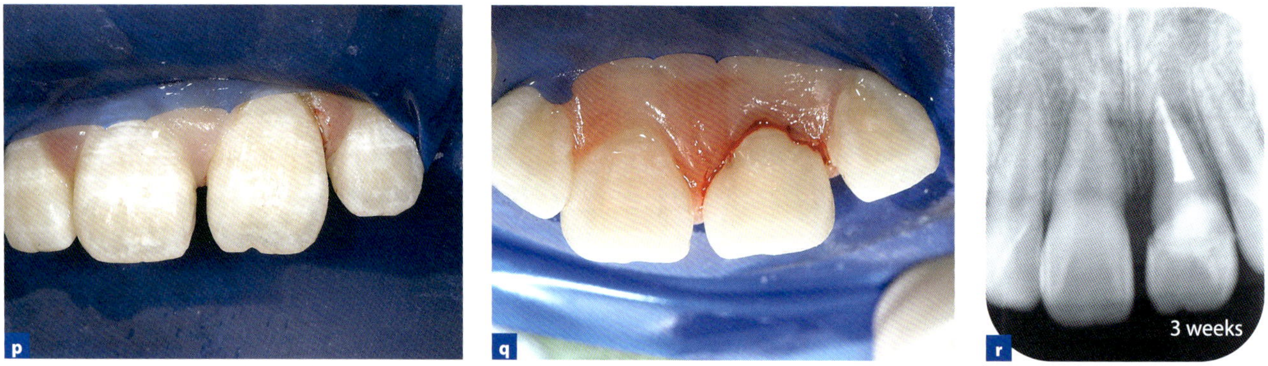

Fig 10-3p to 10-3r Immediately after bonding the enamel shell to the tooth with CR.

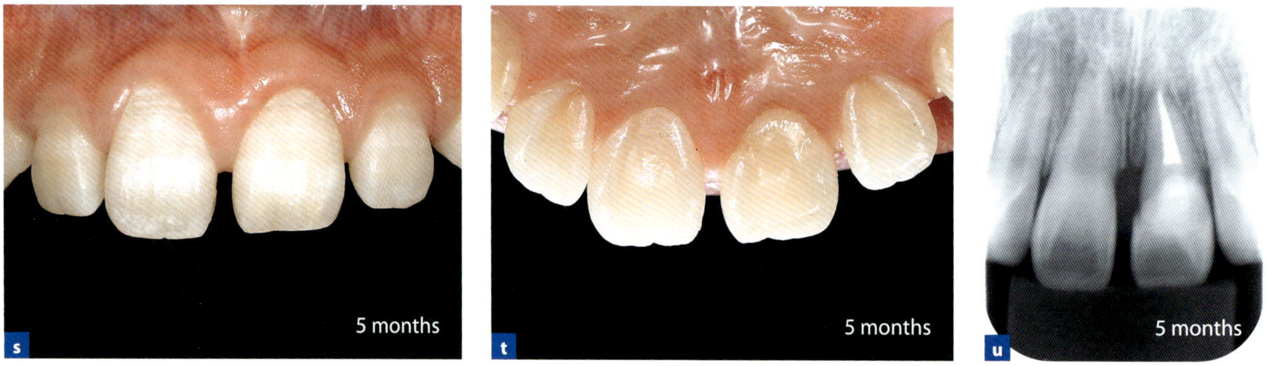

Fig 10-3s to 10-3u Five months after surgery.

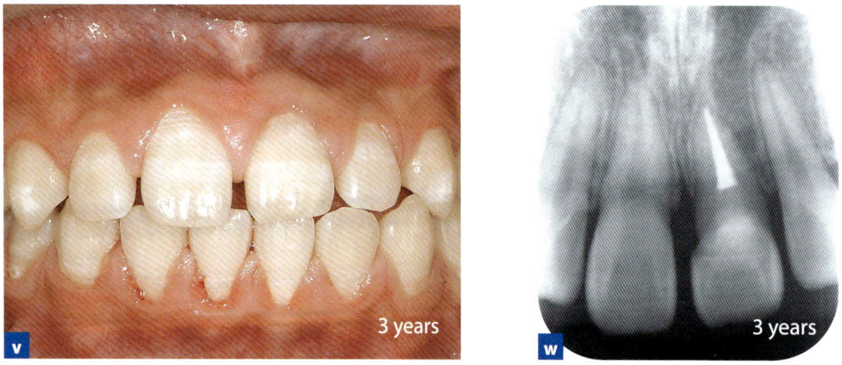

Fig 10-3v and 10-3w Three years after the trauma. The patient was satisfied with the functional and esthetic outcome.

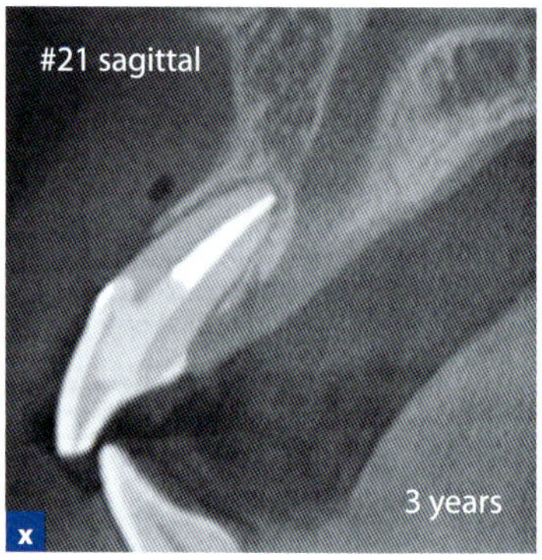

Fig 10-3x CBCT sagittal image 3 years after surgery. There are no apparent abnormalities detected.

Surgical extrusion of a tooth with external resorption ①

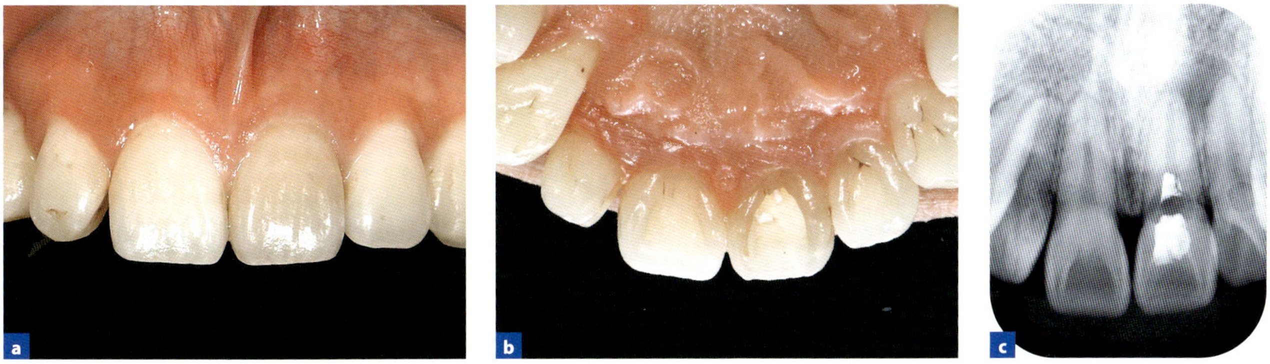

Fig 10-4a to 10-4c Views before treatment of a 20-year-old male who presented with discoloration and discomfort of #21. The radiograph showed evidence of root resorption around the cervical area and periapical radiolucency likely consistent with apical periodontitis.

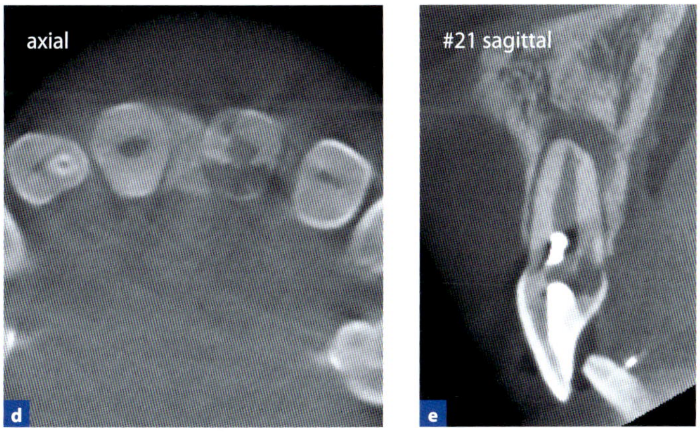

Fig 10-4d and 10-4e CBCT images of #21. The findings show evidence that external root resorption has occurred from the palatal side at the cervical level, and there is evident periapical radiolucency. It was decided that surgical extrusion would be the best way to reestablish biological width and treat the endodontic infection by extraoral apicoetcomy and save the tooth.

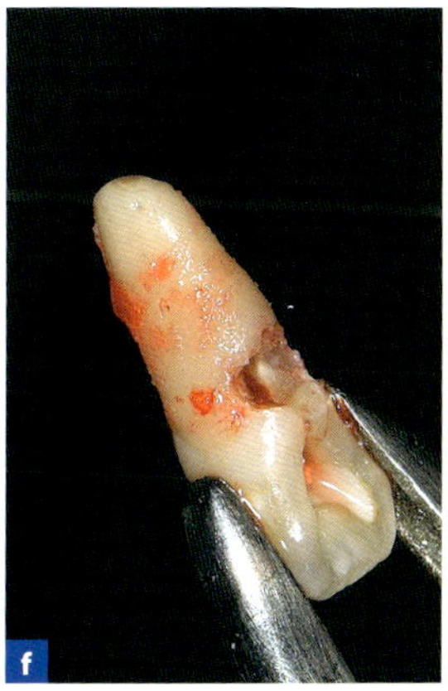

Fig 10-4f Tooth extracted #21 for surgical extrusion.

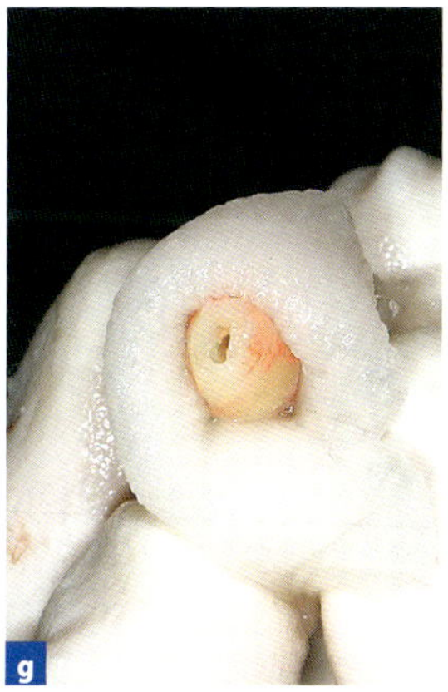

Fig 10-4g Open apex with a likely developed mature biofilm was treated with extraoral apicoectomy and retro filling.

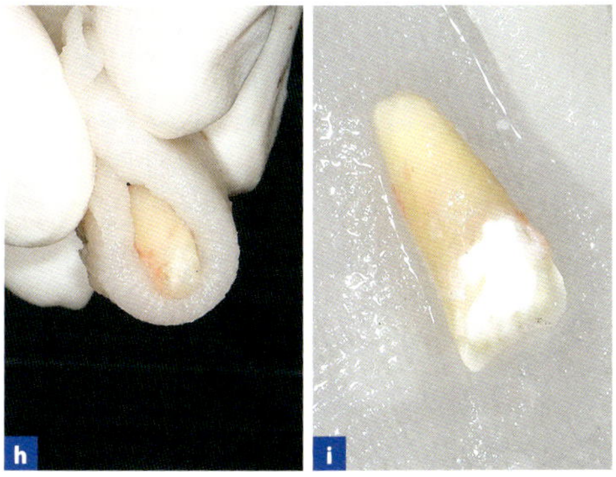

Fig 10-4h Immediately after retro canal filling. The filling material used was a light-cured glass ionomer cement.

Fig 10-4i Crown portion involved in advanced invasive resorption was removed, and the pulp canal was filled with calcium hydroxide preparation temporarily and sealed with conventional glass ionomer cement.

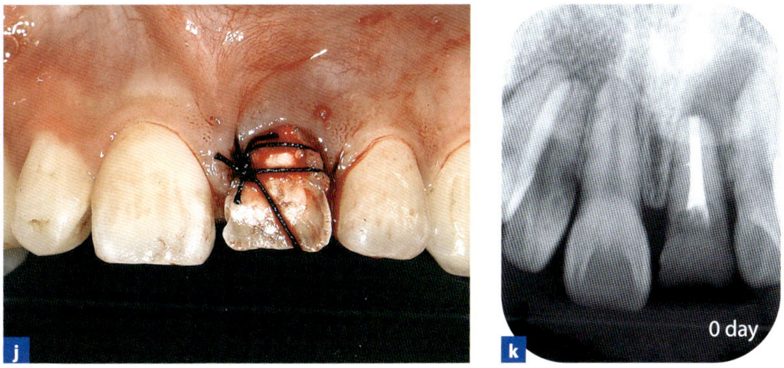

Fig 10-4j and 10-4k Immediate after surgery. The tooth was rotated 180 degrees, and was placed back into the original socket at the desired position so that a certain amount of intact tooth structure could be secured above the bone crest. The gingival flap was sutured and the tooth was fixed with the same suture string.

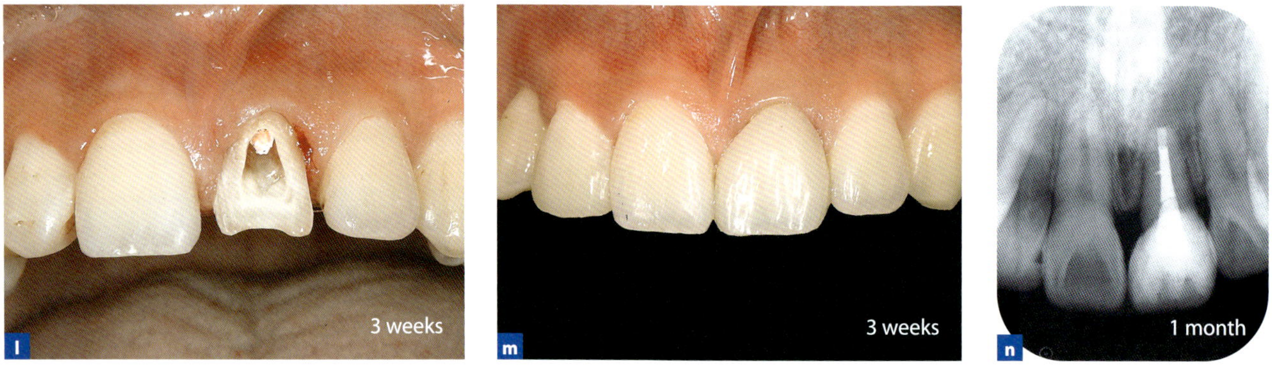

Fig 10-4l Three weeks after surgery. On this day, the calcium hydroxide preparation was replaced with sealer and gutta-percha, and crown restoration with CR (direct method) was performed.

Fig 10-4m and 10-4n One month after crown restoration.

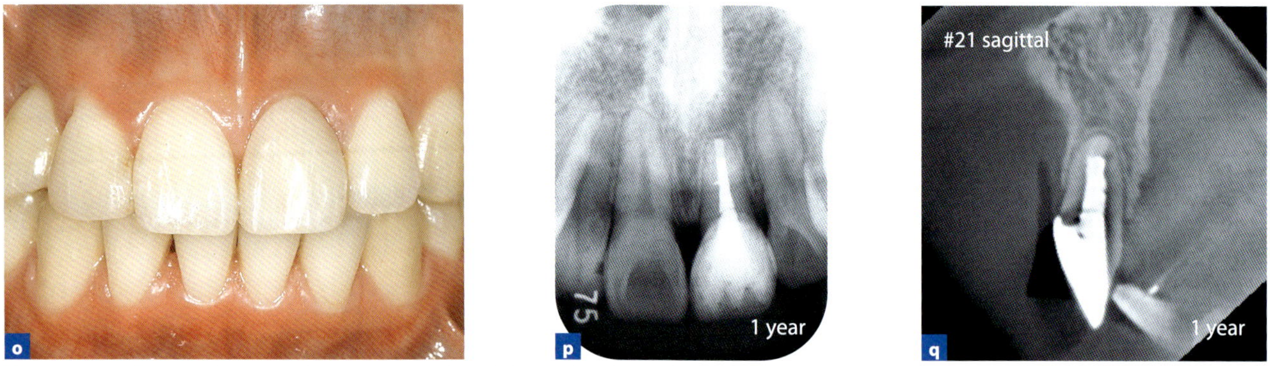

Fig 10-4o and 10-4p One year after surgery. Tooth mobility and probing depths were normal.

Fig 10-4q CBCT sagittal image 1 year after surgery. There is no evidence of root resorption, and a uniform periodontal ligament space is observed all around the root.

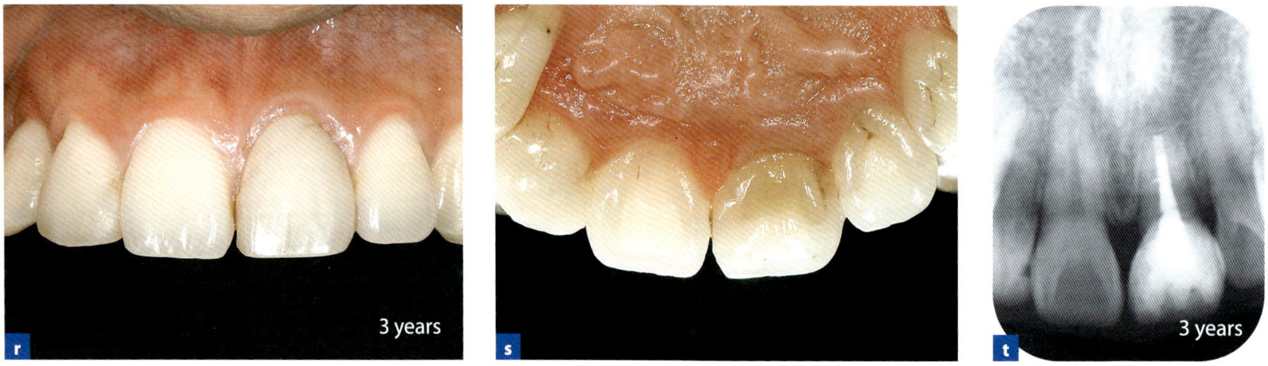

Fig 10-4r to 10-4t Three years after surgery. No problems are observed.

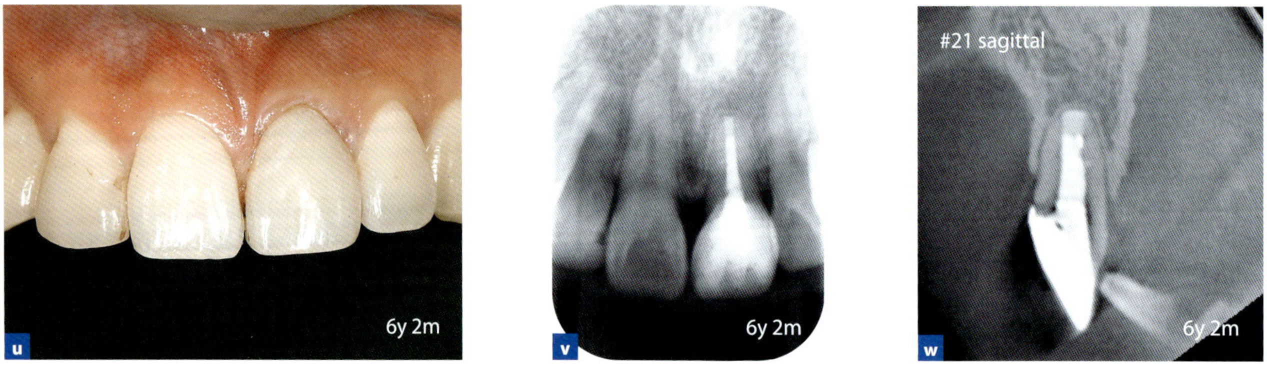

Fig 10-4u to 10-4w Six years and 2 months after surgery.

Surgical extrusion of a tooth with external resorption ② (Fig 10-5)

Fig 10-5 shows a 37-year-old female whose #11 developed invasive cervical resorption. It is difficult to perform crown restoration in this case because the resorption has progressed deep below the bone crest on the mesial aspect (**Fig 10-5a** to **10-5c**). Surgical extrusion was chosen because it was considered difficult to obtain 3 mm or more of healthy dentin above the crest by orthodontic extrusion. By rotating it 90 degrees with the surgical extrusion, enough tooth structure is secured with minimum amount of extrusion (**Fig 10-5d** to **10-5f**). Since the patient was older, there was more time allowed for stabilization and the crown restoration with CR was performed two months after surgery.

Surgical extrusion with surgical up-righting (Fig 10-6)

Fig 10-6 shows a case of a 39-year-old female whose #37 developed advanced secondary caries through the margin of the abutment crown (**Fig 10-6a** and **10-6b**). Since the morphology of the root was simple (single, conical-shaped), surgical extrusion was performed to reestablish the biological width and ferrule (**Fig 10-6c** to **10-6f**). #37 had been tilted before treatment, so the tooth was up-righted with surgical extrusion and socket adjustment and repositioning the tooth with 90 degree rotation. Three months after the surgery a fixed bridge was re-fabricated. The follow-up result after 10 years showed no problems (**Fig 10-6j** to **10-6l**).

Surgical extrusion of a tooth with external resorption ②

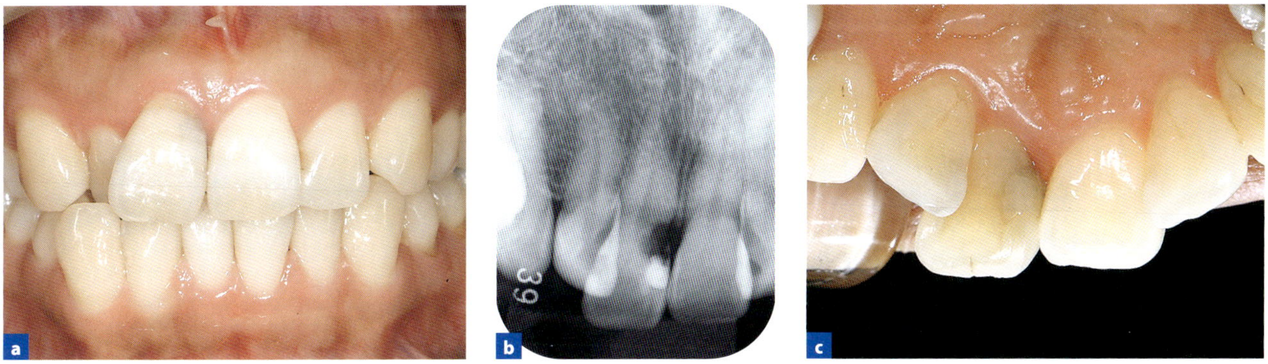

Fig 10-5a to 10-5c Views before treatment of a 37-year-old female. The external root resorption of #11 was progressing during several years observation.

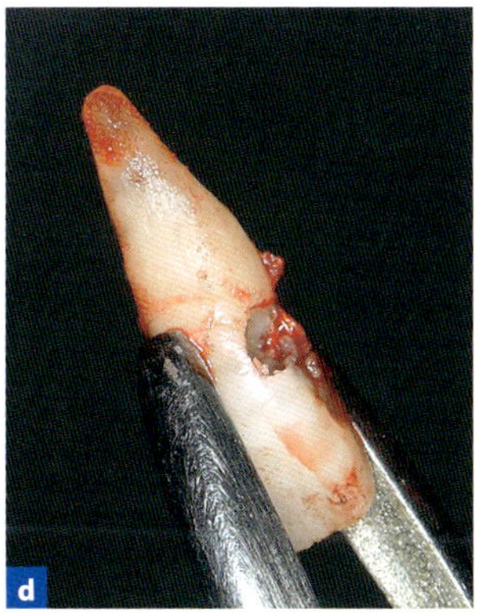

Fig 10-5d Extracted #11. A large resorptive defect was seen on the mesial aspect.

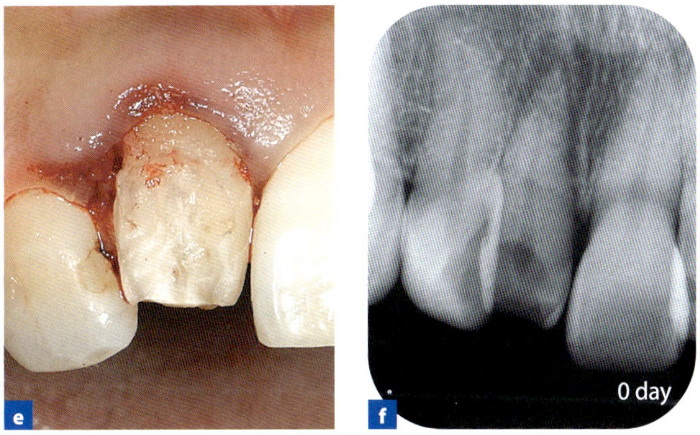

Fig 10-5e and 10-5f Immediately after surgery. The tooth was rotated 90 degrees and placed at the desired extruded position.

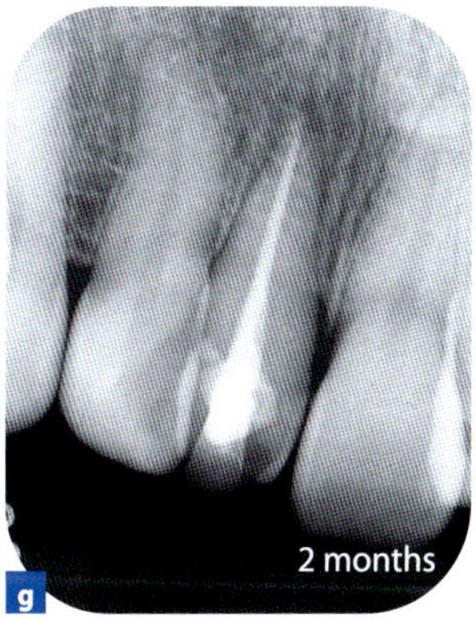

Fig 10-5g After 2 months. Immediately after root canal filling with sealer and gutta-percha.

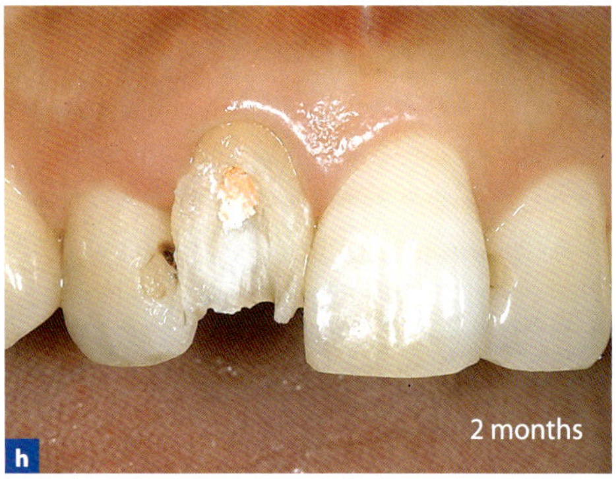

Fig 10-5h The same day as **Fig 10-5g** and immediately before CR restoration of the crown. During the healing period, a temporary crown was attached to the adjacent teeth to maintain esthetics.

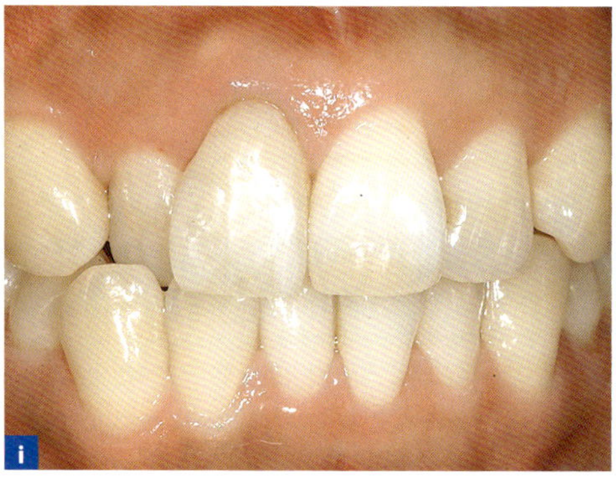

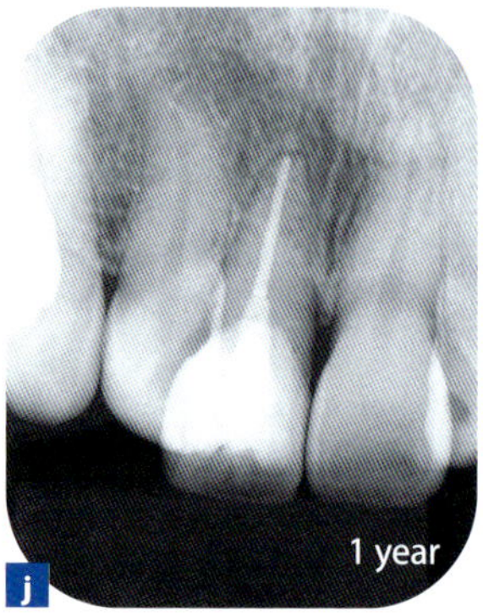

Fig 10-5i and 10-5j One year postoperative.

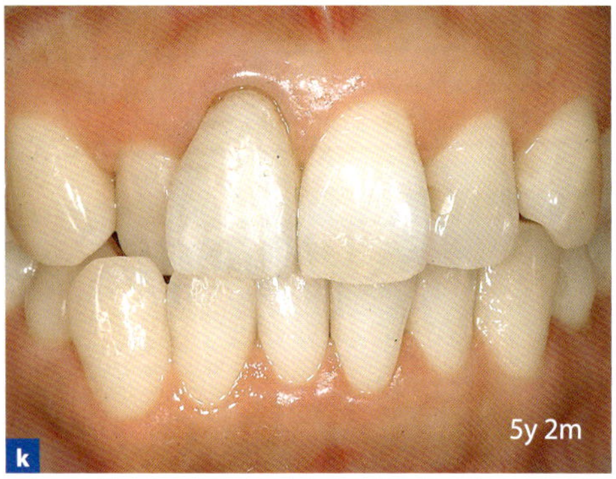

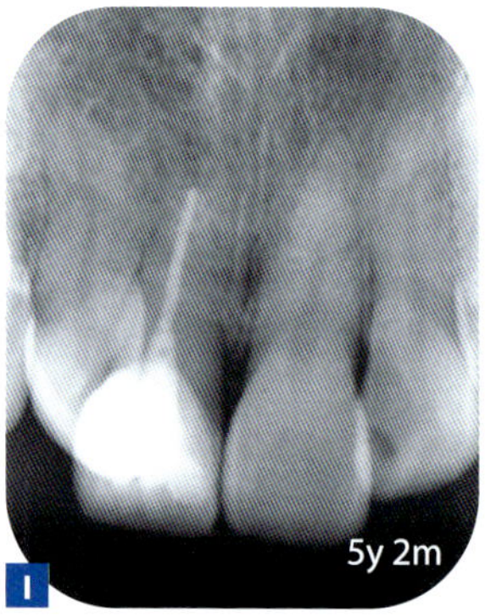

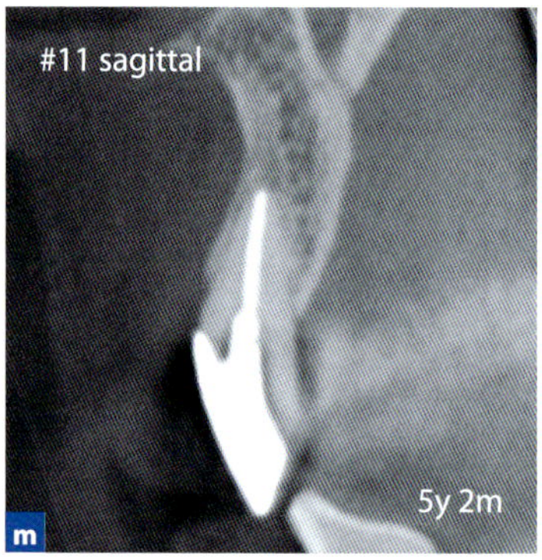

Fig 10-5k to 10-5m Five years postoperative. The CBCT image shows no apparent abnormalities.

Surgical extrusion with surgical up-righting

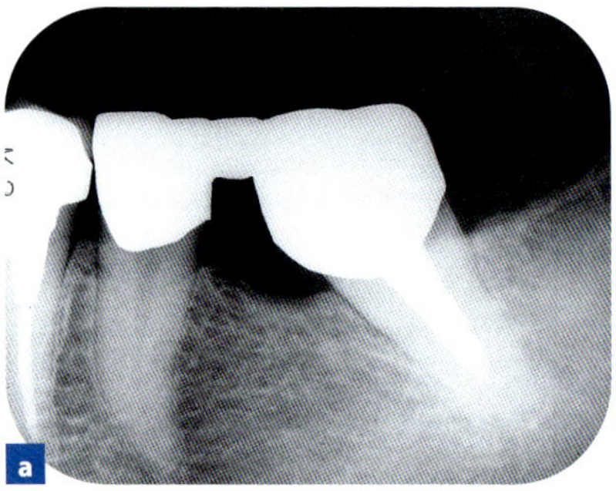

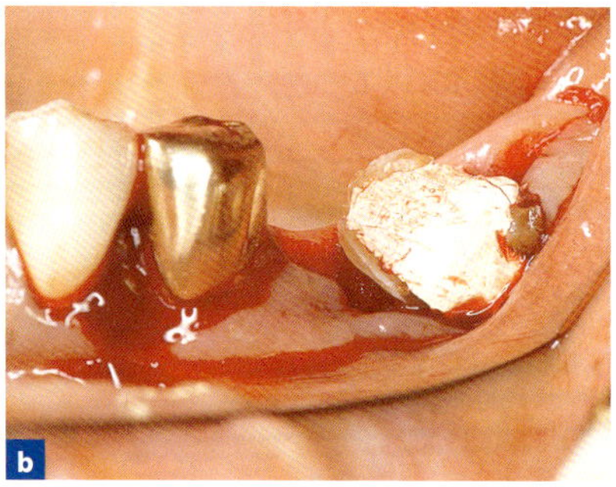

Fig 10-6a and 10-6b Views before treatment of a 39-year-old female whose #37 was involved in deep recurrent caries. Surgical extrusion with surgical up-righting was thought to be appropriate to treat and save the tooth because securing enough tooth structure and correcting the tilting root were necessary.

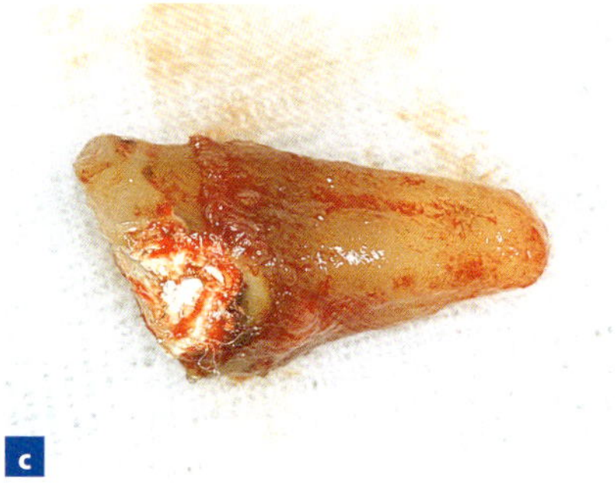

Fig 10-6c Tooth extracted for surgical extrusion.

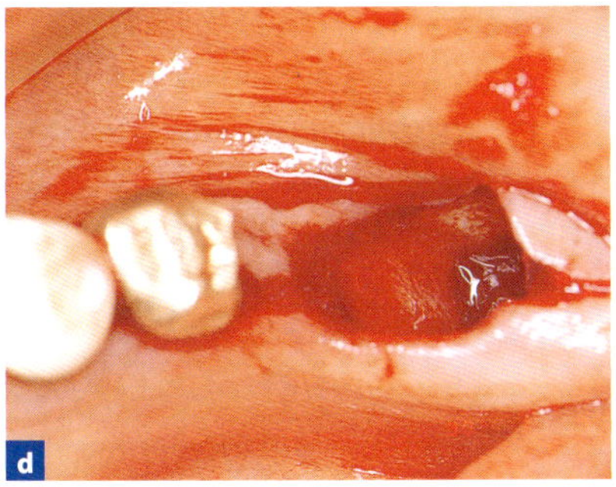

Fig 10-6d New socket was formed within the socket in order to up-right the root.

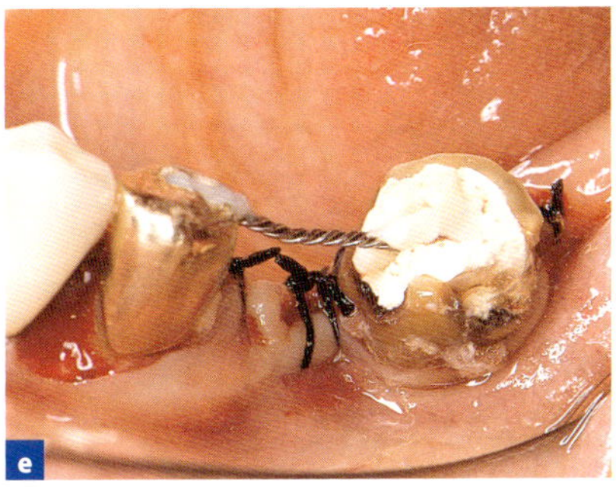

Fig 10-6e Immediately after surgery and fixation. The tooth was rotated 90 so that the buccal surface was positioned on the mesial aspect.

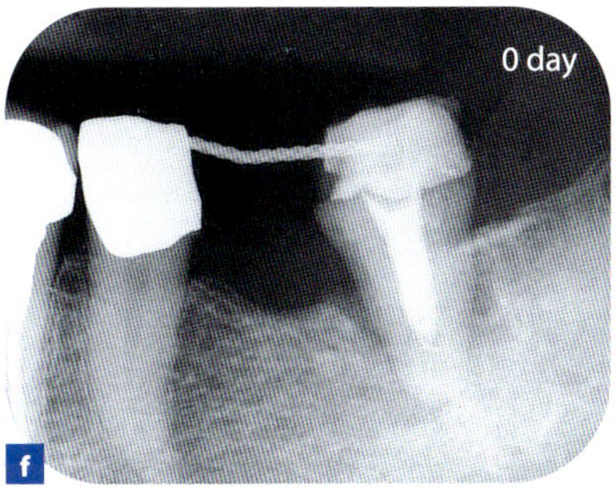

Fig 10-6f Radiograph immediately after surgery.

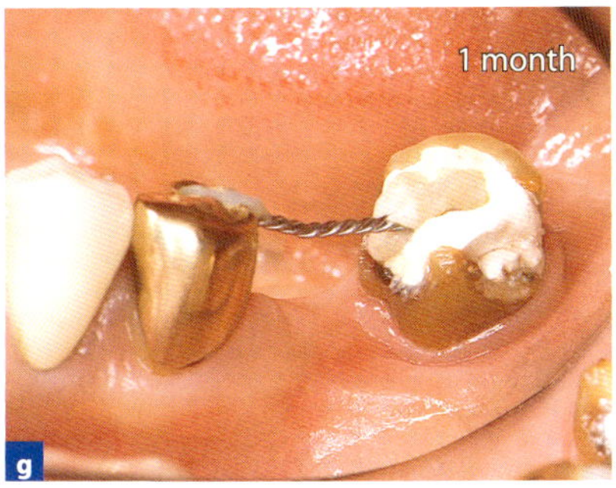

Fig 10-6g One month after surgery.

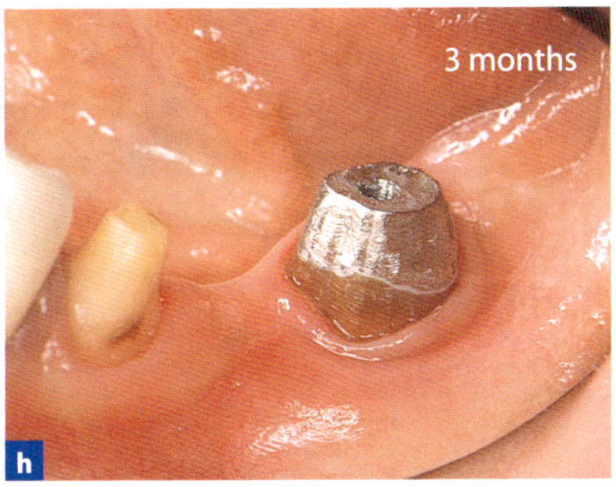

Fig 10-6h Three months after surgery. Just before fabricating a fixed bridge.

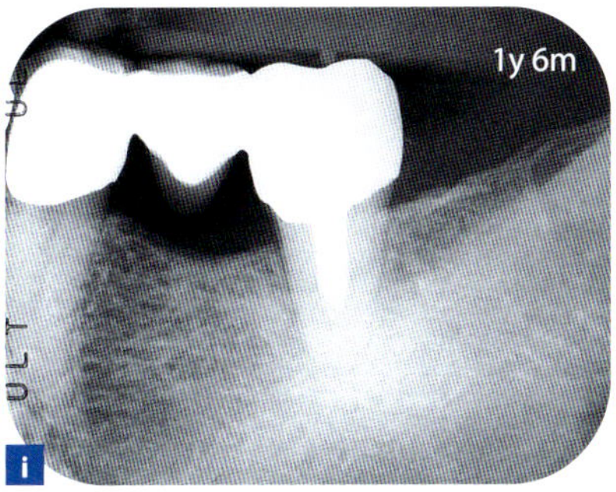

Fig 10-6i Radiograph 1 year and 6 months after surgery. No problems are observed.

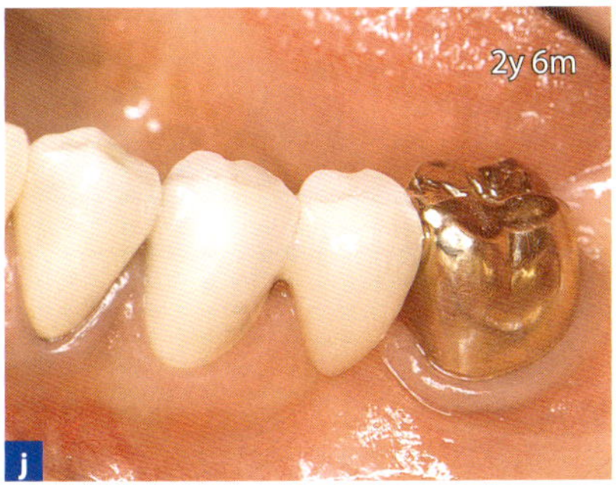

Fig 10-6j Two years and 6 months postoperative.

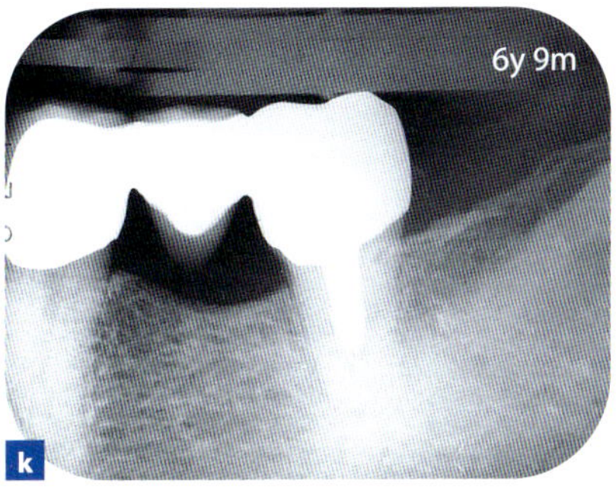

Fig 10-6k Six years and 9 months postoperative.

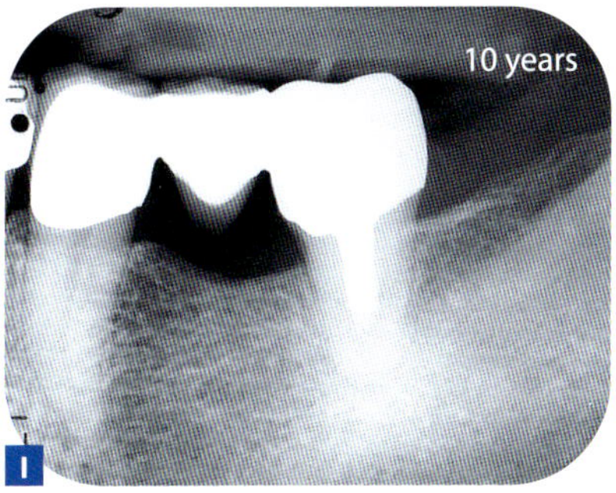

Fig 10-6l 10 years postoperative.

Intentional replantation

Purpose, criteria, and surgical procedures for intentional replantation are almost the same as for surgical extrusion. Intentional replantation[18-22] can be indicated when some of the following criteria are involved and overlapping.

Criteria for choosing intentional replantation

- ☐ When conventional root canal treatment is not successful because of complicated root canal configurations, long posts, broken files, transportation, biofilm, etc
- ☐ When the shape of the root is relatively easy to extract
- ☐ When definitive diagnosis is uncertain and can be verified during the surgical procedure
- ☐ When apicoectomy is difficult because of the position of the tooth
- ☐ If there is no possibility of autotransplantation of the tooth (if there is a good donor available, then transplantation may be the first option)

Case presentations of Intentional Replantation

Intentional replantation of a second molar ① (Fig 10-7)

Fig 10-7 shows a case of a 32-year-old female who presented with the chief complaint of pain to #17 (**Fig 10-7a** to **10-7d**). The pain she was experiencing was very likely due to the continued endodontic pathology from the previously attempted root canal treatment. Orthograde retreatment was initiated but there was transportation of the apical foramen of the mesial root, transportation of the distobuccal root, and overfilling of the palatal root were found, which led to unsuccessful improvement of her symptoms (**Fig 10-7e** to **10-7h**). Therefore, intentional replantation was performed with the patient's informed consent (**Fig 10-7i** to **10-7p**). The patient must be informed about the risk-benefit and cost-benefit of replantation. In this case, based on the findings and location and position of the tooth, apicoectomy would be difficult and likely not successful. The patient should understand that if the tooth

Intentional replantation of a second molar ①

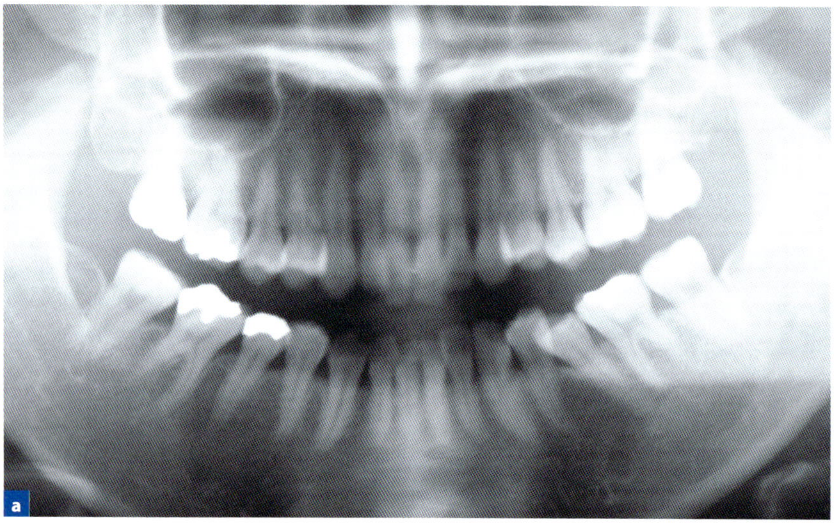

Fig 10-7a to 10-7d Views before treatment of a 32-year-old female. Her chief complaint was pain around #17. The cause of the pain was thought to be caused by the inadequate root canal treatment and apical infection.

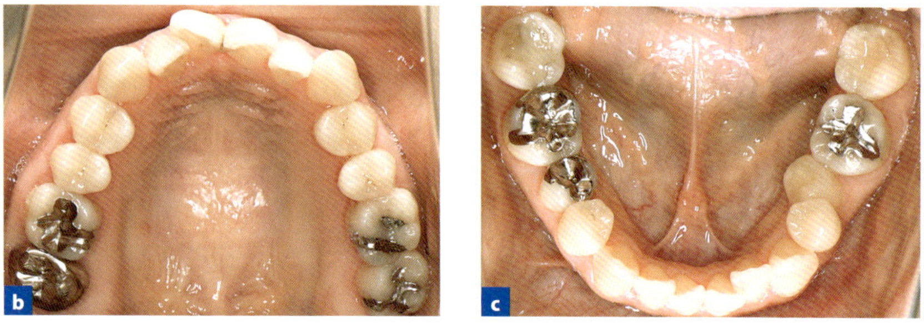

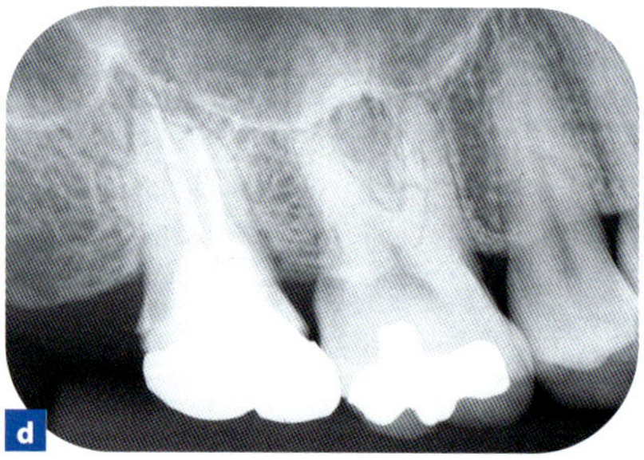

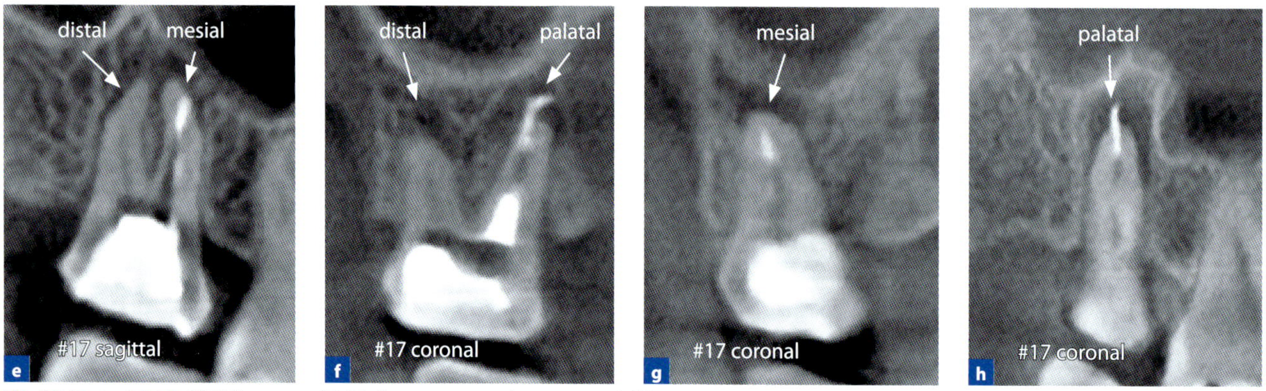

Fig 10-7e to 10-7h CBCT images of #17 after removing the root canal filling materials. Transportation of the apical foramen of the mesial root, zip of the distal root, and overfilling of the palatal root were observed.

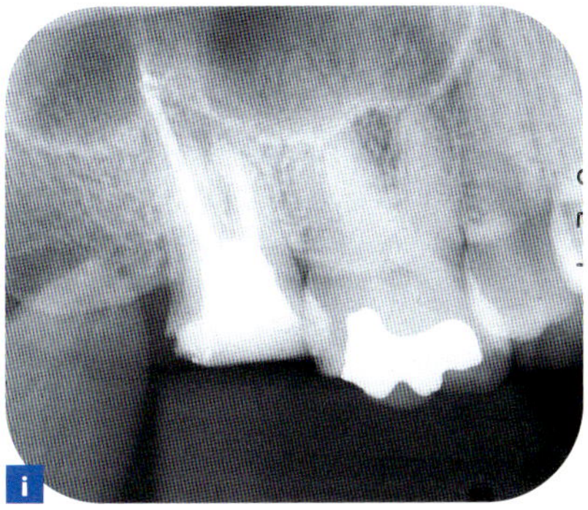

Fig 10-7i Radiograph after root canal filling. Patient's symptoms did not improve.

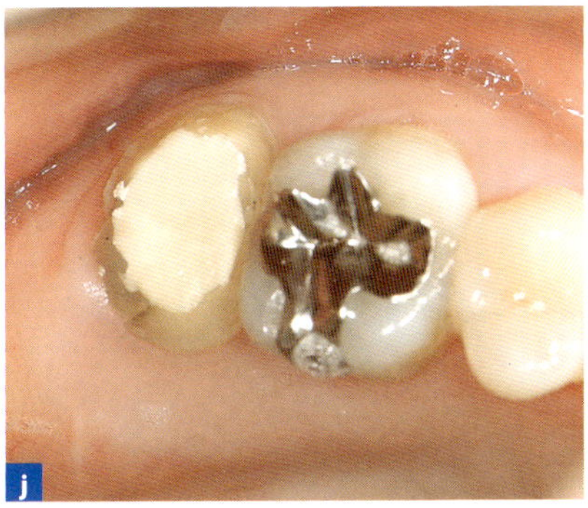

Fig 10-7j View just before intentional replantation.

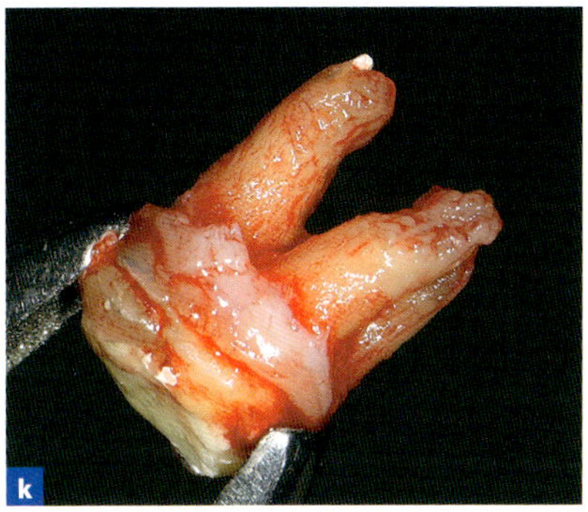

Fig 10-7k Distal view during surgery.

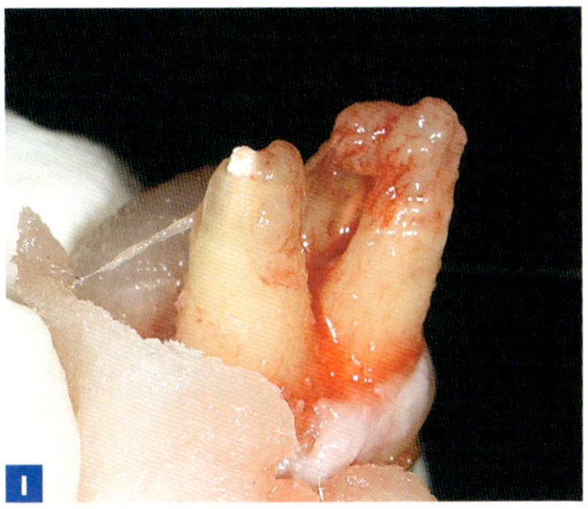

Fig 10-7l Apical view of the roots.

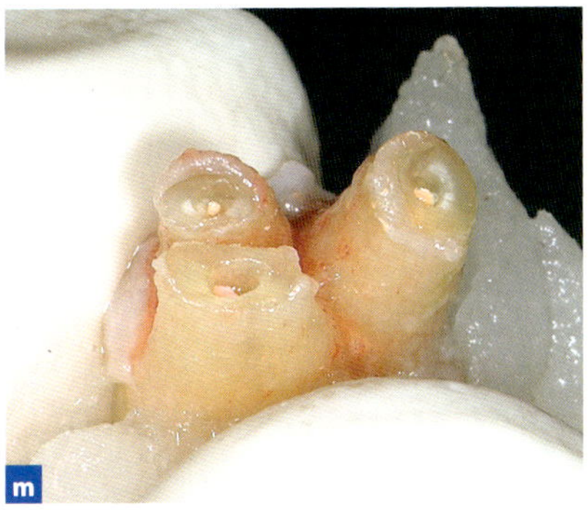

Fig 10-7m After root resection of the apices about 3 mm and root end preparation for retro canal filling.

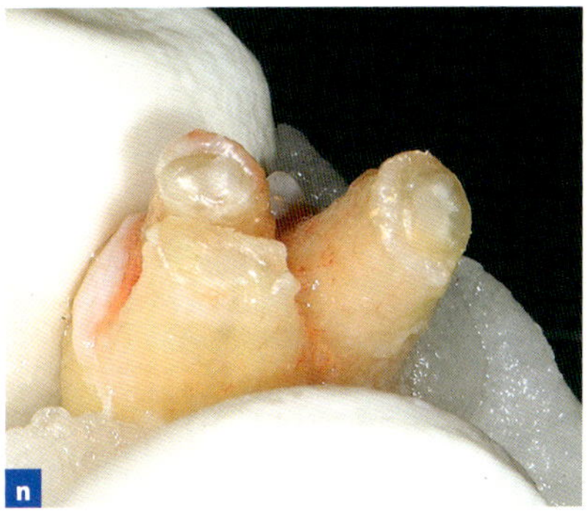

Fig 10-7n After filling with light-cured glass ionomer cement.

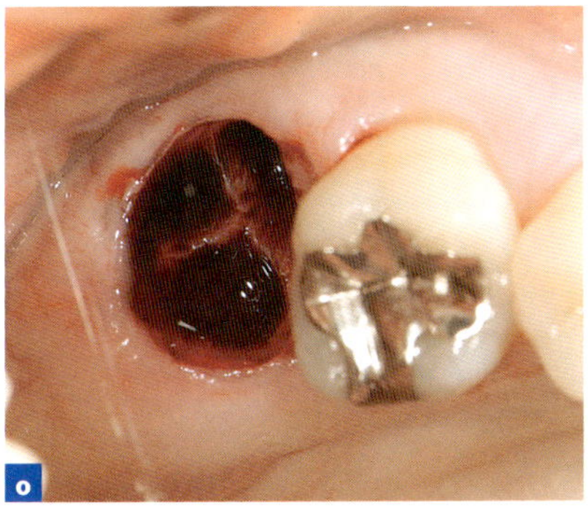

Fig 10-7o Socket after removal of granulation tissue.

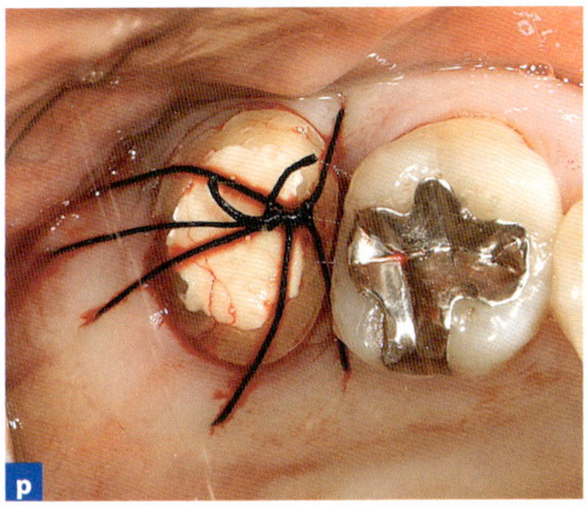

Fig 10-7p Immediately after replantation and fixation with suture. Thereafter the replanted tooth was covered with surgical dressing.

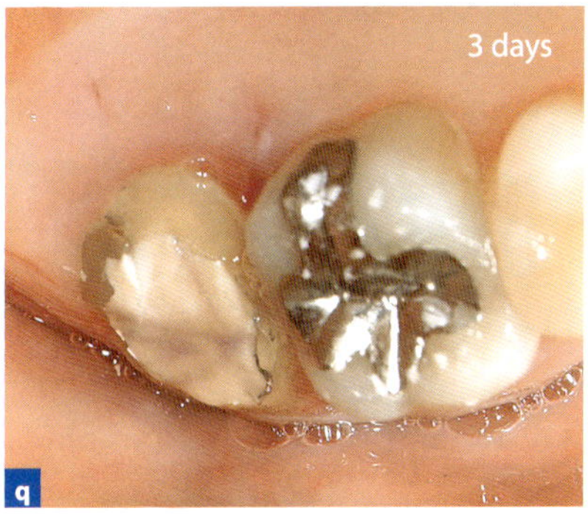

Fig 10-7q Three days postoperative. Immediately after suture removal.

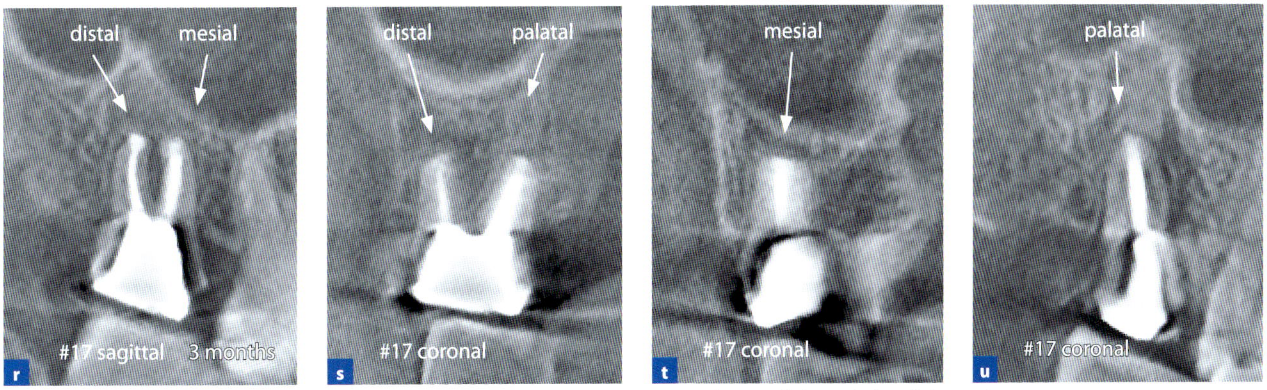

Fig 10-7r to 10-7u CBCT images 3 months after surgery. There is apparent resolution of the apical radiolucencies.

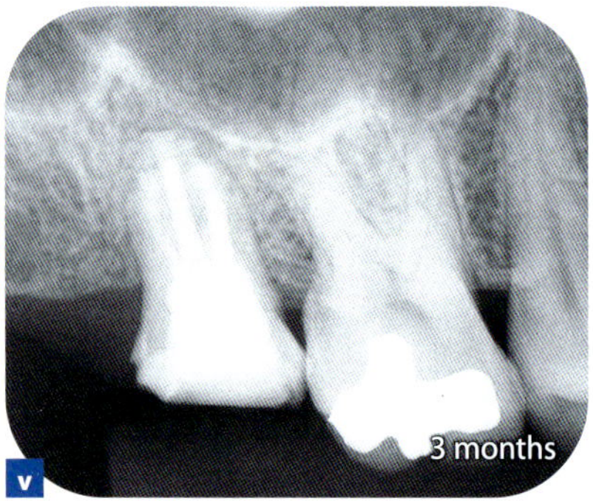

Fig 10-7v Radiograph 3 months after surgery.

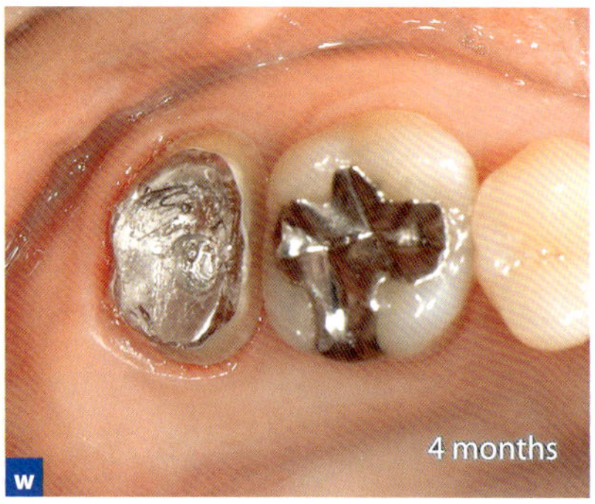

Fig 10-7w View after 4 months. Immediately before placement of a prosthetic crown.

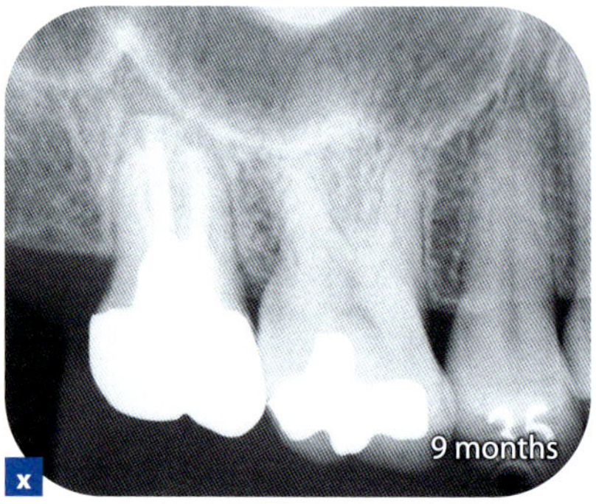

Fig 10-7x Radiograph after 9 months.

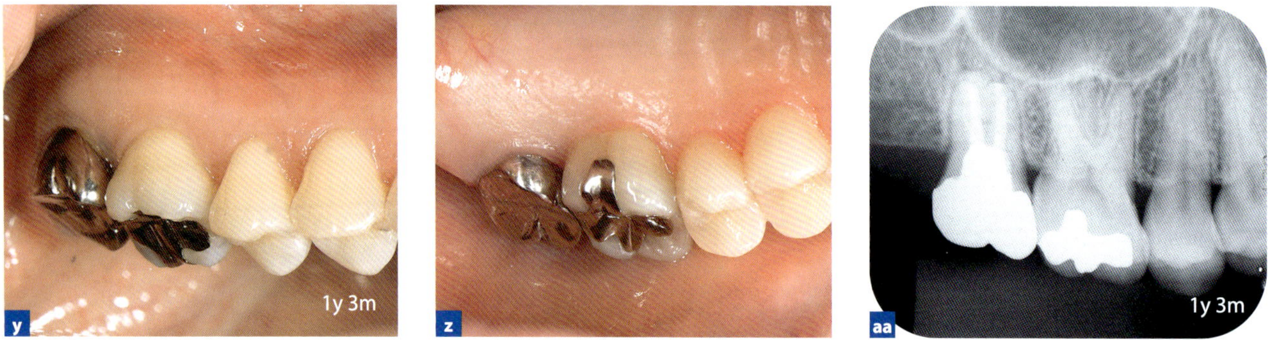

Fig 10-7y to 10-7aa One year and 3 months postoperative.

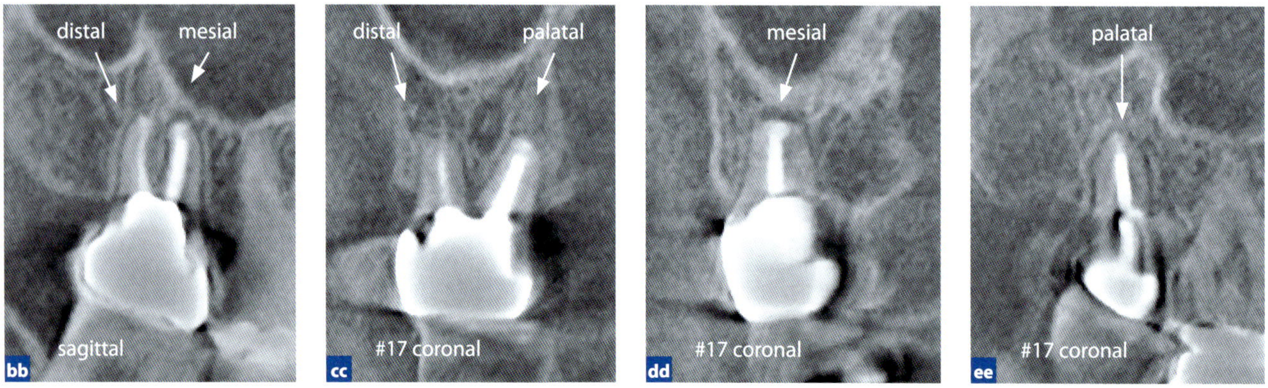

Fig 10-7bb to 10-7ee CBCT images after 1 year and 3 months. No apparent abnormalities such as root resorption are observed.

cannot be extracted well, the treatment may end up being extraction.

Following successful tooth extraction (**Fig 10-7k**), extra-oral apicectomy and retro canal filling were performed (**Fig 10-7l** to **10-7n**). The details on root resection are explained in **Fig 10-2**. The tooth was replanted into the extraction socket where the apical granulation tissue had been cleaned out, and the tooth was fixed with sutures (**Fig 10-7o** and **10-7p**). In this case of intentional replantation, the tooth was stable with suture fixation immediately after surgery because it was placed to the original extraction socket in the original position. Periodontal ligament healing in replantation is very quick(**Fig 10-7q**) (see **Chapter 3**, **Fig 3-1**) and usually, crown restoration is possible a few months after surgery. Periodontal ligament healing was observed on CBCT images taken after 3 months (**Fig 10-7r** to **10-7u**) and the follow-up result showed no apparent abnormalities with evidence of successful healing (**Fig 10-7v** to **10-7ee**).

Intentional replantation of a second molar ② (Fig 10-8)

Fig 10-8 shows a case of a 23-year-old female that presented with a sinus tract on the palatal aspect of #27 (**Fig 10-8a** and **10-8b**). CBCT examination showed inadequate endodontic treatment of all the canals, and re-treatment was indicated (**Fig 10-8c** to **10-8e**). Intentional replantation was chosen because of the complicated root canal morphology, root resorption and surrounding bone loss of the palatal root, large and long post cores, and favorable root morphology for extraction.

Intentional replantation of a second molar ②

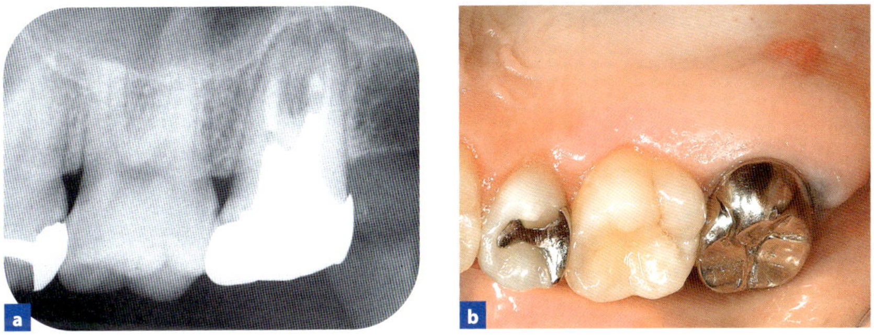

Fig 10-8a and 10-8b Views before treatment of a 23-year-old female. A sinus tract was observed at the apical area of the palatal side of #27, which was thought to be caused by inadequate root canal treatment.

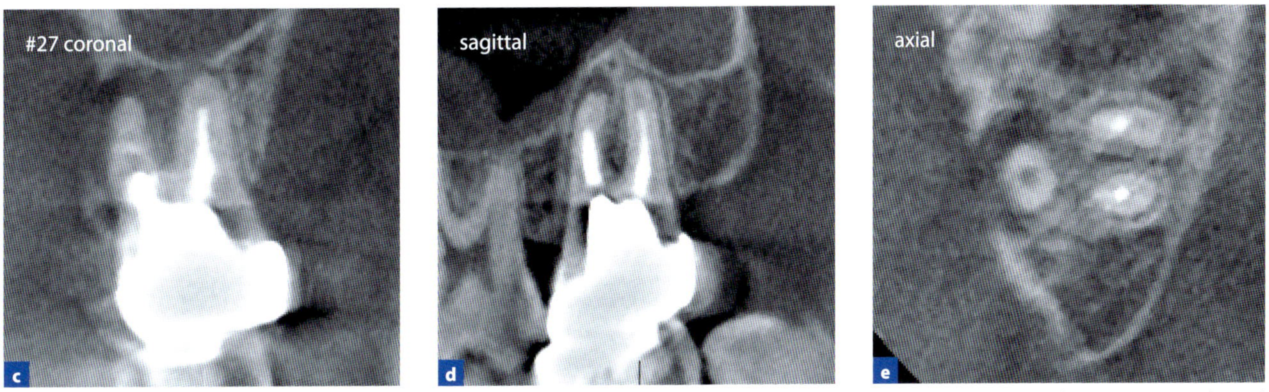

Fig 10-8c to 10-8e CBCT images of #27. Findings show evidence of inadequate treatment on all roots. Intentional replantation was indicated because of the complicated root canal morphology, advanced external root resorption with likely periapical infection in the palatal root, large and long cast post and core attached, and the favorable root morphology for extraction.

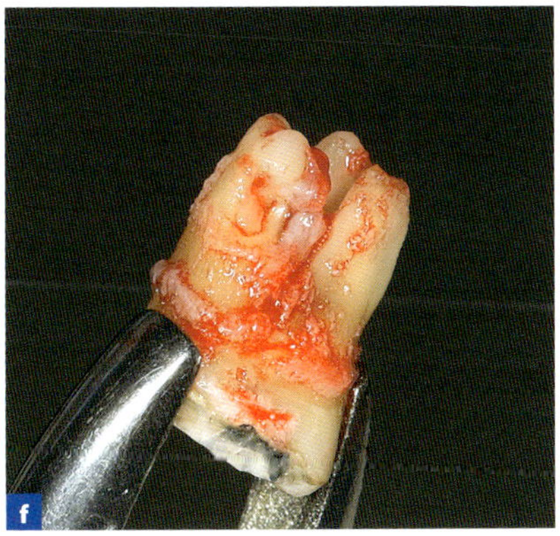

Fig 10-8f Extracted #27.

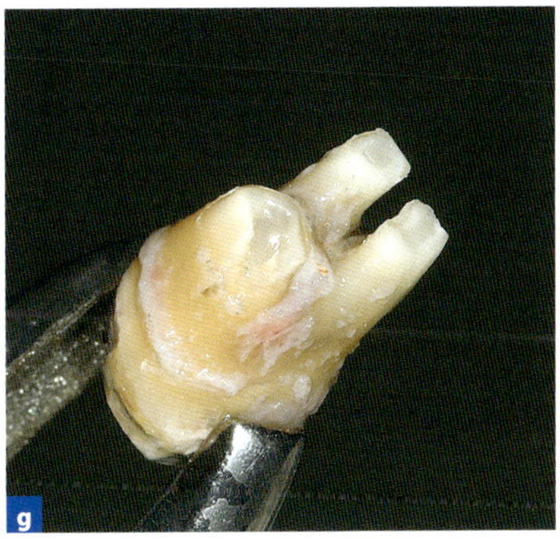

Fig 10-8g After extraoral apicoectomy with retro canal filling.

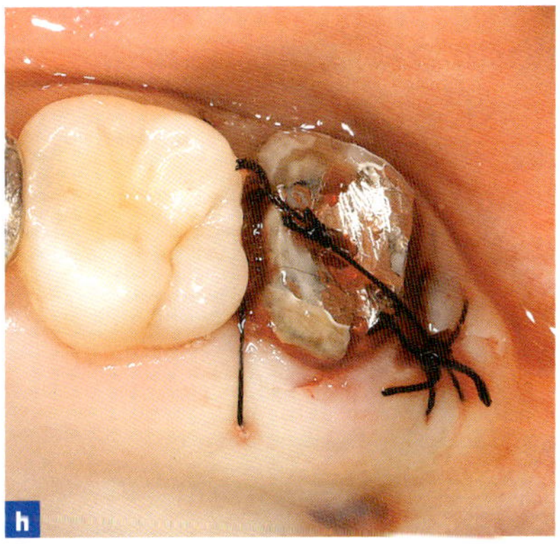

Fig 10-8h After replantation.

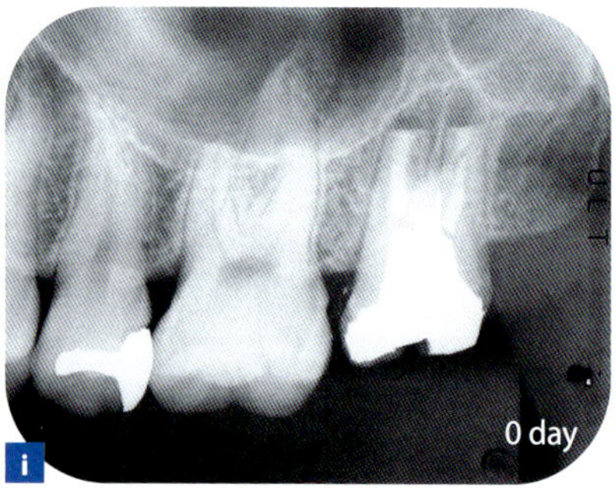

Fig 10-8i Radiograph immediately after replantation.

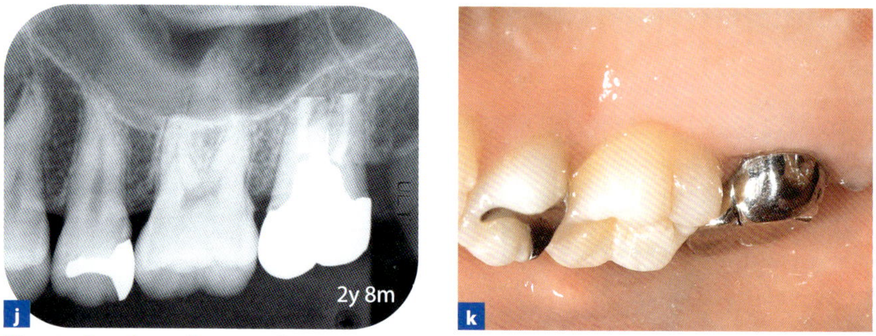

Fig 10-8j and 10-8k Views after 2 years and 8 months.

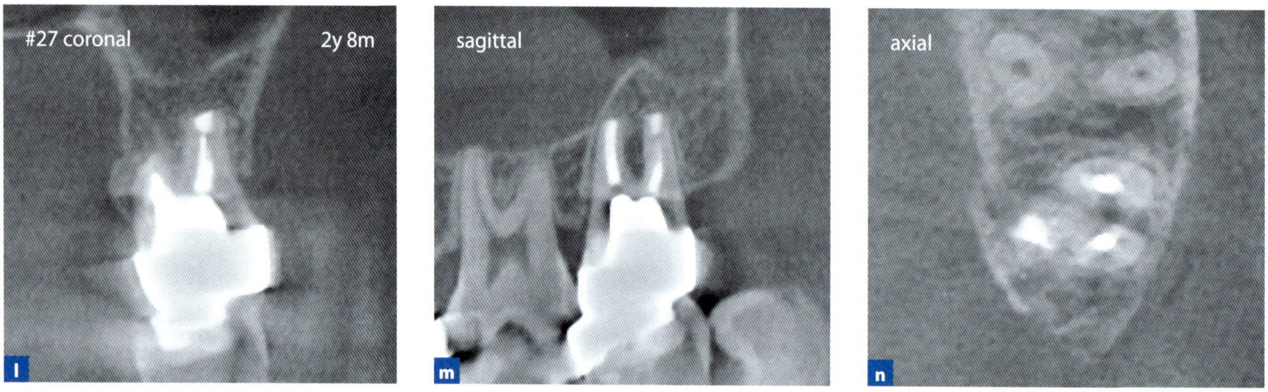

Fig 10-8l to 10-8n CBCT images after 2 years and 8 months. Healing is maintained.

When the actual root was observed extraorally, the mesiobuccal root consisted of two root canal spaces with an isthmus between them (**Fig 10-8f** and **10-8g**). In addition, root resorption or perforation was found on the palatal side of the palatal root. Even under microscope, it is questionable whether such complications can be successfully repaired.

Uneventful healing was observed after the intentional replantation, and the follow-up showed healing with successful outcome (**Fig 10-8h** to **10-8n**).

Endo-perio differential diagnosis case ①

(Fig 10-9)

Fig 10-9 shows a case of a 50-year-old female whose #25 and #27 were scheduled for extraction (**Fig 10-9a** to **10-9c**). Because caries of #25 progressed to the central part of the root, and CBCT study of #27 showed evidence of advanced periodontal bone loss along the mesial aspect (**Fig 10-9d** to **10-9f**) and clinically there was deep probing depth (**Fig 10-9g**).

The two teeth were extracted, but when the extracted #27 was observed carefully, the root was fully covered with connective tissue which was thought to be periodontal ligament (**Fig 10-9h** and **10-9i**). This finding suggested that the large bony defect along the mesial aspect was more likely from an endodontic origin.

Therefore, extraoral apical root resection and retro canal filling were performed (**Fig 10-9j**), and the tooth was replanted to the original socket where the granulation tissue had been cleaned out (**Fig 10-9k**). Because the mesial bony defect was large, the defect was filled with a mixture of bone substitutes 'Bio-Oss'® (Geistlich) and 'Ora Graft'® (Life Net Health) (**Fig 10-9l**). Since no problems were observed after 3 months, a fixed bridge was fabricated between #24 and #27 (**Fig 10-9m** to **10-9p**). A CBCT examination 10 months after surgery showed evidence of normal periodontal ligament healing around the root (**Fig 10-9q** to **10-9s**).

This case demonstrates that clinical probing and CBCT imaging and interpretation cannot determine the status of the periodontal ligament. Therefore, in order to avoid misdiagnosis and tooth extraction, intentional replantation and inspection of the tooth/root can lead to a definitive diagnosis and treatment that can save the tooth.

Fig 10-10 to **10-11** shows cases in which intentional replantation was the best (and perhaps the only) treatment option to save the tooth.

Endo-perio differential diagnosis case ②

(Fig 10-10)

Fig 10-10 shows a case of a 35-year-old female who presented to our clinic in hopes of saving her tooth #27 (**Fig 10-10a** to **10-10c**). Several other clinics she visited before told her the tooth was hopeless and that it should be extracted.

Endo-perio differential diagnosis case ①

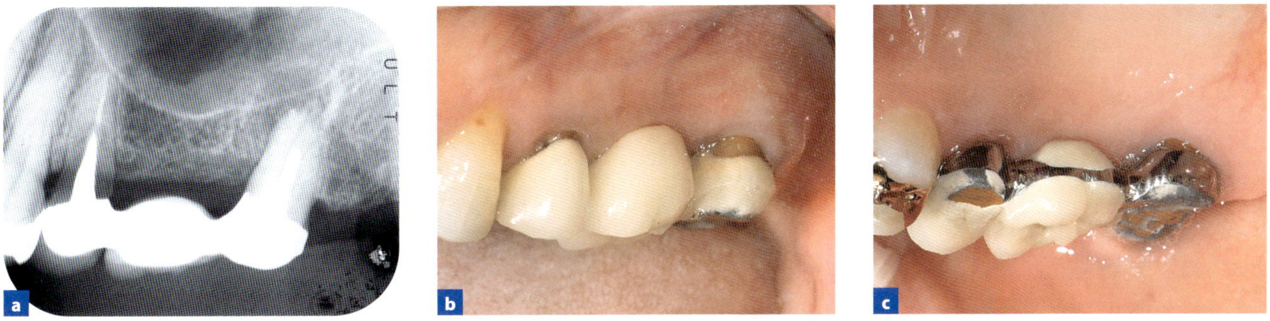

Fig 10-9a to 10-9c Views before treatment of a 50-year-old female. #25 developed significantly deep caries and #27 had an extensive bony defect on the mesial aspect.

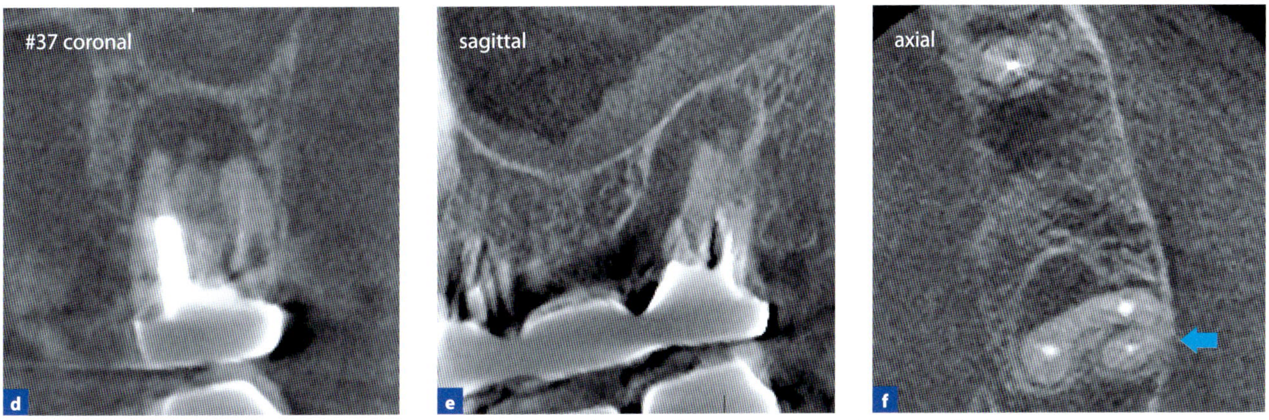

Fig 10-9d to 10-9f CBCT images before treatment. A large bony defect is observed on the mesial aspect of #27.

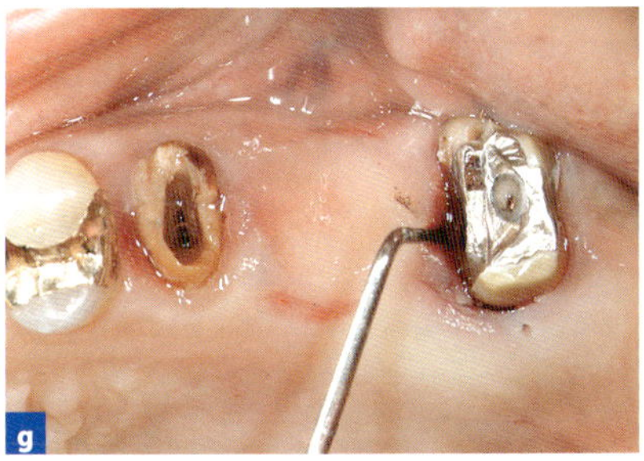

Fig 10-9g Before extraction of #25 and #27. Since the probing was deep and wide along the mesial aspect, it was considered the bony defect was caused by periodontitis.

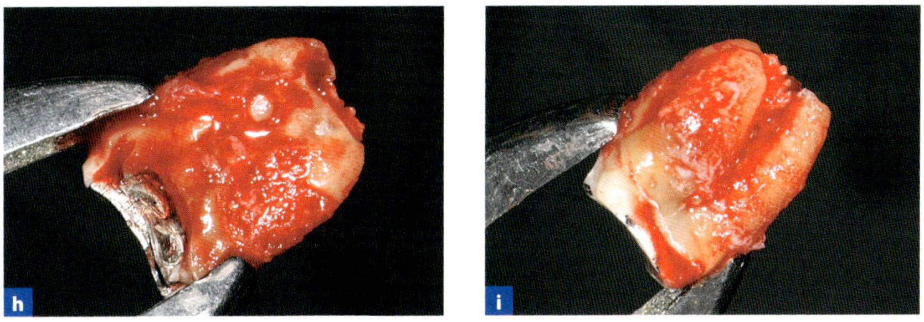

Fig 10-9h and 10-9i #27 extracted. It appeared that the periodontal ligament had been preserved on the entire root surface which indicated that the defect and infection on the mesial aspect was more likely to be of endodontic origin.

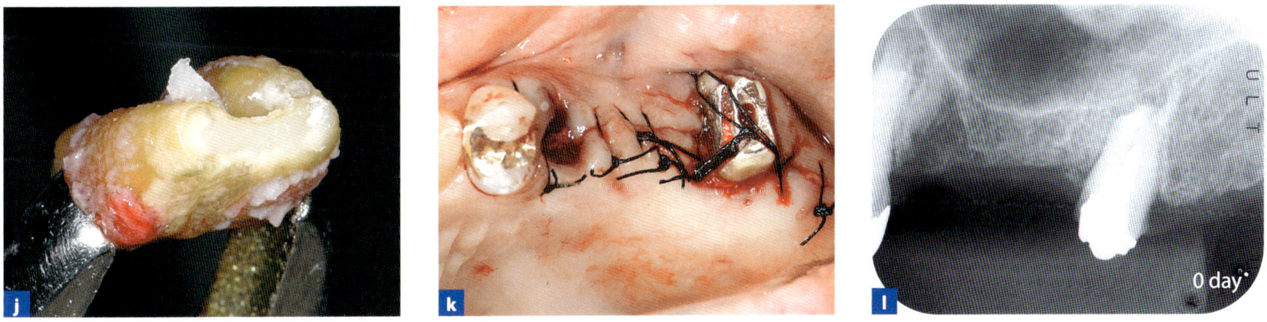

Fig 10-9j After apical root resection and retro canal filling.
Fig 10-9k After replantation. The tooth was replanted in the extraction socket after the granulation tissue had been excavated.
Fig 10-9l Radiograph immediately after replantation. Since the bony defect was large, the defect was filled with a mixture of bone substitutes 'Bio-Oss®' (Geistlich) and 'Ora Graft®' (Life Net Health).

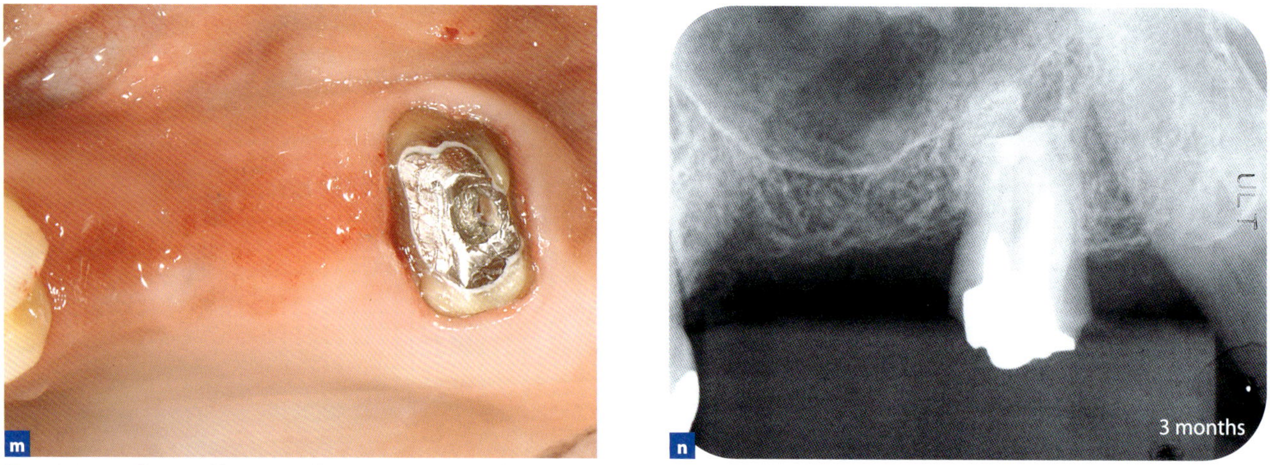

Fig 10-9m and 10-9n Three months postoperative. Healing seems to be progressing smoothly.

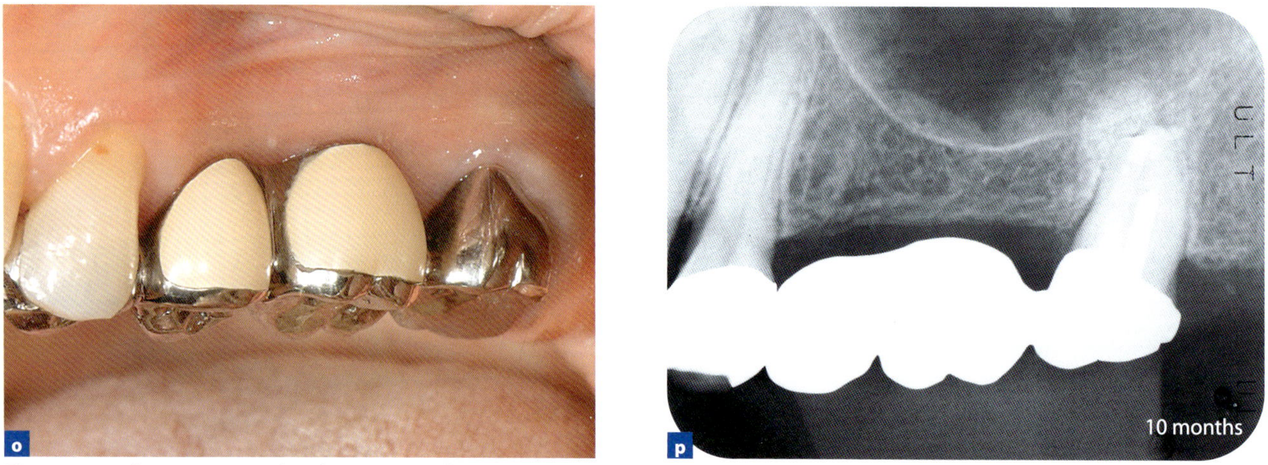

Fig 10-9o and 10-9p 10 months after surgery. A fixed bridge between #24 and #27 had been fabricated 4 months after surgery.

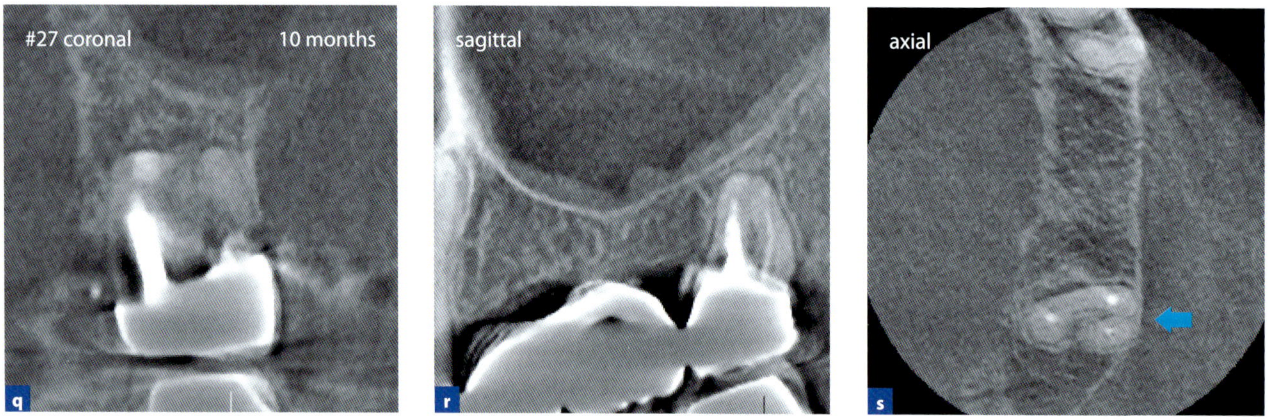

Fig 10-9q to 10-9s CBCT images after 10 months. There is apparent intact lamina dura around the root.

Most of the surrounding bone of #27 was gone, especially on the palatal and distal aspect. In addition, the CBCT findings shows evidence of partial loss of the floor of the maxillary sinus with thickening of the mucosa (**Fig 10-10d** to **10-10f**). At first glance, the prognosis seems hopeless . However, as discussed in the case of **Fig 10-9**, the possibility of preservation is not zero. The final judgement should be made after confirming whether or not the periodontal ligament appears intact (attached to the root) upon visual inspection after the tooth is extracted. If periodontal ligament remains on the root surface, it can be diagnosed that the surrounding bone loss is more likely due to endodontic pathology and extraoral root apicoectomy can be performed.

After informed consent, the tooth was extracted first. Fortu-

Endo-perio differential diagnosis case ②

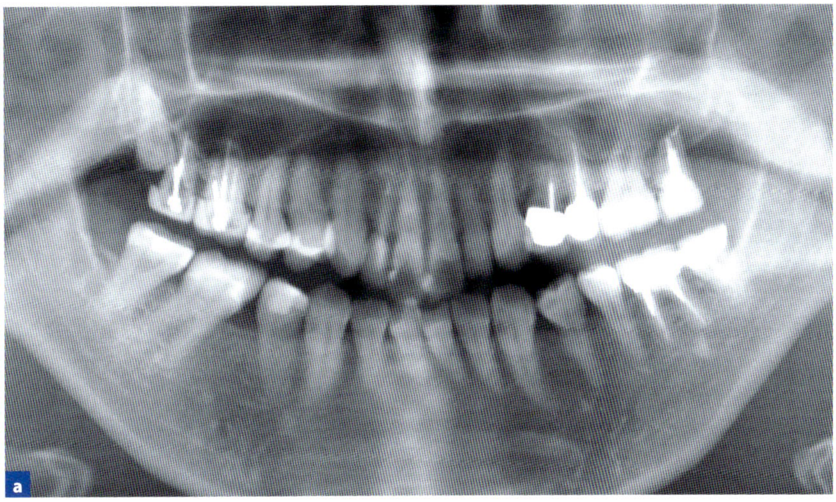

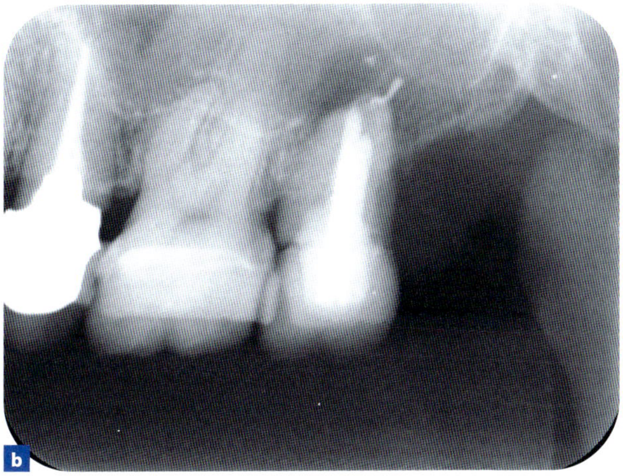

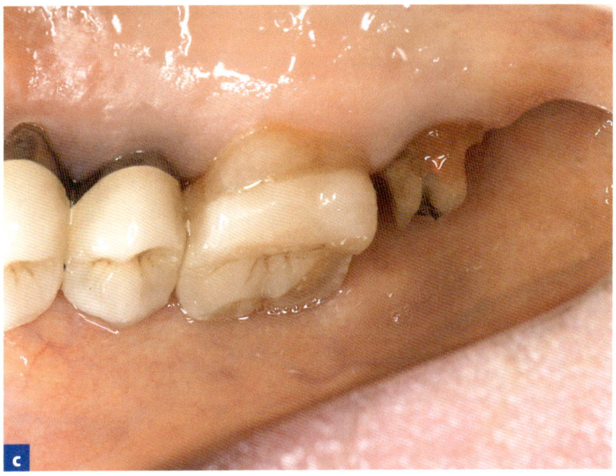

Fig 10-10a to 10-10c Views before treatment of a 35-year-old female who presented with the hope of saving her tooth #27. She was told by several dentists that prognosis was hopeless and so she presented for another opinion.

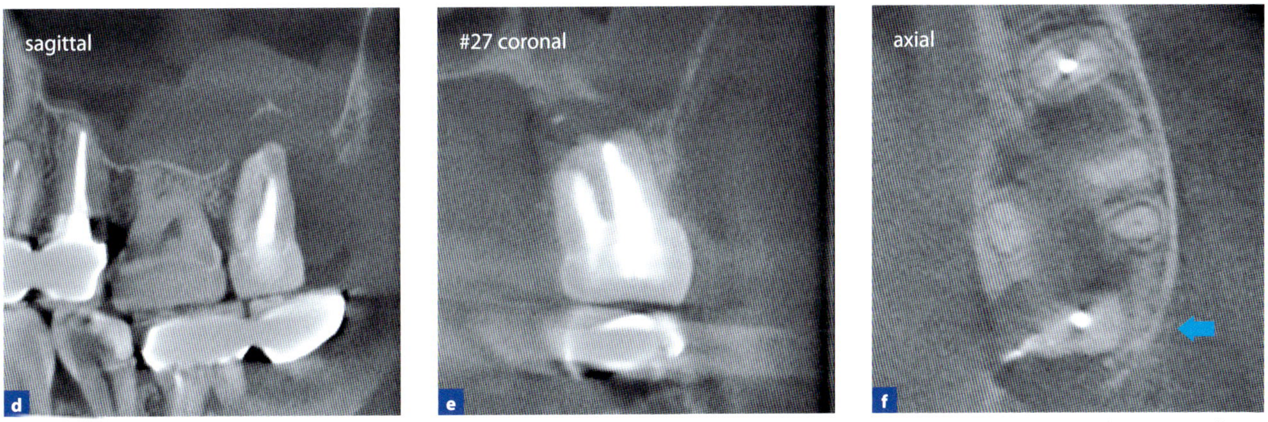

Fig 10-10d to 10-10f CBCT images of #27 before treatment. Findings suggest that most of the surrounding bone has been lost, especially on the palatal and distal sides. In addition, there was apparent perforation of the floor of the maxillary sinus and the sinus mucosa was thickened. At a glance, it seemed that the prognosis was hopeless. However, intentional replantation was suggested as an option.

nately, connective tissue attachment was preserved around the root (though the amount of coverage was lower), and the infection was diagnosed as mainly endodontic in origin. Therefore, the tooth was treated and replanted along with careful excavation of the socket to clean out the granulation tissue (**Fig 10-10g**).

As the 8 months follow-up shows in **Fig 10-10h** to **10-10m**, there was evident osseous regeneration of the large bony defect. Eight years follow-up with CBCT showed healing was maintained (**Fig 10-10n** to **10-10p**).

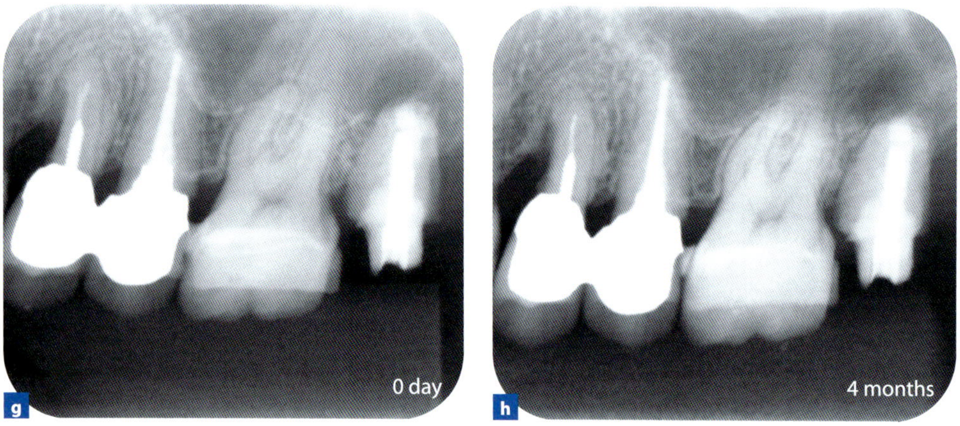

Fig 10-10g Radiograph immediately after intentional replantation of #27. When the tooth was extracted and observed, it was confirmed that there was still some periodontal ligament intact.

Fig 10-10h Four months postoperative. Radiolucency of the bone around #27 is reducing.

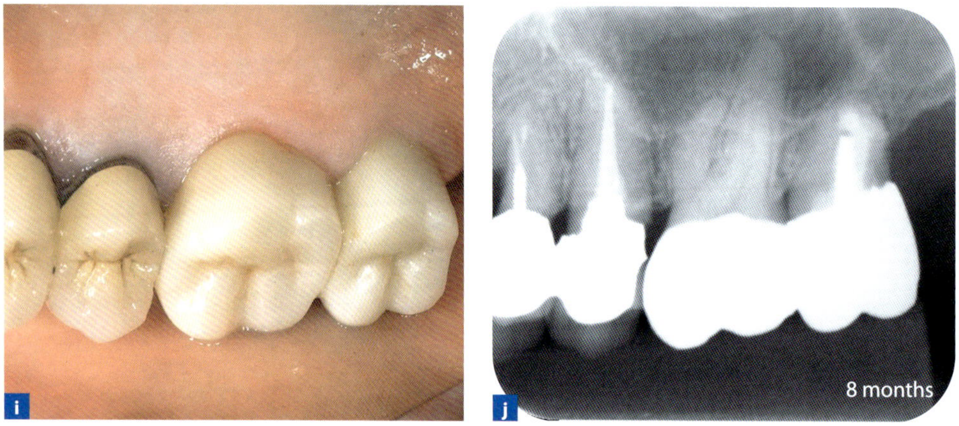

Fig 10-10i and 10-10j Eight months postoperative. Bony defect has disappeared and probing depth is normal.

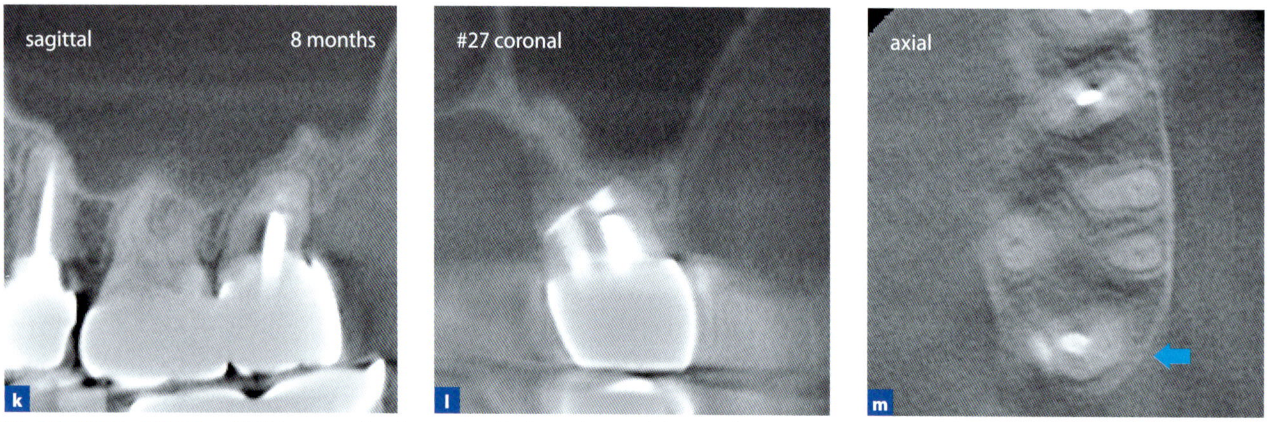

Fig 10-10k to 10-10m CBCT images after 8 months. Findings show evidence of osseous regeneration around #27, and the maxillary sinus appears healed.

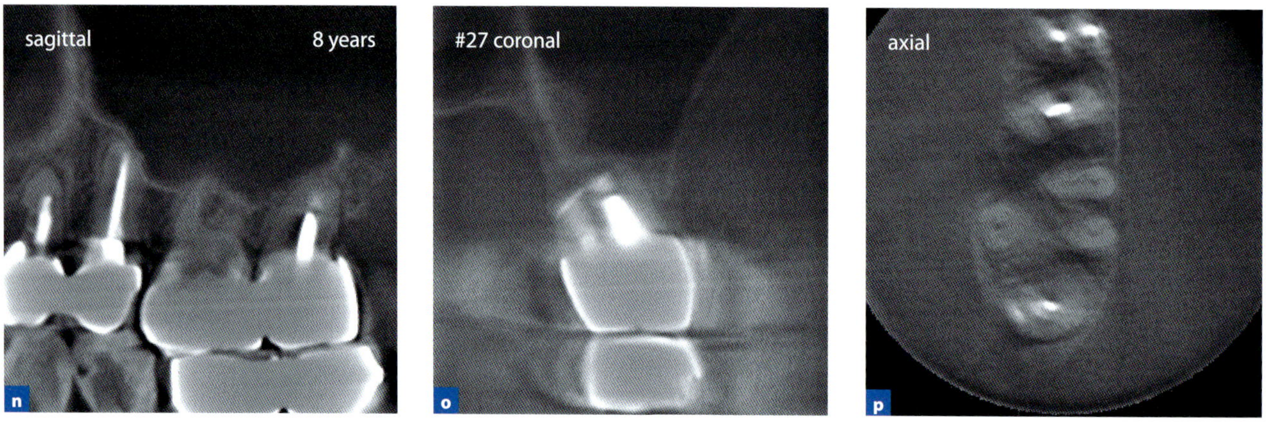

Fig 10-10n to 10-10p CBCT images after 8 years. The bony healing is maintained.

Intentional replantation to treat periodontal pathology (Fig 10-11)

Fig 10-11 shows a case of a 43-year-old male who presented with a chief complaint of pain and mobility of #34 (Fig 10-11a to 10-11h). As can be seen in the radiograph at the first visit, a significant amount of bone loss was observed around the root of #34 (Fig 10-11h), and there was deep probing depths around the tooth. Since #34 responded within normal limits to EPT(+), it was considered that the bony defect was likely to be of periodontal pathology and thus the prognosis was unfavorable. When examining the extracted tooth carefully, there was heavy calculus deposit only on the lingual aspect on the deeper root surface and there was intact, periodontal ligament attached on the other areas of the root (Fig 10-11j to 10-11m). This situation provided some hope in preservation of the tooth because the periodontal ligament remained on the buccal, distal and mesial aspect to some amount, and there was evidence of a thin layer of alveolar bone remaining on the buccal side of #34 as seen in the CBCT images taken immediately after intentional replantation (Fig 10-11v to 10-11x).

Alveolar bone consists of 'tooth-dependent bone volume' that is formed and maintained by teeth with healthy periodontal ligament, and 'tooth-independent bone volume' that is formed and maintained without teeth (Fig 10-A)[23]. When periodontal ligament disappears due to tooth extraction or periodontitis, tooth-dependent bone volume disappears, but tooth-independent bone volume remains. From a clinical point of view, some part of the alveolar bone on the labial side consists of tooth-dependent bone, the approximate volume of which is represented as the red zone shown in Fig 10-A. Tooth-dependent bone volume is lost due to tooth extraction or periodontitis, and cannot be regenerated unless a healthy tooth is transplanted or the periodontal ligament is regenerated. On the other hand, tooth-independent bone volume is maintained even in the absence of teeth.

In this case, the calculus was completely removed extraorally (Fig 10-11n to 10-11q), and the tooth was replanted to the extraction socket where the granulation tissue was excavated (Fig 10-11r and 10-11s). The cervical area of the tooth was closed tightly with the gingival flap and suturing (Fig 10-11s). Since there was no endodontic infection, no apicectomy was performed. No regenerative therapies such as bone grafting materials or growth factors were used.

As the tooth mobility immediately after replantation was very high, wire splinting was performed and maintained for 7 months, which allowed more time for osseous regeneration and stability (Fig 10-11y to 10-11aa). The maximum probing depth reduced to about 4 mm on the lingual aspect and no bleeding on probing was observed. The tooth mobility was almost normal when the wire splint was removed 7 months after surgery.

CBCT examinations after 10 months and 3 years showed evidence that the bone around #34 had healed and was maintained (Fig 10-11dd to 10-11ff, and 10-11jj to 10-11ll). Whether the PDL healing came from new attachment or long junctional epithelial attachment was unknown, but tooth-independent bone was recovered and maintained by removing the biofilm infection on the root surface.

Through this case, it is evident that the removal of infection is fundamental in periodontal treatment. Although various methods have been devised for periodontal regenerative therapies, critical factors for success seem to be related to the configuration of the bony defect and infection control.

Tooth dependent bone volume and tooth independent bone volume

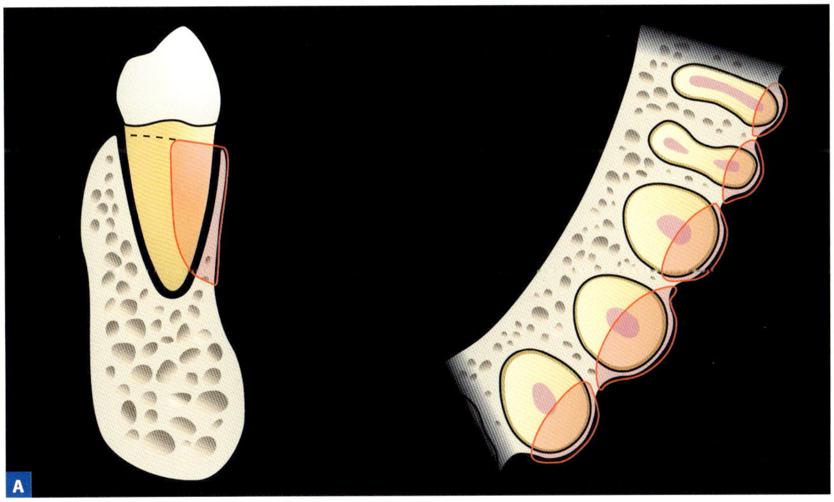

Fig 10-A Alveolar bone is considered to consist of 'tooth dependent bone volume' (red zone) and 'tooth independent bone volume'. If a tooth suffers periodontitis and loses periodontal ligament, tooth dependent bone volume is lost simultaneously but other bone volume can remain depending on the extent of inflammation. Contrarily, tooth independent bone volume can recover without new attachment if infection is controlled.

Intentional replantation to treat periodontal pathology

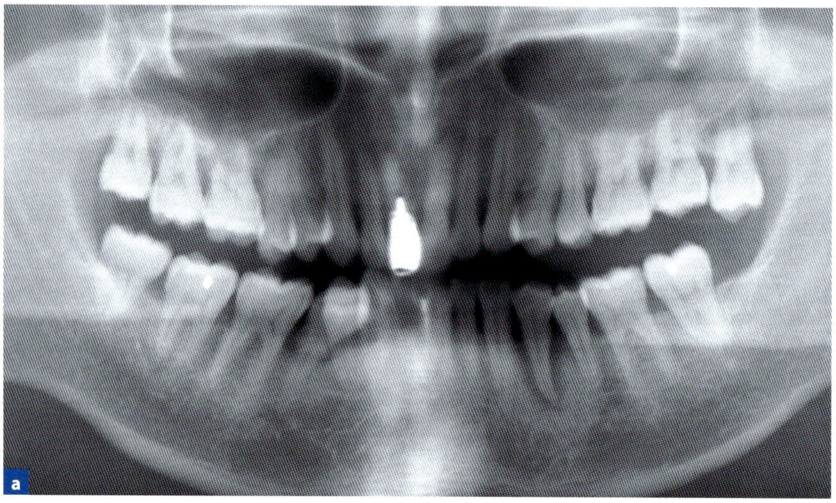

Fig 10-11a to 10-11e Views before treatment of a 43-year-old male who presented with pain, swelling and high tooth mobility of #34.

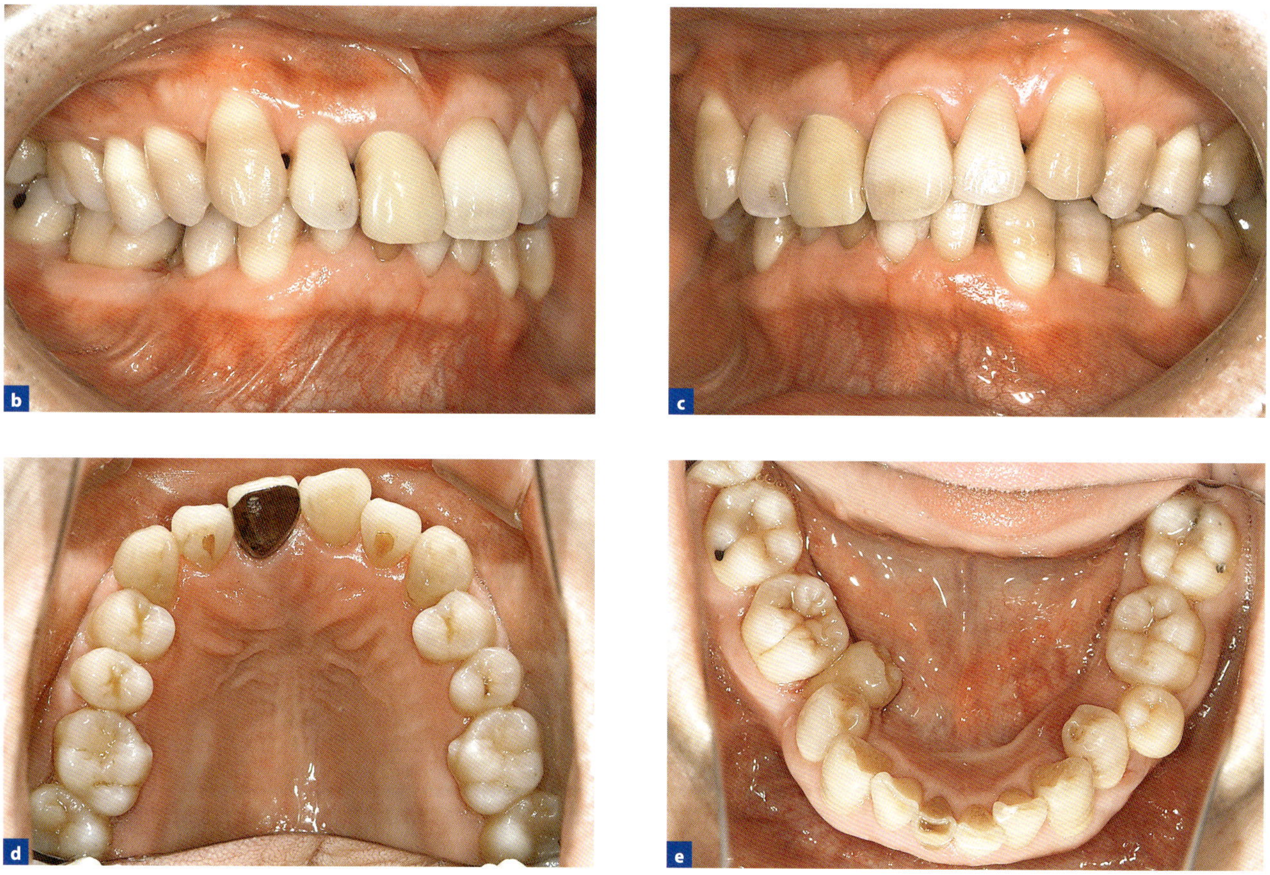

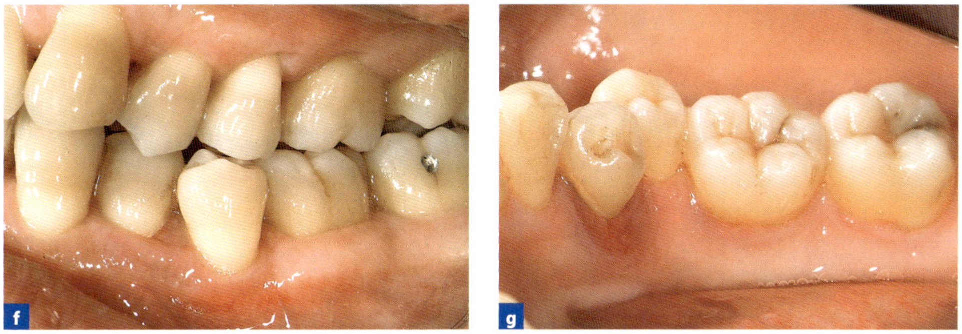

Fig 10-11f Buccal view before treatment.
Fig 10-11g Lingual view before treatment.

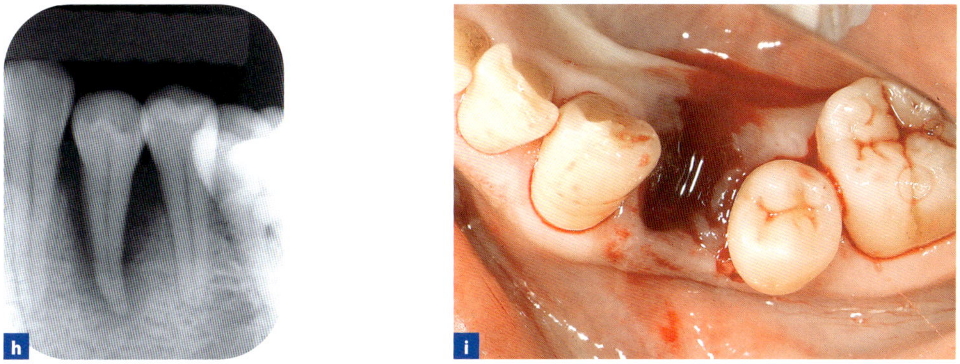

Fig 10-11h Radiograph before treatment. Bone loss has progressed up to the apex of #34 but responded EPT(+). So, it was diagnosed that the bony defect was caused by periodontitis and the prognosis was poor.
Fig 10-11i Extraction socket.

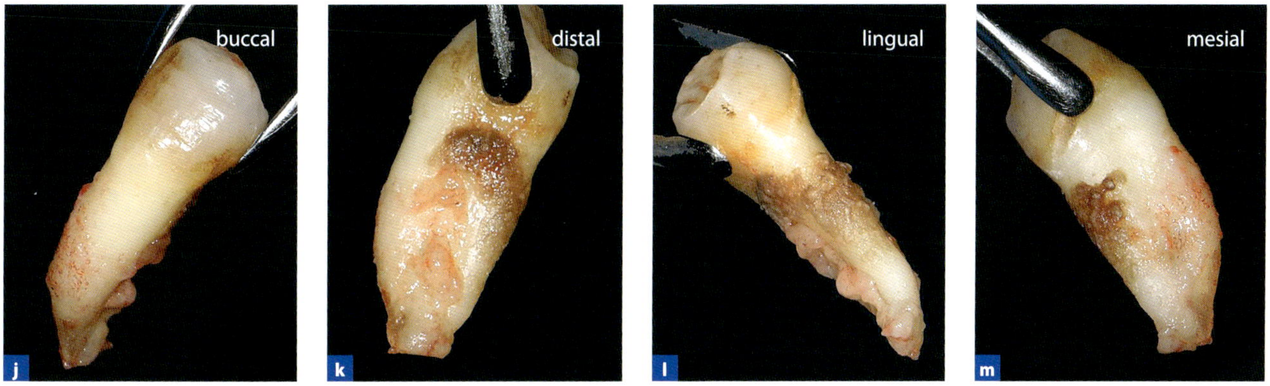

Fig 10-11j to 10-11m Extracted #34. Calculus deposition mainly on the lingual aspect of the root. Periodontal ligament was still intact and attached on the other root surfaces. So, it seemed there was hope that the tooth could be saved by removing the calculus extraorally and replanting the tooth.

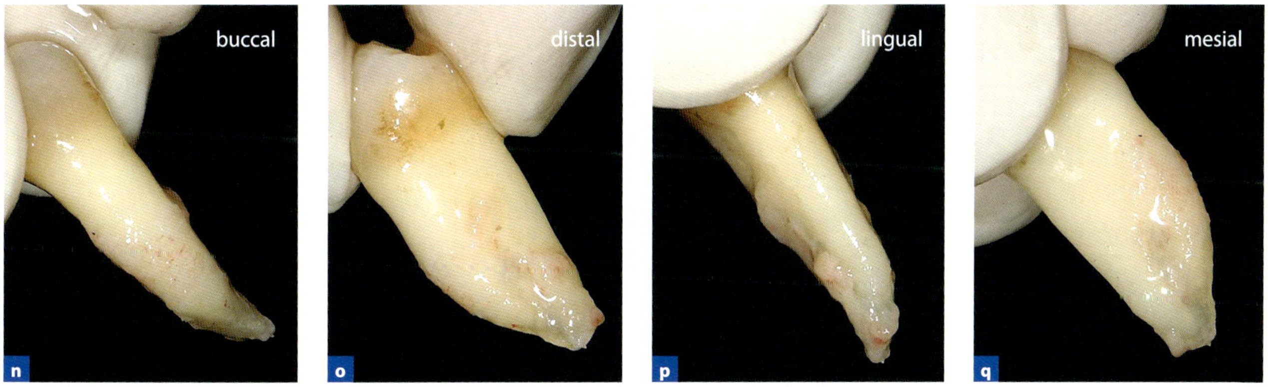

Fig 10-11n to 10-11q Root surfaces after extraoral scaling by an ultrasonic scaler under saline cooling. Care was taken not to damage remaining periodontal ligament.

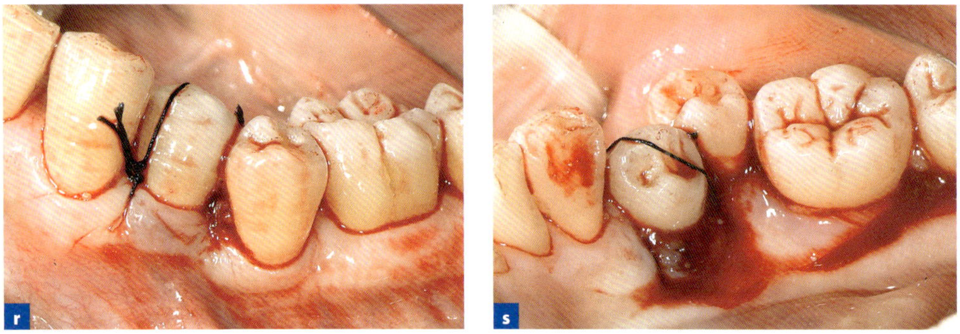

Fig 10-11r and 10-11s Immediately after replantation of #34. The tooth was replanted to the extraction socket after granulation tissue had been excavated. In order to try and seal the cervical area around the root with the gingival flap, the inner marginal epithelium of the extraction socket was turned outward on the lingual side to facilitate closure. Since there was no evidence of root canal infection and periapical pathology, no apicectomy was performed. No regenerative therapies such as bone grafting materials or growth factors were used. After fixation with suture, the replanted tooth was covered with surgical dressing.

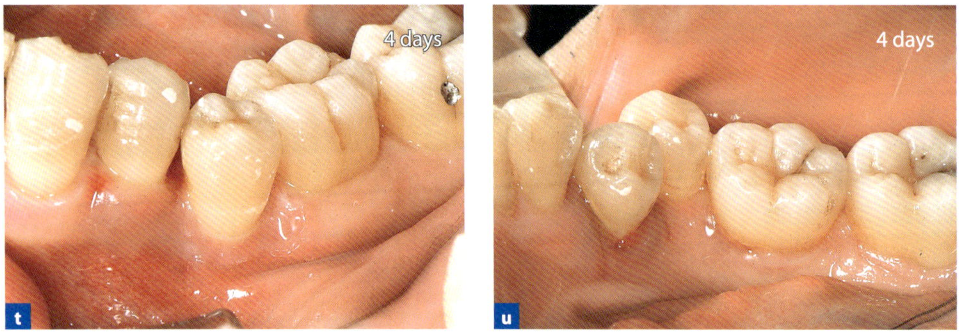

Fig 10-11t and 10-11u Four days after surgery. Immediately after dressing and suture removal. On the same day, the replanted tooth was splinted to the adjacent tooth with wire and adhesive resin.

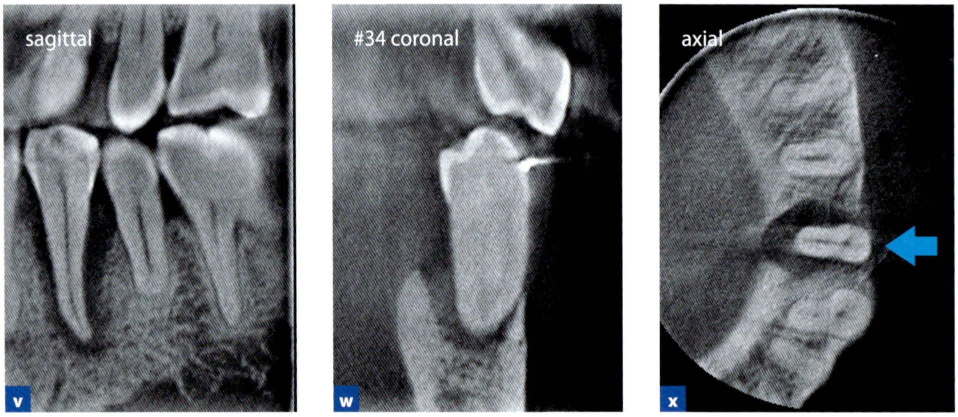

Fig 10-11v to 10-11x CBCT images after 4 days. The mesiodistal and lingual sides of #34 showed bone loss to the apex, but on the buccal aspect, alveolar bone proper derived from the periodontal ligament was maintained, suggesting that the PDL on the buccal root surface was not lost before treatment and bone healing could be expected if inflammation was reduced. In contrast, as mesial, distal and lingual bone consist of tooth-independent bone volume, bone healing could be expected after infection control without new attachment.

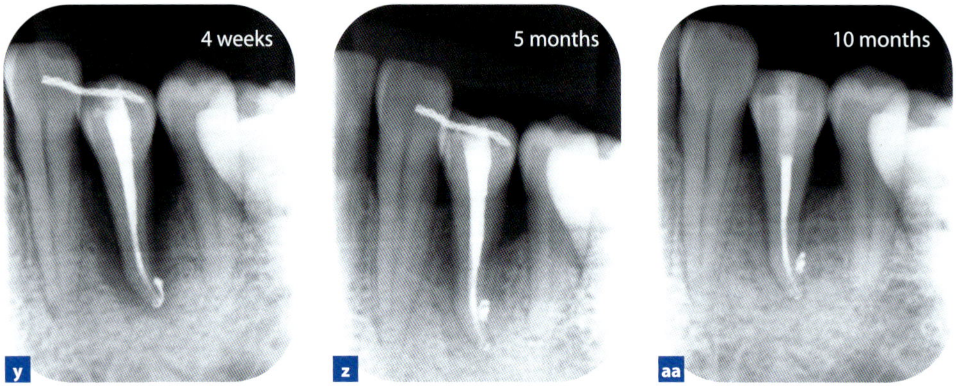

Fig 10-11y Four weeks after replantation. RCT was started 3 weeks after replantation and the root canal was filled with calcium hydroxide preparation 'Vitapex' temporarily.

Fig 10-11z Five months after replantation. Immediately after root canal filling with sealer and gutta-percha.

Fig 10-11aa 10 months after replantation. Wire splinting was removed 7 months after surgery.

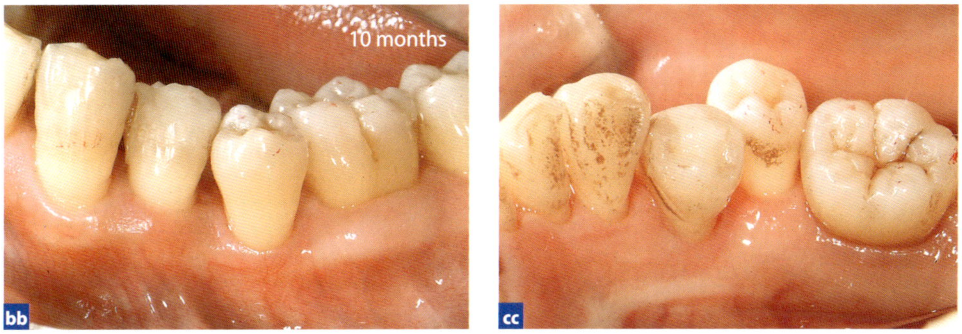

Fig 10-11bb and 10-11cc Oral views after 10 months. Probing depth was 4 mm on the lingual aspect, but on the other aspects it was 3 mm or less. Tooth mobility was normal.

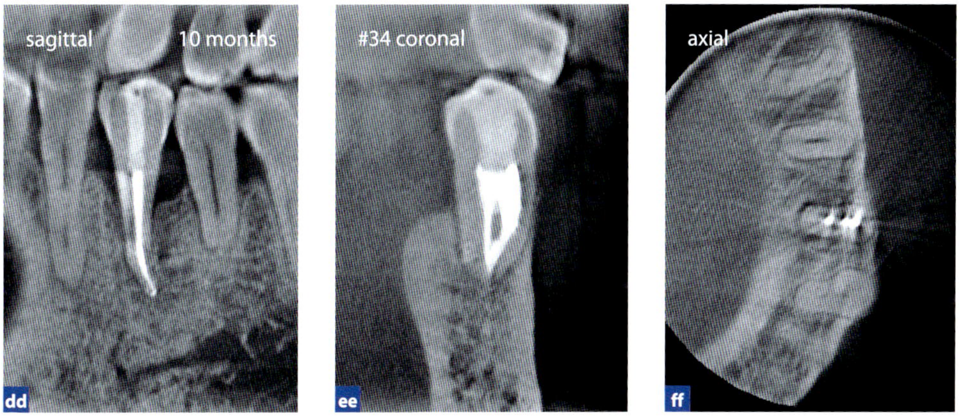

Fig 10-11dd to 10-11ff CBCT images after 10 months. The root of the tooth has been surrounded by new bone.

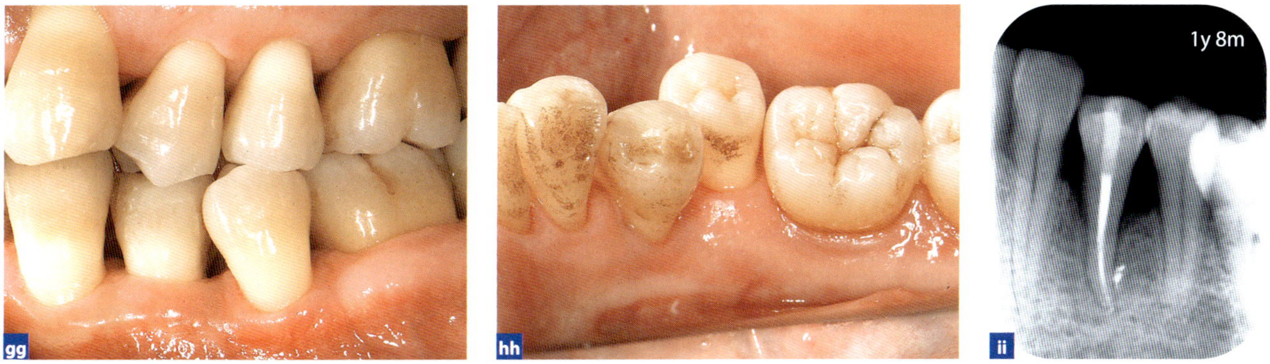

Fig 10-11gg to 10-11ii One year and 8 months postoperative. No problems were observed.

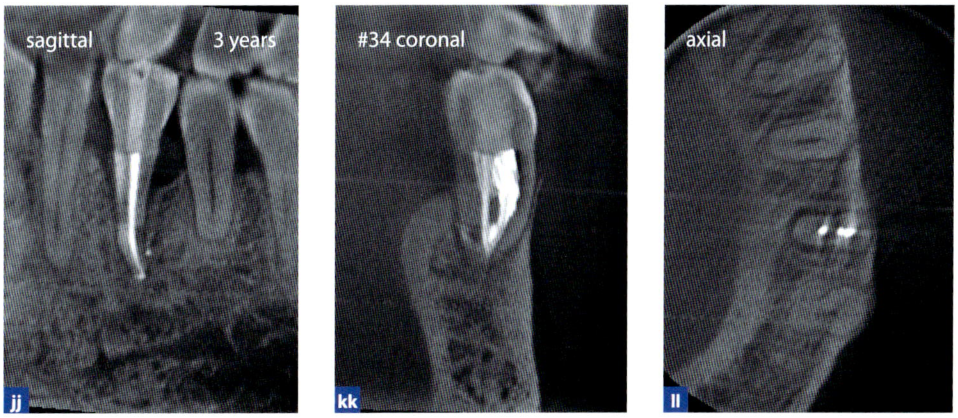

Fig 10-11jj to 10-11II CBCT Images after 3 years. Healing is maintained and there is no significant differences from **Fig 10-11dd to 10-11ff**.

References

1. Gargiulo AW, Wents FM, Orban BJ. Dimensions and relations of the dentogingival junction in humans. J Periodontol. 1961; 32: 261.
2. Maynard JG, Wilson RD. Physiologic dimentions of periodontium significant to the restorative dentist. J Peiodontol. 1970; 50: 170.
3. Ingber JS, et al. The "biologic width": A concept in periodontics and restorative dentistry. Alpha Omegan. 1977 Dec; 70(3): 62-5.
4. Wilson RD, Maynard JG. Intracrevicular restorative dentistry. Int J Periodontics Restorative Dent. 1981; 4 : 34-49.
5. de Waal H, Castellucci G. The importance of restorative margin placement to the biologic width in periodontal health. Part Ⅱ. Int J Periodontics Restorative Dent. 1994 Feb; 14 (1): 70-83.
6. Nevins M, Skurow HM. The intracrevicular restorative margin, the biologic width, and the maintenance of the gingival margin. Int J Periodontics Restorative Dent. 1984; 4 (3): 30-49.
7. Schmidt JC, Sahrmann P, Weiger R, Schmidlin P. R, Walter C. Biologic width dimensions—A systematic review. J Clin Periodontol. 2013; 40: 493-504.
8. Wagenberg BD, Langer B, Eshow RN. Exposing adequate tooth structure for restorative dentistry. Int J Periodontics Restorative Dent. 1989; 9 (5): 322-31.
9. Juloski J, Radovic I, Goracci C, Vulicevic Z. R, Ferrari M. Ferrule effect: A literature review. J Endod. 2012; 38: 11-9.
10. Hempton T, Dominici J. Contemporary crown-lengthening therapy. : a review. J Am Dent Assoc. 2010 Jun; 141(6): 647-55.
11. Fugazzotto P.A, Parma-Benfenati S. Preprosthetic periodontal considerations. Crown length and biologic width. Quintessence Int Dent Dig. 1984; 15: 1247-56.
12. Malmgren O, Malmgren B, Frykholm A. Rapid orthodontic extrusion of crown root and cervical root fractured teeth. Dent Traumatol. 1991; 7 : 49-54.
13. Bach N, Baylard J. F, Voyer R. Orthodontic extrusion: Periodontal considerations and applications. J Can Dent Assoc. 2004; 70: 775-80.
14. Tegsjo U, Valerius-Olsson H, Olgart K. Intra-alveolar transplantation of teeth with cervical root fractures. Swed Dent J. 1978; 2 : 73-82.
15. Kahnberg KE. Intraalveolar transplantation of teeth with crown-root fractures. J Oral Maxillofac Surg. 1985; 43: 38-42.
16. Kahnberg KE. Intra-alveolar transplantation. I. A 10-year follow-up of a method for surgical extrusion of root fractured teeth. Swed Dent J. 1996; 20: 165-72.
17. Das B, Muthu MS. Surgical extrusion as a treatment option for crown-root fracture in permanent anterior teeth: A systematic review. Dent Traumatol. 2013; 29: 423-31.
18. Grossman LI. Intentional replantation of teeth. J Am Dent Assoc. 1966; 72: 1111-8.
19. Bender IB, Rossman LE. Intentional replantation of endodontically treated teeth. Oral Surg Oral Med Oral Pathol. 1993; 76: 623-30.
20. Choi YH, Bae JH, Kim YK, Kim HY, Kim SK, Cho BH. Clinical outcome of intentional replantation with preoperative orthodontic extrusion: A retrospective study. Int Endod J. 2014; 47: 1168-76.
21. Becker BD. Intentional replantation techniques: A critical review. J Endod. 2018; 44: 14-21.
22. Plotino G, Abella Sans F, Duggal MS, Grande NM, Krastl G, Nagendrababu V, Gambarini G. Clinical procedures and outcome of surgical extrusion, intentional replantation and tooth autotransplantation—A narrative review. Int Endod J. 2020; 53: 1636-52.
23. Tsukiboshi M, Tsukiboshi T. Bone morphology after delayed tooth replantation - case series. Dent Traumatol. 2014 Dec; 30 (6): 477-83.

CHAPTER 11

Prognosis

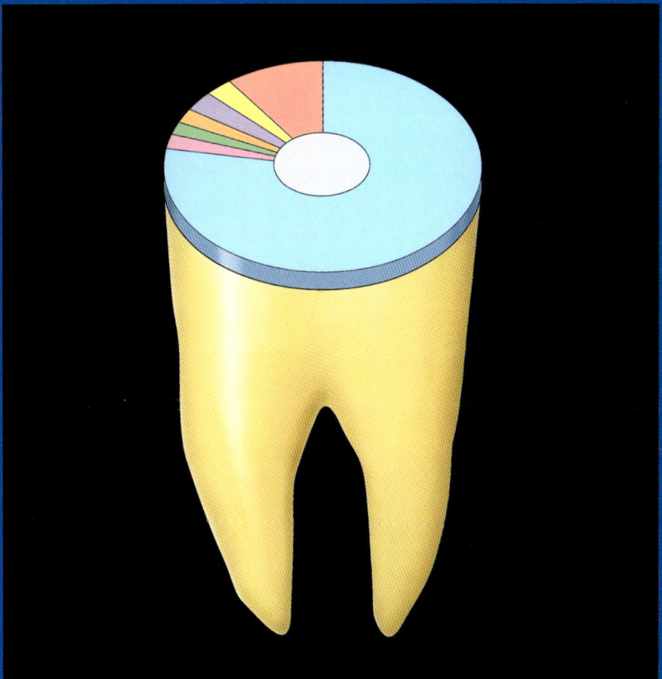

How successful is autotransplantation of teeth? The available data show fairly wide range of success rates. In this CHAPTER, the success of autotransplantation is presented from the author's experience and data collected, as well as from other available studies.

Criteria for Success in Autotransplantation

Success of autotransplantation can be determined on the basis of complete healing (as described in **Chapter 3**) and continued function and maintenance of a healthy tooth-alveolar complex for a long period of time. For instance, in the case of transplantation of immature teeth, criteria for success would be healing of the periodontal ligament without progressive root resorption nor periodontal pocket formation, pulpal healing (revascularization and pulp canal obliteration), root development, and bone healing (**Fig 11-1** and **11-2**). In the case of mature teeth, the criteria would be periodontal ligament and bone healing and successful endodontic treatment (as the pulp is not expected to revascularize and root canal treatment is indicated) (**Fig 11-3**).

Radiographic evidence of success

(1) Normal width of periodontal ligament space around the transplanted tooth.

Long term success of transplantation of an immature tooth ①

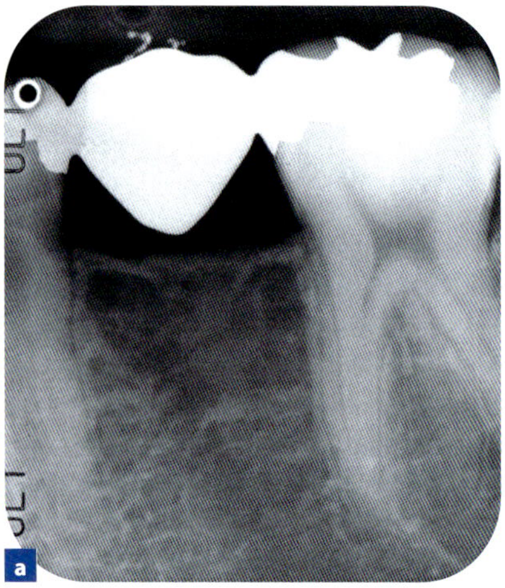

Fig 11-1a Preoperative radiograph of a 16-year-old female congenitally missing #35.

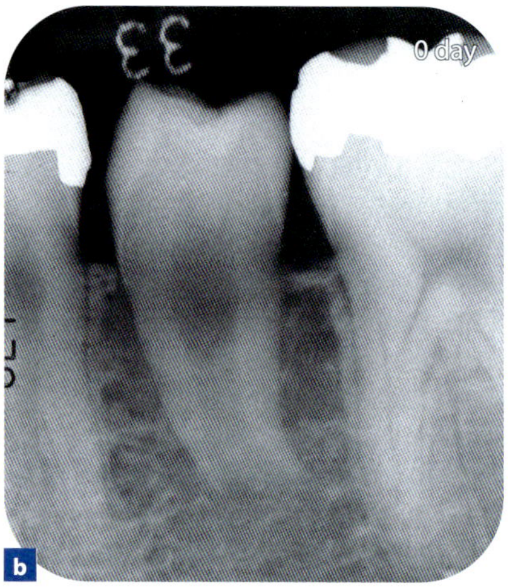

Fig 11-1b Immediately after transplantation of immature #45 to the missing site.

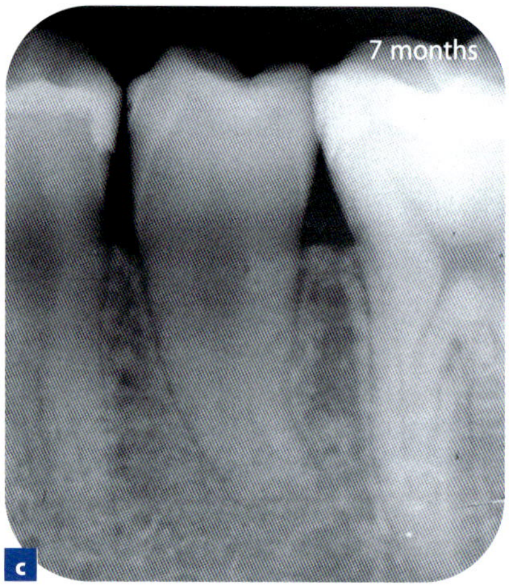

Fig 11-1c Seven months postop. Slight progression of calcification. The transplant responds EPT (+).

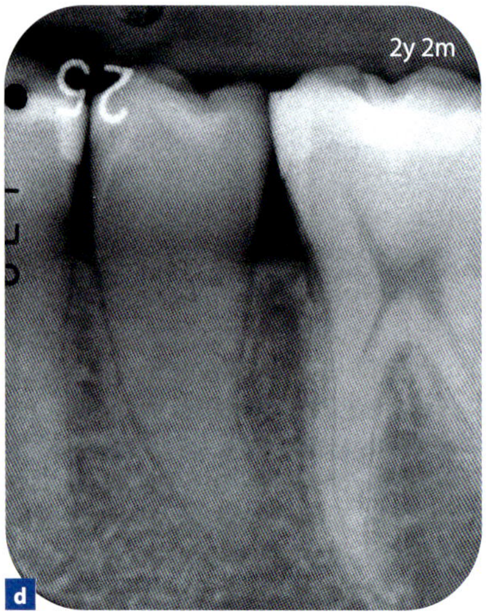

Fig 11-1d Two years and 2 months postop. The canal space shows almost complete calcification and the root development is in its final stage.

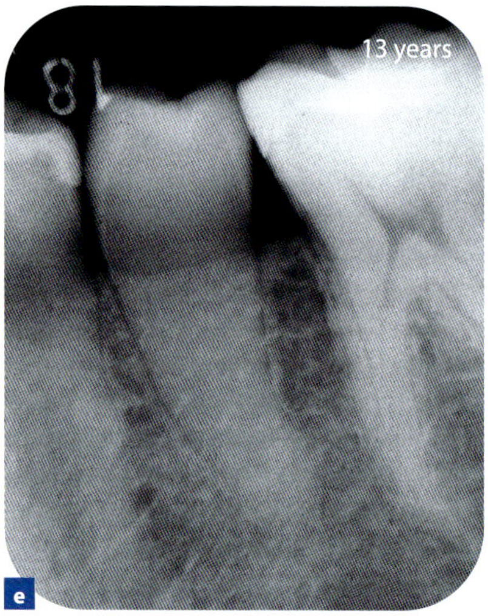

Fig 11-1e 13 years postop. No radiographic changes, but the response to EPT is less.

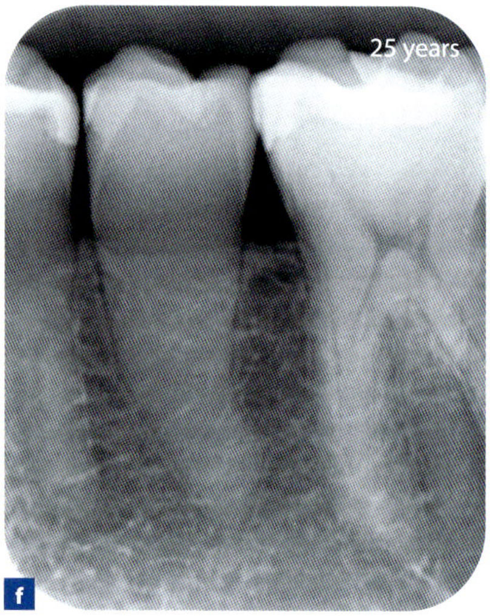

Fig 11-1f 25 years postop. No evident abnormalities are detected.

(2) No evidence of progressive root resorption.
(3) A formation of lamina dura on the side of the recipient socket.
(4) Pulpal healing (pulp canal obliteration) in immature transplant.
(5) Root development in immature transplant although not necessary for long-term success.

Clinical evidence of success

(1) Tooth mobility within normal limits.
(2) Normal percussion sound (no ankylosis).
(3) No evidence of attachment loss (no pocket formation).
(4) No evidence of gingival inflammation.
(5) No patient discomfort.
(6) Normal tooth function.

Histological evidence of success

Histologic evidence of successful transplantation is represented primarily by evidence of restored periodontal ligament fibers that are aligned perpendicular to the root and alveolar bone (see **Chapter 3**). If the fibers are aligned parallel to the root and bone, some may deem it unsuccessful even if the clinical and radiographic evidence indicates healing. However, since such histological examination cannot be performed clinically in most cases, thus histological failure does not necessarily mean clinical failure.

In clinical practice, we may observe some abnormalities such as surface resorption (**Fig 11-4**), the periodontal ligament space that is unclear or has partially disappeared, the delayed emergence of lamina dura, and partial attachment failure or loss (pocket formation), which do not lead to loss of transplanted teeth and continue to be asymptomatic and functional long-term (**Fig 11-5**). Whether or not these conditions should be considered as successful transplantation is a matter of debate, but we would regard them as successful, especially if the patient is satisfied with the result.

Evidence of failure

Fig 11-6 to **11-8** are clinical examples showing that the transplantation failed. Progressive replacement resorption (**Fig 11-6**), delayed inflammatory resorption (**Fig 11-7**, see **Chapter 3**), and advanced deep pockets around the transplant (**Fig 11-8**) are typical examples of failure, although they had fairly long-term survival. The criteria for failure of transplantation are as follows:

(1) Progressive root resorption such as replacement resorption or invasive cervical resorption (**Fig 11-9a**).
(2) Failure to achieve connective tissue attachment soon after transplantation or progressive attachment loss after initial PDL healing (**Fig 11-9b**).

Long term success of transplantation of an immature tooth ②

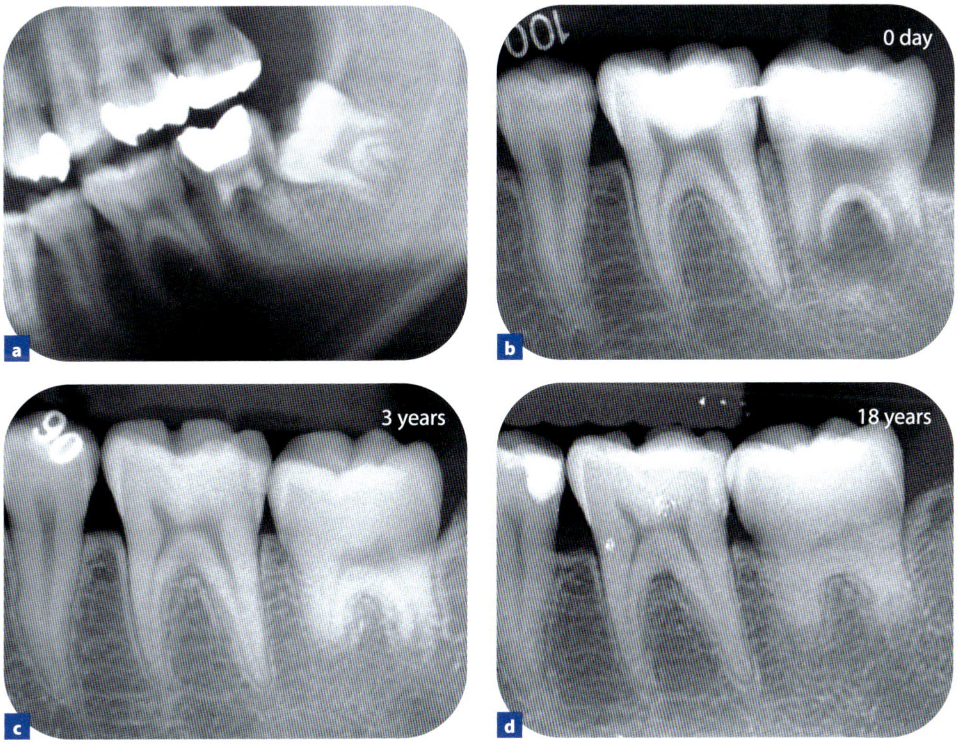

Fig 11-2a Before treatment of a 17-year-old female.
Fig 11-2b Immediately after transplantation. #38 was transplanted to #37 site.
Fig 11-2c Three years postop. Pulp canal obliteration has taken place and responds EPT (+).
Fig 11-2d 18 years postop. The pulp space has continued calcification, and there appears to be slight root development.

Long-term success of transplantation of a mature tooth

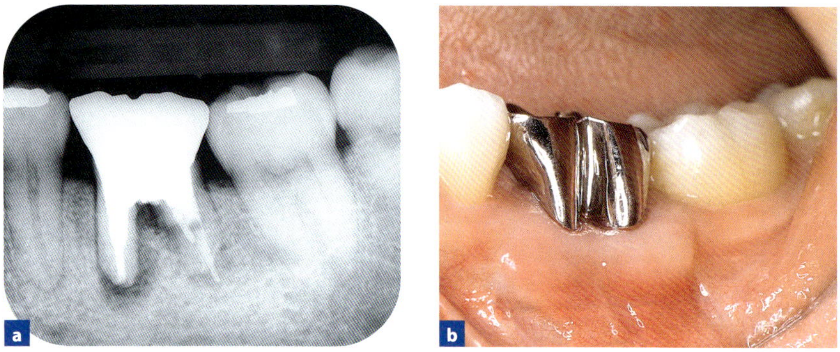

Fig 11-3a, b Preoperative views of a 39-year-old female who is to have #38 transplanted to an unfavorable #36.

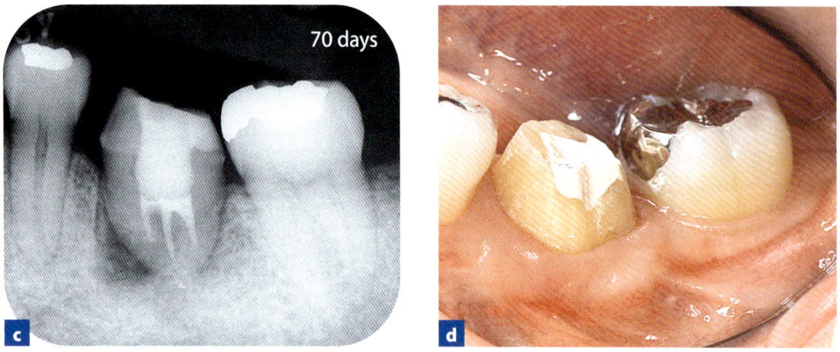

Fig 11-3c, d 70 days after transplantation. Transplantation was performed 2 weeks after tooth extraction. The root canal treatment was finished before transplantation.

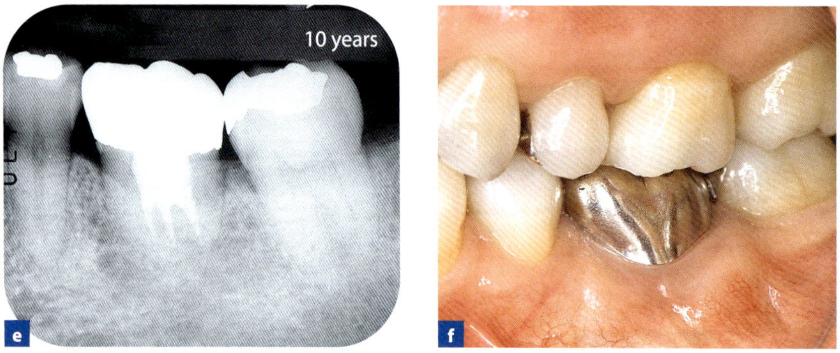

Fig 11-3e, f 10 years after transplantation.

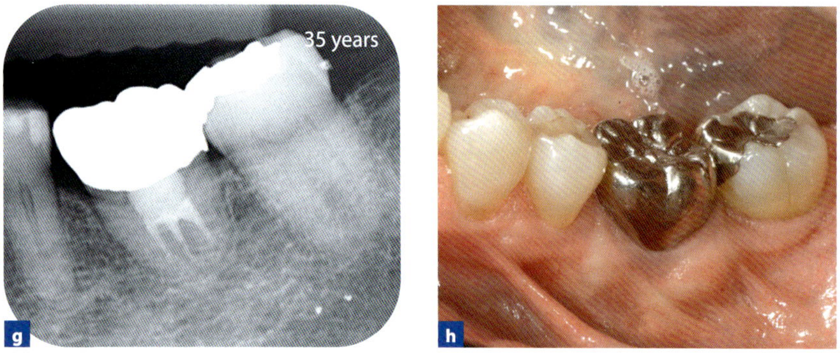

Fig 11-3g, h 35 years after transplantation. There was no evidence of root resorption, and tooth mobility and probing depths were normal.

Surface root resorption (as a successful example)

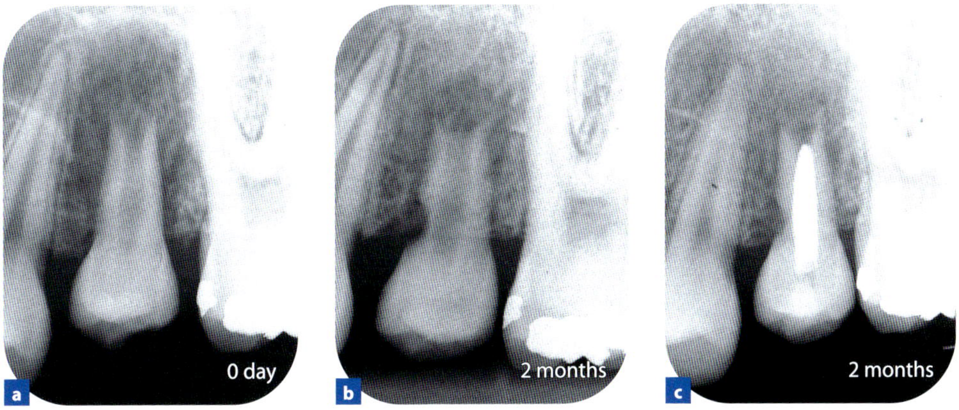

Fig 11-4a A 15-year-old female. Immediately after transplanting a horizontally impacted #25 into the extraction socket of #65.
Fig 11-4b Two months after transplantation. Inflammatory resorption is observed on the mesial aspect.
Fig 11-4c Same day as **Fig 11-4b**. Immediately after root canal treatment of the transplanted tooth (expecting apexogenesis).

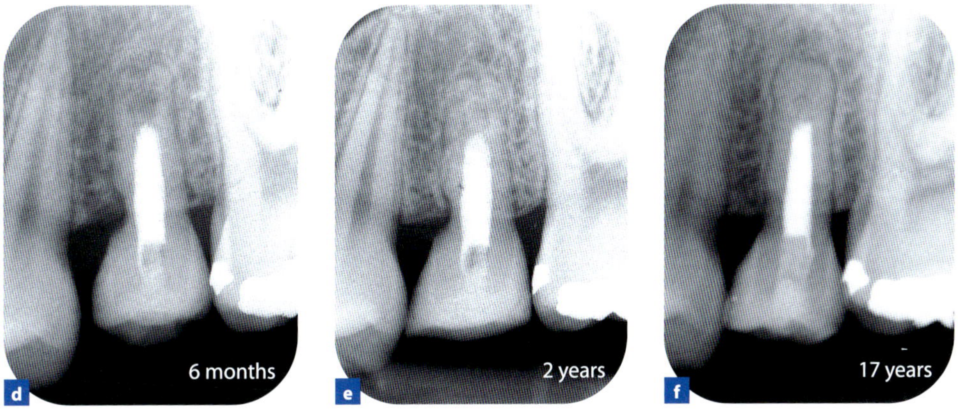

Fig 11-4d Six months postoperative. Root resorption appears arrested.
Fig 11-4e Two years postop. Root resorption continues to be arrested and the root shows evidence of development apically.
Fig 11-4f 17 years postop. The area of previous root resorption is thought to have been repaired by new attachment (see **Chapter 3**).

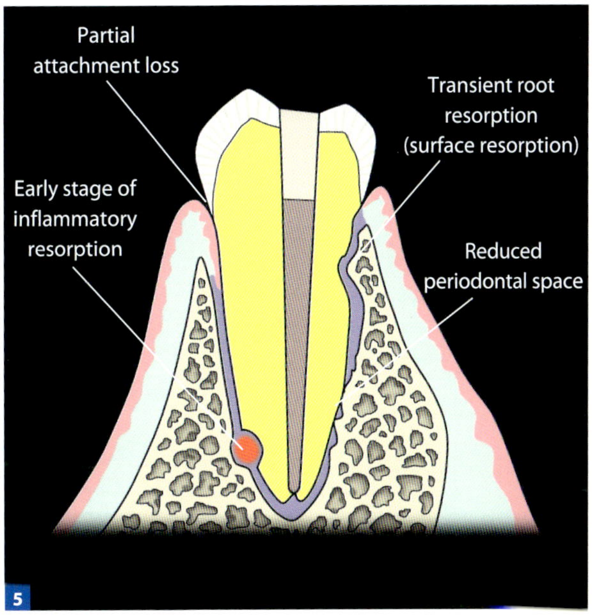

Fig 11-5 Schematic drawing showing clinically acceptable healing. Transient surface root resorption, early stage of inflammatory resorption, partial (maintainable) loss of attachment, and reduced periodontal space are often unlikely progress and should not significantly affect prognosis. Therefore, even if such conditions are observed after transplantation, if it is asymptomatic and functional they should be thought as successful transplantation cases.

Failure of transplantation (replacement resorption/ankylosis)

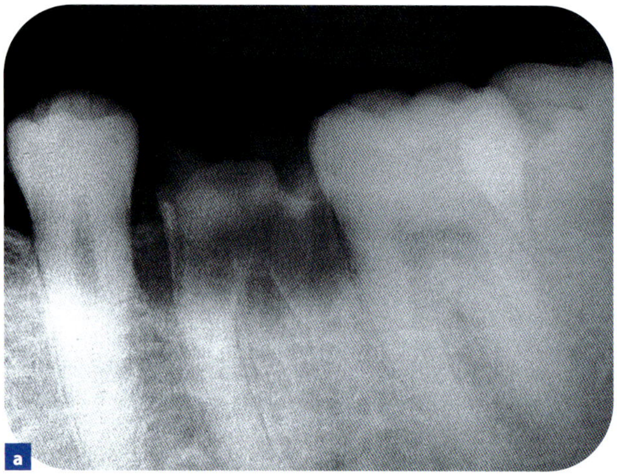

Fig 11-6a Preoperative. A 46-year-old male. #28 is planned for transplantation to the hopeless #36 site.

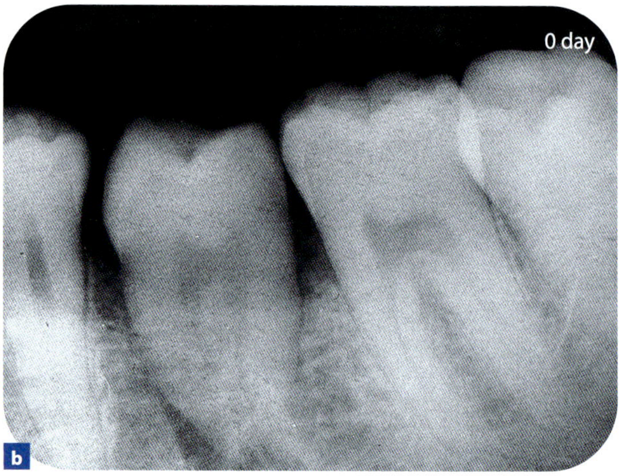

Fig 11-6b Immediately after transplantation.

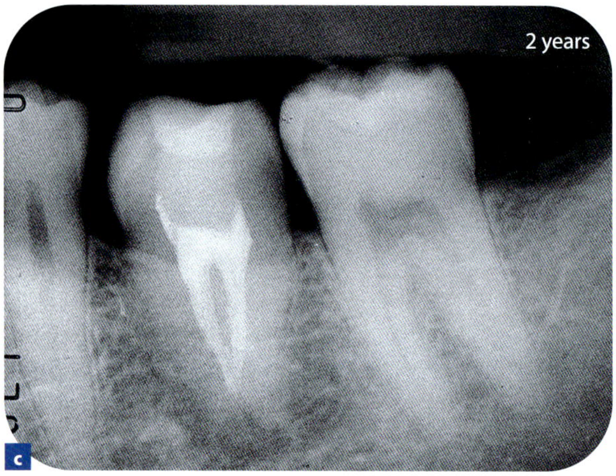

Fig 11-6c Two years postop. There is no evident periodontal ligament space and no tooth mobility is observed clinically.

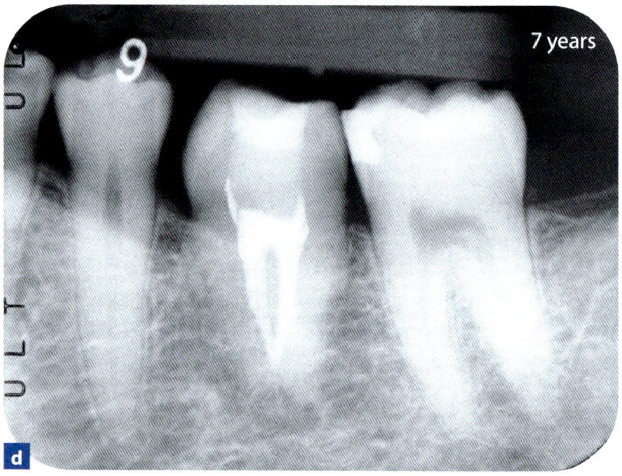

Fig 11-6d Seven years postop. The root appears to be slowly being replaced by bone.

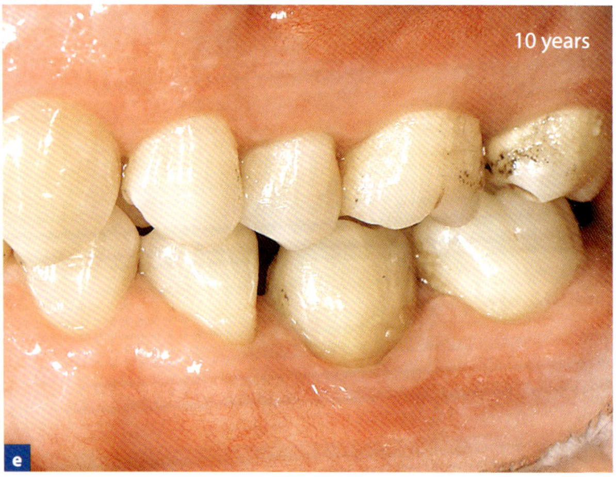

Fig 11-6e Clinical view 10 years after transplantation. The transplanted tooth continues to be asymptomatic, functional and esthetically acceptable to the patient.

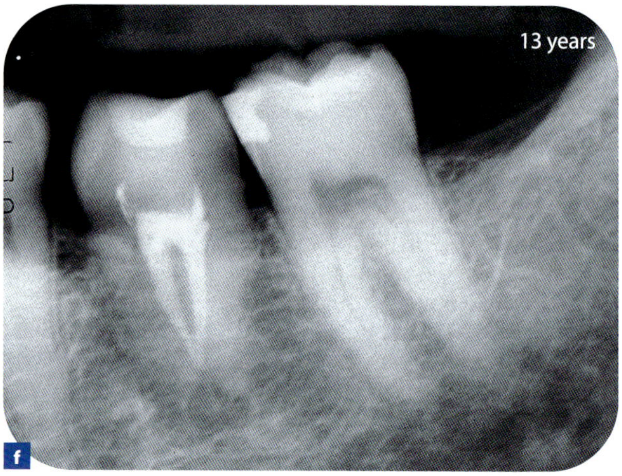

Fig 11-6f 13 years postop. It seems that root resorption progresses extremely slowly in many adults. The transplanted tooth will likely be able to maintain its function as a tooth for the time being, but could be considered a failure of transplantation.

Failure of transplantation (delayed inflammatory resorption)

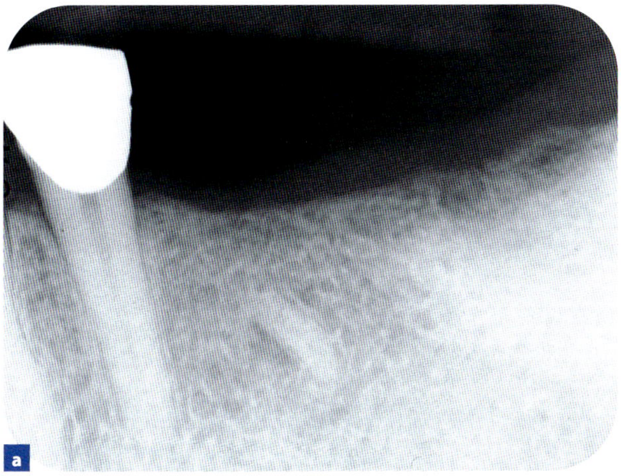

a

Fig 11-7a Preoperative. A 41-year-old male. #28 is planned for transplantation into the edentulous site of #37.

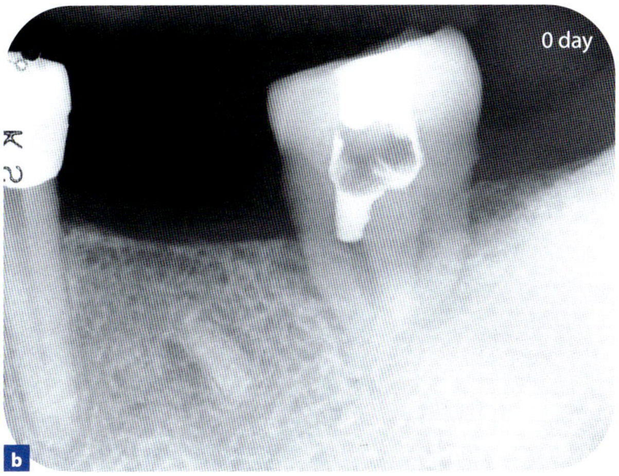

b

Fig 11-7b Immediately after transplantation. Pulp debridement was performed before transplantation.

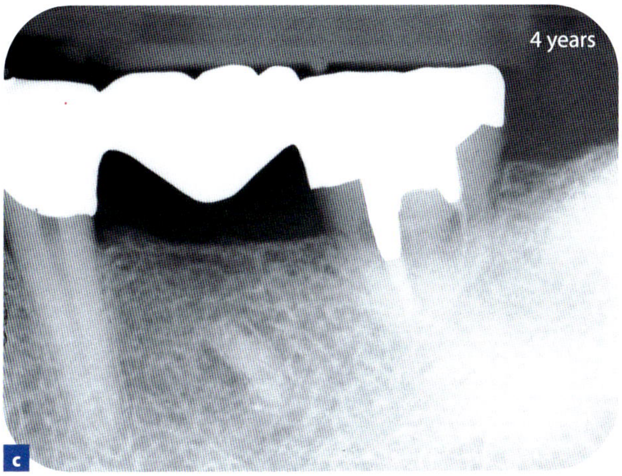

c

Fig 11-7c Four years postop. It appears that there is normal healing.

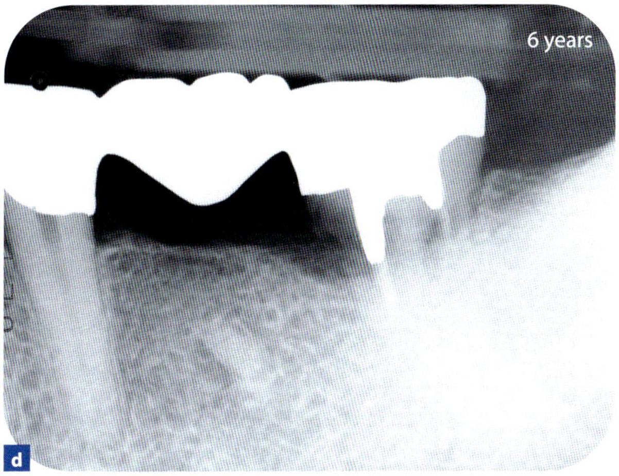

d

Fig 11-7d Six years postop. There is evidence of root resorption on the mesial aspect. It is thought that initial ankylosis turned to infection related resorption (delayed inflammatory resorption).

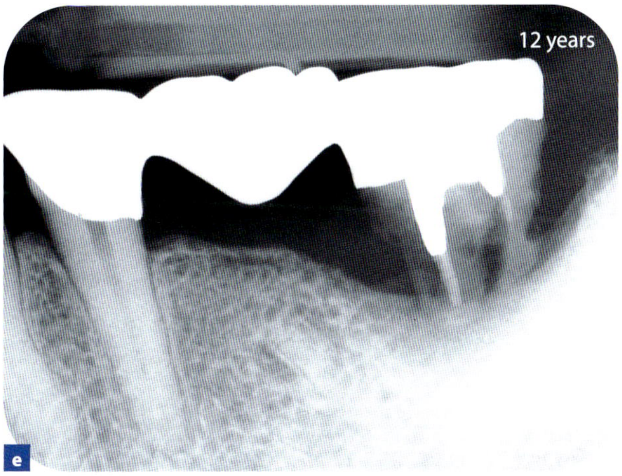

e

Fig 11-7e 12 years postop. Right before the tooth extraction. The tooth remained asymptomatic and functional throughout the 12 years.

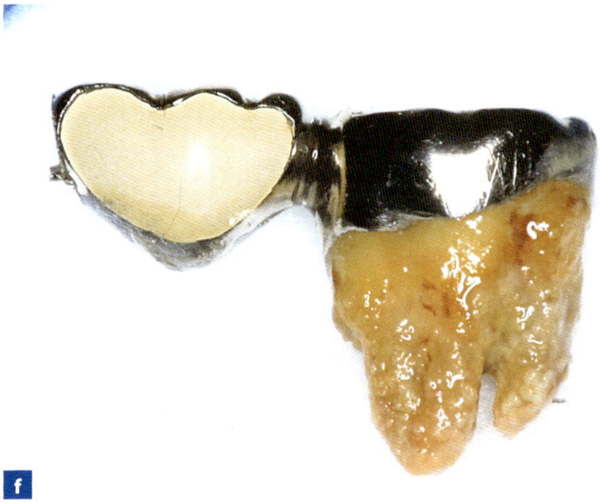

f

Fig 11-7f The extracted tooth. It can be seen that resorption is progressing on the entire surface of the root.

Failure of transplantation (attachment loss)

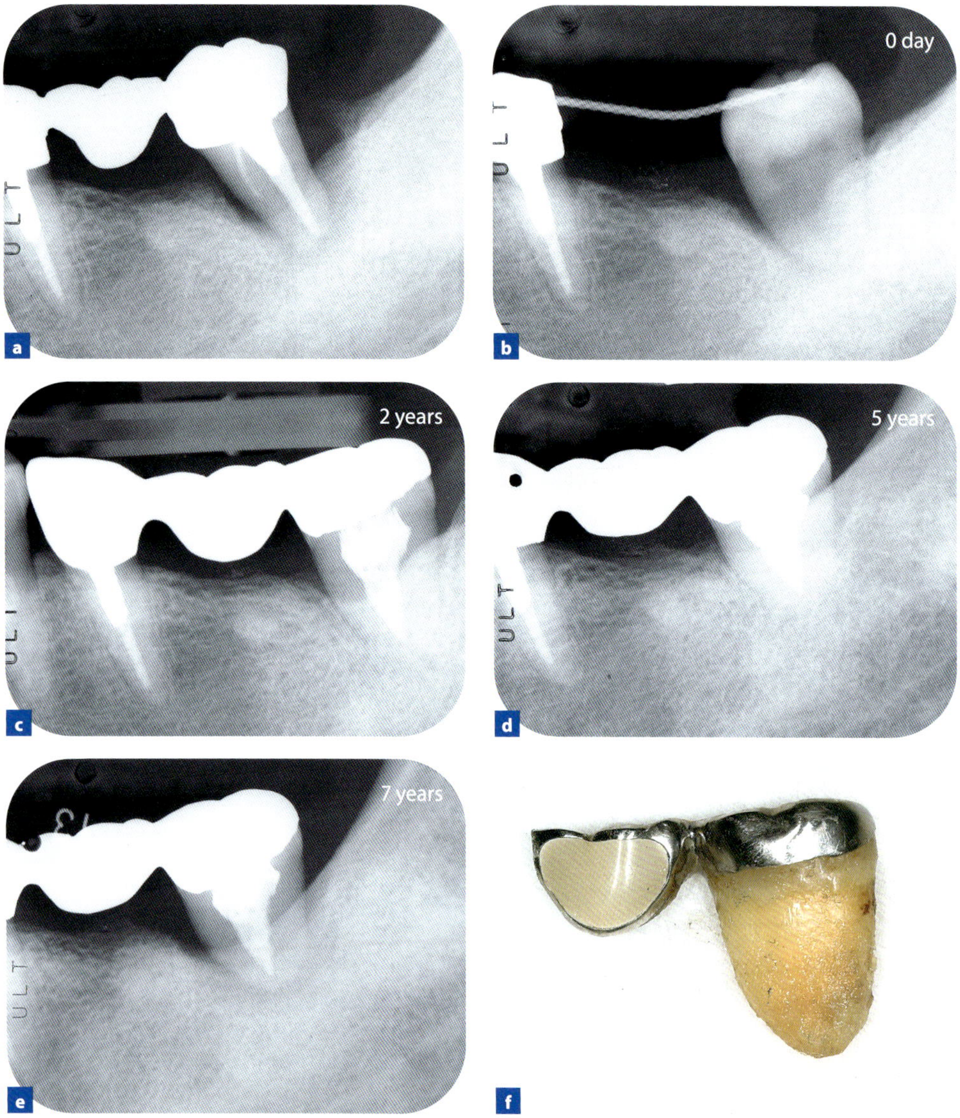

Fig 11-8a Preoperative. A 43-year-old male. #28 is planned for transplantation to #37 which is hopeless because of severe periodontitis.

Fig 11-8b Immediately after transplantation.

Fig 11-8c Two years postop. There seems to be no evident problems.

Fig 11-8d Five years postop. No abnormalities are observed.

Fig 11-8e Seven years postop. Sudden attachment loss (periodontitis) has occurred in the transplanted tooth.

Fig 11-8f The same day as **Fig 11-8e**. Extracted tooth. Although there is no root resorption, there is also no intact periodontal ligament tissue observed.

Schematic drawing showing failures of transplantation

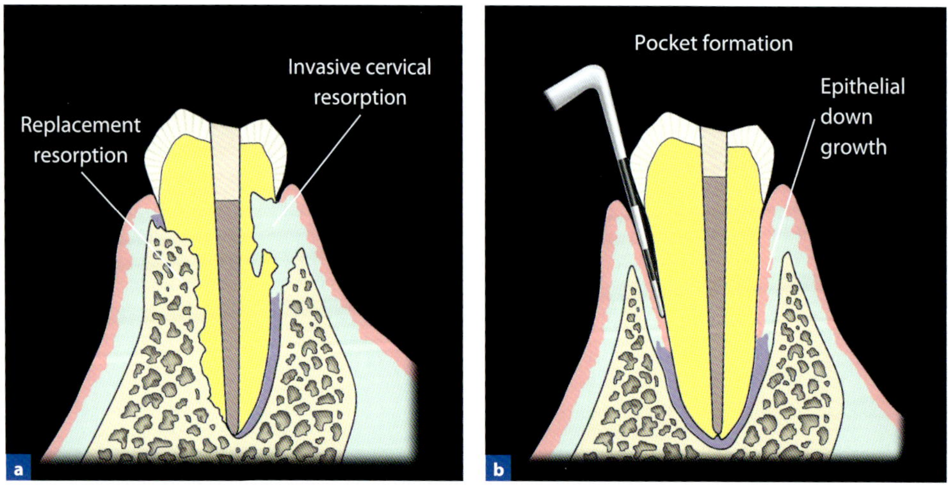

Fig 11-9a Progressive replacement resorption and invasive cervical resorption. Replacement resorption (ankylosis) occurs when the root surface without viable periodontal ligament comes into contact with bone tissue. Invasive cervical resorption[43-46] may occur between the root without viable periodontal ligament and gingival connective tissue.

Fig 11-9b Advanced attachment loss. If the periodontal ligament becomes infected during the healing process after transplantation, epithelial down-growth occurs. Even after initial periodontal healing, attachment loss may occur around transplanted teeth because of periodontitis.

Analysis of Clinical Results from1985-1997

In Tsukiboshi's clinical research in 1990[1], all of the consecutive 190 transplanted tooth which were performed over the 12 years from 1985 to 1997 and were followed up for 2 to 12 years and analyzed. The reasons for transplantation (orthodontics, prosthetics, dental caries, periodontal treatment), the types of transplanted teeth (incisors, canines, premolars, molars), and the ages of patients were diverse. **Table 11-1** to **11-4** and **Fig 11-10** to **11-15** summarizes the survey results from various viewpoints. As shown in **Table 11-1**, the total number of transplanted teeth (not including intra-alveolar transplantation) was 190, and the total number of patients was 166 (57 males, 109 females). The average age of the patient at the time of transplantation was 37 years, and the average follow-up period was 5.6 years. The survival rate was 90%, the success rate was about 80%, and normal healing was about 78% (**Fig 11-10**). The average survival time of the extracted teeth (time from transplantation to extraction) was 6.3 years. Of the extracted teeth, 12 cases were due to attachment loss, 5 were due to root resorption, one was due to progressing dental caries and one was due to root fracture (**Table 11-3**).

Analysis of conventional transplantation

Out of the surviving teeth, 23 cases (12.1%) did not heal normally (**Table 11-1** and **Fig 11-10**). The reasons were as follows: loss of some attachment in 5 cases, inflammatory resorption in 6 cases that were arrested, replacement resorption in 4 cases, and surface resorption (transient root resorption) in 4 cases. Four cases had partial attachment on the distal surface of the second molar. (**Table 11-4**).

Table 11-1 Follow-up results of transplantation (part 1).

Number of patients	166 (males : 57, females : 109)
Age at surgery	14~72 years old (mean : 37)
Follow-up period	2~12 years (mean : 5.6)
Number of teeth	190 (molars : 128, others : 62) (transplanted to extraction sockets : 107) (transplanted to nonextraction sites : 83)
Number of survival teeth	171 (normal periodontal healing : 148) (abnormal periodontal healing : 23)
Number of extraction	19 (All teeth were transplanted to nonextraction sites.) (Mean number of years before extraction : 6.3)

Table 11-2 Number of transplanted teeth and extracted teeth viewing from age.

Age at surgery	Number of teeth	Number of teeth extracted
10~19	9	0
20~29	39	2
30~39	55	2
40~49	49	5
50~59	20	6
60~69	16	3
70~	2	1

Table 11-3 Reasons for extraction of transplanted teeth.

Reasons for extraction	Number of teeth
Attachment loss	12
Root resorption	5
Caries	1
Root fracture	1

Table 11-4 Types of abnormal healing of periodontal ligament.

Types of abnormal healing	Number of teeth
Attachment loss	5
Inflammatory resorption	6
Replacement resorption	4
Surface resorption	4
Failure of reattachment during healing	4

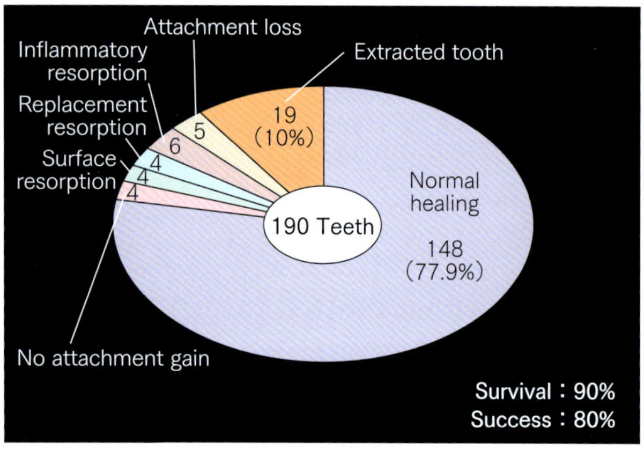

Fig 11-10 Overall survival and success rates of transplantation.*
* Cases of surface resorption are considered successful.

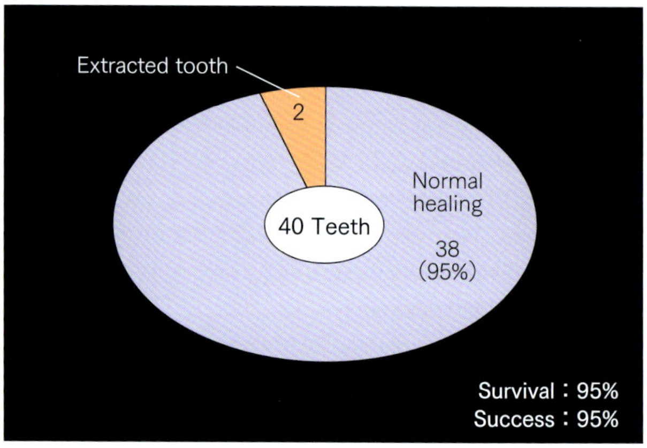

Fig 11-11 Overall survival and success rates of surgical extrusion.*
* Average patient age at the transplantation time is 32; average years of follow-up is 4.5; and transplanted teeth include anterior teeth, premolars, and molars.

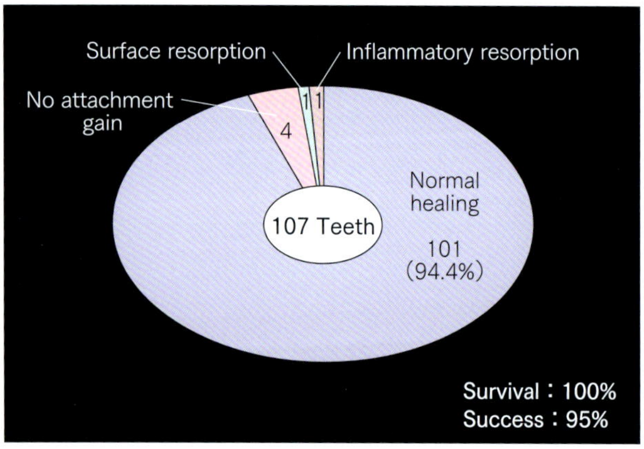

Fig 11-12 Survival and success rates of transplantation to extraction sockets with existing periodontal ligament.

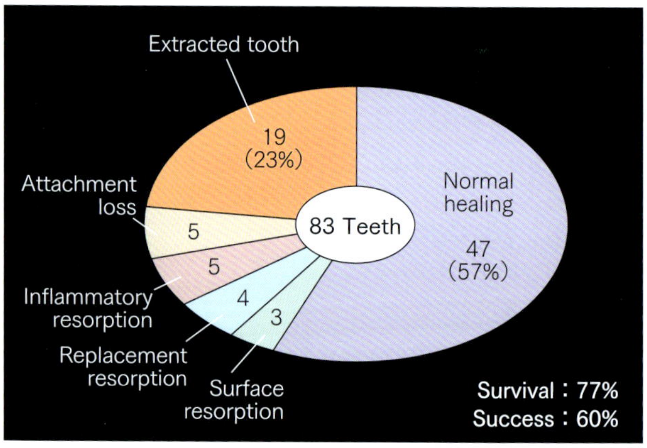

Fig 11-13 Survival and success rates of transplantation to non-extraction sockets (no existing periodontal ligament).

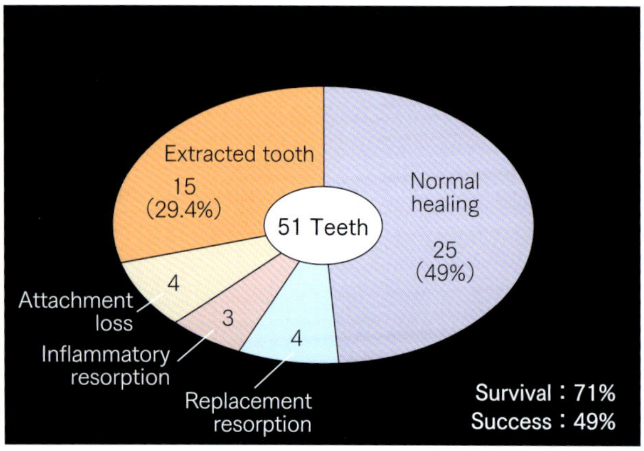

Fig 11-14 Survival and success rates of transplantation to non-extraction sites in patients aged 40 and older.

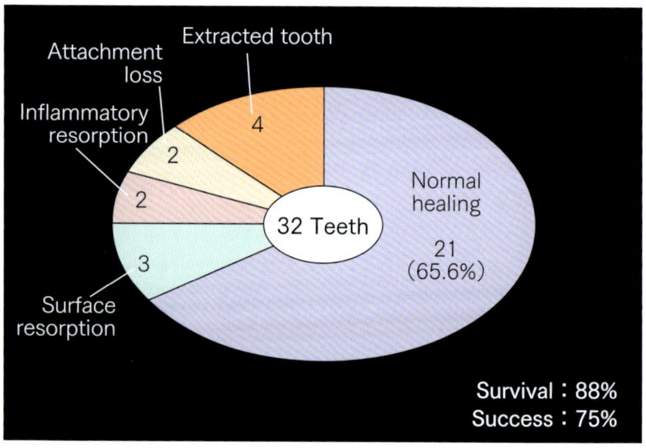

Fig 11-15 Survival and success rates of transplantation to non-extraction sites in patients younger than 40 years.

Transplantation in extraction sockets vs. transplantation in non-extraction sockets

Fig 11-12 is a graph showing the survival rate of teeth when transplanted into an extraction socket (the site where some periodontal ligament likely was present in the recipient site). Transplantation into the fresh extraction socket had a survival rate of 100% and a high success rate of 95% (surface resorption was considered successful). The main reason for failure was attachment loss (in 4 cases) which was considered to be due to the inadequate surgical techniques (see **Chapter 4**). On the other hand, transplantation to non-extraction sites (a site where no periodontal ligament tissue was present in the recipient socket) had a survival rate of approximately 77% and a normal healing rate of approximately 57% (**Fig 11-13**). When the survival rate and success rate are calculated based on age and transplantation into non-extraction sites (newly formed sockets), for those age 40 and older the survival rate is approximately 71% and the success rate is approximately 49 % after an average observation period of approximately 5.6 years (**Fig 11-14**). On the other hand, if transplantation is performed before the age of 40, the survival rate is about 88% and the success rate (superficial resorption is considered successful) is 75% (**Fig 11-15**). So this suggests that the survival and success rate of transplantation are higher when done into the tooth extraction socket and that healing may be more favorable the younger the patient.

Surgical extrusion

Fig 11-11 shows the survival rate and success rate of surgical extrusion (intra-alveolar transplantation) performed by Dr. Tsukiboshi[1]. A total of 40 teeth were treated, the average age of the patients at the time of treatment was 32 years, the average follow-up period was 4.5 years, and the survival rate and success rate were about 95%. Thus, the success rate of surgical extrusion is extremely high.

From the follow-up results of Dr. Tsukiboshi clinical study, it suggests that the age of patient and having periodontal ligament on the recipient site may be important factors that affect the prognosis of transplantation. The recipient site and its periodontal ligament may play a significant role in healing (see **Chapter 3**, compare healing in **Fig 3-1** to **Fig 3-7**).

Analysis of Clinical Results from 2003~2013

Since 1999, based on the above clinical results from 1985 to 1997, the author (Dr. Tsukiboshi) has tried to be more case selective for transplantation performed. In other words, treatment was performed mostly on patients who were no older than 40 years of age and donor teeth were transplanted into existing extraction sockets. The second clinical analysis was performed with 119 patients (129 transplanted teeth) who were followed up for more than 2 years during the 10 years from 2003 to 2013 (**Table 11-5**). The analysis included teeth transplanted before 1999, but most of them were transplanted into extraction sockets. Compared to the previous study, the average age of patients at the time of transplantation was 30.1 years, and the average recall period was 10.2 years. The results showed a survival rate of 94.6% and a success rate of 84.5%. If the patients were no older than 30 years, the success rate was

Table 11-5 Follow-up results of transplantation (part 2).

Number of patients	119
Age of patients at surgery	11~55 years (mean : 30.1 years old)
Follow-up period	2~26 years (mean : 10.2 years)
Number of transplanted teeth	129
Survival rate	94.6%
Overall success rate	84.5%
Success rate of patients no older than 30 years	90.0% (the number of teeth : 60)
Success rate of patients older than 30 years	79.7% (the number of teeth : 69)
Success rate of immature teeth	95% (the number of teeth : 21)

90.0 %. However, if the patients were older than 30, the success rate was 79.7% even though transplantation was performed into extraction sockets. This would suggest that the patient's age at the time of transplantation is a significant predictor of success. This can possibly explain the success rate of 95% for transplantation of immature teeth (21 transplants) that were followed up in this study.

Survival and success rates of tooth transplantation in the literature

It is not easy to determine the success rate of transplantation by reviewing the literature related to prognosis because there was no common defined criteria for success. **Table 11-6** to **11-9** show the prognosis of transplantation of molars, premolars, canines, and incisors based on data from several studies[2-34]. It is possible to calculate survival rates from these tables. However, the success rate of transplantation would be extrapolated based on the healing or non-healing of the periodontal ligament. Therefore, it is important to consider that the rates of periodontal ligament healing may have included cases in which there was evidence of transient root resorption. According to those results, the periodontal ligament of immature teeth heals more quickly and without evidence of any root resorption compared to that of mature teeth; therefore survival and success rates of immature teeth are higher than those of developed teeth. Furthermore, the predictability of transplantation varies depending on the root shape; prognosis for transplantation of premolars was highest and lowest for canines.

The reason for the different success rates found among the studies may be explained by many factors such as the different

Table 11-6 Follow-up results of transplantation of third molars. *Modified from reference[2]

	Years of follow-up (range/mean)	Patient age (range/mean)	Number of Teeth	Root* devel-opment	Survival rate (%)	PDL** healing
Nordenram, 1963[3]	0.5~7	13~22 (17.2)	61	I	79	85
Galanter & Minami, 1968[4]	1~10	15~23	31	I	74	94
Andreasen, et al., 1970[5]	0.7~6	13~23 19~46	18 56***	I C	95 96	94 21
Singh & Dudani, 1970[6]	(4.0)	13~17	25	I		
Hovinga, 1986[7]	2~10 (6.0)	14~21 (17.5)	16	I	100	100
Nethander, et al., 1988[8]	1~5	13~65 (30.7)	57****	I	89	79
Andreasen, 1990[9]	0.5~20 (4.7)	15~21	151	I, C	96	81
Schutz, et al., 2013[10]	2.2	–	57	I	100	94.7

* Immature third molar = I
* Mature third molar = C
** Periodontal ligament healing without evidence of root resorption
*** Impacted third molar with endodontic treatment at the time of transplantation.
**** Examples in which all transplantations were performed in a two-step procedure.

Table 11-7 Follow-up results of transplantation of premolars. *Modified from reference[2]

	Years of follow-up (range/mean)	Patient age (range/mean)	Number of Teeth	Root devel-opment	Survival rate (%)	PDL healing
Slagsvold & Bjercke, 1974[11], 1978[12]	3~13 (6.2)	8~19 (11.8)	34	I, C	100	94
Kristerson 1985[13]	1~18 (6.3)	10~58	82 18	I C	96 78	89 50
Andreasen, et al., 1990[14~17]	5	9~31	317 53	I C	95 98	99 60
Jonsson, et al., 2004[18]	2.5~22.3 (10.3)	–	40	I, C	92.5	92.5
Plakwicz, et al., 2013[19]	0.5~6.5 (3)	9.8~17 (12.7)	23	I, C	100	91.3

I: Incomplete root tooth. C: Completed root tooth.

types of teeth that were transplanted, patients' ages, and the methods and level of the treating clinician. Overall, it appears that survival rates vary from 74% to 100% and success rates from 50% to 100%.

Factors affecting the prognosis of tooth transplantation

Here we will discuss the major factors thought to affect the prognosis of transplantation: (1) donor teeth, (2) recipient sites, (3) patients, and (4) operators.

(1) Donor teeth factors

Periodontal ligament

The most critical factor for success is that there is healthy periodontal ligament attached to donor teeth and after healing it remains functional. Necrosis or mechanical loss of periodontal ligament leads to root resorption (ankylosis or inflammatory resorption) or incomplete attachment with epithelial downgrowth. These will typically lead to failure (see **Chapter 3**).

Root morphology

Root morphology can affect the success in 2 ways: the difficulty and potential damage during the extraction process, and the shape and match between donor teeth and recipient sites.

Table 11-8 Follow-up results of transplantation of canines. *Modified from reference[2]

	Years of follow-up (range/mean)	Patient age (range/mean)	Number of Teeth	Survival rate (%)	PDL* Healing(%)
Thonner, 1971[20]	(5)	–	51	98	69
Cook, 1972[21]	0.5~4	13~27	27	96	67
Reade, et al., 1973[22]	0.3~5	12~50	50	100	56
Lovius, et al., 1974[23]	Min.1.5	10~27 (16)	35	97	49
Moss, 1975[24]	1~10	–	100	100	72
Okasala & Kallioniemi, 1977[25]	4~7	13~43	60	88	25
Altonen, et al., 1978[26]	0.5~2 (1.5)	13~47 (25.2)	28	86	25
Hardy, 1982[27]	1~9	13~30	81	91	61
Reade & Hall, 1982[28]	0.5~9	13~43 (20)	131	90	34
Hall & Reade, 1983[29]	–	–	–	–	–
Ahlberg, et al., 1983[30]	(6)	16~56 (27.5)	33	88	25
Lownie, et al., 1986[31]	0.5~4	12~28	35	88	81
Fagade & Gillbe, 1988[32]	0.2~16	11~35 (17)	200	–	24
Patel, et al., 2011[33]	14.5	13~42.1 (21.8)	63	83	38

* Exclude signs of root resorption.

Table 11-9 Follow-up results of intra-alveolar transplantation in anterior region.

	Years of follow-up (range/mean)	Patient age (range/mean)	Number of Teeth	Survival rate (%)	PDL* Healing(%)
Tagsjö, et al., 1987[34]	4 (4.0)	9~33 (15.0)	56	91	88

Teeth with multiple roots, roots with excessive cementum, or curved roots that could involve periodontal ligament injury or partial root fracture during extraction pose higher risks. Sometimes it is impossible to extract these teeth without damaging them to such a degree that they cannot be used. A multiple-rooted tooth with a short root trunk or a single-root tooth with a deeper concavity around the cervical area make it difficult to close the flap tightly around the tooth without leaving space. As a result, primary healing around the cervical area can be less predictable (see **Chapter 4**).

Functional teeth/non-functional teeth

It has been suggested that the periodontal ligament maintains its normal width and structure by applying functional pressure. Therefore, it has been suggested that when a non-functional tooth such as an impacted tooth is used as a transplant, a sufficient amount of healthy periodontal ligament may not adhere to the root at the time of extraction, resulting in a decreased prognosis for transplantation[2].

Immature tooth/mature tooth

Looking at the studies of Kristerson[13] and Andreasen[14-16] (**Table 11-7**), it can be considered that the degree of root development, that is, whether the root formation is incomplete or complete, affects the success rate of transplantation. The clinical result of Tsukiboshi[1] suggests that there is a decreased success rate when transplantion is performed into a non-extraction socket at an older age. Therefore, it seems likely that the prognosis of transplanting mature teeth is lower than that of immature teeth. However, a slightly higher success rate has been shown for transplantation of mature teeth into extraction sockets, and thus the success rate does not depend only on the degree of completion of the root. In addition, root length and root morphology may be factors affecting the prognosis of transplantation of mature teeth (longer teeth and more complex root morphology are more likely to damage the periodontal ligament during extraction).

Vital pulp /non-vital pulp

In transplantation of immature teeth, pulpal healing can be expected (see **Chapter 3**). It is unclear whether these teeth have a different prognosis compared with non-vital teeth (endodontically treated teeth). Although there seems to be no logical difference in the healing of periodontal ligament and gingival tissues, it is easier to extract immature donor teeth than mature ones, and in these cases the age of patients are younger, and ability of wound healing is higher.

When transplanting immature teeth, it is necessary to carefully monitor pulpal healing. If infection occurs in the pulp space, it may cause inflammatory resorption and periapical lesions[35]. Other concerns on non-vital teeth include increased possibility of secondary caries and root fracture.

Fixation method and duration

There is some evidence that replanted teeth are more likely to develop resorption if they have been rigidly splinted for long periods of time[36]. Though this is an important consideration, one must also consider the need to stabilize transplanted teeth until attachment is adequate, which will depend on the fit between the donor tooth and the recipient site. High mobility after transplantation during the initial healing phase may increase the likelihood of failure in achieving functional attachment (PDL healing).

Timing and magnitude of occlusal force

There is no data on how early how much occlusal force transplanted teeth can withstand. However, applying excessive occlusal force at an early stage may likely lead to increased risk of complications (i.e. loss of reattachment). From authors' experience point of view, in most cases patients are allowed to start chewing gradually after about one month after transplantation.

(2) Recipient site factors

Adaptation between donor teeth and recipient sockets

If viable periodontal ligament remains attached to the entire root surface, one can expect healing/attachment to take place predictably between the donor and recipient socket regardless of the spacing and compatibility between the two[37]. However, if donor teeth are forced into tight recipient sockets, the periodontal ligament may be damaged. Moreover, during extraction there is always some degree of damage to periodontal ligament, so the following clinical situations should be considered;

① **The distance between the walls of recipient sockets and root surfaces of donor teeth:**

If the distance is close, it will take less time for bony tissue to reach the root surfaces; therefore, ankylosis at the site of any areas with injured periodontal ligament is more likely. If the distance is greater, repair of periodontal ligament (new attachment) can take place before bony tissue reaches the roots.

② **Large recipient site**

If the recipient site is too large, gingival connective tissue may have an opportunity to invade the space between the wall of the bone and the root surface. This may cause a delay in bony healing.

Bone morphology

In actual practice, it is safer to assume that periodontal ligament of transplanted teeth cannot always make and/or maintain bone unless there is a certain amount of bone width and height around it (see **Chapter 3**). Therefore, the recipient socket bone should be wide and deep enough to accommodate donor teeth. Also, as discussed in **Chapter 4**, when transplanting horizontally impacted third molars to the adjacent second molar sites, the impacted position of third molars may affect healing.

Depth of socket/transplantation

It has been suggested that the depth of transplantation does not affect prognosis when transplanting intact teeth with incomplete root formation[14-17]. However, when transplantation is performed on the recipient side where the alveolar ridge has been largely resorbed due to periodontitis, etc., it is advised to place donor teeth slightly deeper and allow them to erupt naturally or orthodontically.

Periodontal ligament of recipient sites

It is well-known that periodontal ligament attachment to donor teeth plays an important role in successful outcomes, whereas periodontal ligament of recipient sites has been thought to have little influence. However, clinical follow-up results have suggested that presence of periodontal ligament in recipient sockets may play an important and positive role in wound healing with transplantation. As indicated in **Chapter 3**, immediate transplantation, surgical extrusion, and intentional replantation have higher success rates when teeth are transplanted in sockets with remaining periodontal ligament. Moreover, periodontal ligament healing seems to be quicker and smoother in cases of replantation, while development of structurally normal and functional periodontal ligament alignment may not always occur when the tooth is transplanted in newly formed sockets without remaining periodontal ligament (see **Chapter 3**). Based on this data, it can be concluded that prognosis likely improves when teeth are transplanted into recipient sites with remaining periodontal ligament.

Gingival adaptation

The first critical point for successful healing is the primary closure of the wound by adaptation of a gingival flap around the transplanted tooth as previously discussed. Tight flap adaptation promotes reattachment between the periodontal ligament of the transplanted teeth and the gingival connective tissue, which prevents microbial invasion into the recipient sockets. Infection can devitalize the periodontal ligament and causes attachment loss. Therefore, when recipient sockets are much larger than the size of donor teeth, establishing primary closure will be difficult and thus immediate transplantation is usually not indicated. Sufficient gingival keratinized tissue will regenerate 3 to 4 weeks after extraction at recipient sites, at which time transplantation can be performed.

Attached gingiva

Although it has not been definitively determined whether presence of attached gingiva is necessary for successful transplantation, it is thought that having some attached gingiva around a transplanted tooth is favorable to both the wound healing at the initial stage of transplantation and the long-term maintenance of gingival closure.

(3) Patient factors

Age

Clinical observation indicates that prognosis is better results in younger patients. This may be related to better healing capacity and robustness of the periodontal ligament. In the authors' observation, even transplantation to non-extraction sites (surgically prepared sockets) in patients 30 years or younger have a good prognosis. The two typical age-related problems that are observed are the higher incidence of transient root resorption in younger patients such as inflammatory resorption and the higher rate of attachment loss or ankylosis in order patients.

Antibiotics

There is no strong evidence supporting use of oral antibiotics before and after transplantation and its affect on the prognosis. At the present time, it is advised that the dentist assess each patient and administer antibiotics and other drugs as they would for other dental surgeries.

Systemic diseases and habits

Diabetes and smoking appear to increase risk for developing periodontal pathology[38, 39]. Abnormal metabolic conditions or particular habits that suppress immunity or delay healing can lower the prognosis for transplantation.

Compliance (maintenance)

Patient compliance is one of the most important factors for all successful dental treatments[40]. Regular maintenance visits and good oral hygiene play very important roles in achieving desired results.

(4) Operator factors

Technique

Dentists wishing to perform transplantation must develop skills and expertise in such areas as surgical extractions for both the unrestorable tooth and donor tooth, preparation of the recipient site, and tissue management.

Supportive therapy for oral prophylaxis

Dental caries and periodontal disease are caused in large part by poor oral hygiene. Patients should be motivated to engage in oral prophylactic activities and given instructions on proper at home care. Long-term success will be improved by continued recall visits and maintenance with cleanings (supportive periodontal therapy).

Criteria for Choosing Cases for Successful Transplantation

As discussed above, many factors will affect the prognosis of transplantation. Even more recent systematic reviews have not suggested the critical factors to assure 100% success rate[41, 42]. From authors' experience and point of view, the following key points should be implicated for better prognosis:

1. Preserve as much periodontal ligament on donor teeth. Viable and healthy periodontal ligament attached to the transplanted tooth is an essential condition for success.
2. Immature donor teeth will generally have a better prognosis than mature donor teeth.
3. Having viable and healthy periodontal ligament on recipient sockets may improve prognosis.
4. The younger the patients are, the better prognosis. If the patient is younger than 30 years old, the survival rate of the transplanted tooth can be very high.
5. The less complicated the root shape, the better the prognosis.
6. Minimizing the extraoral working time and reducing the number of donor tooth try-ins by using replicas will enhance the success rate.

Poor case selection will likely lead to poor prognosis, and good case selection leads to predictable, successful results. Even when prognosis may be difficult to predict, transplantation should always be considered. Even in some such instances, transplantation may still be the best answer[47, 48].

References

1. Tsukiboshi M. Autotransplantation of teeth. Chicago: Quintessence Publishing, 2001: 156-9.
2. Andreasen JO. Atlas of replantation and transplantation of teeth. Philadelphia: W B Saunders, 1992.
3. Nordenram A. Autotransplantation of teeth. Acta Odontol Scand. 1963; 21 Suppl: 33.
4. Galanter DR, Minami RT. The periodontal status of autografted teeth. A pilot study of thirty-one cases. Oral Surg Oral Med Oral Pathol. 1968 Aug; 26(2): 145-59.
5. Andreasen JO, Hjørting-Hansen E, Jølst O. A clinical and radiographic study of 76 autotransplanted third molars. Scand J Dent Res. 1970; 78(6): 512-23.
6. Singh KK, Dudani IC. Autogenous transplantation of developing mandibular third molars. J Indian Med Assoc. 1970 Aug; 42(8): 199-212.
7. Hovinga J. Autotransplantatie van kiemen van derde molaren. Resultaten van voortgezette observatie. Ned Tijdschr Tandheelkd. 1986 Jun; 93(6): 235-7.
8. Nethander G, Andersson JE, Hirsch JM. Autogenous free tooth transplantation in man by a 2 -stage operation technique. A longitudinal intra-individual radiographic assessment. Int J Oral Maxillofac Surg. 1988 Oct; 17(5): 330-6.
9. Andreasen JO. Third molar autotransplantation, relation between successful healing and stage of root development at time of grafting. Presented at the annual meeting in Scandinavian Association of Oral and Maxillofacial Surgeons, Aug 15-19, Nyborg, Denmark, 1990.
10. Schütz S, Beck I, Kühl S, Filippi A. Results after wisdom tooth transplantation. A retrospective study. Schweiz Monatsschr Zahnmed. 2013; 123(4): 303-13.
11. Slagsvold O, Bjercke B. Autotransplantation of premolars with partly formed roots. A radiographic study of root growth. Am J Orthod. 1974 Oct; 66(4): 355-66.
12. Slagsvold O, Bjercke B. Applicability of autotransplantation in cases of missing upper anterior teeth. Am J Orthod. 1978 Oct; 74(4): 410-21.
13. Kristerson L. Autotransplantation of human premolars. A clinical and radiographic study of 100 teeth. Int J Oral Surg. 1985 Apr; 14(2): 200-13.
14. Andreasen JO, Paulsen HU, Yn Z, Ahlquist R, Bayer T, Schwartz O. A long-term study of 370 autotransplanted premolars. Part I. Surgical procedures and standardized techniques for monitoring healing. Eur J Orthod. 1990 Feb; 12(1): 3 -13.
15. Andreasen JO, Paulsen HU, Yu Z, Bayer T, Schwartz O. A long-term study of 370 autotransplanted premolars. Part Ⅱ. Tooth survival and pulp healing subsequent to transplantation. Eur J Orthod. 1990 Feb; 12(1): 14-24.
16. Andreasen JO, Paulsen HU, Yu Z, Schwartz O. A long-term study of 370 autotransplanted premolars. Part Ⅲ. Periodontal healing subsequent to transplantation. Eur J Orthod. 1990 Feb; 12(1): 25-37.
17. Andreasen JO, Paulsen HU, Yu Z, Bayer T. A long-term study of 370 autotransplanted premolars. Part Ⅳ. Root development subsequent to transplantation. Eur J Orthod. 1990 Feb; 12(1): 38-50.
18. Jonsson T, Sigurdsson TJ. Autotransplantation of premolars to premolar sites. A long-term follow-up study of 40 consecutive patients. Am J Orthod Dentofacial Orthop. 2004 Jun; 125(6): 668-75.
19. Plakwicz P, Wojtowicz A, Czochrowska EM. Survival and success rates of autotransplanted premolars: a prospective study of the protocol for developing teeth. Am J Orthod Dentofacial Orthop. 2013 Aug; 144(2): 229-37.
20. Thonner KE. Autogenous transplantation of unerupted maxillary canines. A clinical and histological investigation over five years. Dent Pract Dent Rec. 1971 Mar; 21(7): 251-7.
21. Cook RM. The current status of autogenous transplantation as applied to the maxillary canine. Int Dent J. 1972 Jun; 22(2): 286-300.
22. Reade P, Monsour A, Bowker P. A clinical study of the autotransplantation of unerupted maxillary canines. Aust Dent J. 1973 Oct-Dec; 18(5): 273-80.
23. Lovius BB, Atherton JD, Wynne TH, Finch LD. Autogenous tooth transplantation: a clinical and histological investigation. Br J Orthod. 1974 Jan; 1 (2): 27-33.
24. Moss JP. The indications for the transplantation of maxillary canines in the light of 100 cases. Br J Oral Surg. 1975 Mar; 12(3): 268-74.
25. Oksala E, Kallioniemi H. A longitudinal clinical and radiographic study of autotransplantation of the maxillary canine. Proc Finn Dent Soc. 1977 Jun; 73(3): 117-25.
26. Altonen M, Haavikko K, Malmström M. Evaluation of autotransplantations of completely developed maxillary canines. Int J Oral Surg. 1978 Oct; 7 (5): 434-41.
27. Hardy P. The autogenous transplantation of maxillary canines. Br Dent J. 1982 Sep 7 ; 153(5): 183-6.
28. Reade PC, Hall GH. A clinical study of the autotransplantation of maxillary canine teeth. In: Riviere GR, Hildeman WH, eds. Oral immunogenetics and tissue transplantation. New York, Amsterdam, Oxford. Elsevier/North Holland, 1982: 291-300.
29. Hall GM, Reade PC. Root resorption associated with autotransplanted maxillary canine teeth. Br J Oral Surg. 1983 Sep; 21(3): 179-91.
30. Ahlberg K, Bystedt H, Eliasson S, Odenrick L. Long-term evaluation of autotransplanted maxillary canines with completed root formation. Acta Odontol Scand. 1983; 41(1): 23-31.
31. Lownie JF, Cleaton-Jones PE, Fatti P, Lownie MA. Autotransplantation of maxillary canine teeth. A follow-up of 35 cases up to 4 years. Int J Oral Maxillofac Surg. 1986 Jun; 15(3): 282-7.
32. Fagade OO, Gillbe GV, Wastell DG. Radiographic pattern of root resorption in autotransplanted maxillary canines. J Dent. 1988 Apr; 16(2): 80-4.
33. Patel S, Fanshawe T, Bister D, Cobourne MT. Survival and success of maxillary canine autotransplantation: a retrospective investigation. Eur J Orthod. 2011 Jun; 33(3): 298-304.
34. Tegsjö U, Valerius-Olsson H, Frykholm A, Olgart K. Clinical evaluation of intra-alveolar transplantation of teeth with cervical root fractures. Swed Dent J. 1987; 11(6): 235-50.
35. Andreasen JO. The effect of pulp extirpation or root canal treatment on periodontal healing after replantation of permanent incisors in monkeys. J Endod. 1981 Jun; 7 (6): 245-52.
36. Andreasen JO. The effect of splinting upon periodontal healing after replantation of permanent incisors in monkeys. Acta Odont Scand. 1975; 33: 313-23.
37. Andreasen JO. Periodontal healing after replantation and autotransplantation of incisors in monkeys. Int J Oral Surg. 1981 Feb; 10(1): 54-61.
38. Emrich L, Shlossman M, Genco R. Periodontal disease in non-insulin dependent diabetes mellitus. J Periodontol. 1991; 62: 123.
39. Akef J, Weine F, Weissman D. The role of smoking in the progression of periodontal diseases. A literature review. The compendium of continuing education in dentistry. 1992; 13: 526.
40. Wilson TG Jr. Dental maintenance for patients with periodontal diseases. Chicago; Quintessence Pub, 1989.
41. Akhlef Y, Schwartz O, Andreasen JO, Jensen SS. Autotransplantation of teeth to the anterior maxilla: A systematic review of survival and success, aesthetic presentation and patient-reported outcome. Dent Traumatol. 2018 Feb; 34(1):20-7.
42. Machado LA, do Nascimento RR, Ferreira DM, Mattos CT, Vilella OV. Long-term prognosis of tooth autotransplantation: a systematic review and meta-analysis. Int J Oral Maxillofac Surg. 2016 May; 45(5): 610-7.
43. Heithersay GS. Treatment of invasive cervical resorption: An analysis of results using topical application of trichloracetic acid, curettage, and restoration. Quintessence Int. 1999 Feb; 30(2): 96-100.
44. Heithersay GS. Invasive cervical resorption: an analysis of potential predisposing factors. Quintessence Int. 1999 Feb;30(2):83-95.
45. Mavridou AM, Bergmans L, Barendregt D, Lambrechts P. Descriptive Analysis of Factors Associated with External Cervical Resorption. J Endod. 2017 Oct;43(10):1602-10.
46. Patel S, Kanagasingam S, Pitt Ford T. External cervical resorption: a review. J Endod. 2009 May;35(5):616-25.
47. Barendregt D, Andreasen JO, Leunisse M, Eggink E, Linssen M, Van der Weijden F, Louropoulou A. An evaluation of 1654 premolars transplanted in the posterior region-A retrospective analysis of survival, success and complications. Dent Traumatol. 2023 Jul;39 Suppl 1 :50-62.
48. Louropoulou A, Andreasen JO, Leunisse M, Eggink E, Linssen M, Van der Weijden F, Barendregt D. An evaluation of 910 premolars transplanted in the anterior region-A retrospective analysis of survival, success, and complications. Dent Traumatol. 2024 Feb;40(1):22-34.

CHAPTER12

In-house 3D replica fabrication and digital simulation using a free software

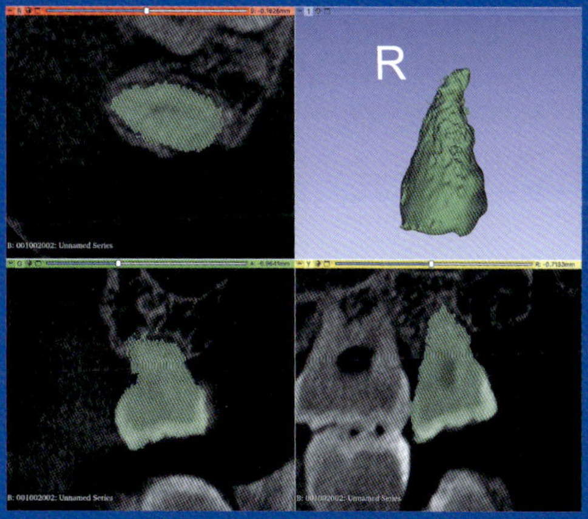

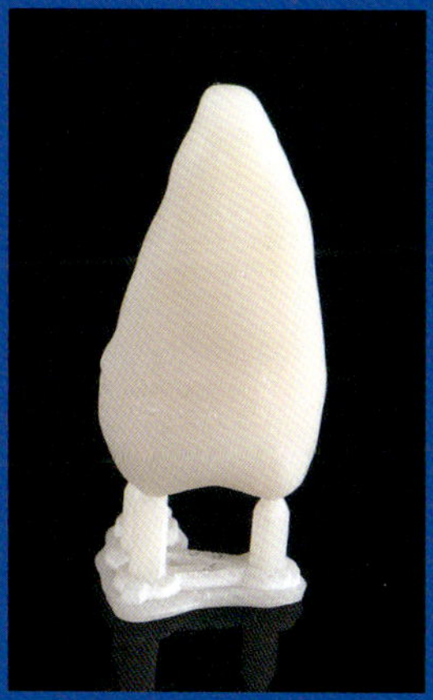

In this chapter, digital workflow of making a 3D replica from the patient's DICOM data as well as digital simulation of autotransplantation is discussed. 3D replicas help to decrease as much extra-alveolar time of the donor tooth as possible, resulting in less damage to the PDL cells on the root. In addition to that, digital simulation can show which bone volume to remove and where the donor tooth can be positioned prior to the actual surgery.

The workflow shown in this chapter utilizes free software, making it easier and more accessible. It offers a convenient and efficient way to prepare and execute autotransplantation of teeth that can further improve the prognosis of these cases.

Installation of the free application

A necessary application is 3D Slicer[1] (**Fig 12-1**), a free and open-source platform for analyzing medical image data. 3D Slicer can be downloaded from [https://download.slicer.org/]. It runs on any Windows, Mac, or Linux computer that was released in the last 5 years and requires memory of more than 4GB (8GB or more is recommended). For more information, refer to the website for the system requirements for running this application.

As 3D Slicer is currently not approved for clinical use and is intended for research use, its use should be under the responsibility of the clinician with the consent of the patient.

Installation of a free application

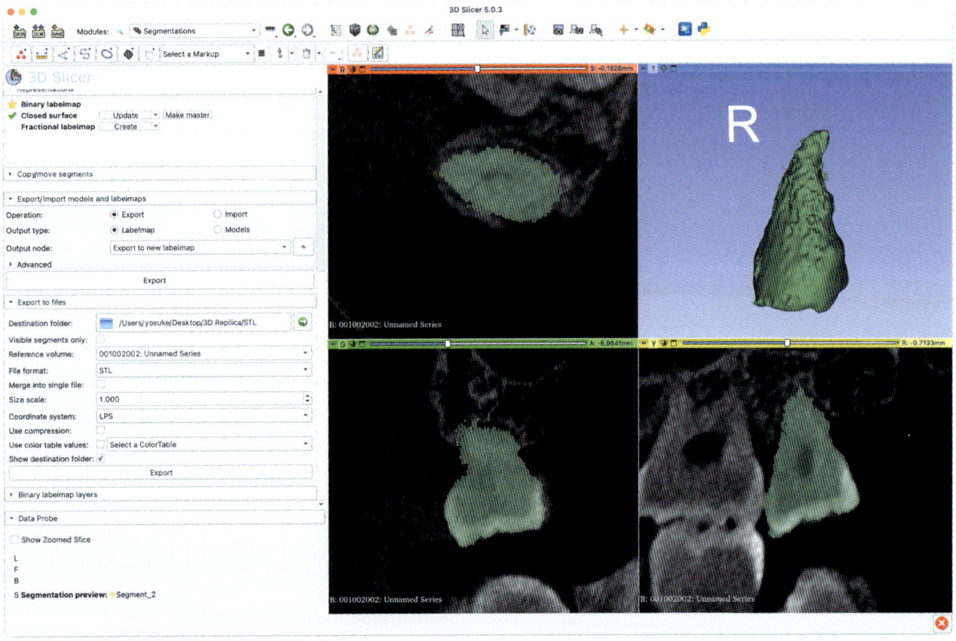

Fig 12-1 Installation of a free application. User interface of 3D Slicer on Mac.

Importing CBCT data into 3D Slicer

DICOM stands for Digital Imaging and Communications in Medicine and is the standard for the communication and management of medical imaging information and related data. The steps to import and load CBCT DICOM data are as follows

1) After taking CBCT, export it as DICOM file and move it into the computer on which 3D Slicer is installed.
2) Launch 3D Slicer application (**Fig 12-2a**, the version shown here is ver. 5.0.3).
3) Click [① Add DICOM Data or the DCM icon] in the upper left to open DICOM database (**Fig 12-2a**).
4) [② Drag-and-drop the DICOM files] to the application window (**Fig 12-2b**).
5) Check if the CBCT data is on the DICOM database, and [③ Double-click it] to load the data object into the scene (**Fig 12-2c** and **12-2d**).

Importing CBCT data into 3D Slicer

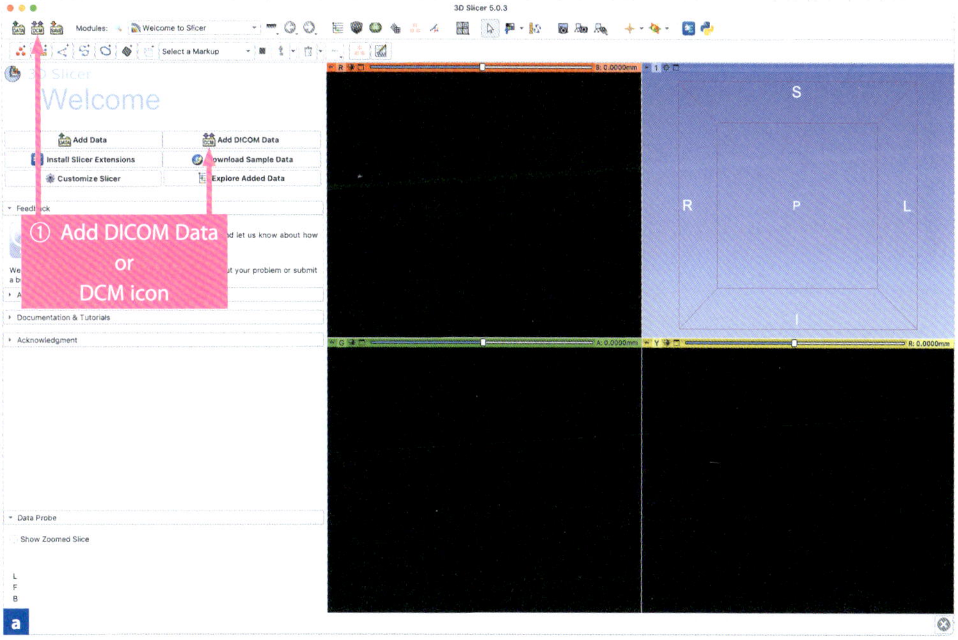

Fig 12-2a Importing CBCT data into 3D Slicer. Launch 3D Slicer application. Click [① Add DICOM Data or DCM icon] to open DICOM database.

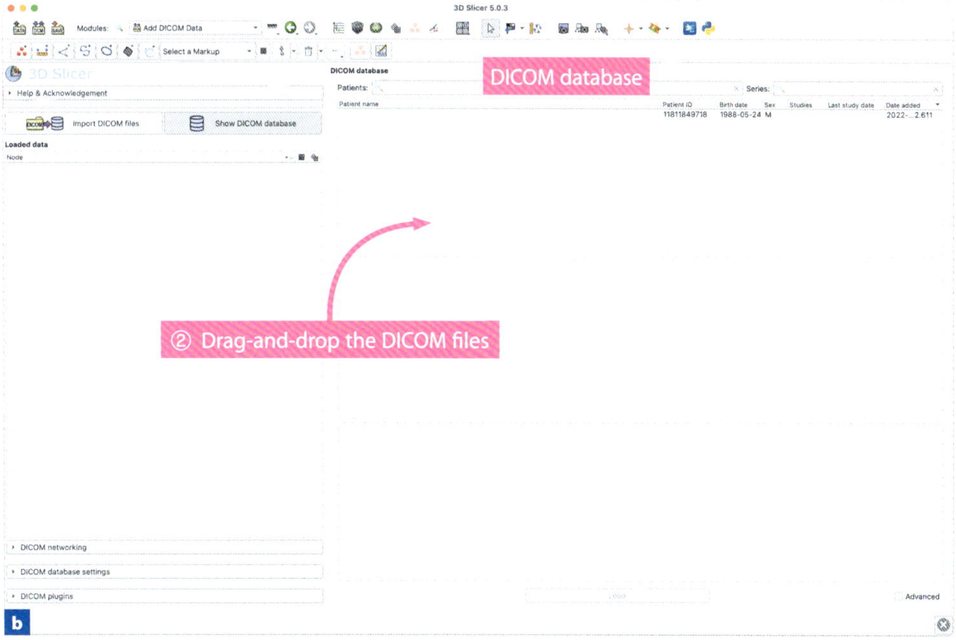

Fig 12-2b [② Drag-and-drop the DICOM files] to the application window.

Donor tooth segmentation

Segmentation is done to delineate the region of the donor tooth for the transplantation and to obtain three-dimensional data that will match the size and anatomical shape of the actual donor tooth. 3D Slicer has many modules for manipulating segmentations; the "Segment Editor" module is useful to create and edit segmentations from images using manual, semi-automatic, and automatic tools[2]. The steps for tooth segmentation are as follows

1) Select [① Segment Editor] from the drop-down list of the Modules on the upper left to launch the Segment Editor (**Fig 12-3a**).
2) Click the [② +Add] TWICE and confirm that [③ green (Segment_1) and yellow (Segment_2) segments] are displayed (**Fig 12-3b**).
3) Click [④ Paint] in the Effects on the left (**Fig 12-3b**).
4) [⑤ Adjust the brush size], and [⑥ paint the donor tooth structure in green and the surrounding area in yellow to make the boundaries clear] (**Fig 12-3c**). It is recommended

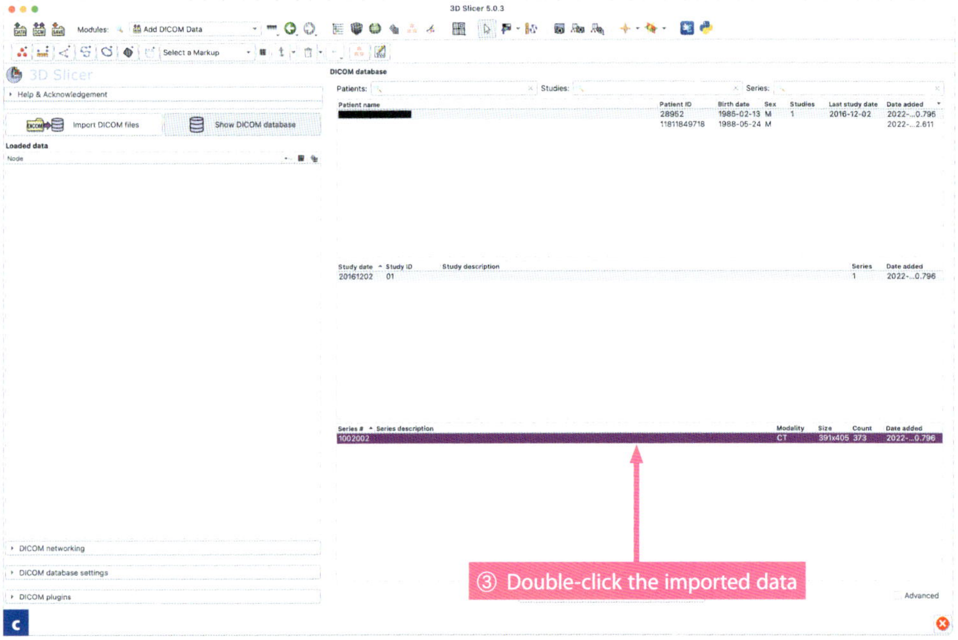

Fig 12-2c Check if the CBCT data is on the DICOM database, and [③ double-click it] to load the data object into the scene.

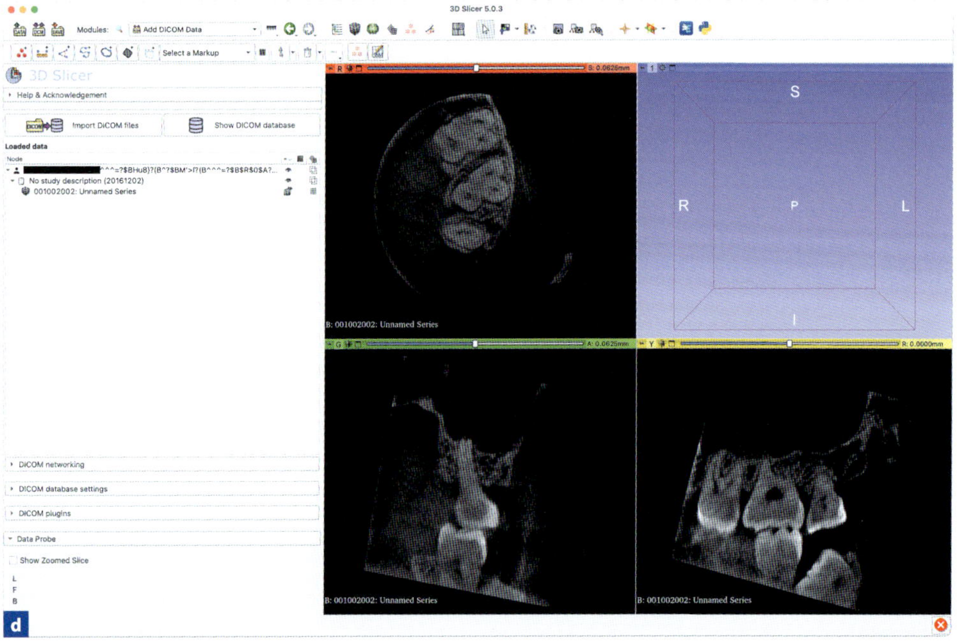

Fig 12-2d Loading the data is done.

to paint the tooth outline in all 3 planes, and make sure that colors don't overlap each other. For a multi-rooted tooth, each root should be painted. After the painting is done, click [⑦ Grow from seeds] (**Fig 12-3c**).

5) Click [⑧ Initialize] to start semi-automatic segmentation of the donor tooth based on the colors painted. The tooth structure will become filled in with green (**Fig 12-3d**).

6) Click [⑨ Show 3D] to display the segmented tooth data in the upper right viewer. If you are satisfied with the results, click [⑩ Apply] to finish segmentation (**Fig 12-3e**).

7) Click the arrow mark to go to the [⑪ Segmentations module] (**Fig 12-3f**), select a destination folder in the "Export to files" section, and click [⑫ Export] below the "Export to files" section (**Fig 12-3g**). The [.stl] file of the donor tooth is now created and this data will be used to create the 3D print.

Donor tooth segmentation

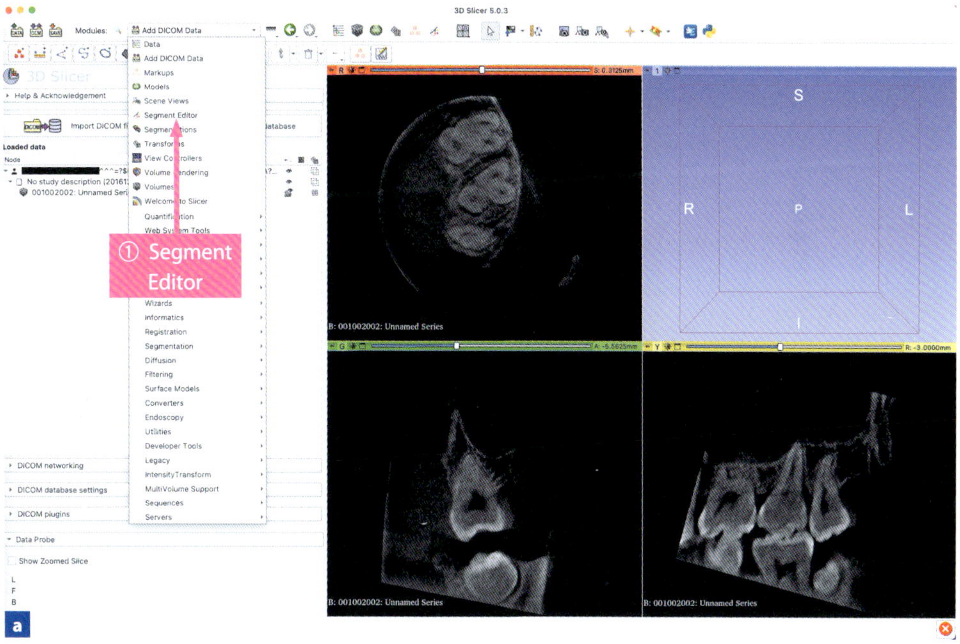

Fig 12-3a Select [① Segment Editor] from the drop-down list of the Modules.

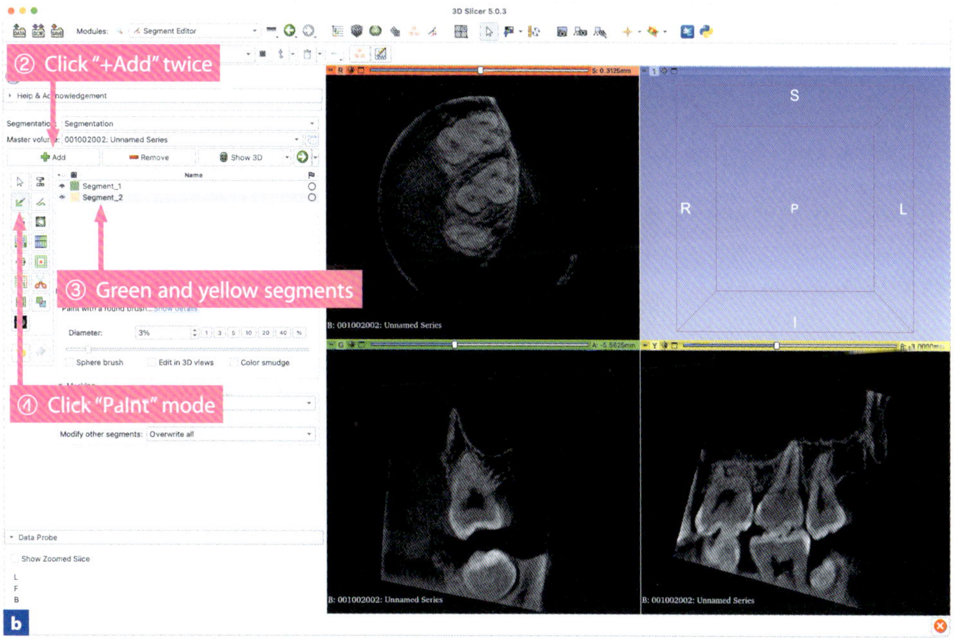

Fig 12-3b Click the [② +Add] TWICE and confirm that [③ green (Segment_1) and yellow (Segment_2) segments] are displayed. Then, click [④ Paint] in the Effects.

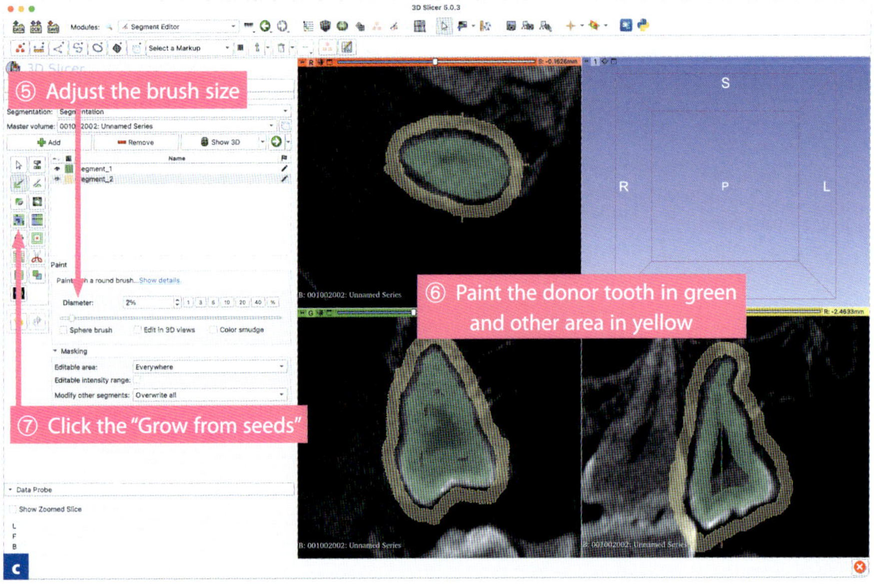

Fig 12-3c [⑤ Adjust the brush size], and [⑥ Paint the donor tooth structure in green and the other area in yellow to make the boundary clear]. After the painting is done, click [⑦ Grow from seeds].

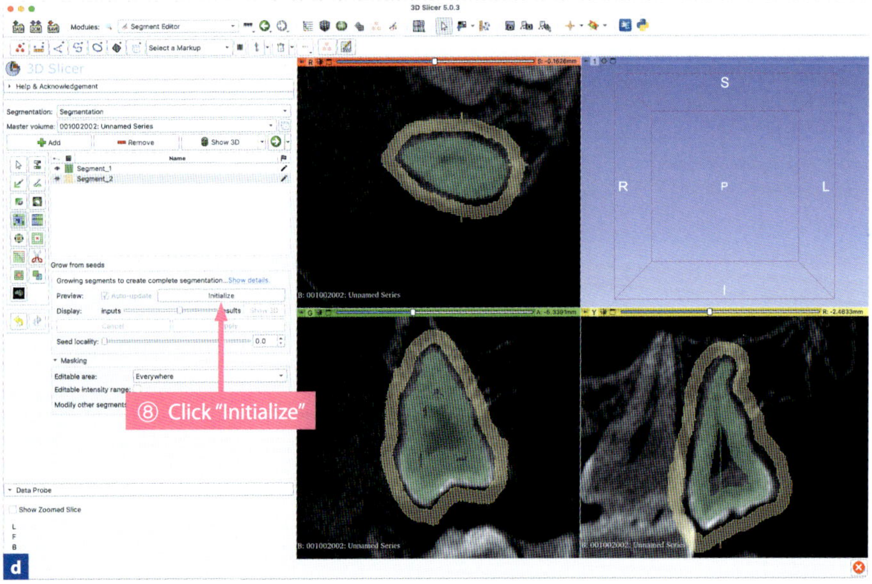

Fig 12-3d Click [⑧ Initialize] to start semi-automatic segmentation of the donor tooth.

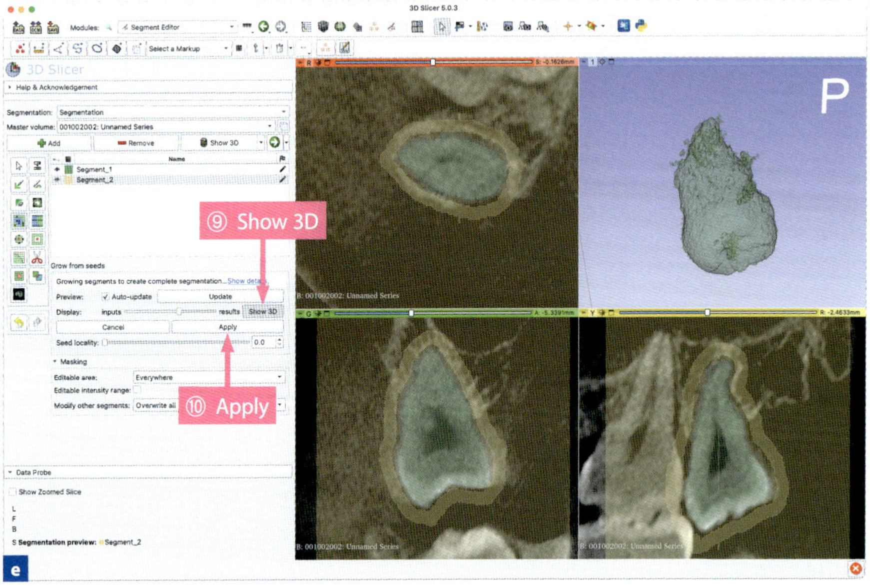

Fig 12-3e Click [⑨ Show 3D] to display the segmented tooth data in the upper right viewer.
Then, click [⑩ Apply] to finish segmentation.

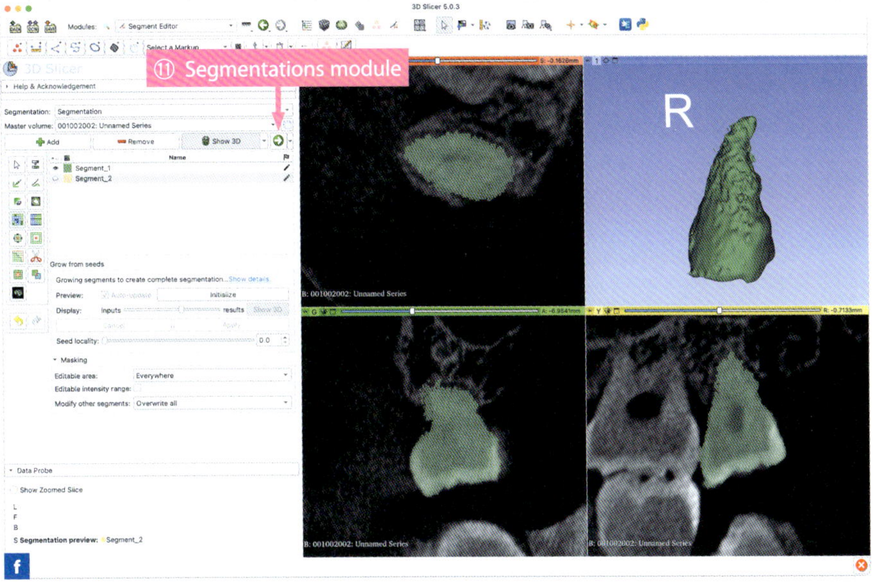

Fig 12-3f Click the arrow mark to open the [⑪ Segmentations module].

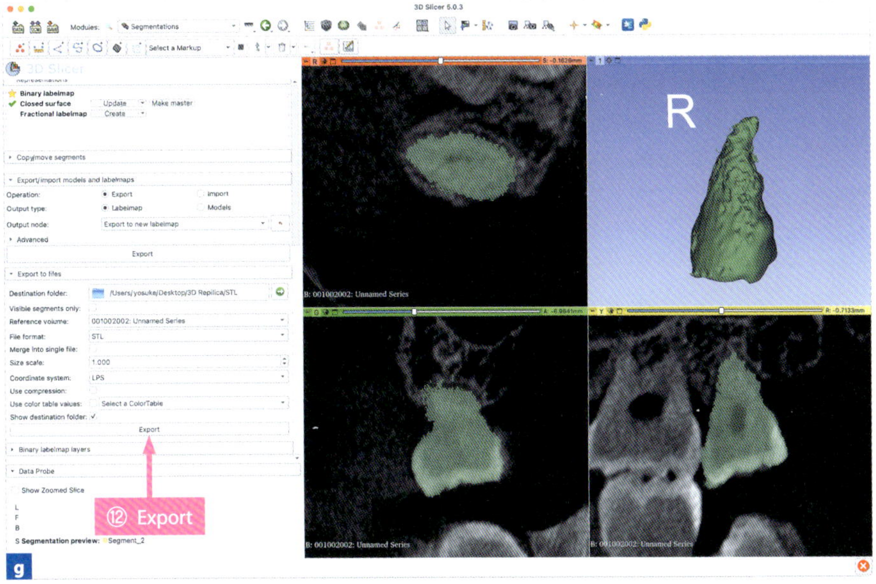

Fig 12-3g Select a destination folder and click [⑫ Export] in the "Export to files" section.

3D printing

After the 3D data of the donor tooth is obtained, it will be imported into a slicing software to translate the [.stl] data into a 3D-printable one. Printing time depends on the size of your object, the materials used, and your printer. The 3D-printed replicas must be sterilized before autotransplantation.

It is encouraged that 3D replicas with and without raft are printed[3] (**Fig 12-4a** and **12-4b**). Raft and supports attached to the replica can ease the try-in procedure during surgery (**Fig 12-4c**); the replica without the raft and supports (or you can also detach them from the replica after try-in is complete) allows us to make sure the replica tooth is placed deep enough so to avoid or minimize any occlusal adjustment when the actual donor tooth is transplanted.

Digital simulation of autotransplantation

One of the advantages of digital dentistry is digital treatment planning before surgery. In autotransplantation, the position of the transplanted donor tooth is important because it should be embedded in the bone housing as much as possible[3]. This treatment planning enables us not only to simulate appropriate three-dimensional donor tooth position, but also to help determinate whether the donor tooth and the recipient site are indicated for autotransplantation or not. Autodesk Meshmixer, a free and popular CAD software, is necessary for simulation (download it from [https://meshmixer.com/]).

1) Launch 3D Slicer. Select "Segment Editor" from the drop-down list of the Modules in the same way as in **Fig 12-3a**. Segment the recipient bone as well as the adjacent teeth using [① Threshold] in the Effects on the left (**Fig 12-5a**). After adjusting the upper and lower threshold to segment the target area enough, click [② Apply] to finish. Export the data in the same way as in **Fig 12-3f** and **12-3g** to create a [.stl] file of the recipient site.
2) Launch Meshmixer, and [③ Import the replica tooth data and the recipient data] (**Fig 12-5b**).
3) Select the tooth data and click [④ Edit→Transform] to move and rotate it so that it's located properly in the bone housing (**Fig 12-5c**). Click [⑤ Accept] to finish simulation. In this example, the simulation reveals that there is some bony dehiscence on the buccal side while not on the lingual side (**Fig 12-5d**).

3D printing

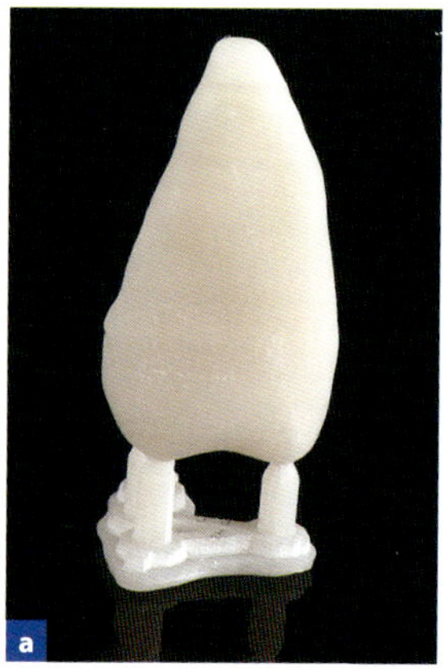

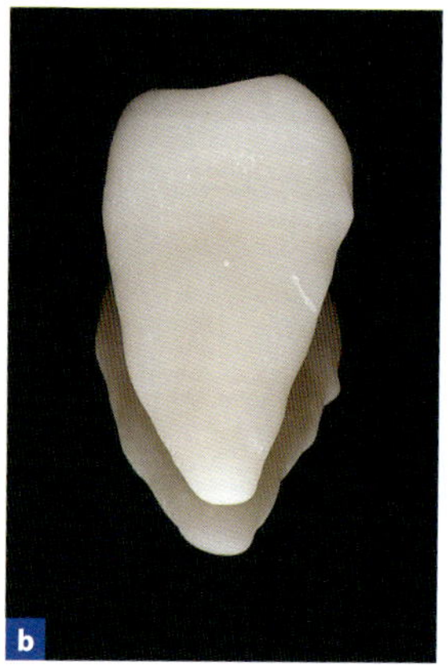

Fig 12-4a The 3D replica with raft and supports. (The replica data is different from one created in **Fig 12-3a** to **12-3g**.)
Fig 12-4b The other 3D replica without raft and supports.
(Raft is a flat base convenient for printing a 3D replica, and supports are connections between the replica and the raft.)

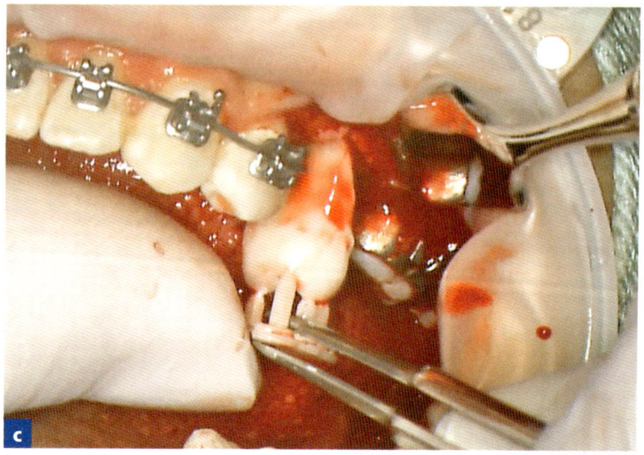

Fig 12-4c Try-in procedure during surgery facilitated by raft and supports.

Digital simulation of autotransplantation

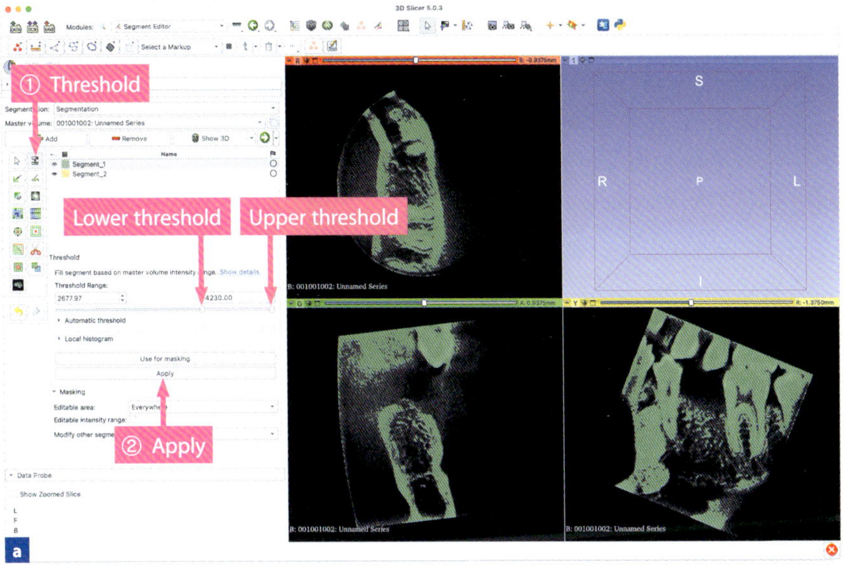

Fig 12-5a Segment the recipient bone including the adjacent teeth using [① Threshold] in the Effects. Click [② Apply] to finish.

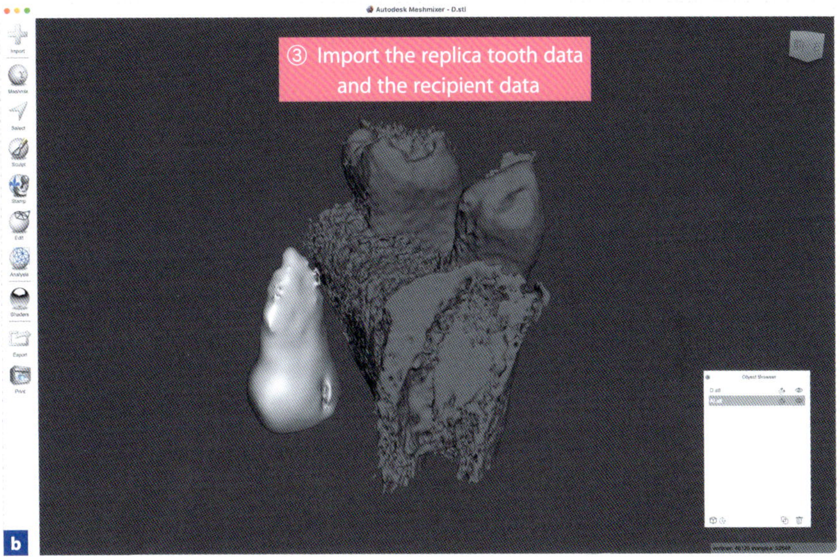

Fig 12-5b Launch Meshmixer, and [③ Import the replica tooth data and the recipient data].

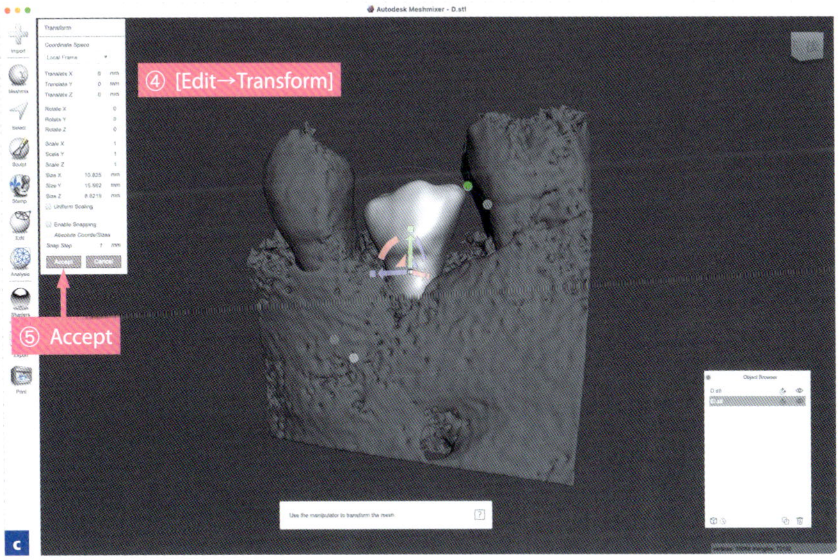

Fig 12-5c Select the tooth data and click [④ Edit → Transform] to move and rotate it. Click [⑤ Accept] to finish.

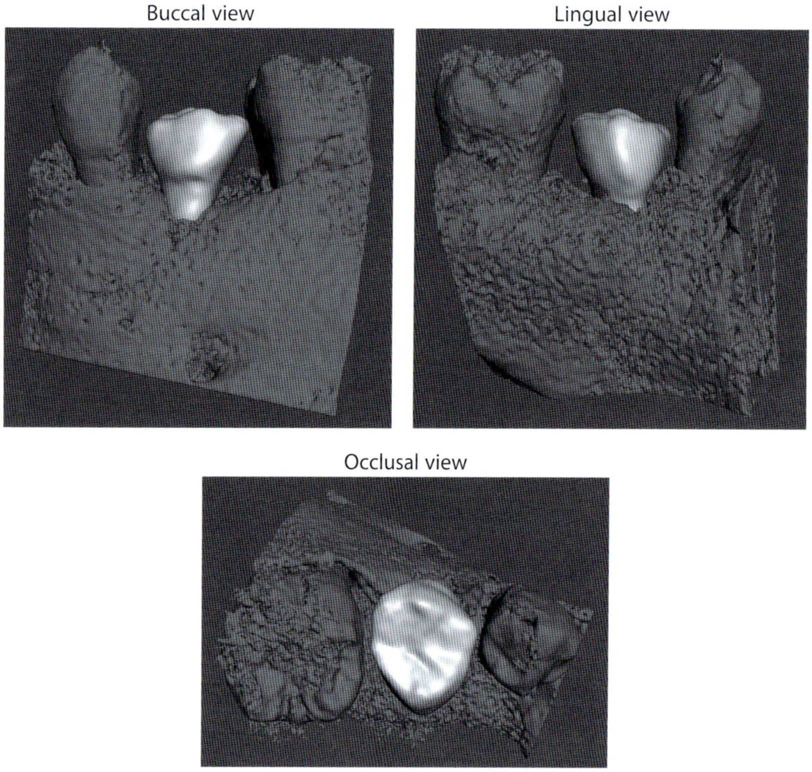

Fig 12-5d Top left (buccal view), there is a bony dehiscence; Top right (lingual view), the root is embedded in the bone housing; bottom (occlusal view), the crown is positioned properly in bucco-lingual direction.

References

1. Fedorov A, Beichel R, Kalpathy-Cramer J, Finet J, Fillion-Robin J-C, Pujol S, Bauer C, Jennings D, Fennessy F, Sonka M, Buatti J, Aylward S, Miller JV, Pieper S, Kikinis R. 3 D Slicer as an image computing platform for the Quantitative Imaging Network. Magn Reson Imaging. 2012 Nov; 30(9): 1323-41.

2. Pinter Cs, Lasso A, Fichtinger G. Polymorph segmentation representation for medical image computing. Comput Methods Programs Biomed. 2019 Apr; 171: 19-26.

3. Tsukiboshi M, Tsukiboshi C, Levin L. A step - by step guide for autotransplantation of teeth. Dent Traumatol. 2023 Jul; 39 Suppl 1 : 70-80.

A

adjustment of the socket **101**
advantages and disadvantages of transplantation **8**
alveolar bone healing **53**
alveolar bone proper **17, 54**
alveolar mucosa **17**
alveolar process **17**
ameloblastin **52**
ameloblasts **14**
amelogenin **52**
analysis of donor teeth **98**
analysis of recipient sites **98**
ankylosis **30, 34, 93, 248, 250**
ankylosis-related resorption **30**
antibiotic administration **104**
antigen-presenting cells **35**
apexification **46, 117**
apexogenesis **47**
apicoectomy **218**
attached gingiva **17**
attachment loss **250**
Autodesk Meshmixer **266**

B

B lymphocytes **35**
B7 **35**
basal bone **17**
bell stage **14**
biologic width
(supracrestal tissue attachment) **16, 17, 38, 215**
Bio-Oss **233**
bone graft material **61, 63**
bone resorption in delayed replantation **57**
bone resorption-promoting factors **32**
bony housing **61**

C

calcium hydroxide **47**
calculus **239**
Cap stage **14**
capillary vessels **42**
CD28 **35**
cementoblasts **15, 16, 54**
cementum **17, 54**
class II MHC **35**
classification of autotransplantation of teeth **72**
classification of Moorrees **43**
classification of root development **49**
classification of root resorption **31**
COE-PAK **124**
compromised surgical extrusion **94**
congenitally missing second premolars **152**
congenitally missing teeth **188, 189**
connective tissue graft **210**
conventional transplantation **72, 73**
coupling phenomenon **30**
crown-root fracture **87, 89**
cytokines **32**

D

definitive diagnosis of traumatized teeth **83**
delayed inflammatory resorption **249**
delayed inflammatory root resorption **37**
delayed transplantation **98, 100, 110**
dental follicle **14, 54**
dental ledge **14**
dental papilla **14**
dentin **54**
dentin and enamel formation **14**
dentin-like hard tissue **44**
development of teeth and periodontal tissues **14**
development of tooth germ **14**
developmental stages of roots **43**
diamond-coated forceps **122**
DICOM data **103, 260**
digital simulation **266, 267**
discrepancy **102**
disinfection **100**

E

ectopically erupted premolar **179**
enamel matrix **14**
enamel projection **79**
enamelin **52**
endo-perio differential diagnosis **232**
epithelial down-growth **250**
epithelial rests of Malassez **16**
examination and diagnosis **98**
external root resorption **225**
extraoral scaling **239**

F

factors affecting the prognosis **254**
fibroblasts **54**
fixation of the transplant **104**
follow-up results of intra-alveolar transplantation **255**
follow-up results of transplantation **251**
follow-up results of transplantation of canines **255**
follow-up results of transplantation of premolars **254**
follow-up results of transplantation of third molars **254**
forming a new socket **100**
free gingiva **17**

G • H

gingivectomy **91**
glass ionomer cement **124**
healing of alveolar bone **52**
healing of gingiva **38**
healing of pulp **43**
healing with inner periodontal ligament **45**

Hertwig's epithelial root sheath **15, 54**
Hertwig's epithelial sheath **39, 45, 47, 49, 54**
horizontally impacted mandibular third molars **80**

I

IL-1 **32**
immediate transplantation **99, 100**
implant **78, 90, 91**
importing CBCT data into 3D Slicer **261**
indications and criteria for conventional transplantation **74, 75**
indications and criteria for intentional replantation **85**
indications and criteria for intra-alveolar transplantation **81**
indications for "Intra-alveolar transplantation" **82**
infection related resorption **249**
inflammation-related resorption **30**
inflammatory resorption **30, 31, 34, 36**
informed consent **7**
infra-occlusion **91, 196**
inner enamel epithelium **14**
inner PDL **45**
installation of a free application **260**
insufficient buccolingual width of bone **102**
intentional replantation **73, 227, 228**
interleukin 1 **32**
internal bleaching **185**
intra-alveolar transplantation **72, 73**
invasive cervical resorption **199, 250**
ischemic change **42**

J • L

junctional epithelium **16**
juvenile periodontitis **146**
lateral canals **218**
limited drying or removal of the periodontal ligament **28**
limited orthodontic treatment (LOT) **81**
lineage of osteoclasts **32**
lingual buttons **124**
long connective tissue attachment **38**

M

macrophages **35**
maintenance **111**
mandibular horizontally impacted third molars **79**
Maryland bridge **174**
maxillary impacted third molars **79**
macrophage colony stimulating factor **30**
MCSF **30, 32**
MCSF receptor **32**
mechanism of inflammatory resorption **35**
mechanism of new attachment **28**
mechanism of pulp healing **42**
mechanism of replacement resorption **31**
mechanism of root resorption **30**
Meshmixer **266**
monocytes **32**

N

natural movement of transplanted teeth **108**
necrosis of pulp **46**
neural crest **14**
neural crest cell **14**
new attachment **26, 27, 37**
non arrest **49, 50**

O

occlusal adjustment **104**
odontoblasts **15**
ontogenesis of osteoclast **35**
ontogenesis of periodontal tissues **54**
Ora Graft **233**
oral hygiene instruction **98**
orthodontic extrusion **87**
orthodontic movement of transplanted teeth **108**
orthodontic treatment **100**
osteoblasts **16, 32, 54**
osteoclast precursors **30**
osteoclasts **32, 33**
osteoinductive ability of periodontal ligament **54**
outer enamel epithelium **14**

P

parathyroid hormone **32**
partial arrest **49, 50**
partial obliteration **42**
partial PCO **39**
PCO **39, 44, 84**
PDL **54**
periodontal ligament **16, 17**
PGE_2 **32**
porykaryotic (multi-nuclear) osteoclasts **33**
precursors of osteoclasts **32**
preoperative administration **100**
preparation of the recipient socket **100**
primary closure **98**
procedures of surgical extrusion **214, 216**
prostaglandin E_2 **32**
PTH **32**
pulp canal obliteration **39, 44, 84**
pulp healing **41**
pulpal healing **39, 40**
purposes of surgical extrusion **215**

R

raft **266**
RANK **30, 32**
RANKL **30, 32**

reattachment 20
reattachment in replantation 20
reattachment in transplantation 22
regeneration of capillaries 39
relationship between periodontal ligament of the donor tooth and horizontal bone regeneration 63
relationship between pulp healing and root length 51
relationship between vertical and horizontal alveolar bone growth with tooth eruption 55
repair-related resorption 30
replacement 250
replacement resorption 30, 31, 34, 57, 248
replica 98
restorative treatment 100
restorative treatment of transplanted teeth 111
retro canal filling 217, 218
revascularization 39
root canal therapy 46
root canal treatment for transplanted teeth 108
root development 40, 41, 49
root development after transplantation 51
root morphology of donor teeth 79
root resorption 30
round bur for drilling 101
ruffled border 32, 33

S

sagittal images of CBCT of maxillary central incisors at different ages 56
Segment Editor 262
segmentation 262
sequence and procedures of conventional transplantation 98
sequence of treatment 8
Sharpey's fibers 15, 16
sinus elevation 102
sinus floor elevation 117, 140
sinus lift 74
sinus mucosa (Schneiderian membrane) 117
soluble RANKL 35
space closure 92
splinting with bonded wire 105
spontaneous eruption 64
stellate reticulum 14
success rate 251
success rates of surgical extrusion 252
success rates of transplantation 252
Super Bond 105, 107, 124
supernumerary premolar 174, 175
supports 266
supracrestal tissue attachment (biologic width) 16, 17, 38, 215
surface resorption 30, 31, 37
surgical dressing 104, 124
surgical extrusion 73, 83, 88, 214
surgical instruments 121
surgical procedures 100
surgical reposition 84
surgical round bur 121
surgical up-righting 72, 73, 82, 226
survival of the periodontal ligament 29
survival rate 251
suture fixation 104, 217
suturing the flaps 104

T

T lymphocytes 35
three-dimensional bone regeneration around a transplanted tooth 59, 60
timing of root canal treatment 99
tooth dependent bone volume 237
tooth independent bone volume 237
total arrest 49, 50
total obliteration 42
total PCO 39
transportation 218
trimming of gingival tissue 102
try-in 101, 102, 103
Twisted wire 7 105, 107, 124

V

vacuolation in cytoplasm 33
vascular dentin 44
vitamin D3 32
Vitapex 48, 113, 117, 161

W • X • Z

walking bleach 185
X Desmo Tool 1 123
Zip 218

Other

3D printing 266
3D replica 103, 197, 260
3D Slicer 260
[.stl] data 266

Author biographies

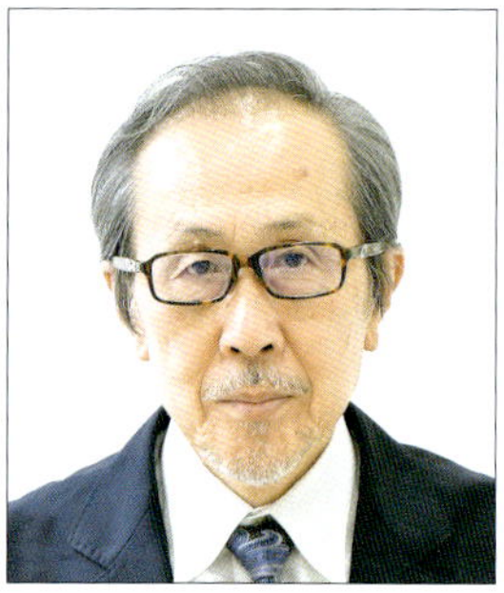

Mitsuhiro Tsukiboshi DDS, PhD

1952 Birth in Aichi, Japan
1977 Graduation of the Osaka University School of Dentistry
1981 Graduation of the Post Graduate of the Graduate School of Medicine, Kyoto University
1982 Chairman of Tsukiboshi Dental Clinic
1998 Lecturer of Loma Linda University in USA
2009–2010 President of International Association of Dental Traumatology
2012 Adjunctive assistant professor of Western University in USA
2014 Part-time lecturer of Osaka University School of Dentistry
2015 Clinical professor of Tohoku University School of Dentistry

Major Publications

Tsukiboshi M, Oka K. Periodontology and Periodontics. Quintessence Publishing, 1992.
Tsukiboshi M. Treatment planning for traumatized teeth. Quintessence Publishing, 1998.
Tsukiboshi M. Autotransplantation of Teeth. Quintessence Publishing, 1999.
Tsukiboshi M, Fukunishi K, Nakata K. Biology Based Endodontics. Quintessence Publishing, 2000.
Tsukiboshi M, Tsukiboshi C. Minimal Tooth Movement. Quintessence Publishing, 2003.
Tsukiboshi M. Treatment planning for traumatized teeth 2nd edition. Quintessence Publishing, 2009.
Tsukiboshi M, Fukunishi K. Biology Based Endodontics 2nd edition. Quintessence Publishing, 2010.
Tsukiboshi M, Izumi H. Composite and Esthetic Restoration. Quintessence Publishing, 2012.
Tsukiboshi M. Autotransplantation of Teeth 2nd edition. Quintessence Publishing, 2014.
Tsukiboshi M. Periodontology & Periodontics. Quintessence Publishing, 2018, 2019.
Tsukiboshi M, Tsukiboshi C, Tsukiboshi Y. Minimal Tooth Movement 2nd edition. Quintessence Publishing, 2021.
Tsukiboshi M, Fukunishi K. Biology Based Endodontics 3rd edition. Quintessence Publishing, 2021.
Tsukiboshi M. Justice in Dentistry. Quintessence Publishing, 2023.

Quintessence Publishing Co., Ltd.
3-2-6, Hongo, Bunkyo-ku, Tokyo 113-0033, JAPAN
Tel: +81-3-5842-2270
Fax: +81-3-5800-7597
URL: www.quint-j.co.jp
Printing and Binding: Sun Art Printing Co., Ltd. Osaka
Printed in Japan
ISBN 978-4-7812-1008-7 C3047